The New Midwifery

For Churchill Livingstone:

Commissioning Editor: Inta Ozols
Project Development Manager: Mairi McCubbin
Project Manager: Jane Shanks
Designer: Judith Wright, George Ajayi

The New Midwifery
Science and Sensitivity in Practice

Edited by

Lesley Ann Page BA MSc RM RN RNT RMT

The Queen Charlotte's Professor of Midwifery Practice, Head of the Centre for Midwifery Practice,
Thames Valley University and Queen Charlotte's and Hammersmith Hospital, London, UK

Associate Editor

Patricia Percival BappSc(Nsg) BappSc (Mid) MAppSc PhD RN RM CHN FRCNA

Formerly Post Gaduate Coordinator, School of Nursing, Edith Cowan University,
Perth, Western Australia

Foreword by

Sheila Kitzinger MLitt MBE

Honorary Professor, Thames Valley University;
Writer and Social Anthropologist, Oxford, UK

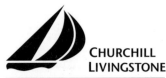

CHURCHILL
LIVINGSTONE

EDINBURGH LONDON NEW YORK PHILADELPHIA ST LOUIS SYDNEY TORONTO 2000

CHURCHILL LIVINGSTONE
An imprint of Harcourt Publishers Limited

First published 2000

ISBN 0 443 05572 6

British Library Cataloguing in Publication Data
A catalogue record for this book is available from the British
Library

Library of Congress Cataloging in Publication Data
A catalog record for this book is available from the Library of
Congress

Note
Medical knowledge is constantly changing. As new
information becomes available, changes in treatment,
procedures, equipment and the use of drugs become
necessary. The editor, contributors and the publishers have,
as far as it is possible, taken care to ensure that the
information given in this text is accurate and up-to-date.
However, readers are strongly advised to confirm that the
information, especially with regard to drug usage, complies
with the latest legislation and standards of practice.

The
publisher's
policy is to use
**paper manufactured
from sustainable forests**

Printed in China

Contents

Contributors

Jean Chapple MB ChB MCommH FFPHM MFFP DRCOG DCH FRCP
Consultant in Perinatal Epidemiology and Senior Lecturer, Department of Epidemiology and Public Health, Imperial College, London, UK
7 A public health view of the maternity services

Pauline Cooke MSc RGN RSCN RM ADM PGCEA
Associate Dean of Midwifery and Child Health, Wolfson Institute of Health Sciences, Thames Valley University, London, UK
6 Providing one-to-one practice and enjoying it

Joanna C. Girling MA MBBS MRCP MRCOG
Consultant Obstetrician and Gynaecologist, West Middlesex University Hospital, Isleworth, UK
15 Physical adaptations to pregnancy

Deborah Harding RM RN MA
Licensed Midwife, Midwifery Care Associates, White Rock, Canada
3 Making choices in childbirth

David Harvey MB FRCP FRCPCH
Professor of Paediatrics and Neonatal Medicine, Imperial College School of Medicine, Queen Charlotte's and Chelsea Hospital, London, UK
16 The newborn

Janet Hirst MSc RN RM
Lecturer in Midwifery, Division of Midwifery, University of Leeds, Leeds, UK
13 Dimensions and attributes of caring: women's perceptions

Eileen Hutton OBE
Immediate Past-President, The National Childbirth Trust, London, UK
Introduction: setting the scene

Anna Kessling MB ChB PhD
Professor of Community Genetics and Director, Kennedy Galton Centre, Northwick Park Hospital, Harrow, UK
14 The beginning of life

Christine McCourt BA PhD
Senior Lecturer in Health Services Research, Thames Valley University, London, UK
10 Becoming a parent
12 Social support in childbirth
13 Dimensions and attributes of caring: women's perceptions

Barbara C. Mills MN PhD RPsych
Psychologist in private practice, Vancouver, Canada
11 The growth of human love and commitment

Wolfgang Müller MRCPCH
Specialist Registrar in Paediatrics, The Royal London Hospital, London, UK
16 The newborn

Lesley Ann Page BA MSc RM RN RNT RMT
The Queen Charlotte's Professor of Midwifery Practice, Head of the Centre for Midwifery Practice, Thames Valley University and Queen Charlotte's and Hammersmith Hospital, London, UK
Introduction: setting the scene
  1 Putting science and sensitivity into practice
  2 Using evidence to inform practice
  5 Keeping birth normal
  6 Providing one-to-one practice and enjoying it
  11 Section on 'Implications for the midwife'
  13 Dimensions and attributes of caring: women's perceptions

Patricia Percival BAppSc(Nsg) BAppSc (Mid) MAppSc PhD RN RM CHN FRCNA
Previously Post Graduate Coordinator, School of Nursing, Edith Cowan University, Perth, Western Australia
  6 Providing one-to-one practice and enjoying it
  8 Exploring new worlds of midwifery
  10 Becoming a parent
  12 Social support in childbirth
  17 Caring for the baby

Lee Saxell RM MA
Practising Independent Midwife, Vancouver, Canada
4 Risk: theoretical or actual?

Jane Sandall BSc MSc PhD RN RM HV
Reader in Midwifery, St Bartholomew School of
Nursing and Midwifery, City University, London, UK
8 Exploring new worlds of midwifery

Trudy Stevens MSc MA(Cantab) RM RN
Research Midwife, The Centre for Midwifery Practice,
Thames Valley University, London, UK
8 Exploring new worlds of midwifery

B. Gail Thomas MSc PGCEA RN RM ADM
Dean of Midwifery and Child Health, Wolfson
Institute of Health Sciences, Thames Valley University,
London, UK
9 Be nice and don't drop the baby

Di Watt BSc PhD
Reader in Anatomy and Deputy Head of Division
(Teaching), Department of Neuromuscular Diseases,
Imperial College School of Medicine, London, UK
14 The beginning of life

Foreword

Throughout history and in cultures across the globe a midwife has never been just a technician; someone who manipulates a round object out of a small hole. She stands at the meeting place of life and death and the crossing point of generations. She works with both physiological and spiritual aspects of the process of coming into being.

This has been recognised in traditional cultures, where the midwife uses her empirical skills, enacts prayers and rites that make the way safe, and choreographs the birth drama and the interaction of everyone taking part in it. The midwife's tasks are multi-dimensional. They involve hands-on diagnosis, treatment, massage and giving comfort, together with understanding of the psychology of pregnancy and birth and awareness of relationships and their effect on a woman's ability to open her body and give birth.

Today the midwife's role is multi-dimensional, too. She must have up-to-date knowledge of birth-related research and the knowledge to evaluate it. She needs to be reflective about midwifery and obstetric practice in the light of this research. Her practice must be evidence-based. At the same time she works not only in a bio-medical framework but with emotional and social aspects of birth. She needs the skills and integrity to meld the art and the science of midwifery. She then gives each woman not only her knowledge, but the personal warmth and caring that makes her a skilled companion and friend.

Any woman who has had midwife care will tell you that it is not just a question of what a midwife knows and how clever she is that matters, but who she is as a person. Research on women's birth experiences reveals that it is the quality of the relationship between a woman and her midwife that is the single most important factor in being able to look back on birth as a satisfying experience (Audit Commission, 1997; Green, Coupland & Kitzinger 1998; McCourt, Page, Hewison & Vail 1998; Simkin 1992). All this research bears out a major theme in the pages of *The New Midwifery*, and mothers' accounts of their feelings about their midwives are remarkably similar.

It was Albert Einstein, I believe, who once said, 'Not everything that can be counted counts, and not everything that counts can be counted.' The quality of the relationship between a woman and her midwife is difficult to evaluate in numerical terms. But this is a vital element in a positive birth experience.

In all cultures the roots of midwifery lie in a one-to-one relationship between a woman and a midwife who is well known in the community and has a life-long relationship with the family, the mother and the child she has helped into the world. In Guatemala, for example, the midwife is the 'grandmother of the umbilical cord' and, as in many other societies, by her participation in a major event in the life of the family she becomes, as it were, a member of that family. No one needs to plan for this in a peasant society. It just happens. It is much more difficult in post-industrial society, where contacts between people are constantly shifting, ephemeral and superficial, and where close bonds tend to be restricted to the nuclear family, immediate peer groups which are formed in a school or leisure activity, and, perhaps, one segment of the work-place.

My own research in a major English teaching hospital revealed that it is often difficult for a woman to get to know her midwife or for a midwife to get to know the woman for whom she is caring (Kitzinger 1998). Women who have fragmented care describe feeling 'confused' and 'bewildered'. This reduced their sense of being in control and undermined their self-confidence. Some felt 'abandoned': 'I was disappointed that the first midwife had to go off shift and leave 50 minutes before the baby was delivered, as I had built up trust in her and had a rapport with her. I didn't have the opportunity to do this with X in the second stage of labour.' A woman who had a previous still-birth said: 'One midwife who knew my history might have made a great difference. They were complete strangers. You ought to know your midwife.' Women who did not know the names of their midwives tended to have a more negative experience of birth, particularly when they had five or more midwives. (This may be correlated with length of labour, and numbers are too small to come to definite conclusions.) Those who had a positive experience usually knew the names of their midwives. They said: 'It was great to have the midwife as my friend'; 'A positive experience was dependent on having the midwife of my choice who I had built up a relationship with and had confidence in. This can be very hit or miss depending on who is on call. I was lucky.'

It is difficult for any midwife to give focused care when she has to rush from one patient to another and relies on an epidural and an electronic fetal monitor to take her place. Women said: 'We had one midwife covering four women, all close to delivery'; 'I was left alone for 35 minutes plus while being monitored in the admission room. By the time the midwife returned I was 9 centimetres dilated.' One woman said that each time another midwife put in an appearance she did a vaginal examination: 'It was the worst and most traumatic aspect of the birth'. Women commented on the lack of shared information between midwives and inadequate hand-over between shifts. They had to explain their priorities, if there was time and they had the courage to do so, to each different midwife.

In many hospitals there is a shortage of midwives. As a result, women encounter a wide range of 'team members' and care is thinly spread between a vast number of staff: 'The room felt like Clapham Junction with people bursting in and out and a ward round coming in unannounced'; 'There was a constant stream of registrars, consultant, house officers, anaesthetists and students in and out of the room all the time'; 'I felt desperately the victim of lack of communication. There were too many people.'

Even women who had satisfying birth experiences were appalled at conditions on post-natal wards: 'All I ever kept hearing was, "Oh, sorry, we are just too busy at the moment."' They had little help with breastfeeding and what there was of it was often incorrect. Many received conflicting advice: 'I found it very confusing to have different advice from a huge number of midwives'; 'I never saw the same midwife twice'. A woman whose baby became severely dehydrated while with her on the ward said that the midwives had no time to help her. When conditions are like this women may be discharged without breastfeeding having been established, with low self esteem and, in one woman's words, 'totally exhausted.' One result is distress after childbirth increasingly recognised as post-traumatic stress disorder (Kitzinger 1992).

Discussion about standards of midwifery care has to take place in the context of the pressures put on midwives within rigid hierarchical structures that are ill-adapted not only to the needs of the mothers and babies but also to those of the midwives themselves. This is why midwives should study also the politics of maternity care, how institutional systems work, how power is exercised, and ways in which competing claims for territorial control operate.

Then they will be able to join with childbearing women to create a system in which the new midwifery, described in detail in this ground-breaking book, can develop and flourish.

Sheila Kitzinger

REFERENCES

Audit Commission 1997 First class delivery: improving maternity services in England and Wales. HMSO, London

Green J, Coupland V, Kitzinger J, 1988 Great expectations: a prospective study of women's expectations and experiences of childbirth. Child Care and Development Group, Cambridge

McCourt C, Page L, Hewison J, Vail A 1998 Evaluation of one-to-one midwifery: women's responses to care. Birth 125:2

Simkin P 1992 Just another day in a woman's life? Part II: Nature and consistency of women's long-term memories of their first birth experiences. Birth 19:2

Kitzinger S 1998 Having a baby in a major teaching hospital: some women's experiences. Unpublished

Kitzinger S 1992 Birth and violence against women: generating hypotheses from women's accounts for unhappiness after childbirth. In: Roberts H (ed), Women's health matters. Routledge, London

Preface

Two revolutionary changes are occurring in midwifery in Britain and other parts of the world. The first is the fundamental reform of the maternity services to more woman-centred and family-centred care. As part of this change, many countries are moving midwifery away from institutional acute care services to a primary care base, and increasing the responsibility and authority of midwives to recognize their role as autonomous practitioners.

The idea of 'woman-centred care' is simple. It means putting individual women and their families to the centre of care and meeting their individual needs. Such simple ideas are, however, often difficult to put into practice. In order to develop woman-centred care, a number of changes are required, including organizational change, different attitudes, different approaches and a new knowledge base. To provide woman-centred care also requires particular relationships between women and their midwives. An important aspect of woman-centred care is doing everything possible to ensure that the care provided for each woman is beneficial. Thus this approach requires an understanding of the potential benefits and risks of particular treatments and forms of care. Scientific knowledge is required in order to give sound information, make good clinical decisions and to support the family in decision-making. Midwives therefore need personal sensitivity and scientific understanding.

This reform of the maternity services, which includes changes in the structure and culture of care, will require that midwives take on far greater clinical responsibility than ever before and that they practise in different ways.

The second big change in midwifery that is occurring in Britain and many other parts of the world is the move towards university-level education for entry to the register of midwives. A large number of midwives are also moving on to postgraduate education. The move to higher levels of education requires a strong knowledge base, and the ability to learn and make independent enquiry at a high level.

The change in midwifery is profound. It is in fact a new midwifery. This new midwifery holds dear the central values of midwifery, of being 'with the woman' and respecting normal birth. However, to put these values into practice in today's world, where midwives often work in institutions and are part of complex health care services and where so much knowledge is available, requires rethinking, rediscovering and reforming practice.

The basis of the new midwifery is an ability to be sensitive to the individual needs of each woman and her family, and to form and work from a relationship with individual women. It also requires an ability to use scientific knowledge to ensure that care is likely to be of benefit for each woman. In short, midwives need to bring together personal sensitivity, scientific understanding, the ability to continue learning and effective clinical skills. They need to bring both science and sensitivity into practice.

Such changes require a new book for midwives who are practising the new midwifery. This book aims to illustrate new approaches to care. It starts intentionally with a true-life birth story, illustrating a way of being sensitive to individual needs while using best evidence to inform decisions.

The book is divided into three sections that reflect the areas that are core to the new midwifery practice:

- effective and appropriate care
- transition to parenting
- physical adaptation and growth in pregnancy, birth and early life.

The chapters in the first section all contribute to the idea that we should ensure that care is beneficial and avoids harm. These chapters give methods of integrating sound evidence with personal preferences, and of finding, appraising and using evidence. Guides to aspects of evidence-based care and primary and secondary research are included.

The second section recognizes that having a baby is a social as well as a physical process. Thus, important outcomes of care include the protection of personal and family integrity, a sense of having been cared for and the recognition that this is a time of transition in taking on the responsibility of caring for the newborn baby. Midwives need an understanding of and insight into the development of attachments between baby and parents, the psychological adaptation to pregnancy and birth, and the effects of social relationships and human support on pregnancy and birth. These chapters weave together the concepts of care, social support, transition and the growth of human love.

The third section provides information regarding the physical changes that are part of the mother's physiological adaptation to support the life of her baby, and about conception, birth and the development of the baby into early life. This information is an important part of the scientific knowledge base of midwifery. The book concludes with teaching plans to help midwives to teach parents about the care of the newborn.

This book is essential reading for all student midwives, midwives studying for higher degrees and any midwives wishing to review and improve their practice to ensure that they are in line with current thinking and approaches to care.

London, 1999   Lesley Ann Page

Acknowledgements

As always, when such profound changes are reflected in a book, there are a number of individuals who should be credited with the developments on which it is based. I feel I stand on the shoulders of giants. The work of such people as Professor Sheila Kitzinger, Baroness Cumberlege, Professor Anne Oakley, Professor Iain Chalmers, Professor Murray Enkin and Professor Marc Kierse provided an invaluable platform for all who wish to improve maternity care. Much of the book, particularly chapter 2, is framed by the work of Professor David Sackett, Dr Muir Gray and their colleagues, who have provided a useful and practical approach for practitioners in their development of evidence-based health care. In addition, there is a whole network of committed midwives, doctors, consumer groups and others who are working to improve the maternity services. I have met many of them in many parts of the world and am indebted to them for their work and their support.

I am also grateful to a number of people for their assistance with the book. These include Dr Patricia Percival for her help in critiquing and editing many of the chapters and for advice on the book in general, and Merle Mullings for her help in organizing, communicating with authors and general support and encouragement. Jane Young proved invaluable in the preparation of the manuscript and tables. Dr Bernd Wittmann and Gail Thomas gave detailed honest and informed advice on Chapter 1, while Dr Mark Starr provided detailed advice and feedback on Chapter 2. Georgina Going of the Imperial College School of Medicine Library at Queen Charlotte's and Chelsea Hospital provided information on searching Medline, and Alison Pearce helped with library searches. Mairi McCubbin, project development manager, has been patient and understanding.

Dr Christine McCourt stepped into the breach with an extra chapter and patiently supported other activities in our Centre while I was immersed in the writing and organization of the book. Bianca Lepori informed my ideas on arranging the room for labour. Thames Valley University gave me time for preparation of the book and has provided both freedom and a supportive environment for the development of ideas and practice over 7 years. My work with The Hammersmith Hospitals NHS Trust has both inspired and informed me. Throughout the book's preparation, Dr Mark Starr provided encouragement, support, ideas and challenging but loving criticism.

Specific thanks go, too, to the Reverend Louise Mangan Harding for her advice on Chapter 3, and to Mary Sharpe for making such detailed notes on her experience, as a midwife, of continuity of care.

Above all, however, my thanks go to the many women and their families in whose care I have been involved over the years and from whom I have learned so much, in particular Jane Phillips, who has kindly given permission for her story to be published in Chapter 1, and Tess McKenney.

Permission to reproduce photographs

Marcia May provided the photographs for Figs 5.1(A) and (B), and I am most grateful to Professor Uwe Kitzinger who took and gave to me the other photographs in Chapter 5.

Permission to reproduce materials

I am grateful to the following publishers for permission to reproduce materials and figures.

Appleton Lange Ltd for permission to reproduce Figure 15.1 from Ganong F W (ed) 1989 Review of medical physiology, 14th edn. Fig. 28.1, page 459, 'Conducting systems of the heart'.

Blackwell Science Ltd for permission to reproduce Figure 15.2 from Passmore 1980 Companions in medical studies, 2nd edn; and Figure 15.5 from Hytten F E & Chamberlain G (eds) 1980 Clinical physiology in obstetrics.

BMA Publishing Group for Box 3.3 and other textual material based on Greenhalgh T 1997 How to read a paper. BMA Publishing, London

British Journal of Obstetrics and Gynaecology for a

structured abstract from Rosenthal A, Patterson-Brown S 1998 Is there an incremental rise in the risk of obstetrical intervention with increasing maternal age? Vol 105, pp1064.

The Cairns Library Oxford for the teaching materials 'Searching narrower searching wider - worksheet' 1997.

Churchill Livingstone for Figure 2.1 p 45; Table 3a 1.26; paragraph 2 p120 to end of first para p12; Table 3b 1.2 page 121; Table 3b4.1 page 147; and an adaptation of Table 1.2 p 27 from Sackett D L, Scott Richardson W, Rosenberg W, Haynes RB 1997 How to practice and how to teach EBM. From Gray M 1996 Evidence based health care, text on problems of searching for evidence has been adapted into a table. Also, a Figure from Hey E 1971 The care of babies in incubators. In: Gardiner D and Hull D (eds) Recent Advances in Pediatrics, 4th edn. pp 171–216.

Cold Spring Harbor Laboratory Press for Figure 1, p103 from Born G V R, Dawes G S, Mott J C and Widdicombe J G 1954 Changes in the Heart and Lungs at Birth.

Department of Pathology, University of Washington, Seattle, for permission to reproduce Figure 4.1, which is copyright © 1995 Department of Pathology, University of Seattle, obtained from the Cytogenetics Gallery on the website http://www.pathology.washington.edu/Cytogallery

MIDIRS for permission to reproduce parts of the Informed Choice leaflets for Professionals, including leaflets on Epidurals, Position in Labour and Support during Childbirth.

Portland Press for permission to reproduce Figure 15.3 from MacGillivray I, Rose G A & Rowe B 1969 Clinical Science 37:395–407, © Biochemical Society and the Medical Research Society.

Radcliffe Medical Press Oxford Definitions from Strauss S, Badenoch D, Richardson Scott W, Rosenberge W, Sackett D L 1998 Practising evidence based medicine. Tutor's manual, 3rd edn.

Royal College of Obstetricians and Gynaecologists for permission to reproduce Table 15.1 from RCOG 1995 Recommendations for thromboprophylaxis at caesarean section.

Update Software Oxford, for Meta Views on Electronic Fetal Monitoring from Thacker S B and Stroup D F 1998 Continuous electronic fetal monitoring. The Cochrane Library

Lesley Ann Page

My special and heartfelt thanks to Arthur Nions for his support and practical help during the various stages of writing and editing this book. I also sincerely acknowledge the National SIDS Foundation of Australia and Rebecca Glover who so willingly shared their excellent illustrations.

Patricia Percival

Introduction: setting the scene

Lesley Ann Page   Eileen Hutton

A midwife is a person, usually a woman, who attends other women in pregnancy, at childbirth and during the early weeks of family life. Beyond this simple function lies a wealth of art and science, knowledge and expertise, attitudes and approaches that provide a unique and irreplaceable approach to care. The essence of midwifery is the assistance of women around the time of childbirth in a way that recognizes that the physical, emotional and spiritual aspects of pregnancy and birth are equally important. The midwife provides competent and safe physical care without sacrificing these other aspects. In her everyday and intimate connection with birth, the midwife is the guardian of one of life's most important events, possibly the most important one of our lives and of our society. The midwife is both friend and expert in her relationship with the woman.

We had, until recently and with a few exceptions, lost sight of the purpose and potential of midwifery. Now, there have been a number of fundamental changes, most backed by government, in many parts of the world, to renew the profession. This renewal requires a transformation, preserving the unique aspects of the knowledge, skills and values of midwifery and making them relevant to modern-day society.

Those changes in midwifery which have occurred in a number of countries, including Britain, parts of Canada, New Zealand and Australia, share a common approach, an approach referred to as 'woman-centred care'. The recognition that the central and unifying value of midwifery is to meet the needs of women and their families around the time of birth represents an important change in power relations, attitude and approach. To a great extent, this shift may reflect the changing role of women in society.

The renewal of midwifery as a profession, then, will depend to a great extent on finding out what women want from midwives. This renewal is happening on two levels: between groups of women in society, and between individual midwives and the women for whom they are caring. Thus, we start our introduction by asking the question, what do women want from midwives? We will then briefly discuss what will be required from midwives in the years to come as they renew their practice, knowledge, skills and commitment to meet the needs of women and their families around the time of the birth of their babies.

WHAT DO WOMEN WANT FROM MIDWIVES?

A survey to discover women's views in relation to the new maternity hospital being built in Bath was undertaken in 1970 (Dawson et al 1971). This involved a 1 in 10 sample of all the women who had given birth in the Bath area hospitals over the 2 previous years and was carried out via face-to-face interviews. A questionnaire covered such matters as what women wanted in antenatal clinics, how many beds there were in a ward, preferences for baths or showers, priorities for postnatal facilities (for their 10-day stay) and so on. At the end of the questionnaire, the women were invited to say whether there was anything else they wanted to add. This often led to comments such as, 'Well, of course, it's not really about buildings is it? It's about the way you're treated.' The women would then go on to give a full account of how they had been treated. Most of the comments related to midwives, women variously being full of appreciation for the throughtful and kind treatment that they had received, or full of dissatisfaction as they recalled thoughtless or insensitive treatment. 'Getting more staff is more urgent than a new building', was quite a common comment, and the staff whom the women wanted more of were midwives.

Drawing on labour reports sent in to National Childbirth Trust (NCT) antenatal teachers found that the situations in the labour and delivery wards helping to reduce women's distress and raise their pain thresholds could be summed up as: 'Midwives and doctors who are kind, encouraging and interested in the woman as a person; who are very good at explaining what they are doing; those who treat their patient as an adult; those who can sense the excitement and the feeling of a uniquely important event for this particular mother and father' (Micklethwait 1975).

A (1987) series of NCT discussion groups at which women were invited to recall their best and worst memories of pregnancy, labour and early postnatal days gave a clear picture of the importance of mid-

wives and the value placed on good midwifery care (Hutton 1988). Particularly when discussing labour, the word 'midwife' kept cropping up in the discussions. Women who had known their midwives before going into labour said how important this had been; those who had felt that their midwives were really interested in helping them to have the sort of birth they wanted were full of appreciation; and the feeling of having a midwife's undivided attention was also important and appreciated, special mention being made of midwives who had stayed beyond the end of their shift until the baby was born. The importance of relationships with midwives was also indicated by the adverse effects on women when good relations had broken down.

In 1990, asked specifically to discuss midwives, groups of NCT members remarked on the contribution that midwives had made to their care (Hutton 1995): encouraging them to have a positive attitude to pregnancy; supporting them through a good birth experience; and helping them get off to a happy start with their babies. There was much enthusiasm for the midwife as the first point of contact for a pregnant woman. Women wished that the system would at least allow midwives to spend more time with them and at best allow them to provide total antenatal care unless there was reason to refer. Continuity of care from midwives during pregnancy, birth and the postnatal period was high on the list of wants, and there was considerable demand for midwives to attend for more than the first 10 postnatal days. They wanted support from midwives in obtaining domino deliveries and home births; they wanted midwives rather than doctors to do any necessary stitching of episiotomies.

Aware of the demands that they were making, these women were explicit that they wanted midwives to have more power and authority, a high public profile and higher status; to have outlets for stress and support in dealing with stress; to be better paid, and for the NHS to employ them in greater numbers. Women also wanted all midwives to have the example of good management from a manager who was a practising midwife.

In its written evidence to the House of Commons Select Committee on Health in 1991, the NCT had much to say about midwives:

- that the role of the midwife should be clarified, emphasized and advertised;
- that a midwife should be the central care-giver during the antenatal, intrapartum and postnatal periods;
- that a woman should be able to consult with a

midwife in the community to book a home birth without first having to be referred by her GP;

- that midwives should be able to refer women directly for screening during pregnancy and directly to a consultant obstetrician at any time during pregnancy or labour, should a complication occur;
- that, in the interests of user satisfaction, cost-efficiency and job satisfaction on the part of the midwife, the knowledge and expertise of midwives should be used to the greatest advantage;
- that maternity units should not institute a policy of early discharge unless there are enough community midwives to give women appropriate and adequate clinical support at home;
- that women who have not required medical care during labour or postnatally should be discharged by a midwife.

Submitting written evidence to the Expert Maternity Group in 1993, the NCT pressed for expectant women to be given full information early in pregnancy about such things as the foods and drugs they should avoid, the choices available for place of birth and policies in local units. This paper again stressed the importance of midwives having the professional freedom and responsibility to provide individualized, ongoing care for women in the belief that caseload practice would increase the likelihood of women's wishes being respected. Women writing to the NCT were still commenting on the need to have more time for discussion with health professionals and were reporting a perceived shortage of midwives available during labour and for postnatal visits.

Members who served on Maternity Services Liaison Committees were asked to report to the NCT's Maternity Services Committee in 1997. Coming from all regions of England, their reports showed varying standards of care. Some writers were happy with the calibre of local midwives, saying that antenatal care and care in labour had improved in the wake of *Changing Childbirth* (Department of Health 1993), especially in relation to communication and information-giving. There were, however, many adverse comments about midwifery staffing levels – particularly in relation to postnatal care.

This 30-year span shows a consistent and persistent desire on the part of women to have sufficient time with familiar, sensitive, well-informed and skilled midwives who are able to provide the necessary level of information and support to meet the needs of the individual woman.

WHAT DOES THIS MEAN FOR MIDWIVES?

These apparently simple desires are reflected in a number of other surveys and reports. However, we should not be deceived by their apparent simplicity into thinking that it will be easy to meet them. A frequent response from midwives in discussing the changes that are being made to provide woman-centred care is that this is the way in which midwifery was practised 20 or 30 years ago. This is to some extent true, but it denies the importance and extent of the changes that have occurred in society and in most health services over recent decades.

The renewal of midwifery will require a rediscovery of much that has been important to midwives in the past, but midwifery will need to be reshaped and reconsidered so that midwives may provide the best care in our current social context. This context is far from easy and is changing rapidly. Moreover, unless we recognize the extreme constraints that many maternity services place on our ability to meet the apparently simple needs of women as outlined above, we will not be able to give women what they need and want.

In such rapidly changing times, it sometimes helps to concentrate on some simple ideas and clear values. Renewing midwifery, and putting science and sensitivity into practice, is based on some very simple ideas. The birth of a baby is a fundamental life transition in which the experience may influence the whole life of the baby and the family, and future generations. For the woman, it is a physical journey requiring physical adaptation, discomfort and arduous work. It will also be a journey of discovery of intense and often new emotions, which most often involves love and incredible tenderness for her child. For the mother and father, it is a journey to a new life of different roles and responsibilities, a new life requiring adaptation and sacrifice. For the baby, it is entry to the world and to all the possibilities of new life.

In some parts of the world, the birth of a baby is often a journey to death for the mother, and many babies are conceived or born to die. In the industrialized world, pregnancy and childbirth are comparatively safe but are often treated as increasingly high risk. More and more women in the Western world give birth through an operation, either caesarean, forceps or vacuum extraction. Midwives face different problems depending on where they practise, and midwives have an important role in reducing these problems.

Wherever she practices, the midwife is a friend and guide on this journey, with knowledge and expertise, and the ability to support the woman and her family, while helping them to choose their own ways and make their own decisions. Such a friend requires many qualities, including knowledge, skill and commitment. Fundamental to the role is the sensitivity to respond to women and their families as individuals, to understand the experience and to possess sensitivity to the significance of birth. The journey may lead to healthy fulfilled life or to ill-health, handicap and unhappiness. The midwife plays an important part in influencing the outcome.

Renewing midwifery requires a different approach to care. It will require change, questions and challenge. This book is intended as an aid to midwives in developing this new approach, an approach that requires personal sensitivity, an understanding of the science that forms the basis of modern-day care and an understanding of the meaning of pregnancy and birth in modern-day society. Importantly, it will require the ability to think, to learn, to make decisions and to question. The days are gone when one book could answer all the questions and tell a midwife all she needed to know. This book is not expected to be a comprehensive encyclopaedia but is intended to illustrate an approach to care and to be a source book for a number of the topics that are important to midwifery practice. The integration of science and sensitivity in practice is the crux of the new midwifery. We hope that this book helps you put science and sensitivity into your practice.

REFERENCES

Dawson J, Hutton E, Chatfield C 1971 Maternity services in Bath. National Childbirth Trust, London
Micklethwait P 1975 The aims, objectives and future development of the National Childbirth Trust. Paper presented to RCOG meeting, October
Hutton E 1988 The importance of the midwife. Midwives Chronicle (Sept): 273–4

Hutton E 1995 What women want from midwives, obstetricians, general practitioners, health visitors, anaesthetists. National Childbirth Trust, London
Department of Health 1993 Changing childbirth: the report of the expert maternity group, vol. 1. HMSO, London

Effective and appropriate care

The new midwifery requires an understanding of the profound and longlasting consequences of birth. In this section, the chapters show how sensitivity to individual women and their families may be integrated with scientific understanding to provide care that is both effective and appropriate, in other words, care in which midwives do the right things, in the right way, for individual women and their families. Ways of finding and assessing evidence, integrating it into practice and applying it to individual women are described in detail. Giving families the best start in life requires an understanding that we may do harm as well as good, so the questions 'Is what I am doing likely to do more harm than good, and am I spending my time doing the right things?' are important. As well as looking theoretically at issues such as how we best involve women in shared decision-making and how we assess risk, practical advice is given. In addition, the importance of the midwife as guardian of the normal is emphasized, and a practical approach to keeping birth normal is illustrated. The new midwifery depends on a different approach and different structure of practice; ways of doing this so that it is enjoyable not only for women, but also for midwives are described. Finally, moving from the particular to the general, the final two chapters examine a public health perspective, that is, a concern with the health of populations rather than individuals. The final chapter in this section examines the process of research, why we should do it, where research questions come from and the politics of midwifery research.

1

Putting science and sensitivity into practice

Lesley Ann Page

JANE'S CARE STORY

Jane was expecting her seventh baby. By most risk assessment scales, this grand multiparity would put her at risk of postpartum haemorrhage. In most settings, a hospital birth would be indicated. However, Jane and her husband wanted their baby to be born at home. This situation presents the midwife with a clinical dilemma. Having given birth to her last two babies at home and her older children in hospital, Jane felt that there were considerable advantages to her and her family of staying at home. In her own words (Page et al 1997):

What appeals to me about home birth? A number of factors – each insignificant on its own, but together they make a recipe for confidence. You are already in the right place when labour starts and can arrange things around as you will want them. Life can carry on as normal with very little upset, which is an important stabilizing factor with other children around … Before a home birth I would never have dreamed that I could get through labour without pain control. At home I didn't need anything. The breathing I had learned was enough.

In these simple and homely words, Jane described what was important to her about the birth of her baby. Other women may want different things: some a hospital birth and technological support, others something in between. What is important is that, as midwives, we get to know what is important to each woman and use that understanding to inform our care. This chapter uses Jane's care story to illustrate an approach to practice that responds to the personal needs of women. It is an approach recognizing that the birth of a baby is one of the most important experiences of life, an experience that has profound and longlasting consequences. This approach encourages women to become involved in making decisions about their care. It acknowledges that maternity care may do harm as well as good, however well intentioned, and thus requires that decisions are based on good infor-

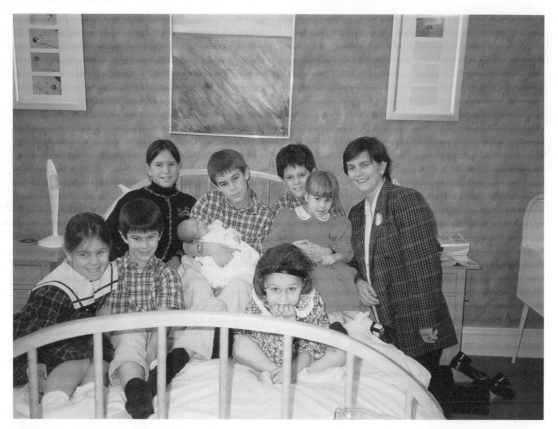

Figure 1.1 Now there are eight. Following the care story described, Jane gave birth to her eighth child; this picture was taken at the time of Jack's baptism. Back, from left: Hannah, Jonathan with Jack, Sam, Esther and Jane Phillips. Front: Miriam, Tim and Megan.

mation. This information includes sound evidence when it is available.

This approach, which integrates sensitivity to the individual woman and her family with scientific understanding, arises from a relationship between the woman and her midwife. This relationship is both personal and professional, often being like a friendship, but a friendship with a purpose. The midwife is an expert who uses her skill, knowledge, understanding and commitment to the women in her care in order to support them around the time of the birth of their babies. Through a relationship of trust, the midwife works with the woman, integrating this personal sensitivity and scientific understanding in a way that gives the mother and her family the best possible start to this new life.

This best start includes achieving optimal physical and emotional health, and helping the mother and her family to feel strong, competent and loving in the care of their baby. It also includes having the family leave the maternity services with good memories of their care around the time of birth, no matter what the course of events has been (Fig. 1.1).

PUTTING SCIENCE AND SENSITIVITY INTO PRACTICE

The ideas in this chapter are influenced by a number of new ideas that have developed towards the end of the 20th century. These ideas are expressed in publications such as *Changing Childbirth* (Department of Health 1993) and *Effective Care in Pregnancy and Childbirth* (Chalmers et al 1989), and are part of the more general movement toward evidence-based health care and medicine (Gray 1997, Sackett et al 1997).

Changing Childbirth

Changing Childbirth, the report of the Expert Maternity Group, published by the Department of Health for

England (1993), became policy for the maternity services soon after it was published (NHS Executive Letter 1994). It describes a number of important principles for maternity care. In short, the report calls for 'woman-centred services', that is, the creation of maternity services that meet the needs of individual women and their families. As well as providing clear principles, the report gives a number of strategic targets for achievement and lists 10 indicators of success. In brief, the report calls for the three Cs of continuity, choice and control; women should have continuity of carer, be in control and have choices in their care.

The first and foremost principle of *Changing Childbirth* and the principle most salient to this chapter reads (p. 8):

> The woman must be the focus of maternity care. She should be able to feel that she is in control of what is happening to her and able to make decisions about her care, based on her needs, having discussed matters fully with the professionals involved.

Effective Care in Pregnancy and Childbirth

The publication of this seminal two-volume set (1989) was influential in the movement to encourage an evaluation of treatments and forms of care to see whether or not they were likely to be beneficial or harmful. Systematic reviews and meta-analyses were used to synthesize high-quality evidence about the effect of a number of interventions on particular outcomes. Conclusions were drawn from the evidence, which were then categorized into the following:

- forms of care that reduce negative outcomes of pregnancy and childbirth;
- forms of care that appear promising but require further evaluation;
- forms of care with unknown effects, which require further evaluation;
- forms of care that should be abandoned in the light of the available evidence.

These volumes gave rise to the development of a database of evidence called *The Cochrane Library*, an electronic publication which is updated quarterly (Update Software 1998).

We need knowledge of the effects of care, this knowledge being 'an essential prerequisite if the choices made by individuals about care are to be properly informed' (Chalmers et al 1989, p. 1466). The development of care during pregnancy and childbirth has witnessed not only important advances, but also some tragic disasters (Silverman 1980); those who provide care owe it to their clients to consider carefully how best to maximize the former and minimize the latter (Chalmers et al 1989, p. 3). This knowledge is gained by giving 'careful consideration to the strengths and weaknesses of the various kinds of evidence on which they base their conclusions'.

Similarly, evidence-based clinical practice involves the 'patient' in decisions about care. Gray describes evidence-based practice as 'the judicious use of the best evidence available so that the clinician and the patient arrive at the best decision, taking into account the needs and values of the individual patient' (Gray 1997). In such a way, care will become *appropriate* to the individual woman. Sackett et al (1997) describe four sources of information for making evidence-based clinical decisions. The four sources of information described by Sackett et al (1997) and Gray (1997) are:

- individual values and preferences;
- information from the clinical history and examination;
- information from the best available evidence;
- the context of care.

EVIDENCE-BASED MIDWIFERY

Evidence-based midwifery draws on the principles of *Changing Childbirth, Effective Care in Pregnancy and Childbirth* and evidence-based medicine. Evidence-based midwifery is a process of involving women in making decisions about their care and of finding and weighing up information to help make those decisions. Evidence-based midwifery is founded on an understanding that not only physical safety, but also the personal integrity of the mother, baby and family are important outcomes. Our concern is not only with the short-term outcomes, but also with an understanding that care may affect the family in a number of important ways for many years to come. Outcomes such as the form of feeding, emotional well-being and the love between mother, baby and family are of fundamental importance and are likely to affect the individuals involved for a lifetime. Birth is the most formative event of life, and sensitivity to the potential influence of care is crucial to evidence-based midwifery.

THE FIVE STEPS OF EVIDENCE-BASED MIDWIFERY

In this chapter, I propose five steps that need to be taken to practise evidence-based midwifery. These are described in detail in relation to Jane's care and then later in the chapter with respect to another clinical situation. These steps will help bring together sensitivity to individual needs and the use of scientific evidence in practice.

The five steps are as follows:

1. finding out what is important to the woman and her family;
2. using information from the clinical examination;
3. seeking and assessing evidence to inform decisions;
4. talking it through;
5. reflecting on outcomes, feelings and consequences.

These five steps will be used to tell Jane's care story, each being illustrated with examples from practice. You will remember that Jane was expecting her seventh baby and wished for a home birth. Jane's experience of home birth was similar to that of a large proportion of the women in the study of Chamberlain et al (1997). As Oakley (1997, p. 187) comments, reporting the women's follow-up survey of this large study.

There is a contrast between accounts of hospital care that seems to remain impersonal despite the improvements of recent years and accounts of birth at home, which lead most who have experienced it to regard it as a marvelous experience.

There are a number of assumptions about a woman expecting her seventh baby. Foremost of these is the assumption that the probability of postpartum haemorrhage is greater. Turnbull & Chamberlain (1989, p. 868) state that 'grand multiparae are prone to postpartum haemorrhage. One possible explanation is that with increasing multiparity there is an increasing amount of fibrous tissue in the myometrium hindering effective contraction of the uterus'.

In addition to postpartum haemorrhage, a number of other serious adverse outcomes have been attributed to grand multiparity. When a perception of added risk is combined with a generally held assumption that home birth is less safe than hospital birth, there is likely to be considerable pressure, on both mother and midwife, to have the woman give birth in hospital. This care history, then, is one of the most controversial examples of evidence-based midwifery I can provide.

Step 1: Finding out what is important to the woman and her family

Providing personal care requires that we understand the values, anxieties, hopes and dreams of the woman expecting a baby. We need to start finding out what is important to the woman right at the beginning of care.

It is, of course, far easier if the midwife has a continuous relationship with the woman, when this becomes a more natural process of getting to know each other.

In practice, we always seek the best outcomes. These will depend on the personal values and preferences of the family. Safety is, of course, an important underlying principle of maternity care. Mortality is, naturally, one of the most important outcome measures. However, the issue of safety may, as the expert maternity group commented, 'become an excuse for unnecessary interventions and technological surveillance which detract from the experience of the mother'; one example of this has been the excessive reliance on electronic fetal monitoring that is common in most maternity services. Different things will be important to different women. One woman may place great value on the avoidance of analgesia in labour, while another may wish, above all else, for a pain-free labour. It is of paramount importance that the issue of safety is not used to restrict women's choices or their ability to be in control of decisions.

Open-ended questions such as 'Tell me how you feel about being pregnant?' 'What is important to you about your care/the birth of your baby?' and 'Where would you like your baby to be born?' will usually start to clarify what the woman wants and feels. With Jane, such questions were much more a part of natural conversation than a formal interview (Page et al 1997).

I had been her midwife three times before and saw the family occasionally between pregnancies. My visits to her were in her own home, and although not long (we were both too busy), they were relaxed. We had become friends and had developed what Freeley (1995) described as 'the shorthand of a working friendship'. Although I knew Jane well, it was important to check out my assumption that she would want this baby at home. So, early on, we talked about her preferences for place of birth and why it was important to her. It was clearly a deeply felt preference. In addition, she had always made it apparent that she and her husband felt that it was important for parents to take responsibility for making decisions about their children. They were active in the work of founding a school in which parents would be involved and active in the education of their children. In this choice of place of birth, and their need to make their own decisions, they were therefore reflecting some of their core values, the need to take responsibility for the health and welfare of their children. The domination of such values gives them added weight. If, for example, Jane had felt less strongly about having her baby at home, this would carry less weight when balancing all the factors to make a decision.

Step 2: Using information from the clinical examination

The second source of information that should be taken into account when the woman and her midwife weigh up the merits of particular courses of care is the clinical history and clinical examination. Information from these is important in interpreting the evidence and determining any increased probability of adverse outcome. With respect to general health, at a minimum the following questions should be answered by a clinical examination.

General questions

History

- Is the mother generally healthy and well nourished?
- Is she a smoker?
- Is there a habitual use of drugs or heavy alcohol consumption?
- Is there any history of illness that may be relevant?
- Is the mother well supported?
- Is she generally confident and how does she feel about pregnancy and birth?
- Are there any previous obstetric problems?

Clinical

Is the mother generally healthy?

- Are the blood pressure and urine tests for protein within normal limits?
- Are the heart and lungs normal?
- Are there any signs of disease or abnormal conditions?
- Is the fetus healthy?
- Is the baby well grown, and was growth constant?
- Is there consistent fetal growth as measured by fundal height measurements and or ultrasound scans?
- Is the baby active?
- Is the fetal heart reactive to stimulation?
- Is there a lot of amniotic fluid?
- Is it clear of meconium?

Case-specific questions

In addition to general questions to be answered by all clinical examinations, there will be specific questions for each situation, for example with regard to the probability of postpartum haemorrhage:

- Is the mother obese?
- Is the baby excessively large (over 4 kg)?
- Is there a history of postpartum haemorrhage?
- What is the haemoglobin level?

It was easier to answer the questions from the history in Jane's situation because I knew her so well. She was a healthy and self-confident woman, and had experienced no problems in her previous pregnancies or births. She had none of the clinical risk factors for postpartum haemorrhage. In addition to the answers to these questions, I took into account the fact that Jane had always had short labours, with strong contractions. At the end of her pregnancy, her haemoglobin levels were normal. The baby was active and, according to fundal height measurements, had grown consistently, being estimated to be of an average size. Neither was the fetus estimated to be large for dates by Jane's scan and abdominal palpation. All of these were reassuring factors in assessing the health of the baby before labour started.

Step 3: Seeking and assessing evidence to inform decisions

In Jane's situation, major questions fell around two key areas: *place of birth* and the increased probability of adverse outcome because of *grand multiparity*. Three general questions were important:

1. What is the evidence on the relative safety of different places of birth?
2. Is there an increased probability of any adverse outcome in Jane's case?
3. In particular, is there an increased probability of postpartum haemorrhage?

Place of birth. Home birth remains one of the most contentious issues in maternity care in much of the Western world. Considerable uncertainty exists surrounding the comparative safety of home and hospital birth. One complicating factor when looking for information on the safety of home birth is that many studies include both unplanned and unbooked cases in the out-of-hospital category. The outcomes of such births are generally poor, and their inclusion in studies of home birth skews the results. Nevertheless, such studies have been presented as evidence of the lack of safety of home birth.

A recent study illustrates the poor outcomes from unplanned, unbooked out-of-hospital births. In the UK's Northern Region Perinatal Mortality Survey (Northern Region Perinatal Mortality Survey Coordinating Group 1996), which took place between 1981 and 1994, the overall perinatal mortality rate for births occurring outside hospital was over four times higher than the average for the total population (38.7 versus 9.7 deaths per 1000 births). However, of the 134 perinatal deaths, only three had occurred in women with planned home deliveries. The others had either been planned for hospital (64 out of 134) or had not been planned at all (67 out of 134).

The best way to research the relative safety of home versus hospital birth would be to conduct a randomized controlled trial (RCT). Conducting a study of this sort would involve many practical problems, and there is considerable debate about the feasibility and advisability of using an RCT to evaluate the outcomes of home birth (Dowswell et al 1996, Macfarlane 1996, Newburn & Dodds 1996, Raisler 1996, Settattree 1996, Wiegers et al 1996a, Young 1996, Chamberlain et al 1997). One problem is that, given the low mortality rates in most developed countries, a trial would need to be very large (e.g. encompassing over 20 000 participants) in order to answer questions about safety. Given the current organizations of maternity care, a trial of this size would be almost impossible to mount. Some attempts are being made to conduct RCTs in which the outcome measures do not include mortality. Olsen (1997a) has proposed criteria for reviewing RCTs comparing home with hospital birth.

We must at this point rely on non-RCT evidence to form opinions about the relative safety and merits of different places of birth. Recent high-quality studies indicate that, for low-risk women, planned home births are no less safe than planned hospital births. It is instructive to look at a number of recent studies in some detail (Table 1.1).

Olsen (1997b) compared the outcomes of planned home births (backed up by a modern hospital system) with those of planned hospital births for women with similarly low-risk pregnancies. He completed a meta-analysis of six controlled observational studies that included the perinatal outcomes of 24 092 selected and primarily low-risk pregnancies. The results were analysed to shed light on both mortality and morbidity. Confounding was controlled through restriction and matching, or in the statistical analysis. The characteristics of the studies included in Olsen's review are shown in Table 1.1. Together, these studies provide data on over 24 000 low-risk pregnancies.

The UK Northern Region Perinatal Mortality Survey was a retrospective follow-up study of 558 691 newborns registered to mothers living in a health region of North England between 1981 and 1994. The Weigers et al (1996b) study was, in contrast, a prospective cohort study of mothers in the Gelderland province of the Netherlands. Of the women studied, 1140 had chosen home birth and 696 hospital birth.

Chamberlain et al (1997) aimed to obtain a contemporary account of booked home births from midwives and from the women having babies in the UK during the year 1994. This was a prospective study of all women who were booked for home birth at 37 weeks gestation, irrespective of where the birth actually took place. Those planning home birth were matched with women of similar background, resident locality, age group, parity and obstetric history who at 37 weeks had planned to have their baby in hospital. Data were collected on 7571 women who had planned to give birth at home, as well as on 1600 who had not planned to give birth at home. In total, the study includes over 60% of all home births in 1994.

The Ackerman et al (1996) study similarly was a follow-up prospective cohort study with matched pairs (489 versus 385). The study was situated in Switzerland.

None of these studies found an increase in the perinatal death rate in planned home births, and there is no indication that home birth is less safe for low-risk women than hospital birth, at least when the back-up of a modern hospital system is available (Table 1.1).

Interestingly, there appear to be a number of benefits to home birth. Intervention rates were significantly lower, and there were significantly fewer low Apgar scores in the home birth groups than in the control groups (Ackermann et al 1996, Olsen 1997b, Wiegers et al 1996b). There was a slightly higher intervention rate in the births planned for home but occurring in hospital than in the matched controls. However, these controls in themselves have a lower rate of intervention than average (Chamberlain et al 1997).

It is important to note that these studies must be interpreted with caution. In general, women having home births are well educated and healthy, and this may be a major factor influencing the outcomes of such studies. We must also be careful in generalizing from the results of population-based studies, particularly those carried out in other countries or communities, in which risk assessment and the management of home births may differ. On the other hand, it is important to remember that the hospital may introduce factors into care that may constitute a risk. As Campbell & MacFarlane (1996) note,' the iatrogenic risk associated with institutional delivery may be greater than any benefit conferred'.

As Olsen (1997b, pp. 9–10) comments, it cannot be claimed 'that birth in hospital is safe for all babies – nor can it be claimed that home birth is safe for all babies'.

Grand multiparity.   In Jane's case, the decision about place of birth was complicated by the fact that she had given birth to more than five babies. Did she then have a higher chance of adverse outcome because of her 'grand multiparity'? There is a long-held belief that

Table 1.1 Recent home birth studies

Author	Participants	Number of participants	Objective	Methods	Outcome measures	Results
Olsen (1997a)	Selected low-risk women (Wisconsin, USA; England; Netherlands; Tennessee, USA; Western Australia; Switzerland)	24 092	To compare outcomes of planned home births with those of hospital births for women with similarly low-risk pregnancies	Meta-analysis of studies meeting predesignated criteria	Perinatal and maternal mortality	Not significantly different between two groups OR = 0.87; 95% CI = 0.54–1.41
					Apgar scores	Lower frequency of low Apgar scores in the home birth group OR = 0.55; 95% CI = 0.41–0.74
					Severe lacerations	Lower frequency in home birth group OR = 0.67; 95% CI = 0.54–0.83
						Fewer in home birth group Statistically significant
					Induction	OR = 0.06–0.39
					Augmentation	OR = 0.26–0.69
					Episiotomy	OR = 0.02–0.39
					Operative vaginal birth	OR = 0.03–0.42
					Caesarean section	OR = 0.09–0.31
Northern Region Perinatal Mortality Survey Coordinating Group (1996)	Registered newborns to mothers living in a health region of Northern England between 1981 and 1994	558 691	To document the outcome of planned and unplanned births outside hospital	Confidential review of every pregnancy ending in stillbirth or neonatal death in which plans had been made for home delivery, irrespective of where delivery eventually occurred (Part of a sustained collaborative survey of all perinatal deaths)	Perinatal death: booked/delivered home booked for home all births	Estimated perinatal mortality among women booked for home birth 3/1733 (1.7/1000 births) 14/2888 (4.8/1000 births) 5405/558 691 (9.7/1000 births) Independent review suggested that 2 out of 14 deaths might have been averted by different management. (Both occurred in hospital)

(Cont'd)

Table 1.1 Recent home birth studies (*cont'd*)

Author	Participants	Number of participants	Objective	Methods	Outcome measures	Results
Wiegers et al (1996b)	Midwives Women with low-risk pregnancies who had planned to give birth at home or in hospital (Netherlands)	97 midwives 1836 women	To investigate the relationship between the intended place of birth (home or hospital) and perinatal outcome in women with low-risk pregnancies after controlling for parity and social, medical and obstetric background	Analysis of prospective data from midwives and their clients in 54 midwifery practices in the province of Gelderland, Netherlands	Perinatal outcome index based on 'maximal result with minimal intervention' (incorporating 22 items on childbirth, 9 on the condition of the newborn, 5 on the mother after birth)	No relationship between planned place of birth and perinatal outcome in primiparous women when controlling for a favourable or less favourable background In multiparous women, perinatal outcome was significantly better for planned home births than for planned hospital births, with or without control for background variables
Ackermann et al (1996)	Women opting for home delivery versus women opting for hospital delivery (Zurich, Switzerland 1989–92) (self-selected low-risk group with good health)	489 versus 385	To assess procedures and outcomes in deliveries planned at home versus those planned in hospital among women choosing the place of delivery	Follow-up prospective cohort study with matched pairs	Need for medication and incidence of interventions during delivery	Home birth group needed significantly less medication and fewer interventions
					Medication expulsion period	OR = 0.46 (0.33–0.64; 95% CI)
					Analgesia	0.16 (0.07–0.33)
					Induction	0.18 (0.06–0.43)
					Caesarean section	0.45 (0.19–1.00)
					Forceps, vacuum extraction	0.41 (0.14–1.04)
					Episiotomy without lesion	0.09 (0.04–0.18)
					Apgar score	Mean Apgar score at 5 minutes significantly higher (but cord pH lower) in home birth group 9.26 (0.90) to 9.08 (0.64) $P < 0.05$

(Cont'd)

Table 1.1 Recent home birth studies (cont'd)

Study		Numbers	Purpose	Design	Outcome measure	Result
Chamberlain et al (1997)	All women, booked at 37 weeks gestation, having been booked for home birth irrespective of where birth took place (61.35% of all home births in England in 1994) Both groups privileged socially and biologically Home birth group even lower risk	7571 home (5971 planned, 1600 unplanned) 4700 hospital controls	To obtain a contemporary account of booked home births from midwives and from women having babies in the UK during 1994	Prospective study of all women booked at 37 weeks, matched with women of similar characteristics	Duration of labour	No difference
					Intact perineum	6.22 (3.05 to 14.31); *P* <0.001
					Maternal blood loss	No difference
					Perinatal morbidity and death	No difference
						Perinatal death recorded in 1 hospital delivery, 1 home delivery (overall perinatal mortality 2.3/1000)
					Birth weight	No difference
					Gestational age	No difference
					Clinical condition	No difference
					Intervention rate	Lowest in home-booked, home-delivered women. Higher in hospital-booked, hospital-delivered women
					Spontaneous cephalic: home booked, hospital booked	4390 (94.1%) 3005 (89.6%) *P* <0.0001
					Assisted vaginal: home booked, hospital booked	115 (2.4%) 180 (5.4%)
					Caesarean: home booked, hospital booked	94 (2.0%) 139 (4.1%)
					Induction: home booked, hospital booked, home planned, hospital delivered	(0.2%) (19%) (29%)

(Cont'd)

Table 1.1 Recent home birth studies (cont'd)

Author	Participants	Number of participants	Objective	Methods	Outcome measures	Results
					Pain relief none: home planned hospital planned	798 (17.1%) 287 (8.6%)
					Apgar score Apgar below 7 at 1 min + at 5 min: home booked, home delivered	4.1% (N = 157 at 1 min) 0.7% (N = 23 at 5 min)
					hospital planned, hospital delivered	9.3% (N = 308 at 1 min) 1% (N = 24 at 5 min)
					home planned, hospital delivered	12.1% (N = 89 at 1 min) 2% (N 14 = at 5 min) P < 0.001 for 1-min Apgar scores P < 0.0016 for 5-min Apgar scores

OR = odds ratio; CI = confidence interval.

there is a greater chance of adverse outcome in 'grand multiparous' woman. In particular, many believe that such a woman has a higher probability of postpartum haemorrhage.

Framing clear questions

In this situation, I thought it was important for both Jane and me to find out whether or not current evidence supported the link between grand multiparity and an increased risk of postpartum haemorrhage. Sackett et al (1997) recommend that the first step in finding evidence-based information to inform decisions is to frame a clear question that will help in a literature search. The questions with regard to Jane's care were as follows:

- Is there a higher probability (chance) of adverse consequences because of her grand multiparity?
- Is there an increased probability (chance) of postpartum haemorrhage for a woman who is gravida 8 para 6 (i.e. 8 pregnancies with 6 babies born after 24 weeks' gestation)?
- Are there any other factors that would increase the probability of postpartum haemorrhage?

Searching for the evidence

I looked for studies in the following categories:

- risks of grand multiparity;
- factors associated with postpartum haemorrhage.

For this, population-based studies describing the prevalence of particular conditions in a defined group of women were needed. I asked the Midwives Information Resource Service (MIDIRS) to do a standard search for 'Grand multiparity and postpartum hemorrhage'. I searched using the MIDIRS database at two separate times, once around the time of Jane's pregnancy (Page et al 1997) and later to update the information for this book, using the abstracts provided to decide which would be useful. Studies from extremely poor, non-industrialized countries where there was a poorly developed health service (e.g. Nigeria) were omitted. Eleven relevant studies on grand multiparity and adverse outcome were discovered, as were four additional studies that concentrated on risk factors for postpartum haemorrhage (Table 1.2).

The studies presented in Table 1.2 were conducted in a number of different countries with different social, religious and economic conditions. The settings included Israel (Eidelman et al 1988, Seidman et al 1988, Goldman et al 1995, Kaplan et al 1995), the United Arab Emirates (Hughes & Morrison 1994), Saudi Arabia (Al-Sibai et al 1987, Fayed et al 1993), Malaysia (Tai & Urquhart 1991), Hong Kong (King et al 1991), England (Henson et al 1987) and the USA (Toohey et al 1995).

The dramatically different features of these countries and their health care systems must be taken into account when considering the results. Care must be taken not to make assumptions about the conditions in the different countries. Two of the studies took place in relatively affluent countries: England and the USA. Both, however, included immigrant women from deprived home countries – Bangladesh (Henson et al 1987) and a Hispanic population living in California (Toohey et al 1995).

Participants and methodology. Goldman et al (1995) aimed to evaluate the management of grand multiparous patients in contemporary obstetrics and to assess whether grand multiparas were still at risk. Their study was conducted over 3 years (1988–90) in Jerusalem. The participants included primiparous women, multiparous women (2–3 deliveries) and grand multiparous women (five or more deliveries). It was a retrospective cohort study, comparing the grand multiparous women with the two control groups that were randomly selected. Statistical analysis was by the chi-square test. There was no adjustment for other factors that might have affected the study group.

Kaplan et al (1995) investigated the perinatal and obstetric complications of women delivering for the tenth or more time ('grand-grand multiparas', in whom parity ranged from 10 to 19), compared with the general population, between January 1990 and June 1994 in Israel. Tests of statistical significance were applied.

Toohey et al (1995) compared the incidence of intrapartum complications among grand multiparous women (para >5) with that of age-matched controls who were multiparous (2–4 births). This was a low socioeconomic Hispanic group of women living in California who delivered between July 1989 and September 1991.

Hughes & Morrison aimed to document the reproductive performance of grand multiparous women receiving modern antenatal care through cross-sectional study. Participants included grand multiparous women delivering after the 20th week of pregnancy after seven or more viable pregnancies and all para 1–6 mothers. A total of 2784 multiparous women were studied. Of these, 882 were grand multiparas. The highest parity in this series was 17, that is, the eighteenth pregnancy. Of this grand multiparous group, 22.8% were in the 40+ age range.

Fayed et al (1993) studied the obstetric performance

Table 1.2   Adverse outcomes in studies of grand multiparity

Authors	Participants	Number of participants	Objectives	Methods	Outcome measures	Results
Goldman et al (1995)	Primiparous women	622	To evaluate the management of GMs in contemporary obstetrics and to assess whether GMs are still at risk	Retrospective study of 1700 women in 5th or more delivery compared with 2 control groups (both randomly chosen) Statistical analysis by chi-square test No adjustment for other factors affecting study group	Age	Significantly higher in GMs
	Multiparous women (2–3 deliveries)	735			Pre-term	No difference
					Post-term	No difference
	Grand multiparas (GMs) (5 or more deliveries) Range 6–10 (9.1% >10)	1700			Small-for-gestational-age	No difference
					Polyhydramnios	No difference
					Oligohydramnios	No difference
	Study conducted over 3 years 1988–90, Jerusalem				Perinatal death	No difference
					Fetal distress	No difference
					Multiple births	No difference
					Placenta praevia	No difference
					Placental abruption	No difference
					Cord prolapse	No difference
					Macrosomia	Higher in multiparas and GMs than primiparas Primiparas 83 (13.3%) Multiparas 102 (13.9%) $P = 0.001$ GMs 406 (23.9%) $P = 0.001$
					Maternal death	None
					Rupture uterus or bladder	None
					Postpartum haemorrhage: primiparas multiparas GMs	23 (3.7%) 17 (2.3%) 82 (4.8%) $P = 0.004$
					C/S: primiparas multips GMs	Significantly fewer 103 (16.6%) 83 (11.3%); $P = 0.001$ 116 (6.8%)
Kaplan et al (1995)	Women delivering for 10th time or more (grand grand multiparas) between 1 January 1990 and June 30 1994 Parity range 10–19 Israel	420	To investigate perinatal and obstetric complications of women delivering for the 10th or more time	Retrospective study and comparison with control group from general population No control or adjustment for confounding variables	Age	Average age 9.98 years older than average parturient Range 10–19
					Parity Low birth weight	Significantly lower rate 3523 ± 591 g versus 3400 g ($P < 0.005$)
					Vertex Breech	99% (higher) 1% versus 3% control group ($P < 0.05$)

(Cont'd)

Table 1.2 Adverse outcomes in studies of grand multiparity (cont'd)

Study	Setting/population	Aim	Sample	Methods	Outcomes	Results
Toohey et al (1995)	Largely low socio-economic Hispanic in California, USA. All delivering between July 1989 and September 1991	To compare intrapartum complication incidence among GMs with that of age-matched control multiparous women	382 GMs (>para 5) 382 age-matched controls (para 2–4)	Case control study of GM (>5) with age-matched multiparous women (parity 2–4) Control subjects selected by identifying next delivery of index case of age-matched multipara Intrapartum complications most associated in the literature reviewed Analysis: Tests of significance applied. Reanalysis for control of confounding variables and to see whether enough distinction between study group and controls	C/S Pathological presentation Instrumental deliveries Maternal hypertension Gestational diabetes Twins Antepartum complications No prenatal care Macrosomic Operative delivery Placental abruption Dysfunctional labour Fetal malpresentation Postpartum haemorrhage defined as drop of ≥ 8% from admission haematocrit Shoulder dystocia Patients transfused Uterine rupture Maternal deaths Meconium staining Apgar score mean rates Neonatal deaths Intrauterine fetal death	No significant difference No significant difference No significant difference No significant difference No significant difference Slightly higher No difference GMs significantly higher GMs 11% multiparas 16% GMs 55 (14.4%); multiparas 79 (20.7%) $P < 0.05$ No significant difference No significant difference No significant difference No significant difference No significant difference No difference None None No difference No difference 2 in study group 1 in control population GM 14 Multiparas 8 CI 95%; OR 1.78 (0.69–4.69)

(Cont'd)

Table 1.2 Adverse outcomes in studies of grand multiparity (cont'd)

Authors	Participants	Number of participants	Objectives	Methods	Outcome measures	Results
Hughes & Morrison (1994)	GM mothers delivering after 20th week of pregnancy after 7 or more viable pregnancies, and all para 1–6 mothers in Tawam hospital 1990–92 United Arab Emirates Parity range 7–14+	2784 multiparas 882 GMs	To document the reproductive performance of GMs receiving modern antenatal care	Cross-sectional study of multiparous and grand multiparous mothers	Age	Youngest GM 23 22.8% of GMs >40 years
					Highest parity	17 483 (53%) over 35 years
					Major outcome events documented:	
					Antenatal	Minimal difference
					Peripartum	Minimal difference
					Neonatal	Minimal difference
					Gestational diabetes	Higher rate GMs 15 (5.2%) Non-GMs 14 (2.2%)
					Pre-existing diabetes	GMs 14 (4.8%) Non-GMs 7 (1.1%)
					Birth weight > 4 kg	GMs 95 (106/1000) Non-GMs 104 (54/1000)
					Stillbirth rate	GMs 7 (7.7/1000) Non-GMs 21 (10.8/1000)
					Neonatal deaths (early)	GMs 6 (6.7/1000) NGMs 8 (4.2/1000)
						GM *Non-GM*
					Induced	105 (11.9%) 160 (8.4%)
					Instrumental	14 (1.6%) 15 (0.8%)
					Elective C/S	9 (1.0%) 20 (1.1%)
					Emergency C/S	57 (6.5%) 91 (4.8%)
					Retained placenta/ postpartum haemorrhage	15 (1.7%) 19 (1.0%)

(Cont'd)

Table 1.2 Adverse outcomes in studies of grand multiparity (*cont'd*)

Study	Subjects	Numbers	Aim	Methods	Outcome measure	Results
Fayed et al (1993)	Dependants of the Ministry of the Interior being cared for in Security Forces Hospital, Riyadh, 1 June 1986 to 31 May 1991. Mothers of 10 or more controls parity 2–5	228 versus 3349	To study obstetric performance and outcome of patients of extreme multiparity (10 or more)	All records examined for obstetric characteristics and fetal outcome. Analysis included Mann-Whitney U test, OR 95% CI interval. Mansel–Haanssel extension summary with calculated under OR	Mean social class	Similar (no social class IV or V)
					Incidence of hypertension	Significantly higher in para 10 group > 35 years: 34 (16%) versus 20 (14.2%)
					Anaemia and diabetes Prematurity Prolonged gestation Breech presentation Malpresentation Twin pregnancy Placenta praevia Placental abruption	No significant difference
					C/S	Significantly higher in para 10 group: 52 (22.8%) versus 372 (11.1%) OR 2.4 (95% CI)
					Instrumental delivery	Lower in para 10 group
					Incidence meconium-stained amniotic fluid Postpartum haemorrhage Perinatal mortality rate Congenital fetal anomaly Fetal distress Second stage of labour	No significant difference
					Third stage of labour	Significantly longer: Mean 9.4 versus 8.3 (< 0.05)
					Large-for-gestational-age baby	No significant difference
					Small baby-for-gestational-age	Significantly higher in para 10 patients: 25 versus 15.5 OR 2.5 (95% CI 1.6–3.9)
					Ruptured uterus	No significant difference
					Maternal mortality	None
						None

(Cont'd)

Table 1.2 Adverse outcomes in studies of grand multiparity (*cont'd*)

Authors	Participants	Number of participants	Objectives	Methods	Outcome measures	Results
Tai & Urquhart (1991)	Women aged less than 35 years of parity 5 and above who delivered during a 1-year period at the University Hospital Kuala Lumpur from 1 January 1988 to 21 December 1988	477	To compare GMs aged 25–34 years with women having second baby	Study group identified from computerized obstetric data bank	Anaemia	Significantly more common with increasing parity Controls 145 (12.8%) versus 76 (18.7%) versus highly parous 21 (29.6%) P < 0.05
	Control group all women less than 35 years having second baby same period of time	1135		Study groups divided into highly parous groups (parity 5 and 6; N = 406) and very highly parous group (para 7 and above, N = 71)	Pre-eclampsia Raised blood pressure	No difference between control group and para 5 and 6 Significant difference between para 7 and above group versus controls 8 (11.3%) versus 41 (3.6%) P < 0.000001
					Diabetes Impaired glucose tolerance Malpresentation Antepartum haemorrhage Retained placenta Induction of labour	No difference
					Preterm	Women of 7 or above significantly more likely to deliver preterm – (< 37 weeks) 9 (12.7%) versus 56 (4.9%) (P < 0.000001) – and very preterm (34 completed weeks) than women of lower parity 11 (15.8%) versus 43 (3.8%) P < 0.000005
					Baby weighing less than 2.5 kg	Very high parity: 127 (11.2%) versus 38 (9.4%) versus 18 (25.3%) P < 0.000005

(*Cont'd*)

Table 1.2 Adverse outcomes in studies of grand multiparity (cont'd)

Study	Description	Number	Method	Outcome	Result
				Very large babies (>4 kg)	No increase
				Abnormality	No difference
				Caesarean delivery	
				Breech delivery	Similar
				SUD	
				Forceps or ventouse	Women of parity 5 and above significantly less likely to need: 43 (3.8%) versus 3 (0.7%) versus 1 (1.4%) $P<0.01$
				Maternal death	None
				Perinatal death	Greater to mothers of para 7:14 (1.2%) versus 6 (1.5%) versus 3 (4.2%) ($P < 0.05$) No difference between para 5 and 6 group and controls
King et al (1990)	Women delivering after 5 or more viable pregnancies. Comparison group: rest of hospital during period of 1984–88 in Hong Kong. Highest parity 11, average parity 6	168 / 29 048	Hospital records of GMs for (1984–88) studied compared with rest of hospital. None given	Hypertension	Lower in GMs 6 (3.7%) versus 7.5%
				Antepartum haemorrhage	3 (1.8%) versus 3.4%
				Anaemia	Higher 14 (8.5%) versus 7.5%
				Antenatal gestational diabetes	10 (6.1%) versus 5.1%
				Spontaneous vaginal delivery	Higher: 141 (86%) versus 64.5%
				Forceps and ventouse	Lower: 4 forceps, 4 ventouse (5.5%) versus 20%
				Caesarean delivery	14 (8.5%) versus 15.5%
				Vaginal breech	None
				Uterine rupture	Only 1
				Primary postpartum haemorrhage (due to trauma of genital tract)	1
				Perinatal mortality rate	Nil

(Cont'd)

Table 1.2 Adverse outcomes in studies of grand multiparity (*cont'd*)

Authors	Participants	Number of participants	Objectives	Methods	Outcome measures	Results
Seidman et al (1988)	Mothers giving birth in Bikin Cholin Hospital, Israel between January 1984 and June 1986	5916	None given	Records of all women delivered in Bikur Cholin Hospital, Israel between January 1984 and June 1986	Diabetes mellitus	More common < para 7 0.6% 2–6 0.7% >7 2.3%; $P<0.001$
	More than 7 infants	893 (13%)		were analysed. Cases divided into two study groups.	Chronic hypertension	Correlated with age rather than GM
				Group 1: GMs having given birth to 7 or more infants. Group 2: having given birth to 2–6 infants	Abnormal placentation including placenta praevia Placenta accreta Placental abruption Postpartum haemorrhage Anaemia Need for oxytocin induction or augmentation Blood transfusion Malpresentation Rupture of membranes Vacuum and forceps extraction	No difference
				Statistical analysis chi-square. Perinatal factors found to differ when subjected to more analysis	Uterine rupture	None
					C/S	Significantly less common: GM group 9.6 versus 9.3 versus 13.1 χ^2 9.51; P 0.01
					Use of demerol	
					Meconium-stained amniotic fluid	No difference
					Abnormal fetal heart rate patterns	
					Low Apgar score	No difference
					Perinatal mortality	No difference
					Large gestational age baby	9.8% versus 11.1% versus 21.7% χ^2 54.3; $P <0.001$
					Small-for-gestational age babies	Significantly more common in low-parity group
					Preterm and post-term	No difference

(Cont'd)

Table 1.2   Adverse outcomes in studies of grand multiparity (cont'd)

Study	Population	Number		Study type	Outcome	Results
Eidelman et al (1988)	Mothers including (11.5%) who were GMs (after 20 weeks after 5 or more previous pregnancies in hospital in Jerusalem)	7785 including 889 GMs	Not given	Retrospective review of records	Hypertension Diabetes Uterine atonia Antenatal/postnatal haemorrhage C/S Stillbirth Congenital malformation	No increase in incidence
					Neonatal deaths	GMs significantly lower Non-GMs 21 (3 per 1000 live births) GMs 1 (1.1) $P < 0.01$
					Stillbirth Lower low birth weight rate Admission to special care baby nursery Multiple birth and trisomy 21	No difference 451 (65) versus 28 (31) Significant 543 (78) versus 20 (22) Higher incidence 62 (9) versus 22 (24) $P < 0.01$
					Forceps and vacuum	Non-GMs 420 (6.1%) GMs 24 (2.7%) $P < 0.01$
					Maternal deaths C/S Prolonged labour	None No difference 174 (2.4) versus 5 (0.6) $P < 0.01$
Al Sibai (et al) 1987	Saudi Arabia Women with 7 or more pregnancies beyond 28 weeks Youngest age 22 para 7, oldest age 51 para 19	1330	None given	Retrospective survey of pregnancies beyond 28 weeks	Iron deficiency anaemia	High in GMs 221 (16.6%) versus 409 (3.5%)
					Diabetes mellitus	64 (4.8%) versus 327 (2.8%)
					Postpartum haemorrhage	86 (6.5%) versus 362 (3.1%)
					Breech presentations	93 (7.0%) versus 315 (2.7%)
					Unstable lie	74 (5.6%) versus 140 (1.2%)

(Cont'd)

Table 1.2 Adverse outcomes in studies of grand multiparity (*cont'd*)

Authors	Participants	Number of participants	Objectives	Methods	Outcome measures	Results
					C/S	152 (11.4%) versus 1040 (8.9%)
					Uterine rupture	2
					Perinatal mortality rate	62/1000 in GMs 21/1000 in rest of hospital
					Maternal mortality	One mother died
Henson et al (1987)	Pregnancies progressing beyond 28 weeks, London GM group included large group of Bangladeshi women	216 versus 216		Retrospective case control comparison of GM pregnancies progressing beyond 28 weeks compared with control group of lesser parity matched by age and ethnicity	Antenatal complications	No difference
					Perinatal mortality	Significantly higher in GMs GMs 9 Controls 1 $P < 0.01$ (Perinatal mortality higher in previous pregnancies in GM group)
					Postpartum haemorrhage (>500 ml)	Significantly higher in GMs GMs $N = 5$ Controls $N=0$ ($P <0.01$)
					Postpartum anaemia and blood transfusion	Same in both group
					Maternal mortality	No deaths in either group

C/S = caesarean section; OR = odds ratio; CI = confidence interval.

and outcome of 228 patients of extreme multiparity (mothers of 10 pregnancies or more) against a control group of 3349 women of parity between two and five in a hospital in Saudi Arabia. Stratified sampling was used to adjust for confounding variables. Analysis combined crude calculated odds ratios and tests for significance.

Tai & Urquhart (1991) compared a parous group of women aged less than 35 years, para 5 and 6 (N = 406), and a very highly parous group of women less than 35 years of age (para 7 and above) (N=71), with all women under 35 having their babies in the same period of time (1.1.88–21.12.88). Tests of statistical significance were applied and relative risks with confidence intervals calculated. This study took place in Malaysia but consisted of a highly mixed race group of women.

King et al (1991) compared the outcomes of all grandmultiparous (over para 5, average parity 6 and highest parity 11) women who gave birth in a hospital in Hong Kong over the 5-year period 1984 to 1988 inclusive with the rest of the hospital population (168 [0.57%] versus 29 048 deliveries). No tests of significance were applied.

Seidman et al (1988) studied the population of the Bikin Cholin Hospital Jerusalem between January 1984 and June 1986. This study included 5916 deliveries, 893 (13%) of the mothers being over para 7. This was an ultra-orthodox Jewish community that the authors believed would have avoided the confounding variables of low income, mixed race and low income. The women in this population were relatively young (39.8% being above 35-years of age).

Eidelman et al (1988) studied a population of 7785 women in Jerusalem. This population comprised 889 (11.5%) grand multiparas. Of these grand multiparas, 23% were in their ninth delivery or more. Seventy-eight per cent of the population were of social class 1–3, and 35% were over 35 years. Tests of statistical significance were applied.

Al-Sibai et al (1987) surveyed 1330 grand multiparous women who were para 7 or more and compared outcomes with those of the rest of the population (N=11 687) between January 1982 and December 1986 in the Al-Khoban University teaching hospital in Saudi Arabia. The mean age was 34.6 years, and the oldest participant was para 19 at the age of 51 years. No tests of statistical significance were applied.

Henson et al (1987) undertook a retrospective study of 216 grand multiparae and compared them with controlled patients who were matched for maternal age and ethnic origin. Tests of statistical significance were applied. There was no adjustment or analysis for confounding variables. Grand multiparity was

defined as five previous pregnancies progressing beyond 28 weeks.

Results. Of the 11 studies, four reported an association between grand multiparity and adverse outcome in the intrapartum period (see Table 1.4 below). Of these Al-Sibai et al (1987) reported increased rates of stillbirth, perinatal mortality, postpartum haemorrhage, breech presentation, unstable lie, uterine rupture, caesarean section and maternal mortality in the grand multiparous group. Henson et al (1987) found a higher rate of perinatal mortality and postpartum haemorrhage in the grand multiparous group, while Tai & Urqhart (1991) reported a higher rate of perinatal mortality, low birth weight and preterm delivery in the over para 7 group. Goldman et al (1990) found an association between grand multiparity and postpartum haemorrhage (not defined).

Assessing the evidence

There is an inherent problem with interpreting the results of any population-based study with an individual in mind. This problem is particularly marked when studies have been situated in different locations with different health care systems and different populations. Because grand multiparity is so uncommon in much of the industrialized world, much of the research has been undertaken among populations of women, and in places, that are very different from Jane and her place of care. Table 1.3 reports on the validity of studies of grand multiparity.

Moreover, the outcomes of grand multiparity are very likely to be confounded by other factors that affect outcomes, for example age and chronic medical conditions, socio-economic status and having had a number of previous pregnancy losses. One of the factors that is likely to affect outcome is the management and quality of care. Especially in relation to postpartum haemorrhage, this can range from very aggressive treatment, including routine intravenous oxytocin, to the physiological management of third stage. Few studies give enough detail to understand the type of care provided. In addition, facilities vary from one institution to another, and few reports give any description of facilities available or of routine management. It was important, then, to make some assessment of the quality of the studies.

Sackett et al (1997, p. 86) propose three major questions for assessing evidence on prognosis before it is applied in practice:

1. Are the results of this prognosis study valid (i.e. close to the truth)?

Table 1.3 Validity of studies of outcomes of grand multiparity

Author (Population)	Matched or random control	Prestudy intentions on outcomes	Analysis or adjustment for confounding variables	Numbers and precision
Eidelman et al (1988) (Jerusalem)			For maternal age in relation to trisomy 21	778 versus 5889
Toohey et al (1995) (Hispanic community, USA)	Matched	Yes	Reanalysis for confounding variables	382 grand multiparas and 382 age-matched multiparous women Power calculations included P value, confidence intervals and odds ratios
Fayed et al (1993) (Riyadh, Saudi Arabia)		Predesigned data collection sheet	Stratified sampling and analysis	237 of para 10 or more versus 19 756 Power calculations Tests for significance, odds ratio and confidence interval
Tai & Urquhart (1991) (Kuala Lumpar)	Controls all women 25–34 years	Yes		477 versus 1135 statistical significance, relative risk and confidence intervals
Seidman et al (1988) (Israel)			Factors found to differ; reanalysed to determine relationship, age and parity	893 versus 5916 Chi-square tests for significance
Henson et al (1987) (Bangladeshi community, UK)	Matched age ethnicity			216 versus 216
Goldman et al (1995) (Jerusalem)	Controls randomly selected			1700 versus 622 + 735 Chi-square test for statistical significance
Kaplan et al (1995) (Israel)		Yes		420 grand grand multiparas versus rest of population Chi-square test for statistical significance
Hughes & Morrison (1994) (United Arab Emirates)		Yes		882 versus 2784 No tests of significance
King et al (1991) (Hong Kong)				168 versus 29 048
Eidelman et al (1988) (Jerusalem)		Yes	Analysis by social class Ethnic background	7785 of which 889 (11.5%) grand multipara Chi-square test Significance $P < 0.05$,
Al-Sibai et al (1987) (Saudi Arabia)				1330 versus 11 687 No tests of significance

2. Are the valid results of this prognosis study important?

3. Can you apply this valid important evidence in caring for your patient?

Criteria for validity of the studies. As with any study, there are a number of general questions to be asked with regard to the validity of prognostic studies. Is the study likely to be biased? Is it powerful enough to detect any difference. Are estimates of differences precise and not likely to be the result of chance? Has confounding been controlled for?

Adapting some of the criteria for validity proposed by Sackett et al (1997), I assessed the studies against five criteria:

• *A study group compared with a control group, which may be matched, specified or random. A control group* acts as a basis for comparison with groups who do not have the condition being studied. RCTs, in which people are randomly assigned to the study group or the control group, are the least likely to be biased, but it is not always possible to assign study participants randomly, and matched or specified groups are often used instead in an attempt to control for bias.

- *A pre-study intention of the outcomes to be measured.* The outcomes to be studied should be specified in advance because a study that looks for any differences is likely to find some simply by chance.
- *An analysis or adjustment for confounding variables.* This aims to determine whether or not the condition being studied is causally related to outcomes or whether they are associated with other variables (e.g. a number of previous perinatal losses when the perinatal mortality rate is high; see, for example, Henson et al 1987).
- *Number.* The study should be powerful enough to detect any important differences, and tests of significance should be applied to ensure that differences do not arise by chance alone. Studies of prognosis may give a relative risk or odds ratios, indicating precision in measurement.
- *What are the characteristics of the population studied?* Is this likely to affect the outcomes?
- *Were objective criteria applied in a blind fashion?* Some element of interpretation is always necessary in taking data from records. Blinding the auditor guards against his or her being influenced in this interpretation.
- *Was a defined representative group of patients assembled at a common (usually early) point in the course of the disease?* Prospective studies are less likely than retrospective studies to be biased.

Are the results of these studies on grand multiparity valid?

Was there a control group and was it restricted or matched? In pregnancy, the adverse outcomes that are likely to occur in grand multiparous women are also possible in women of lower parity so a basis for comparison is necessary to determine any increase in risk. The question is, then, how much more probable is this adverse outcome in grand multiparity than in lower-parity women? For this reason, control groups are necessary. Control groups are most useful when they are comparable for other relevant factors in the study group. Thus, matched case controls are likely to be the most useful studies. For a number of the studies, the control was the rest of the population (Al-Sibai et al 1987, Eidelman et al 1988, Tai & Urquhart 1991 [all women having a second baby], Fayed et al 1993,

Hughes & Morrison 1994 [cross-sectional], Kaplan et al 1995, King et al 1991). Seidman compared two groups: women having given birth to seven or more infants and women having given birth to 2–6 infants.

Only the studies of Henson et al (1987; on age and ethnic origin) and Toohey et al (1995; age matched) had matched controls and that of Goodman et al (1995), controls who were randomly selected. The studies defined grand multiparity in a number of ways, from more than 5 live births after 20 weeks to more than 10 live births. Within these studies, there was a wide range in parity.

Was there a clear pre-study intention of outcomes to be measured? *Were there clear definitions?* Only seven of the studies gave prespecified outcome measures or clear objectives. One study involved no tests of significance.

Was there an analysis or adjustment for confounding variables? Reports claiming one subgroup of patients has a different prognosis from others should ensure that the outcome is not being distorted by the unequal occurrence of another prognostic factor (Sackett et al 1997, p. 89). This is particularly important in grand multiparity, where other factors that are prognostic of poorer outcome (for example, socio-demographic characteristics) may confound the study. Sackett et al recommend looking for an adjustment for other prognostic factors. This adjustment is evident in stratified analyses (e.g. were older women more likely to have hypertension?; was macrosomia associated with higher rates of postpartum haemorrhage?) and multiple regression analyses (that could take into account age and economic factors). Of the studies described, only a few undertook any kind of analysis or adjustment for the control of confounding variables. Such studies included those of Eidelman et al (1988; maternal age and trisomy 21), Toohey et al (1995), to address whether or not there was enough distinction between study group and controls, Fayed et al (1993), who stratified women for example according to age in relation to hypertension and fetal weight, and Seidman et al (1988), who submitted the four perinatal factors that were found to differ significantly to further analysis in an attempt to determine the relationship between maternal age and parity.

Were the numbers powerful enough to detect a difference in the outcomes? It is important to remember that these studies may not be powerful enough (e.g. large enough) to reach any firm conclusions about the prevalence of the less common but clinically highly important complications, such as maternal mortality or uterine rupture.

Only two studies reported the use of power calculations. Where these are not reported, it is difficult to know whether the lack of a significant finding is the result of insufficient numbers, particularly when the incidence of a particular outcome is rare.

What are the characteristics of the population being studied? This question has been addressed above. In general, the characteristics of the populations are likely to have affected the outcome.

Were objective criteria applied in a blind fashion? None of the studies reported blinding for the audit of records. The criteria for multiparity and postpartum haemorrhage varied between studies.

Was a defined sample of patients assembled at a common (usually early) point in the course of their disease? None of the studies was prospective.

Applying these criteria, I could find no evidence from the strongest of these studies to support the assumption that postpartum haemorrhage is more probable in women who are grand multiparous.

Are the valid results of this study important? Table 1.4 shows the findings with respect to adverse outcomes.

Measures include maternal and perinatal death, and trauma including uterine rupture, as well as other life-threatening conditions. One of the studies (Al Sibai 1987) reports an increased incidence of perinatal mortality postpartum haemorrhage and uterine rupture. Henson et al (1987) show an increased incidence of perinatal mortality and postpartum haemorrhage, and Goldman et al (1995) reports an increased incidence of postpartum haemorrhage.

Let us look at the incidence of these outcomes and what the authors have to say about them. In Al-Sibai et al's (1987) study, the perinatal mortality rate was 62 per 1000 in the series compared with 21 per 1000 in the general hospital population. There were 50 stillbirths and 32 neonatal deaths. Of the 50 stillbirths, 41 occurred in the antenatal period. The description of this group indicates a high rate of macrosomia, a large number of congenital abnormalities and medical problems. There was one maternal mortality, which occurred in a woman who was gravida 11, para 10, and who had never attended the antenatal clinic; she suffered intrauterine death and, following a number of complications, died, probably of infection. The incidence of postpartum haemorrhage was double that seen with other deliveries. This may have been associated with the high incidence of large babies, macrosomia and induction reported in the study. There were four uterine ruptures, two being associated with obstructed labour and two with induction. The rate of trauma or adverse outcome in this population appears to be generally high. This raises a number of questions about the population and management of care in this study.

Henson et al's (1987) study reports a very high rate of perinatal mortality of 31.8 per 1000 compared

with 4.1 per 1000 in the controls. There were 5 stillbirths and 4 neonatal deaths in the group of grand multiparas and 1 neonatal death among the controls. Two of the neonatal deaths were caused by rhesus iso-immunization. There was a high rate of previous perinatal death in the grand multiparous group, which had a high number of Bangladeshi women who had lost babies in Bangladesh before moving to London. Henson et al also report a higher rate of postpartum hemorrhage. A blood loss of more than 500 ml occurred in five grand multiparae (out of a total of 216) but no controls. However, the incidence of blood transfusion and anaemia was similar in both groups. The similar rates of anaemia and blood transfusion might indicate that the blood loss was within the physiological range.

Tai & Urqhart's (1991) evidence suggests that the perinatal deaths in the highest parity group are most probably a function of low birth weight and preterm labour.

Thus, although these studies show an increased incidence of the most important outcomes, the higher rate may be a result of confounding by other factors.

The Goldman study (Goldman et al 1995) reports a significantly different, higher rate of postpartum haemorrhage associated with grand multiparity (see Table 1.2 above). Postpartum haemorrhage is not defined, and there is no control for possible confounding variables in this study. It is possible that the higher incidence of macrosomia in the grand multiparous group is associated with the higher rate of postpartum haemorrhage.

Can you apply the results to the patient in your care? The three studies reporting adverse outcomes in association with grand multiparity are likely to be confounded by other factors occurring independently of the grand multiparity.

All the studies reviewed were based on populations of women who differed in ethnicity, location and cultural characteristics. Many of the studies indicate a perinatal mortality rate that is far higher than that of the UK overall, indicating some fundamental difference in either the population or the care provided. It is difficult to know how far it is appropriate to apply the findings in this particular situation. There was very little similarity between the populations described and Jane. Thus, any application of findings from these studies to Jane's situation could be made only with great caution, although overall the findings indicated that, in healthy, higher socio-economic group women, where relevant factors had been controlled for, there was little evidence of an association between grand multiparity and adverse outcome in the intrapartum period.

Table 1.4 Summary of studies showing adverse outcomes associated with grand multiparity

Adverse outcome	Higher in grand multiparas	No statistically significant difference or outcome	Not reported
Hypertension	Al Sibai*, Goldman* (age higher), Fayed (age confounding factor), Tai* (in highly parous group), Seidman (age confounding factor)	Eidelman, Kaplan, Tai, King (lower rate) Toohey, Hughes & Morrison	
Diabetes	Al-Sibai*, Goldman (age higher), Hughes & Morrison* (age higher), King*, Seidman	Eidelman, Kaplan, Fayed, Tai, Seidman, Toohey, King	
Antenatal haemorrhage	Al-Sibai*	Eidelman, Kaplan, Henson, Fayed (placenta praevia or placental abruption), King (lower rate), Seidman (no difference in abnormal placentation)	Goldman, Toohey, Tai, Hughes & Morrison
Increased multiple births	Eidelman, Kaplan, King	Goldman, Hughes & Morrison, Fayed	Al-Sibai, Seidman, Toohey, Fayed, Kaplan, Tai
Caesarean section	Al-Sibai*, Fayed (in para >10 group) (instrumental delivery lower)	Eidelman, Hughes & Morrison, Kaplan, Toohey (decreased), Tai (includes instrumental delivery), King (including instrumental delivery), Seidman (less common; including instrumental delivery and use of pain relief), Goldman, Henson	Toohey
Breech presentation	Al-Sibai*	Eidelman, Kaplan (lower), Toohey, Fayed, Tai, King, Seidman, Hughes & Morrison	Goldman
Unstable lie or transverse, malpresentation	Al-Sibai* et al, King, Hughes & Morrison	Kaplan, Fayed, Tai, Henson, Eidelman, Toohey, Seidman	Goldman
Uterine rupture	Al-Sibai et al*	Goldman, Hughes, Seidman, Henson, Fayed, King, Toohey, Eidelman	Kaplan, Tai, Hughes & Morrison
Spontaneous vaginal delivery rate		Kaplan (higher rate), Toohey (higher rate), Tai, King, Goldman (higher rate)	Fayed, Seidman, Eidelman, Hughes & Morrison
Fetal distress		Goldman, Toohey (Apgar), (Fayed), Seidman (but more meconium), Eidelman (admission to SCBU), Hughes & Morrison	Kaplan, Tai, King
Postpartum haemorrhage	Al-Sibai* and Henson** (defined as >500 ml). Postpartum anaemia and blood transfusion Goldman* (age of grand multiparas higher)	Stones at al, Vivien, Begley, Combs, Toohey, Fayed, Tai (retained placenta), King (intravenous ergot with anterior shoulder), Seidman, Eidelman, Hughes & Morrison	Kaplan
Low birth weight	Tai* Seidman* (increased with high parity and high maternal age)	Eidelman, Henson (lower rate), Goldman, Kaplan (lower rate), Fayed, Seidman	Al-Sibai, Goldman, Toohey, Hughes & Morrison

Table 1.4 Summary of studies showing adverse outcomes associated with grand multiparity (*cont'd*)

Adverse outcome	Higher in grand multiparas	No statistically significant difference or outcome	Not reported
Increased still birth rate	Al-Sibai*	Eidelman, Hughes & Morrison (Lower for grand multiparas) King, Toohey	Goldman, Fayed, Kaplan, Tai
Increased neonatal mortality rate		Eidelman (lower rates) King (morbidity), Hughes & Morrison	Al Sibai, Fayed, Kaplan, Tai, Seidman
Increased perinatal mortality rate	Al-Sibai*, Henson**, Tai* (mothers of para 7 and above)	Eidelman, Goldman, Toohey***, Fayed, Tai (no difference para 5 and 6 and controls), King, Seidman	Kaplan, Hughes & Morrison
Maternal mortality	Al-Sibai et al	Eidelman, Goldman, King, Tai, Toohey, Fayed	Kaplan, Seidman, Hughes & Morrison
Congenital malformations		Eidelman, Fayed, Tai, King	Al-Sibai, Goldman, Toohey, Kaplan, Seidman, Hughes & Morrison
Trisomy 21	Eidelman*		Al-Sibai, Goldman, Kaplan, Toohey, Fayed, Tai, King, Seidman, Hughes & Morrison
Large-for-gestational-age babies	Goldman*, Seidman*, Fayed, King	Kaplan, Toohey, Tai, Hughes & Morrison	Eidelman
Preterm	Tai* (for over para 7)	Goldman, Seidman, Henson, Toohey	Kaplan, King, Eidelman
Post-term		Goldman, Fayed, Seidman, Tai	Hughes & Morrison, Kaplan, Toohey, King, Eidelman
Anaemia	Al-Sibai*, Tai*, King*, Hughes & Morrison	Toohey, Fayed, Seidman, King	Goldman, Kaplan, Eidelman

Hughes & Morrison: Minimal differences in major antenatal, peripartum and neonatal outcome events.
*Indicates no analysis for confounding variables.
**Indicates control for age and ethnicity but not social class (this study included a large group of Bangladeshi women). Perinatal mortalities of previous pregnancies significantly higher in grand multiparas.
***Intrapartum fetal death.
All references are listed at the end of the chapter.

From the general studies of grand multiparity and postpartum haemorrhage, I moved to a review of the studies of risk factors for postpartum haemorrhage.

Postpartum hemorrhage

Four studies of factors associated with postpartum haemorrhage have been reviewed (Table 1.5), all calling into question a relationship between grand multiparity and a greater probability of postpartum haemorrhage.

One study was an RCT to evaluate active versus physiological management of the third stage of labour. From the data collected from the physiologically man-aged group, the factors that increase the risk of postpartum haemorrhage were identified. The authors of the study concluded that postpartum haemorrhage fell with increasing parity and was highest in primiparous women (Begley 1991).

In a case control study of 9598 deliveries to find risk factors for postpartum haemorrhage, there was an association with nulliparity (an adjusted odds ratio of 1.56) but no association with grand multiparity (Combs et al 1991).

In a retrospective review of data relating to 37 497 women in London, intrinsic factors associated with significant risk factors (99% confidence intervals) were

Table 1.5 Studies to identify risk factors for postpartum haemorrhage (PPH)

Authors	Participants	Number of participants	Objectives	Methods	Risk factors	Results
Begley (1991)	Two groups of women who participated in a randomized controlled trial, Ireland	705 versus 724		Part of randomized controlled trial to evaluate active versus physiological management of 3rd stage of labour. Identification of risk factors associated with PPH from data	Risk factors in physiologically managed third stage of labour. Midwife's skill. Primagravidas	Primagravidase versus other parities 11.9% versus 7.1% Significant difference (Z = 2.83; P > 0.005)
					Mean blood loss	Fell with increasing parity 263 ml in primigravidae to 109 ml in para 5. Active group. No difference between primigravidas and others
					Second stage > 40 min	Significantly increases risk of excessive blood loss + PPH
					Weight of the baby	(P < 0.05) but not active group
					Highest PPH rate	13.4% in group where baby weighed more than 4001–4500 g
Combs et al (1991)	Women having vaginal deliveries	9598	To identify risk factors for PPH	Case control study to identify risk factors for PPH. Three controls matched to each case. Multiple logistic regression used to control for co-variance between predictor variables	Prolonged 3rd stage	PPH occurred in 374 cases (3.9%)
					Pre-eclampsia	Adjusted OR 7.56
					Mediolateral episiotomy	OR 5.02
					Previous PPH	OR 4.67
					Twins	OR 3.55
					Arrest of descent	OR 3.31
					Soft tissue lacerations	OR 2.91
					Augmented labour	OR 2.05
					Forceps or vacuum delivery	OR 1.66
					Asian	OR 1.66
					Hispanic ethnicity	OR 1.73
					Midline episiotomy	OR 1.66
					Multiparity	OR 1.56
						OR 1.45

(Cont'd)

Table 1.5 Studies to identify risk factors for postpartum haemorrhage (PPH) (cont'd)

Authors	Participants	Number of participants	Objectives	Methods	Risk factors	Results
Stones (1993)	North West Thames region, London	37 497	To identify intrinsic factors associated with significant risk ratios (89% CI)	Factors associated with PPH analysed using data related to 37 497 women in one region in London	Placental abruption	*OR significant risk ratios (99% CI)*
						12.6 (7.61–20.9)
					Placenta praevia	13.1 (7.47–23.0)
					Multiple pregnancy	4.46 (3.01–6.61)
					Obesity	1.64 (1.24–2.17)
	Complicated by haemorrhage of 1000 ml or more	498 (1.3%)			C/S versus spontaneous vaginal delivery	8.84 (6.74–11.6)
					High parity	No association
					Retained placenta	13.7 (5.92–31.8)
					Induced labour	2.22 (1.67–2.96)
					Episiotomy	2.06 (1.36–3.11)
					Birth weight	
					4 kg or more	1.90 (1.38–2.60)
					Blood loss over 1000 ml	
					Retained placenta	13.7 (5.92–31.8)
					Induced labour	2.35 (1.11–4.98)
Tsu (1993)	Two groups of women Group 1: PPH (500–800 ml) after normal vaginal delivery. Group 2. normal	151	To identify risk factors for PPH	Date abstracted from medical records Relative risks estimated by multivariate logistic regression (part of longer study)	Low parity	Para 1 and 2: 70% greater incidence
					Advanced maternal age (35+)	Over 35: 2.5 times greater risk
	unassisted delivery without PPH	299			Antenatal hospitalization	3 or 4 times greater risk
	Similar socio-economic, height and weight measurements Harare, Zimbabwe				History of poor maternal and perinatal outcomes	2 times greater risk
					Borderline anaemia	No association
					Grand multiparity	No association

OR = odds ratio; CI = confidence interval; C/S = caesarean section.

identified. There was no association with high parity (Stones et al 1993).

Tsu undertook a study of two groups of women, one group consisting of those with postpartum haemorrhage after a normal vaginal delivery and the other of women with a normal unassisted delivery without postpartum haemorrhage. The women shared similar socio-economic characteristics and height–weight measures. Relative risks were estimated by multivariate logistic regression. The study called into question the significance of grand multiparity. The significantly elevated crude risks for high parity seen in these data virtually disappear once they are adjusted for maternal age (Tsu 1993).

Assessing the evidence for validity and importance. None of the studies reviewed demonstrated a direct association between grand multiparity and a higher probability of postpartum haemorrhage.

Can you apply this valid, important evidence about prognosis in caring for your patient? The largest study (Stones et al 1993) was conducted in a substantial region of London. It included 37 497 women and was the most likely of all the studies to have participants who would be like Jane in a number of ways.

Reaching conclusions

I could find no sound evidence to support the belief that grand multiparity on its own is a predictor of severe adverse outcome and the four studies of postpartum haemorrhage indicated no association between grand multiparity and postpartum haemorrhage. None of the risk factors for postpartum haemorrhage identified by these studies (weight of baby, ethnicity, previous postpartum haemorrhage and pre-eclampsia for example; Table 1.6) applied to Jane. Given her clinical history of short labours and strong contractions, I decided that Jane did not have a higher probability of postpartum haemorrhage than other less parous women in the population.

Step 4: Talking it through

Individual women will differ in the amount of detail they want to consider with regard to information taken from evidence. Some, for example, may lead the search for evidence themselves and approach health care professionals with searches of databases and the Internet. Others may leave it up to their professional carers to stay up to date and informed on recent evidence. Women need information, and they should be given every chance of asking questions and requesting help with interpreting information. For some topics,

aids such as the MIDIRS informed choice leaflets may be helpful. However, there are a number of topics for which no materials are available.

Jane knew of my search for evidence on grand multiparity. I told her of my interpretation that I had found no evidence to support the belief that grand multiparity was in itself a cause of adverse consequences and that I did not believe her to be in a high-risk group.

Step 5: Reflecting on feelings, outcomes and consequences

Much of my care of Jane was against usual practice. Usual practice nowadays is dominated by routines of technological intervention and hospital care, and frequent medical treatment. As in any walk of life, there is likely to be difficulty in challenging the usual way of doing things, difficulty in doing something a little different. Such care is likely to attract attention and scrutiny. This is particularly so if there are adverse outcomes, which are always possible no matter how low the probability. It is important therefore to document discussions, decisions, actions, treatments and rationale very carefully in the medical records.

One of the difficulties for any midwife who is trying to use evidence in practice is that the perspective of research, which is a more distant perspective of populations of people, is very different from the perspective of any midwife in practice. The midwife in practice is not making a population-based assessment but an assessment for an individual, with more direct consequences. For example, although perinatal mortality rates may be so low that any differences arising from place of birth are likely to be small (MacFarlane 1996), the possibility of death of the mother or baby is of enormous consequence for the parents and their carer(s). In practice, an individual is not a statistic.

The decisions to be made by a midwife who wishes to meet the individual needs of women and to avoid unnecessary intervention are finely tuned. There has to be enough confidence not to overdiagnose complications, but the decisions should be made within the parameters of safety while recognizing that there is no such thing as absolute safety. These decisions are also made in a system in which intensive surveillance and hospital birth are the norm. There is little tolerance for any decision that upsets these norms, even when there is no indication of a problem. Once there is any indication of a potential problem, however slight, it becomes difficult to find any support for the decision to continue to avoid technological intervention and transfer to hospital.

Jane went into labour at term early in the evening.

Table 1.6 Factors associated with postpartum haemorrhage

Factor	Yes (Author)	No (Author)
Midwife's skill	Begley	
Primigravida	Begley, Combs et al	
Low parity	Begley, Tsu	
Long second stage	Begley	
Episiotomy	Begley, Combs et al	
Heavy baby	Begley, Stones et al	
Prolonged third stage	Combs et al	
Pre-eclampsia	Combs et al	
Previous postpartum haemorrhage	Combs et al	
Multiple pregnancy	Combs et al, Stones et al	
Arrest of descent	Combs et al	
Lacerations	Combs et al	
Augmented labour	Combs et al	
Caesarean	Stones et al	
Forceps or vacuum delivery	Combs et al, Stones et al	
Asian	Combs et al	
Hispanic	Combs et al	
Ethnicity	Combs et al	
Midline episiotomy	Combs et al	
Placental abruption	Stones et al	
Placenta praevia	Stones et al	
Obesity	Stones et al	
Grand multiparity	Al-Sibai et al, Goldman et al, Henson et al	Begley, Combs et al, Eidelman et al, Fayed et al, Hughes & Morrison, Kaplan et al, King et al, Seidman et al, Silva, Stones et al, Toohey et al, Tsu
Retained placenta	Stones et al	
Induction with oxytocin	Stones et al	
Pyrexia in labour of 38°C or more	Stones et al	
Prolonged labour	Begley, Stones et al, Tsu	
Smoker	Stones et al	
Young age	Begley	
High age	Tsu	
Antenatal hospitalization	Tsu	

All references are listed at the end of the chapter.

On arrival at her house, all was going well. Her baby continued to be active, and contractions were regular, ranging from mild to moderate in intensity. Jane was still feeling that to stay at home was the right decision for her. However, early in labour, her membranes ruptured spontaneously and there was meconium in the amniotic fluid, which was greenish brown with no particulate matter. There was, however, copious amniotic fluid, and on auscultation the fetal heart was reactive, with a rate of between 120 and 140. Accelerations occurred with movement. These are reassuring signs.

Because of the meconium-stained amniotic fluid, I suggested that we might want to transfer to hospital.

The decision was upsetting to both Jane and John. The ambulance was ordered, and the hospital was warned of our intention to transfer. This set up another cycle of decision-making that is described below.

MANAGING JANE'S CARE IN HOSPITAL

Step 1: Finding out what is important to the woman and her family

When we arrived in hospital, it became more important than ever to ensure that Jane and John's feelings and values continued to be taken into account. The transfer to hospital sets up a round of negotiations with other midwives and doctors, and in most hospitals, meconium in the amniotic fluid means that the situation will be treated as high risk. Jane did not want unnecessary intervention and wished to go home as soon as possible after birth. Such a situation sometimes becomes a balancing act between meeting usual practices half way and respecting the woman's wishes. I suggested that we do some electronic fetal monitoring and then go back to intermittent auscultation if all was well.

Referrals may take considerable negotiation skills. On arrival, I spoke to the senior doctor, giving all the details of the situation. He advised me that Jane was at high risk of postpartum haemorrhage and that she should have an intravenous catheter inserted in case intravenous fluids were required. I informed him of my interpretation of the evidence but asked Jane how she would feel about the procedure. She declined with great certainty.

Step 2: Using information from the clinical examination

After transfer, a reassessment of the condition of mother and baby is always required. On Jane's arrival at the hospital, an admission trace was reactive and reassuring. Following that, the fetal heart was monitored using a Doppler device every 15 minutes, for a full minute during and following the contraction and following every contraction in second stage (Royal College of Obstetricians and Gynaecologists 1993).

When I made my reassessment, I had a number of questions in mind. These included:

1. How was Jane's general health after the transfer: was she excessively tired or anxious?

2. How should assessment for possible fetal compromise be made?

3. Of what significance was the meconium-stained amniotic fluid in this situation?

4. What was the general health of the unborn baby?

5. How far had labour progressed, and how frequent and strong were the contractions?

In answering these questions I took into account the following factors:

- The general health of the mother was good.
- The meconium was thin, and there was copious amniotic fluid.
- The baby had grown well throughout pregnancy and was not small-for-gestational-age (estimated by palpation and ultrasound)
- The baby had been active throughout the pregnancy and in labour
- Both the auscultation and the cardiotocograph indicated that the fetal heart was accelerating with movement and contractions; this reaction is a good predictor of fetal health.
- There were fetal heart accelerations with contractions on intermittent auscultation.
- Labour was progressing well, the contractions were strong and frequent, and labour should not be long.
- The pregnancy was not post-term, and the amount of amniotic fluid was not reduced.

In brief, labour was progressing well, and both mother and baby were healthy and coping well with it.

Step 3: Seeking and assessing evidence to inform decisions

Naturally, in this kind of situation, we cannot 'look things up'. We depend, in acute, urgent situations, on drawing from knowledge already stored in our memories. I have stayed up to date on the literature regarding meconium-stained amniotic fluid partly because of my work as an expert witness.

Nowadays, because the majority of women are quite automatically placed on an electronic fetal monitor, there is little attempt to discriminate between who should and who should not receive continuous electronic fetal monitoring. Although clinically we discriminate between light and heavy meconium staining, all women tend to be treated as if they are in a high-risk group, and continuous electronic fetal monitoring is used.

Meconium

Framing clear questions.   If we are to go beyond the routines of continuous electronic fetal monitoring and suctioning for all babies whose amniotic fluid is stained with meconium, a number of questions must be asked. In relation to Jane's care, the following were relevant:

- Why does the fetus pass meconium in utero?
- What is the prevalence of meconium-stained amniotic fluid?
- Is meconium in the amniotic fluid always a marker of fetal distress?
- Do thin and thick meconium differ in significance and why?

- What is the cause of meconium aspiration syndrome?
- How should the birth be managed?

Using reviews. For the purposes of this section, I have drawn, in the main, on two review papers. A systematic review of the many studies in this area would be very useful but, given the number of papers, is beyond the scope of this chapter. Readers wishing to pursue the issue will find the standard MIDIRS database search useful. A review brings together a number of studies. Reviews are essential for clinicians that wish to go beyond one or two studies to inform decisions but who do not have the time available for doing a complete search. Reviews should, however, be treated with caution as they have the potential to be incomplete and biased. Chapter 2 gives more complete advice on assessing reviews.

Reaching conclusions. Despite evidence to the contrary (as far back as 1925), the presence of any meconium at all in the amniotic fluid is still, in many health services, treated as if it were an independent marker of fetal distress and as if it led directly to meconium aspiration syndrome. In a comprehensive review of the subject, Katz & Bowes (1992) questioned three fundamental assumptions about meconium:

- that the presence of meconium in the amniotic fluid is an independent marker of fetal distress;
- that meconium aspiration primarily occurs when the fetus gasps at birth or in utero, in response to severe asphyxia;
- that meconium aspiration syndrome is the result of the deleterious effect of the inhaled meconium on the neonatal lungs.

In challenging these assumptions, Katz & Bowes review physiology, the aetiology of meconium aspiration syndrome, animal experiments and clinical research.

The fetus is more likely to pass meconium, the contents of the fetal bowel, into the amniotic fluid as it matures. The passage may be physiological or may be caused by a transient episode such as cord or head compression causing a vagal response. Some fetuses with meconium-stained amniotic fluid will be compromised; many will not.

Meconium and fetal distress. The passage of meconium into the amniotic fluid is common at term and frequent in the post-dates pregnancy. It is estimated as occurring in between 12% (Katz & Bowes 1992) and 13% of all live births, increasing to 30% at 40 weeks and 50% at 42 weeks. An increase in incidence to a rate of 26.5% was reported despite there being no increase in the rate of post-date pregnancy (Danelian 1994). The

identification of fetal distress when there is meconium-stained amniotic fluid depends on careful fetal heart monitoring (Katz & Bowes 1992, Danelian 1994).

Do thin and thick meconium differ in significance and why? Thick meconium is thick because it is not diluted with amniotic fluid, either because of oligohydramnios or because the membranes have ruptured. Reduced amniotic fluid both reflects reduced uterine placental sufficiency and predisposes to fetal compromise because of the likelihood of cord compression. Thick meconium is more likely to be aspirated. Ninety-five per cent of cases of meconium aspiration syndrome develops in the presence of thick meconium (Katz & Bowes 1992). Thick meconium is therefore more likely to be associated with fetal distress.

What is the cause of meconium aspiration syndrome? Meconium aspiration is an antepartum intrauterine event, which occurs either with gasping or with deep breathing. Meconium aspiration syndrome is defined as the presence of meconium below the vocal cords. It is estimated to occur in 11–58% (mean 35%) of live births with meconium-stained liqour, approximately equal to 4% of all live births. Whereas it was once believed that meconium aspiration syndrome, a potentially serious condition with an associated mortality of up to 40%, was caused by meconium aspiration, there is now evidence to the contrary. Meconium aspiration syndrome occurs in only 5–10% of infants with meconium below the vocal cords. Meconium aspiration syndrome is initiated by pulmonary vascular disease that is caused by fetal hypoxia and asphyxia. Although the primary cause of the condition is hypoxia or asphyxia, the presence of meconium in the lungs compounds it. Meconium aspiration syndrome is a thus multifaceted condition. Although 5% of cases develop in the presence of thin meconium, the associated respiratory disease is mild.

How should labour and birth be managed? There are three issues in the management of labour and birth. The first concern is whether this fetus is at a higher risk of fetal distress. Katz & Bowes recommend that the identification of high risk should be by clinical observation and selective antepartum testing for reduced amniotic fluid if the fetus is post-term.

Second is the issue of identifying fetal distress, for which Katz & Bowes (1992) advise careful fetal heart rate monitoring when there is meconium-stained amniotic fluid. If the meconium is thick, electronic fetal monitoring is advised (Neilson 1993). It is important to have clear protocols for monitoring the heart and to interpret any changes carefully.

Third, is suctioning of the nasopharynx and trachea justified? Given that aspiration is intrauterine and does not occur during birth, suctioning of the nasopharynx and trachea to prevent meconium aspiration syndrome is not logical. A number of studies have brought into question the efficacy of suctioning these areas. Nor are procedures such as chest-clamping at birth likely to be beneficial. Suctioning, particularly intubation and tracheal suctioning, is likely to be traumatic and to induce bradycardia because of vagal response. The airway may need to be cleared if meconium is obstructing ventilation. Otherwise, suctioning is only recommended if there have been signs of fetal distress (Katz & Bowes 1992, Halliday 1992, Danelian 1994). If there have been signs of fetal distress, a paediatrician should be present for the birth in case resuscitation is required (Danelian 1994).

I decided that, in Jane's case, the meconium was not an indicator of fetal distress. The meconium was thin, there was copious amniotic fluid and the fetal heart rate pattern both on auscultation and in a short period of electronic fetal monitoring showed a number of accelerations, a reactive pattern. It was unlikely also that the baby would suffer from meconium aspiration syndrome. After a 30 minute cardiotocograph, I monitored the heart carefully according to the Royal College of Obstetricians and Gynaecologists (1993). There was no suctioning of baby Esther at birth, and she was discharged home into the care of her family doctor as early as possible.

Step 4: Talking it through

Labour is not the time for detailed conversations! It is certainly far easier if, as I did, the midwife knows the woman ahead of time. By then, some trust should have built up, and the woman and her midwife will have got to know each other. Instant and crucial decisions sometimes need to be made in labour; If the midwife knows the woman's feelings and values, these provide a framework for making such decisions. In this case, Jane and I did not need long conversations, and discussion was in the kind of shorthand that goes on between contractions. Nevertheless, it is important that the woman is involved in making decisions.

Step 5: Reflecting on feelings, outcomes and consequences

Baby Esther was born after a short labour less than 2 hours after admission, with Apgar scores of 9 at 1 minute and 10 at 5 minutes. Mother and baby were both well. No suctioning was performed at birth. Jane wished to go home immediately after birth, and her postpartum recovery was normal.

It can be seen that there were a number of decisions to be made about Jane's pregnancy, labour and birth, most of which were quite complex. This is one of the most complex fields of evidence-based health care because, although a considered judgement can be made on the probability of adverse outcomes, adverse outcomes, including death and cerebral palsy, can never be entirely ruled out. We should not forget, however, that high-quality, sensitive care will make even the most unthinkable outcome – the death of the baby – more bearable. Perhaps what is most important is that parents make a genuine choice. From Chamberlain et al's study (1997, p. 108) one woman who lost her baby said:

> We found the staff all cared for us with real thought and compassion in the most difficult of circumstances. Our main concern now is that we receive a full detailed account of what went wrong with the pregnancy. We hope no information will be withheld, and the truth will help us come to terms with our grief. This was to be our first home birth having experienced three pretty awful hospital experiences previously. I was wonderfully relaxed and well in control of labour with breathing exercises alone. I would recommend a home birth to anybody.

Midwives practising in countries such as the UK and North America need to be aware of the legal context in which they practise. Evidence is not weighted heavily in most legal proceedings; there is greater weight put on professional opinion and usual practice. This is entirely contrary to evidence-based clinical practice, which is a movement away from care based on professional opinion. Ultimately, the midwife is obligated to do the best for the woman in her care and must therefore be guided by the wishes of the woman and good information based on sound evidence. Decisions and the reasons for them should always be recorded in the notes alongside notes of discussion with the parents in case of any future scrutiny of care.

In this situation, I judged that the meconium-stained amniotic fluid was not indicative of fetal distress and would not lead to problems. The decision to transfer to hospital was made on the side of caution. For all of us, the transfer was unpleasant. In common with many women who have planned home birth but need to be transferred, Jane was disappointed by this turn of events (Chamberlain et al 1997). In retrospect, I felt that I might more strongly have encouraged Jane to consider the slight possibility of the need for transfer.

In addition to the disappointment of transfer, Jane found the electronic fetal monitoring uncomfortable, feeling that attention was being diverted from her to the monitor, even though it was only used for 30 minutes.

In conclusion, I had balanced information from the

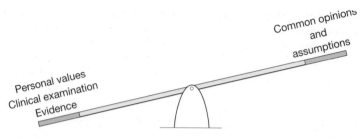

Figure 1.2   Weighing up the evidence.

clinical examination, from the evidence available to me, in the light of Jane and John's values and preferences, and the context of care. The evidence alone is never enough to make decisions about the management of care, individual women are not a population, and clinical factors, particularly in this case a history of good contractions and fast, problem-free labours, need to be borne in mind when making decisions about care (Fig. 1.2).

TRANSLATING PRINCIPLES INTO PRACTICE: A SECOND CARE STORY

This case history considers the application of routines and individual thoughtful practice in the situation of testing for hypoglycaemia in the newborn.

Not all the decisions we make are as urgent or seem as dramatic as those required in Jane's case, but they nevertheless often have important consequences. Sometimes, we may use evidence to inform guidelines for practice or to question routine practice. Much of effective and appropriate care is concerned with the idea that we need to move from set routines towards care that is thoughtful and individual. Many midwives spend most of their professional lives attached to wards in hospital. In this situation, it is all too easy to follow a routine without thought for the individual consequences. Such routines may involve tests, treatments or the organization of care, which are well entrenched and rarely questioned. Such a routine is the test for low blood sugar in newborn babies. In many maternity services, it is common to see babies with heels that are bruised, marked by a number of puncture sites. Such tests are merely screening tests; they are not diagnostic and should be used in conjunction with clinical judgement, and then only in a high-risk population.

It is far easier to follow a well-trodden routine than it is to think about the care we provide, even when such routines fill our days with routine tests or tasks and we should be doing more important things. One of the routines that is common on postnatal wards,

and which should be suspended, concerns the frequent heel pricks and 'BM' testing to screen for hypoglycaemia in babies who are not at risk of newborn hypoglycaemia.

For a few days, I was involved in the care of a woman who gave birth with the assistance of a ventouse extractor. The baby was a good weight and healthy at birth. The mother was determined to breastfeed, although there were some difficulties on the first night because she was so tired after a hard labour. I visited her a few times to support her desire to feed, and although she expressed a number of anxieties, I believed that she and the baby were doing well. The baby was feeding frequently, his positioning was good, and he sucked well. I came to say goodbye to the mother but found that discharge had been delayed because a blood glucose reading had been taken using a test strip, the result being borderline. The ward midwife wished to repeat the test. She had planned to give a bottle-feed if it was borderline again, and discharge might have been delayed. The baby was clinically well. I was aware that although test strip reading, which requires obtaining a blood sample through heel pricks, is undertaken very frequently, it is not without its dangers. It is painful to the baby; the heel often becomes bruised and damaged. At the time of this incident, I had been involved in providing an expert opinion regarding a child who had developed an infection of the calcaneum as a result of a heel prick. In consequence, the growth of the affected foot was limited, it being one size smaller than the other, and the child suffered long-term discomfort. Although such consequences may be rare, they are serious.

I decided that delaying the discharge of the mother and baby, and giving a bottle-feed were more likely to be harmful than beneficial to this family. I suggested to the mother that she should decline the suggested test and spoke to the midwife, who was quite happy to avoid it. Although such decisions are made very quickly, and many of the processes become seemingly 'automatic', the process is made explicit below.

Step 1: Finding out what is important to the woman and her family

Soon after the birth of the baby, I had discussed feeding with the mother. It was clear that there was a strong preference to breast-feed, although this first-time mother was quite anxious about managing to breast-feed successfully. At the time of the proposed discharge, she was excited and eager to go home, where there was plenty of help available.

Step 2: Using information from the clinical examination

I had assessed feeding on several occasions, and the baby was feeding well, that is, frequently with good positioning, sucking well and producing enough wet nappies. The mother, however, was still anxious that the baby was not getting enough milk. The baby was not sleepy. None of the risk factors for a high probability of neonatal hypoglycaemia applied.

Step 3: Seeking and assessing evidence to inform decisions

Framing clear questions

My decision was made very quickly, using knowledge that was 'in my head'. However, to make it more explicit, these are some of the questions that were appropriate:

- Is this baby in a high-risk group for neonatal hypoglycaemia?
- How far out of the range of 'normal' is the test result?
- How reliable are the test and the test result?
- Does the clinical examination show any signs of or risk factors for neonatal hypoglycaemia?
- What are the probable consequences of this test? Is it likely to result in more harm than good?

Searching for evidence

In a few rare situations, guidelines that are evidence based may be available. In this case, there were comprehensive and sound national guidelines to help to answer the relevant questions (National Childbirth Trust 1997).

Assessing the evidence

The guidelines I refer to here are of high quality, showing:

- a clear explanation and rationale;
- a thorough process of discussion and consideration of the evidence;
- agreement by a number of organizations and experts of national standing, including consumer organizations.

Reaching conclusions

Let us now try to answer the questions listed above in relation to this particular baby.

Is this baby in a high-risk group for neonatal hypoglycaemia? The answer to this question is no. According to the statement on hypoglycaemia of the newborn (National Childbirth Trust 1997), the following have a higher incidence of hypoglycaemia:

- a baby who is ill;
- a baby who is small-for-gestational-age;
- a baby born to a diabetic mother;
- a baby who has been born prematurely.

Babies in this group may not have an appropriate metabolic response, which puts them at greater risk.

How far out of the range of 'normal' is the test result? This is a difficult question to answer given that there are insufficient data to compile a normal range of blood glucose concentration for healthy, breast-fed, term newborn infants (National Childbirth Trust 1997). Most definitions of neonatal hypoglycaemia are based on the random distribution of random glucose concentration measured in large populations containing both fed and fasted neonates (Di Giacomo & Hay 1992). In other words, the 'normal' level is uncertain.

How reliable are the test and the test result? The test used is an example of a screening test. A screening test is used to identify potential problems, which are then confirmed by diagnosis. The problems with such tests are that they may result in 'false positives', in other words identifying a problem when there is none, or false negatives, reassuring that there is no problem when there is.

The possibility of such false positives and false negatives occurring is based on the sensitivity and specificity of a test. 'Sensitivity' refers to the proportion of people with the disease who demonstrate positive test results. The higher the sensitivity, the greater the detection of rate and the lower the false negative rate. The specificity of the test is the proportion of people without the disease who have a negative test. The higher the specificity, the lower will be the false positive rate and the lower the proportion of people with the disease who will be unnecessarily worried or exposed to unnecessary treatment (Moore et al 1995).

A third important measure is the predictive value. The positive predictive value of a test is the probability of a patient with a positive test actually having a disease, whereas the negative predictive value is the probability of a patient with a negative test not having the disease.

While the sensitivity and specificity of a test are constant within the populations under test, and generally wherever the test is performed, the predictive value of a test result depends not only on the sensitivity of the test, but also on the prevalence of the condition within the population being tested (Moore et al 1995). Currently used reagent strips have a sensitivity approximating 80% and a specificity in the region of 75% (National Childbirth Trust 1997). In other words, the test is most likely to show an accurate result in terms of making a positive diagnosis if there is a high rate of the condition in the population being tested, which there is not with newborn hypoglycaemia. The higher the sensitivity, the less likely the test is to miss a diagnosis.

Does the clinical examination indicate a diagnosis of hypoglycaemia? The answer here is no as the baby was easy to wake and was feeding well. The National Childbirth Trust guidelines (1997) advise:

The infant who is unwilling to feed or does not wake may be ill. Clinical observation and physical examination are more valuable than blood glucose testing alone in expediting the appropriate investigation and treatment of underlying disease. If there is concern that an infant's feeding pattern is abnormal, underlying illness should be considered and the infant physically examined. If the infant is difficult to wake or shows signs such as hypotonia, jaundice, fever, tachypnoea or peripheral circulatory failure, further investigation including measurement of the blood glucose concentration is appropriate. In these circumstances hypoglycaemia may reflect an underlying illness rather than underfeeding.

What are the probable consequences of this test? We need to be alert to the possibility that screening tests may result in more harm than good. This is an example of a test that has crept into routine practice without evidence to support it. Like the many screening tests, which have become a part of routine care in modern maternity services, it may be justified in populations at risk but not in the population as a whole. Moreover, with regard to screening methods such as enzyme test strips, several studies have demonstrated that these test strips show only a modest correlation to actual blood glucose concentrations obtained by more precise methods. In other words, this test is not only unjustified for a low-risk population, but also provides an unreliable estimate of the blood glucose level.

This is a test that is performed regularly on a number of postnatal wards. Given the scarcity of midwives, and the need for more attention to mothers, such routine or regular testing is a waste of time and resources so it is difficult to see how such tests work their way into routine care. It may have something to do with a general lack of confidence in breast-feeding, or be associated with a lack of confidence in clinical judgement as a way of identifying ill babies. It is possible that the 'busyness' of postnatal wards makes it difficult for midwives to think about what they are doing.

Step 4: Talking it through

I told the baby's mother that I believed the baby was in good health and was feeding well (having watched and assessed feeding on two occasions). There was very little risk of newborn hypoglycaemia. I also checked with the mother, eliciting that she was eager to get home. This conversation was as much about restoring confidence in her feeding as anything.

Step 5: Reflecting on feelings, outcomes and consequences

The practice of screening normal newborn babies is flawed for the following reasons. The currently used reagent strip test has a sensitivity approximating 80% and a specificity of around 75%. There is no substantial evidence that other cot-side tests are any better (Di

---

Pointers for practice

- In order to provide care that meets the parents' most deeply felt needs, and in order to use science, we can in practice never take anything for granted. Putting science and sensitivity into practice relies on the ability of the midwife to think, to ask and to answer questions.
- In this chapter, I have described five steps for ensuring that:
  - the preferences and values of the woman are known and that she is involved in making decisions about her care;
  - harm is, as far as possible, avoided;
  - evidence is sought and assessed;
  - the four sources of information, individual values, the clinical history and examination and strong evidence and policy are taken into account;
  - there is a process of reflection on care.
- The review of evidence outlined in this chapter is provided to give an example of the process. By the time this book goes to print, there may be new evidence available.

Giacomo & Hay 1992). Second, there are insufficient data to compile a normal range for blood glucose concentration for healthy, breast-fed, term normal infants (Di Giacomo & Hay 1992). There is also evidence that healthy, breast-fed, term newborns mobilize alternative cerebral fuels (particularly ketone bodies and lactate) when the blood glucose concentration falls. The measurement of blood glucose concentration alone therefore provides very limited information and may not reflect the adequacy of the cerebral fuel supply (National Childbirth Trust 1997).

Thus, in this case, not only is the test inadvisable, but a number of adverse effects are also likely to arise from performing it:

- going home was going to be delayed;
- the baby was to have two heel pricks;
- the baby would have received a bottle, with the potential for affecting feeding;
- the mother was extremely worried, and the situation was likely to reduce her confidence about breast-feeding even further.

When tempted or asked to undertake routine tests, it is advisable first to pose the following questions to determine whether or not the test is justified and whether the benefits are likely to outweigh the risks or inconvenience:

- What are the probable risks or benefits for this particular woman and baby?
- Are mother and baby in a 'high-risk' group?
- What is the clinical condition?
- What are the mother's feelings about the test?
- What is the prevalence of the condition that is being screened for?
- What are the sensitivity and specificity of this particular test?

In order to provide care that meets parents' most deeply felt needs, and in order to use science, in practice we can never take anything for granted. Putting science and sensitivity into practice relies on the ability of the midwife to think, to ask and answer questions. The next chapter will provide a guide for the skill of finding information.

(The review of evidence provided in this chapter is provided to give an example of the process. By the time this book goes to print there may be new evidence available.)

This chapter is published with the consent of Jane Phillips.

REFERENCES

Ackerman-Liebrich U, Voegeli T, Gunter-Witt K et al 1996 Home versus hospital deliveries: follow-up study of matched pairs for procedures and outcome. British Medical Journal 313: 1313–18

Al-Sibai M H, Rahman M S, Rahman J 1987 Obstetric problems in the grand multipara: a clinical study of 1330 cases. Journal of Obstetrics and Gynaecology 8: 135–8

Begley C M 1991 Postpartum haemorrhage – who is at risk? Midwives Chronicle and Nursing Notes (Apr). 102–6

Campbell R, MacFarlane A 1996 Where to be born: the debate and the evidence. National Perinatal Epidemiology Unit, Oxford

Chalmers I, Enkin M, Kierse M J N C 1989 Effective care in pregnancy and childbirth. Oxford University Press, Oxford

Chamberlain G, Wraight A, Crowley P 1996 Home births. The report of the 1994 Confidential Enquiry of the National Birthday Trust Fund. Parthenon, London

Combs C A, Murphy E L, Laros R K 1991 Factors associated with postpartum haemorrhage with vaginal birth. Obstetrics and Gynecology 77: 69–76

Danelian P J 1994 The significance of meconium in the amniotic fluid. Contemporary Reviews in Obstetrics and Gynaecology 6: 129–32

Department of Health 1993 Changing Childbirth. Part 1. Report of the Expert Maternity Group (Cumberlege report). HMSO, London

Di Giacomo J E, Hay W W 1992 Abnormal glucose homeostasis. In: Sinclair J C, Bracken M B (eds) Effective care of the newborn infant. Oxford University Press, Oxford

Dowswell T, Thornton J G, Hewison J, Lilford R J L 1996 Should there be a trial of home versus hospital delivery in the United Kingdom? British Medical Journal 312: 753–7

Dyack C, Hughes P F H 1996 Why does 'failure' follow 'success'? Factors surrounding caesarean section in grand multipara. Journal of Obstetrics and Gynaecology 16: 151–4

Eidelman A L, Kamar R, Schimmel M S, Bar-on E 1988 The grandmultipara: is she still at risk? American Journal of Obstetrics and Gynecology 158: 389–92

Fayed H M, Abid S F, Stevens B 1993 Risk factors in extreme grand multiparity. International Journal of Gynecology and Obstetrics 41: 17–22

Freely M 1995 Team midwifery – a personal experience. In: Page L A (ed.) Effective group practice in midwifery: working with women. Blackwell Science, Oxford

Goldman G A, Kaplan B, Neri A, Hecht-Resnick R, Harel L, Ovadia J 1995 The grand multipara. European Journal of Obstetrics and Gynecology 61: 105–9

Gray M J A 1997 Evidence-based healthcare: how to make health policy and management decisions. Churchill Livingstone, Edinburgh

Halliday H 1992 Other acute lung disorders. In: Sinclair J C, Bracken M B (eds) Effective care of the newborn infant. Oxford University Press, Oxford

Henson G L, Knott P D, Colley N V 1987 The dangerous

multipara: fact or fiction? Journal of Obstetrics and Gynaecology 8: 130–4

Hughes P F, Morrison J 1994 Grandmultiparity – not to be feared? Analysis of grandmultiparous women receiving modern antenatal care. International Journal of Gynecology and Obstetrics 44: 211–17

Kaplan B, Harel L, Neri A, Rabinerson D, Goldman G A, Chayen B 1995 Great grand multiparity – beyond the 10th delivery. International Journal of Gynecology and Obstetrics 50: 17–19

Katz V L, Bowes W A 1992 Meconium aspiration syndrome: reflections on a murky subject. American Journal of Obstetrics and Gynecology 166: 171–83

King P A, Duthie S J, Ma H K 1991 Grand multiparity: a reappraisal of the risk. International Journal of Gynecology and Obstetrics 36: 13–16

MacFarlane A 1996 Trial would not answer key question, but data monitoring should be improved. British Medical Journal 312: 754

MIDIRS 1997 Midwives Information and Research Service and NHS Centre for Reviews and Dissemination: Informed choice leaflets. MIDIRS, Bristol

Moore A, McQueen H, Gray M 1995 Testing a test. Section 3, p. 1: In: Bandolier, the first 20 issues. Bandolier, Oxford.

National Childbirth Trust 1997 Joint statement. Neonatal hypoglycaemia of the newborn. Guidelines for appropriate blood glucose screening and treatment of breast-fed and bottle-fed babies in the United Kingdom. National Childbirth Trust/British Association of Perinatal Medicine/Neonatal Nurses Association/Royal College of Midwives/Unicef UK/Baby Friendly Initative, London

Newburn M, Dodds R 1996 Such trial should not limit the choices of women who already have a preference. British Medical Journal 312: 756

Neilson J 1993 Cardiotocography during labour: unsatisfactory technique but nothing better yet. British Medical Journal 306: 347–8

NHS Executive (1994) EL(94)9 Women centred maternity services. Department of Health, London

Northern Region Perinatal Mortality Survey Coordinating Group 1996 Collaborative survey of perinatal loss in planned and unplanned home births. British Medical Journal 313: 1306–9

Oakley A 1997 The follow-up study In: Chamberlain G, Wraight A, Crowley P (eds) Home births. The report of the 1994 confidential enquiry by the National Birthday Trust Fund. Parthenon, London

Olsen O 1997a Home vs hospital birth [protocol]. Cochrane Library, Issue 1. Update Software, Oxford

Olsen, O 1997b Meta-analysis of the safety of home birth. Birth 24: 4–13

Page L A, Phillips J, Drife J O 1997 Changing childbirth: changing clinical decisions. British Journal of Midwifery 5(4): 203–6

Raisler J 1996 Evidence from US suggests that trials will not alter obstetric behaviour. British Medical Journal 312: 754

Royal College of Obstetricians and Gynaecologists 1993 Recommendations arising from the 26th RCOG Study Group. In: Spencer J A D, Ward R H T (eds.) Intrapartum fetal surveillance. RCOG Press, London

Sackett D L, Rosenberg W M C, Gray J A M, Haynes R B, Richardson S S 1997 Evidence based medicine: what it is and what it isn't. Churchill Livingstone, Edinburgh

Seidman D S, Armond Y, Roll D, Stevenson D K, Gale R 1988 Grandmultiparity: an obstetric or neonatal risk factor? American Journal of Obstetrics and Gynecology 158: 1034–9

Settatree R S 1996 Mortality is still important, and hospital is safer. British Medical Journal 312: 756–7

Silverman W A 1980 Retrolental fibroplasia: a modern parable. Academic Press, London

Spencer J A D, Ward R H T 1993 Intrapartum fetal surveillance. RCOG Press, London

Stones R W, Paterson, C M, St G Sanders N 1993 Risk factors for major obstetric haemorrhage. European Journal of Obstetrics, Gynecology, and Reproductive Biology 48: 15–18

Tai C, Urquhart R 1991 Grandmultiparity in Malaysian women. Asia-Oceania Journal of Obstetrics and Gynaecology 17(4): 327–34

Toohey J S, Keegan K A, Morgan M A, Francis J, Task S, deVeciana M 1995 The 'dangerous multipara'. Fact or fiction? American Journal of Obstetrics and Gynecology 172: 683–6

Tsu V D 1993 Postpartum haemorrhage in Zimbabwe: a risk factor analysis. Journal of Obstetrics and Gynaecology 100: 327–33

Turnbull A, Chamberlain G 1989 Obstetrics. Churchill Livingstone, Edinburgh

Update Software 1998 Cochrane Library. Update Software, Oxford

Wiegers T A, Keirse M J N C, Berghs G A H, van der Zee J 1996a An approach to measuring quality of midwifery care. Journal of Clinical Epidemiology 49: 319–25

Wiegers T A, Keirse M J N C, van der Zee J, Berghs G A H 1996b Outcome of planned home and planned hospital births in low risk pregnancies: prospective study in midwifery practices in the Netherlands. British Medical Journal 313: 1309–11

Yong G 1996 Uncertainty is likely to persist, but some knowledge would be better than none. British Medical Jorunal 312:755

2

Using evidence to inform practice

Lesley Ann Page

My own interest in what we now call evidence-based care started when I practised as a midwife in Canada, providing care for women and their families through the whole process of pregnancy and birth, for the first time in my experience as a midwife. As I got to know these women as individuals, I became increasingly aware of the importance of doing the right things for them as individuals. Inevitably, as we came to know each other through the course of pregnancy, the parents would start to ask why certain things were undertaken as a routine. Intuitively, I guessed that many of these routines, which were imposed in our large maternity hospital, were unfounded. It was only when I started to search for evidence, so that I could make an argument for abandoning some routines for the women in my care, that I began to realize just how senseless some of the routines were. For example, there was a very strict rule that there was to be absolutely nothing to drink or eat in labour, yet many of the women I cared for wanted the freedom to eat and drink in labour. Thus, I started to investigate the evidence on the topic. This took me many hours. I contacted others who were undertaking research in the area in question, and used the library. Now, with a number of sources of synthesized evidence, the search for evidence is easier in some areas.

There are two questions that every midwife should ask herself, questions fundamental to evidence-based midwifery:

1. Is what I intend to do likely to do more good than harm?
2. Am I spending my time doing the right things?

Once these questions have been asked, a number of changes follow in their wake. First and foremost is the need to be able to 'look things up', that is, to find the best research evidence to answer the questions. The approach that I describe here involves responding to the needs of individuals to ensure that they receive appropriate care and that they benefit from the care provided. Integral to this approach is an awareness of the many important outcomes of maternity care, which include personal and family integrity, and emotional well-being as well as physical outcome. This broadening of goals to go beyond mortality rates as an outcome measure of care makes decisions more complicated, inevitably meaning that the research studies to be considered will be more complex too. Perhaps the most challenging aspect of this approach, however, is the need to weigh up the potential benefits and risks of certain decisions, understanding that there are many 'clinical dilemmas' for midwives.

This has implications for the way in which midwives learn in their basic education programmes and for their continuing education. The skills of lifelong learning and the ability to undertake independent enquiry are crucial. Such a change in orientation also means that we often find ourselves in the situation of challenging longstanding routines in systems that are not easy to challenge. If we know that a routine is likely to harm individuals, it is no longer ethical to undertake it.

EVALUATING CARE AND EFFECTIVE CARE

The drive to improve the safety of birth through hospitalization and the use of technology and medical diagnosis was marked by the imposition of treatments and care that were largely unevaluated. The routine use of shaving and enemas, the routine induction of labour and the move to universal hospitalization for birth are familiar examples of this problem. The publication of the book *Effective Care in Pregnancy and Childbirth* (Chalmers et al 1989) brought about a greater awareness that we should seek to understand the effects of our care through evaluation. This seminal work provided an important foundation for helping to understand the different forms of evidence, and ways of judging the strength of that evidence, which may be considered in deciding the probable effects of care. In addition, the book provided a synthesis of much of the relevant evidence for reference. This was the basic work that led to the present day Cochrane Library (Cochrane Collaboration 1998).

Although the term 'effective' is frequently used, it is a complex concept. One of the difficulties is that different people will have different goals in mind. Moreover, as Chapter 1 reminds us, judgements about the effects of care during pregnancy and childbirth, as in other areas, are neither value free nor situation free: different observers see different problems and often reach different conclusions (Susser 1984, in Chalmers et al 1989). Understanding and evaluating the effects of care is important for a number of reasons. The development of care in pregnancy and childbirth has led to some tragedies (Silverman 1980). In his book, Silverman describes the story of the tragedy of retrolental fibroplasia. This is a dramatic example of the use of a well-intentioned treatment, giving extra oxygen to premature babies, which resulted in great harm: the blindness of some of the large number of babies receiving the treatment. Moreover, we frequently spend our times doing things that may not be helpful, and not doing things that would be more helpful. Take, for example, the routine of taking frequent blood glucose measurements, described in Chapter 1, when we might instead be supporting women in feeding their babies.

The movement towards 'evidence-based health care' (Gray 1997) has been important in helping professionals and others, including policy-makers and managers, to become aware that research is performed to be used. Evidence-based care is about using research rather than doing it. It is a movement away from always doing things in the way in which we were taught and from decisions based on personal opinion. Instead, evidence-based practice requires that we look for and appraise research evidence to inform decisions about tests, treatments, patterns of practice, and policy. Although personal experience is an important basis to understanding what works and why, our personal experience is rarely wide enough to give us objective answers about the effects of particular tests and treatments.

EVIDENCE-BASED CARE

Muir Gray (1997, p. 213) describes evidence-based clinical practice as 'the judicious use of the best evidence available so that the clinician and the patient arrive at the best decision, taking into account the needs and values of the individual patient'. Evidence should be used to inform decisions in a number of areas: policy, guidelines for practice, the appropriate organization of care, public health decisions (about the use of resources, for example), clinical decisions and information to help women's choice, health promotion and education for parenting.

Caring about women and their families requires that we always ask, am I likely to do more good than harm? Chapter 1 described a way of using evidence in practice and described the sources of information used to inform decisions about care. These are:

• individual values or preferences

- the clinical examination
- research evidence
- the context of care.

In that chapter, five steps for the use of evidence in practice were described:

1. finding out what is important to the woman and her family;
2. using information from the clinical examination;
3. seeking and assessing evidence to inform decisions;
4. talking it through;
5. reflecting on outcomes, feelings and consequences.

In this chapter, I focus on the third step: finding and critiquing the evidence. I will describe approaches to asking clear questions, planning a search of the literature and assessing the evidence. I will also define some key terms and give some examples of the assessment of evidence in practice. Although evidence-based midwifery is about using rather than doing research, the same aim of doing primary research applies – the aim of avoiding bias, that is, skewed evidence, in seeking, selecting and assessing evidence.

The process of using evidence in practice includes:

- framing clear and relevant questions that will lead to an effective search;
- planning an efficient search to answer the question;
- assessing and weighing up the evidence.

FRAMING CLEAR QUESTIONS

Midwives in practice will be called on daily to make decisions, together with women, about a number of questions. The questions that arise from practice will range from relatively simple types of question about the effect of a particular treatment on specific outcomes, to more complex ones, including those of the probability of adverse outcomes. Midwives will often be in the situation of weighing up a number of potential risks and benefits.

Clinical and care decisions

Questions concerning care are likely to arise from a number of areas, as outlined below.

1. **How might I best support the childbearing woman and her family?**:
   - a good experience of care;
   - the best organization of midwives;
   - ways in which to enhance social support;
   - the relief of symptoms/comforting;

- where care should be given and who should lead the care (including place of birth);
   - maternal – child attachment.
2. **What do I need to assess, how is it best assessed, what do the findings mean, and are they likely to be 'true'?**:
   - clinical parameters (e.g. weight gain and fundal height measurements);
     - learning needs;
     - parenting abilities.

Significance of clinical findings

Part of an assessment includes the interpretation of screening and diagnostic tests, such as haemoglobin levels and cardiotocography. We need to know how reliable these measures are.

- Screening and diagnostic tests.

Probability of adverse outcome (risk)

1. **How do I best recognize and support 'normal' or physiological processes?**:
   - the length of labour;
   - the duration of pregnancy;
   - indications for intervention.
2. **How may I improve health and prevent problems?**:
   - approaches to health promotion and education;
   - the effects and mitigation of poverty;
   - the effect of lifestyle changes;
   - smoking cessation;
   - the promotion of breast-feeding.
3. **Are any interventions necessary, and how likely are they to be beneficial or to be harmful?**:
   - caesarean and operative delivery;
   - electronic fetal monitoring in labour;
   - episiotomy;
   - the augmentation and acceleration of labour.

Outcomes.   In research, it is common to consider or measure the effect of an intervention on particular outcomes. Given the breadth of our concerns in maternity care, it is important for midwives to consider a range of outcomes in considering questions about care. These include:

- the mortality and morbidity of both mother and baby;
- intervention rates, that is, of caesarean section, operative delivery, epidural anaesthesia and episiotomy;
- measures of emotional well-being, including

memories of care, particularly of labour and birth, postnatal depression and confidence in parenting;
- breast-feeding rates and duration;
- family integrity;
- the security of attachment between mother and baby;
- the relief of the unpleasant aspects of pregnancy and childbirth;
- a knowledge of pregnancy and birth and parenting skills;
- optimal care, for example in confidential reviews of maternal deaths and infant deaths.

Principles of good questions

The skill that is basic to finding the right and best evi-

dence is the ability to ask good questions. Such questions are directly relevant to patients' problems and are phrased in ways that direct one's search towards relevant and precise answers (Sackett et al 1997). In their work, Sackett et al provide a table of four elements of well-built clinical questions. I have modified these components for those working in maternity care, where the frame of reference is different. In the maternity services, the majority of women and families start off by being healthy, and our aim should be to keep them that way. Because of this, the potential for doing harm is greater. One of the problems of maternity care in much of the industrialized world is the routine treatment of all women as if they are high risk with a very high probability of adverse outcome. In fact, the risk of an adverse outcome is lower than it has ever

Table 2.1   Comparisons of good questions. (Adapted from Sackett et al 1997, p. 27 with kind permission)

1. Woman or problem	2. Intervention (cause, prognostic factor, treatment)	3. Comparison intervention (if necessary)	4. Outcome(s)
Tips for building How would I best describe a group of women similar to mine?	Which main intervention or complication or 'risk factor' am I considering?		What can I hope to accomplish? What else would be affected? What is the probability of adverse outcome?
Examples In women in early pregnancy who are vomiting most of the day	Acupressure		lead to a reduction of vomiting and the experience of nausea?
In women without other complications	who are grand multiparous (greater than gravida 5)	when compared with women who are less than gravida 5	is there a greater probability of excessive bleeding, a need for blood transfusion, illness or death?
In women of 26 years of age	who have an amniocentesis for the diagnosis of Down syndrome		what is the probability of miscarriage? What is the probability of Down syndrome? What are the sensitivity and specificity of the test?
In nulliparous women without complications	who have an elective prelabour caesarean section	rather than allowing labour and vaginal birth	what will the effect on perinatal mortality and morbidity, and maternal mortality and morbidity be?
In pregnant women	who are over 40 years old	compared with women of under 40 years of age	is there a greater probability of adverse outcomes (e.g. perinatal mortality and higher intervention rates) as a result of age alone?

been. Thus, many of the questions that midwives ask will arise from the need to determine whether or not a woman is actually in a high-risk group. Or, to put it another way, has she a higher chance than usual of an adverse outcome? If she does, what is the adverse outcome? With this in mind, I have adapted one of the components of Sackett et al's table (Table 2.1).

Exercise

Consider your own practice and think of a number of questions about the routines you undertake. Use the following components:

- How would I best describe a group of women similar to mine?
- Which main intervention risk factor or complication am I considering?
- What is the comparison group or treatment?
- What are the outcomes that I am considering?

For example, you may be looking after a woman who is experiencing leg cramps. The question in this case might be:

In a woman with a normal pregnancy and severe cramps in her leg at night, is extra calcium likely to help, and are there likely to be any side-effects from the extra calcium?

This question may be broken down as follows:

- a group of women like mine = women with normal pregnancy;
- is calcium likely to help? = the intervention;
- compared with exercise only = the comparison treatment;

- the reduction of leg cramps = the desired outcome;
- are there any harmful side-effects of the treatment? = harmful outcomes.

Now, imagine the following situation. Mrs Smith is approaching term. She has prepared a birth plan indicating that she wishes to avoid intervention in labour. At her 39 weeks visit, the fundal height is 39 cm, the fetus is active, the blood pressure is 120/85, and there is no protein in the urine. At this visit, Mrs Smith wonders whether it is enough to listen to the fetal heart regularly or whether she should think about having continuous electronic monitoring.

Using the components from Table 2.1, write a question to guide your search for evidence in the box below. The question might read:

In women at term, with no problems in the pregnancy, would using continuous electronic fetal monitoring, rather than intermittently listening to the fetal heart, lead to lower mortality and morbidity, and how would it affect the intervention rate?

Other types of question

We have started with questions that concern the effect of particular interventions on outcomes of care. Perhaps 12% of our decisions lie in that area. There is, however, a further large and important field for consideration. This encompasses the decisions to be made concerning risk, or the probability of adverse outcome, in particular women. The best way to get started is to use reviews of research, which combine the results of a number of studies. There may be a large number of

Write a question in this box to guide your search for evidence.

individual studies, and the time taken to find and read them all is beyond the capability of most individual clinicians. For example, when Olsen undertook his meta-analysis of the studies of home birth, he found 65 separate studies that met his criteria (Olsen 1997). It is important to check the quality of reviews as they may be biased (see below).

An example of the kind of question that we might be faced with answering was given in Chapter 1, in relation to risk and multiparity. Such questions can be quite complicated. Fortunately, midwives have a very good specialist database service available: the MIDIRS database search service. This provides a list of references and abstracts, helping to identify which papers are likely to be useful and thus saving library time. A list of standard searches is available from MIDIRS, and they will also undertake individual searches. In addition, copies of papers can be obtained from MIDIRS if it is difficult to get them from the library. The most frequently used general resource for finding references is Medline. When finding all the available research in an area is important, some investigators will use a combination of MIDIRS and Medline (see, for example, Olsen 1997).

PLANNING AN EFFICIENT SEARCH

Once you have asked a clear question, it is time to start planning a search. Sackett et al (1997) describe searching for research evidence as an essential clinical skill. Such a skill needs to be efficient enough to accomplish a search to answer a question about clinical practice in the very little time available to midwives. Luckily, there are a number of secondary resources of extracted, synthesized and organized research evidence to make it accessible to professionals and women.

The process of secondary research is guided by the same aim as primary research (actually doing the research): that is, to avoid a biased result that arises from missing important pieces of evidence. It is thus important to use a database of both original (primary) and secondary research. These may be paper based or electronic. One of the important factors is ensuring that the sources are updated regularly so that one is not using out-of-date research.

The need for efficiency is crucial. The amount of information available to health professionals is unmanageable without some system for tracking, retrieving and managing the information found. Greenhalgh (1997) writes that there are over 10 million articles on our library shelves, and 4000 journals are published world wide every month.

There are fortunately some very good specialist resources such as the MIDIRS database service for midwives who wish to track the answer to particular questions. Original research or a synthesis of original research such as a review paper may be used. There are a number of resources of synthesized evidence, for example the Cochrane Library. The source of evidence to be searched will depend very much on the evidence needed. Thus, in planning a search, think about the nature of the question you have asked. If the question is about the effect of certain interventions on the outcome of care, start with the Cochrane Library. This provides overviews or meta-analyses of high-quality research studies, usually randomized controlled trials, from different parts of the world. It is intended to help clinicians as well as researchers, and provides suggestions on implications for practice. It provides a synthesis of studies, giving accumulated results. This is in general more powerful and more informative than looking at individual studies.

In planning a search, there are thus a number of ways to proceed. According to the kind of evidence needed, one may wish to consider the following:

- a database of meta-analyses such as the Cochrane Library;
- leaflets or books that have synthesized research;
- journals of secondary reports of research studies;
- Medline, Cinahl or Embase;
- a specialist service, for example the MIDIRS database search service;
- a search through the journals;
- the Internet;
- books that are referenced and up to date, particularly for understanding physiology.

Research may be published or unpublished. Most professionals in clinical practice need to rely on published information. This can be found in non-peer-reviewed or peer-reviewed journals. Although it is generally accepted that peer review is a method of quality control, a number of questions have been raised about the adequacy of peer review as a mechanism to achieve this.

In addition to looking at the original reports of research in books and journals, there are a number of sources that provide digests of research (e.g. the MIDIRS digest), compilations of references (the MIDIRS standard and individual search databases), a systematic review and meta-analysis of the results of research (e.g. the Cochrane Library) and clinical guidelines based on research (e.g. NHS Wales Health 1998).

The following are examples of sources for searching for and retrieving research. Table 2.2 below gives a description of these databases and some examples.

Table 2.2 Resources for searching for evidence

Source	Availability	Description
Cochrane Library	On CD-ROM and over the Internet	A collection of databases relevant to evidence-based health care. The main sections include: • regularly updated, systematic reviews of the effects of health care • critical appraisals of reviews published elsewhere • a register of controlled clinical trials • a database of articles on the science of reviewing research
MIDIRS digest	Printed digest of articles from journals publishing high-quality research	The editor (always a midwife) selects reports from those which have been scanned. Articles are abstracted or reviewed for presentation in the journal
MIDIRS database searches	Printed results of electronic searches of the MIDIRS database	Standard and individual searches are available. Five hundred English language journals are scanned. These include all midwifery, obstetrics and gynaecology, paediatrics, neonatal and key general medical and consumer journals.
Bandolier	Newsletter (also available on the Internet)	A newsletter containing highlights of health care research and examples of using evidence in practice
Best Evidence and *Evidence Based Medicine*	*Evidence Based Medicine* is published as a journal. *Best Evidence* is available on CD-ROM and includes the articles published in *Evidence Based Medicine*	Reviews, in the form of structured abstracts, of articles whose results are likely to be both true and useful. The purpose is to alert clinicians to important advances. Includes *Obstetrics and Gynaecology*
Welsh office protocols (NHS Wales 1998)	Guidelines and protocols	A systematic summary of evidence in the area of maternal and early child health. A hierarchy of types of evidence is used
Medline	Electronic database	Compiled by the National Library of Medicine of the United States, Medline indexes over 3800 journals published in over 70 countries. Medline is available free of charge over the Internet and on CD-ROM from a number of commercial vendors.
Embase	Electronic database	The database of Excerpta Medica is especially strong on drugs and pharmacology and other biomedical specialties
Cinahl	Electronic database	A nursing and allied health database covering all aspects of nursing, including occupational therapy, health education, occupational therapy, social services in health care and other related disciplines from 1983
DH data	Electronic database produced by the UK Department of Health	Indexes articles covering health service and hospital administration from 1983
Current Contents	Available in both paper and electronic format	Tables of contents of journals, often available before the journals are published. Updated weekly
WHO reproductive health library	Diskette and CD-ROM	An electronic review journal focusing on evidence-based solutions to reproductive health problems in developing countries

In planning your search think about the kind of information you require and the kind of search you need to conduct. For example, your questions may arise in the following areas:

• You have questions about the possibility of enhancing 'attachment' between mother and baby. This might call on qualitative (that is concerned with words) as well as quantitative (that is concerned with numbers) research so you may wish to go to a review such as that in Chapter 11 of this book.

- You have a question about what causes nausea in pregnancy. A physiological explanation might be needed so you may wish to use a resource such as Chapter 15 of this book.
- You wish to give a mother advice on rest and work. In answering the question, 'What should my advice be regarding rest and work', you will draw on a number of different studies. You might want to try the MIDIRS database service.
- You have heard that ginger helps sickness caused by pregnancy. To answer a question about the effect of an intervention on an outcome, about a treatment, the Cochrane Library would be the best source of evidence.
- You often give advice about sore breasts in the postnatal period and wish to find the best treatment and comfort measures. This is a question about finding the most effective treatment, for which the Cochrane Library is the best source of information.

When you search the source for evidence, you may face some basic problems: either there may be so much research that it is difficult to handle it all, or you may find very little. In the case of having too much, it is sensible to limit the research you review. You may wish to cut down the years to encompass only recent studies, or you may wish to limit the research to those who are English speaking, to an area similar to your own or to specific groups of people.

If you find very little or no evidence, it may be necessary to use a different database to make sure that nothing has been missed. There are, however, a number of areas that are underresearched, and this is not an uncommon problem.

In order to make sure that you are getting well-balanced or unbiased information, it is rarely enough to go by one report or the first journal paper you find. However, you can start to build up a list of references from a single paper.

Searching for research is fast becoming a science in itself. When using Medline, for example, the search must be conducted so that it is neither too broad, in which case you will retrieve too many references, nor too narrow in which case you may miss important ones. Greenhalgh (1997, p. 13) describes the 'jungle which calls itself medical literature'. As she notes, you can apply all the right rules for reading a paper, but if you are reading the wrong paper, you might as well be doing something else completely.

Greenhalgh quotes Jewell's three levels of reading – browsing, reading for information and reading for research (Jewell et al 1995). Although there is much enjoyment to be gained from browsing and reading journals and books at random, it is important not to conduct a search to answer specific questions at random.

Muir Gray (1997) describes some of the problems of searching for research and ways of overcoming them. These include a lack of relevant research, the unavailability of unpublished research, the limitations of electronic databases, and misleading abstracts. He provides some useful solutions to these problems (Table 2.3).

Sackett et al (1997) provide a diagram of the steps for getting started on a search (Figure 2.1). They describe the need for a clever search strategy for large databases to be sure that you have retrieved the most relevant citations with a minimum of 'junk' (Greenhalgh suggesting that only 10–15% of the research literature is of lasting scientific value). In order to do this, it is necessary to understand general indexing and search strategies and to think about a specific task.

The most general database is Medline. Greenhalgh (1997) says that most people can learn to carry out a basic search in an hour, but more skilled searching needs further training, and it is best, if possible, to get a skilled librarian (or knowledge manager) to help. A Medline search may have high sensitivity, that is, a high likelihood of retrieving relevant items, and/or a high specificity, that is, the likelihood of excluding irrelevant items (Cairns Library Oxford Teaching Materials on Medline 1998).

Basic medline search

Articles can be traced in two ways: any word listed on the database including words in the title or abstract, the authors' names and the institution where the research was carried out, or through the restricted thesaurus of medical titles known as medical subject headings (MeSH terms).

If possible, have a librarian help you to learn the following skills described in Sackett et al (1997, p. 73):

- the use of natural language (text words) and MeSH headings;
- the identification of MeSH (subject headings; sh) using the thesaurus;
- the use of limiters such as publication type (pt) or publication year (py);
- joining natural language terms (tw) MeSH terms (sh) and limiters such as pt using Boolean operators such as AND, OR or NOT to form methodological filters;
- using * at the end of words to replace characters within words;

Table 2.3 Problems in searching for research and how to overcome them. (Based on Muir Gray 1997, with permission)

Problem	Description	Solution
Lack of relevant research	Only a small amount of high-quality evidence is available on which to base a decision, (unless the decision is about cardiac services)	Use best evidence available rather than best evidence possible
Unpublished evidence	Main source of evidence is published. This is incomplete because much research is not written up for publication, pharmacological companies and other sponsors may not be keen to write up research that may not show the company's products in the most advantageous light, and there is a bias towards publishing positive rather than negative results	Appropriate to search for unpublished literature when doing research, but if a decision-maker or in clinical practice, may be a waste of time
Limitations of electronic databases	Two principle sources are Medline and Embase. They cover only 6000 of the 20 000 journals published worldwide	The use of specialist databases such as the Cochrane Library
Inadequate indexing	Inadequacies of indexing journals and within electronic databases means that, in general, only about half of the trials in Medline can be found even by the best electronic searcher	Use of good search strategy; best strategy is to have an expert searcher, but this is not always possible. Hand-searching of journals and incorporating with a Medline search may add greatly to the number of studies available
Misleading abstracts	Quality of any search is measured by accuracy (the proportion of findable articles that are found) and precision (the proportion of articles that are useful, the rest being 'junk'). Good searching increases accuracy but almost always decreases precision and almost always uncovers junk	Having found the articles, identify and discard 'junk', the simplest way being to read the abstract. Two guidelines for reading abstracts are: 1. If the abstract is unstructured, be suspicious 2. If the abstract highlights negative findings, it may not be biased, but if it highlights positive one's, check the methods section

- the use of 'near 2' or 'near 3' to link words in phrases separated by two or three words.

Sackett et al (1997) emphasize the need to think while undertaking a Medline search. There may be a need to broaden or narrow your search. The Boolean operator OR broadens the search; AND narrows it. The following is the Cairns Library advice (1998) on widening or narrowing your search:

Go wider

- Broaden your question
- Use more search terms – synonyms, related terms, broader or narrower terms
- Use truncation or wildcards in Free Text searches
- Combine terms of related meanings with ORs
- Use a combination of Free Text with Thesaurus searches
- Explode Thesaurus terms
- Add All Subheadings to Thesaurus terms

Go narrower

- Narrow your question!
- Use more specific search terms
- Use only the most relevant terms
- Use a Thesaurus search
- Add specific Subheadings to Thesaurus terms
- Add in terms using AND to represent other aspects of the question
- Try NEAR instead of AND to relate terms more closely (1997)

(Reproduced with kind permission from Robin Snowball, *Widening or Narrowing Your Search*.)

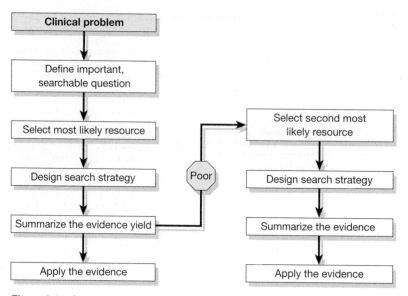

Figure 2.1 General search strategy. (Reproduced from Sackett et al 1997, with permission.)

It may be impossible for clinicians to make a systematic review of all the evidence available in the time available, and in this case, it is important to find good review papers on a topic. You should in this case ensure that the review is not biased.

ASSESSING AND INTERPRETING THE EVIDENCE

Once you have found the appropriate information to answer your question, it is necessary to assess the quality of the information in order to ensure that it is right for your purposes and that it provides valid evidence to answer your question.

There are several good books that provide a structured approach to assessing research reports (see especially Greenhalgh 1997, Muir Gray 1997, Sackett et al 1997). Each book offers a slightly different approach, but all treat the subject in more detail than is possible here.

An essential first step in assessing the evidence is discarding poor-quality or irrelevant reports. Greenhalgh (1997) emphasizes the need to 'trash' papers and suggests that 'some purists would say 99% of published articles belong in the bin' (p. 34). She makes a strong argument that the quality of a paper is best assessed through the methods section and that the article should be 'trashed' on methods alone before looking at the results. Greenhalgh suggests three preliminary and basic questions as a way of getting an orientation to the paper are:

1. Why was the study done, what were the hypotheses, and what were the authors testing?
2. What type of study was carried out (Box 2.1)
3. Was this research appropriate to the broad field of research studied? (Box 2.1).

In order to assess the evidence, Sackett et al (1997) propose the following questions:

- Is it true (valid)?
- Are the valid results important?
- Does it apply to the woman/women in my care?

Validity

In Chapter 8, Sandall et al define internal validity in correlational and experimental research as the extent to which the independent and dependent variables are truly related. In other words, with what degree of assurance may we say that the factor which is being tested (for example, the effect of giving folic acid in pregnancy) causes or is correlated to the outcome being evaluated (the reduction of neural tube defects)?

Validity is related to research design. External validity is concerned with the extent to which the research findings can be generalized to other groups of people in the general population. The type of sample selection is critical to the external validity of the study.

Earlier, we described the many complex questions that arise from midwifery practice. It is important to remember that different questions will be answered with various research methods. Chapter 8 provides a number of different methods for answering different questions. A fundamental point when assessing evidence is to ensure that the methodology is appropriate to the question posed.

Box 2.1 Broad topics of research

Most research studies are concerned with one or more of the following:

- *Therapy* – testing the efficacy of drug treatments, surgical procedures, alternative methods of service delivery, or other interventions. Preferred study design is randomised controlled trial.
- *Diagnosis* – demonstrating whether a new diagnostic test is valid (can we trust it?) and reliable (would we get the same results every time?). Preferred study design is cross sectional survey … in which both the new test and the gold standard test are performed
- *Screening* – demonstrating the value of tests that can be applied to large populations and that pick up disease at a presymptomatic stage. Preferred study design is cross sectional survey
- *Prognosis* – determining what is likely to happen to someone whose disease is picked up at an early stage. Preferred study design is longitudinal cohort study
- *Causation* – determining whether a putative harmful agent, such as environmental pollution, is related to the development of illness. Preferred study design is cohort or case-control study, depending on how rare the disease is … but case reports … may also provide crucial information

Reproduced from Greenhalgh T 1997 How to read a paper, with kind permission from BMJ Books, BMJ Publishing Group.

Importance

Questions of importance are based on numerical data and are related to the size and potential benefits of the effects over time, the probability of outcomes occurring over time, the strength of association between the outcomes (either harmful or good) and interventions, the increased probability of particular outcomes in different groups, and the precision of estimates. Sackett et al (1997) show a way of helping individual professionals to calculate how many people need to be treated to avoid an adverse outcome (number needed to treat; NNT) or to harm one person (number needed to harm; NNH) (see below). Measures of importance, strength of association and precision include relative risks, absolute risk reduction, NNT, NNH, odds, odds ratios

and confidence intervals. Strauss et al (1998, pp. 141–5) define these as follows:

- Odds – a ratio of non-events to events. If the event rate for a disease is 0.1 (10%), its non-event rate is 0.9 and therefore its odds are 9:1. Note this is not the same as the inverse of event rate.
- Odds ratio (OR) – is the odds of having the target disorder in the experimental group relative to the odds in favour of having the target disorder in the control group (in prospective case control studies, overviews) or the odds of being exposed in subjects with the target disorder divided by the odds in favour of being exposed in control subjects (without the target disorder).
- Risk ratio (RR) – is the ratio of risk in the treated group (EER) to the risk in the control group (CER) – used in Randomised Controlled Trials and cohort studies: RR = ERR/CER
- Relative risk reduction (RRR) – the proportional reduction in rates of bad outcomes between experimental and control participants in a trial.
- Absolute risk reduction (ARR) – the absolute arithmetic difference in rates of bad outcomes between experimental and control participants in a trial.
- Number needed to treat (NNT) – the number of patients who need to be treated to achieve one additional favourable outcome, calculated as 1/ARR and accompanied by a 95% confidence interval. If the ARR is 25% 1/25% = 4
- NNH as above but for harm rather than good (e.g. cancer in association with vitamin K).
- Confidence interval (CI) – the range within which we would expect the true value of a statistical measure to lie. The CI is usually accompanied by a percentage value, which shows the level of confidence that the true value lies within this range. For example, for an NNT of 10 with a 95% CI of 5–15, we would have 95% confidence that the true value of NNT values was between 5–15.

Application to families in your care

Questions of application are concerned with the similarity between families in your care and those in the reported research, and of their preferences and values.

Appraising evidence for validity and importance

The assessment of the validity of particular studies will depend on the type of evidence used. Sackett et al (1997) propose the following categories:

- diagnosis
- prognosis
- harm
- therapy
- systematic reviews
- decision analysis
- qualitative research.

I present Sackett et al's (1997) structured questions for

the assessment of quantitative evidence and have based the assessment of qualitative evidence on Greenhalgh's work. I have not presented any information on the assessment of decision analysis.

The following is based on the work of Sackett et al (1997) and Strauss et al (1998), using their categories for structured steps for appraisal. We have summarized many of the suggestions from three sources: Sackett et al (1997), Strauss et al (1998) and the handbook from the 1998 Oxford workshop on teaching evidence-based medicine (University of Oxford 1998).

Diagnosis

One of the most rapidly changing fields of maternity lies in diagnosis and screening, particularly in the antenatal period. Midwives should be able to appraise current evidence and convey the accuracy of results to the women and families in their care. For example, a friend recently telephoned in great distress. She had been rung up on a Friday night to say that her alpha-fetoprotein tests were abnormal and that there was a strong possibility of a problem with the baby. In simply talking to her, I realized that the calculation of gestation might have been wrong by enough days to affect the estimation of normality for her test result. Her midwife who conveyed the worrying news should have understood this. The test result was later interpreted as normal, but my friend and her husband had spent a dreadful weekend, all for nothing.

This area is perhaps one of the most complex, and an understanding of a number of concepts, such as sensitivity and specificity, is crucial not only to interpreting evidence, but also to interpreting test results and understanding their predictive value in practice.

Assessing validity. Sackett et al (1997, p. 82) suggest using the following questions critically to appraise a paper or systematic review on diagnosis for its proximity to the truth:

1. Was there an independent, blind comparison with a reference 'gold' standard of diagnosis?
2. Was the diagnostic test evaluated in an appropriate spectrum of patients (like those in whom it would be used in practice)?
3. Was the reference standard applied regardless of the diagnostic test result?

Was there an independent, blind comparison with a reference 'gold' standard of diagnosis? Two criteria should have been met in order to answer this question in the affirmative. First, the women or babies in the study should have undergone both the diagnostic test in question (for example, nuchal fold scanning for Down syndrome) and the reference (or 'gold') standard of

testing (e.g. amniocentesis for Down syndrome). Second, the person interpreting the tests of one should not know the results of the other, otherwise, consciously or subconsciously, the interpretation might be biased.

It is sometimes difficult to provide reference standards, but a definition of normal has in some way to be agreed. Sackett et al (1997, p. 83) use the diagnostic definition of normal alongside other definitions of normal, that is shown in Box 2.2.

Box 2.2 Six definitions of normal. (Reproduced from Sackett et al 1997, with permission.)

1. *Gaussian*: the mean ± standard deviations. Assumes a normal distribution and means that all 'abnormalities' have the same frequency.
2. *Percentile*: within the range, say, of 5–95%. Has the same basic defect as the Gaussian definition.
3. *Culturally desirable*: preferred by society. Confuses the role of medicine.
4. *Risk factor*: carrying no additional risk of disease. Labels the outliers, who may not be helped.
5. *Diagnostic*: range of results beyond which target disorders become highly probable – the focus of this discussion.
6. *Therapeutic*: range of results beyond which the treatment does more good than harm. Means you have to keep up with advances in therapy.

Was the diagnostic test evaluated in an appropriate spectrum of patients (like those in whom it would be used in practice? For example, if you are asking a question about the use of nuchal fold testing in all age groups of women, you would want it to be tested in a population of all age groups of women.

Was the reference standard applied regardless of the diagnostic test result? Sackett says that when patients have a negative diagnostic test result, investigators are tempted to forego applying the reference standard, and when the latter is invasive (which an amniocentesis is), it may be considered inappropriate to do so.

Sackett suggests that if the report fails one or more of these criteria, you may wish to keep searching.

Is this evidence about a diagnostic test important? Once you have decided on the validity of the report or reports, the above question needs to be answered.

Sackett et al (1997, p. 118) describe what they call 'a modern way of thinking about diagnosis that takes into account both components of evidence based medicine; your individual clinical expertise and the best external evidence'. This includes your assessment of the prior assessment of possibilities before carrying out the test (prior or pretest probabilities) and the ability of the test to distinguish patients with and without the target disorder (sensitivity and specificity, and likelihood ratios). The definitions of these terms are shown in Box 2.3.

Box 2.3   Diagnostic tests: key terms (Reproduced from Sackett et al 1997, with permission.)

Sensitivity: the proportion of people with the target disorder who have a positive test. It is used to assist in assessing and selecting a diagnostic test/sign/symptom.

SnNout: when a sign/test/symptom has a high **s**ensitivity, a **n**egative result rules **out** the diagnosis.

Specificity: the proportion of people without the target disorder who have a negative test. It is used to assist in assessing and selecting a diagnostic test/sign/symptom.

SpPin: when a sign/symptom has a high **s**pecificity, a **p**ositive result rules **in** the diagnosis.

Positive predictive value: the proportion of people with a positive test who have the target disorder.

Negative predictive value: the proportion of people with a negative test who are free of the target disorder.

Likelihood ratio: the likelihood that a given test result would be expected in a patient with the target disorder compared with the likelihood that the same result would be expected in a patient without the target disorder.

Sackett et al (1997, p. 118–21) provide the following example of the results of a systematic review of serum ferritin as a diagnostic test for iron deficiency anaemia. They describe a situation in which there is an estimation that the person has a 50% probability of iron deficiency anaemia, that is, odds of 50–50 that iron deficiency is present. A systematic review gives values for the calculations shown in Table 2.4. The person's ferritin level comes back as 60 mmol/L. Sackett et al describe the calculation (Table 2.5) as follows (1997, pp. 119–21)

Your patient's result places them in the top row of the table, either in cell a or cell b. From that fact you would conclude several things: first, you'd note that 90% of patients with iron deficiency have serrum ferritin in the same range as your patient, $a/(a + c)$, and that property, the proportion of patients with the target disorder who have positive test results, is called sensitivity.

And you might also note that only 15% of patients with other causes for their anaemia have results in the same range as your patient … which means that your patient's result would be about six times as likely (90%/15%) to be seen in someone with, as opposed to someone without, iron deficiency anaemia and that's called the likelihood ratio for a

Table 2.4   Calculation of sensitivity, specificity and likelihood ratio (LR)

	Disease positive	Disease negative
Test positive	a	b
Test negative	c	d
Sensitivity = a/(a+c)	LR = sensitivity = a/(a+c) 1-specificity = b/(b+d)	
Positive predictive value = a/(a+b)	Negative predictive value = d/(c+d)	

Table 2.5   Results of a systematic review of serum ferritin as a diagnostic test for iron deficiency anemia. (Reproduced from Sackett et al 1997, with kind permission)

		Target disorder (iron deficiency anemia)		Totals
		Present	Absent	
Diagnostic test result (serum ferritin)	Positive (<65 mmol/L	731 a	270 b	1001 a+b
	Negative (≥ 65 mmol/L	78 c	1500 d	c+d 1578
	Totals	a+c 809	b+d 1770	a+b+c+d 2579

Sensitivity = a/(a + c) = 731/809 = 90%
Specificity = d/(b+d) = 1500/1770 = 85%
LR+ = sens/(1–spec) = 90%/15% =6
LR– = (1–sens)/spec = 10%/85% = 0.12
Positive predictive value = a/(a+b) = 731/1001 = 73%
Negative predictive value = d/(c+d) = 1500/1578 = 95%
Prevalence = (a+c)/(a+b+c+d) = 809/2579 = 32%
Pretest odds = prevalence/(1–prevalence) = 31%/69% = 0.45
Post-test odds = pretest odds × likelihood ratio
Post-test probability = post-test odds/(post-test odds +1)

positive test result. Furthermore, since you thought ahead of time (before you had the result of a serum ferritin) that your patient's odds of iron deficiency anaemia were 50–50, that's called a pretest odds of 1:1 and as you can see from the formula at the bottom of the table, you can multiply that pretest odds of 1 by the likelihood ratio of 6 to get the post test odds of iron deficiency anaemia after the test: $1 \times 6 = 6$. Since, like most clinicians, you may be more comfortable thinking in terms of probabilities than odds, this post test odds of 6:1 converts (as you can see at the bottom of [Table 2.5]) to a post test probability of 6/(6 +1) = 6/7 = 86%. So it looks like you've made the diagnosis and this diagnostic test looks worthwhile.

Once you have determined validity and importance, the following questions help to determine whether or not you can apply this valid, important evidence to your patient (Sackett et al 1997, p. 160):

● Is the diagnostic test available, affordable, accurate, and precise in your setting?

- Can you generate a clinically sensible estimate of your patient's pre-test probability (from practice data, from personal experience, from the report itself, or from clinical speculation)?
- Will the resulting post-test probabilities affect your management and help your patient? (Could it move you across a test-treatment threshold? Would your patient be a willing partner in carrying it out?)
- Would the consequences of the test help your patient?

Prognosis

Is this question about prognosis valid?   At first, it seemed difficult to equate Sackett et al's (1977) example question of 'How long have I got?' to maternity care. On reflection, it seems that this is a category we usually call risk estimation. Thus converted, an example question might be 'What is the increased probability of postpartum haemorrhage when a woman is gravida 6' (see Chapter 1). In assessing evidence related to prognosis for validity, we need to ask (Sackett et al 1997, p. 86):

1. Was a defined, representative sample of patients assembled at a common (usually early) point in the course of their disease?
2. Was patient follow up sufficiently long and complete?
3. Were objective outcome criteria applied in a blind fashion?
4. If subgroups with different prognoses are identified
   - Was there adjustment for important prognostic factors?
   - Was there validation in an independent group of test set patients?

For example one of the 'old chestnuts' (if the reader will pardon the pun) of maternity care is that older women are at greater risk. This proposition raises its ugly head over and over again. Using age as a prognostic indicator of adverse outcome (in this case, operative birth), let us examine a recent paper. Rosenthal & Paterson-Brown have examined the question of an incremental rise in the risk of obstetric intervention with increasing maternal age. The following is the structured abstract of their paper (Rosenthal & Brown 1998, p. 1064):

Objective   To determine whether increasing maternal age increases the risk of operative delivery and to investigate whether such a trend is due to fetal or maternal factors.

Design   Analysis of prospectively collected data on a maternity unit data base.

Population   6410 nulliparous women with singleton cephalic pregnancies delivering at term (37–42 weeks of gestation), nulliparous women with singleton cephalic pregnancies delivering at term between 1 January 1992 and 31 December 1995.

Setting   The study was undertaken in a teaching hospital. There was a population of 6410. The results showed a positive highly significant association between increasing maternal age and obstetric intervention.

Main outcome measures   Mode of delivery, rates of prelabour caesarean section, induction of labour and epidural usage.

Results   There were a positive, highly significant association between increasing maternal age and obstetric intervention prelabour ($P < 0.001$) and emergency ($P < 0.001$) caesarean section, instrumental vaginal delivery (spontaneous labour $P < 0.001$; induced labour $P = 0.001$), induction of labour ($P < 0.001$). Epidural usage in induced labour and the incidence of small for gestational age newborns did not increase with increasing maternal age ($P = 0.68$ and $P = 0.50$, respectively).

Conclusions   This study demonstrates that increasing age is associated with an incremental increase in obstetric intervention. Previous studies have demonstrated a significant effect in women older than 35 years of age, but these data show changes on a continuum from teenage years. This finding may reflect a progressive, age-related deterioration in myometrial function.

(Reproduced with kind permission from Blackwell Science Ltd.)

A study of this topic is interesting for a number of reasons. First, there is an important danger of the idea that women are at increasing risk of intervention in labour becoming a self-fulfilling prophecy. It is quite likely that attendant anxiety or perception is likely to affect the outcome of labour (and this has not been refuted by this study). Second, there is a great danger of the outcomes of such studies being confounded (that is, being affected by other factors than the one under study, in this case increasing age), for example by the existence of medical problems in subgroups of older women or by the tendency to treat older women as being at higher risk, leading to a higher rate of continuous electronic fetal monitoring, which in itself produces a higher intervention rate. Unfortunately, the authors of this study did not heed the warnings of one of the papers referenced, that such studies require control for confounding variables (Harker & Thorpe 1992).

Rosenthal & Patterson-Brown's study misses a vital component, which is further analysis to control for confounding variables. Let us look at this paper against the framework of two of Sackett et al's (1997) questions:

Was a defined, representative sample of patients assembled at a common (usually early) point in the course of their disease?   This was a retrospective review of what is described as 'prospectively' (although the information was entered onto the database after delivery) routinely gathered data. Information that might help to explain and define some of the measures (for example, the definition and diagnosis of fetal distress) is missing from the data collection. The lack of identification of the women forming the sample at the beginning of the pregnancy and the lack of collection of data to explain the diagnosis of fetal distress weakens the study. There are a number of indications in the report that the population studied may be slightly different from the norm, for example in the description of the intervention rate in the hospital in which the study took place and in the description of the population as having a higher than average age and a larger proportion of 'career women'. This limits the confidence with which we might generalize the findings to other populations because the women in this study may not be representative of women in other populations. The length of follow-up was appropriate in a study that was concerned only with intervention rates.

Were objective criteria applied in a blind fashion? Some of the criteria, for example operative delivery, are objective; others, such as failure to progress and fetal distress, are more subjective measures. There is no clear definition of or criteria for the diagnosis of fetal distress and failure to progress (both of these being prone to bias in clinical interpretation). There is no mention of blinding for interpretation or for analysis. There was also no adjustment for prognostic factors. It is quite probable that increased attendant anxiety is a factor in increasing interventions in older women, and nothing in this study informs us that this is not the case. In studies examining the effect of maternal age on outcome that are adequately controlled for factors which may confound the outcomes, no significant differences are found (Harker & Thorpe 1992). There is no control or reanalysis for such factors (e.g. raised blood pressure). The higher incidence of epidural analgesia in spontaneous labour may well have been an independent factor in increasing the intervention rate. Moreover, there is no mention of the fetal monitoring rate, which is likely to have been higher in this group of women, and which is in itself associated with a higher rate of intervention and a falsely high rate of diagnosis of fetal distress. A number of factors, including mobility and position in labour, may have affected the outcome; but none of these are described in the report.

In addition, the lack of clear definition of failure to progress and fetal distress, which may be highly subjective assessments, is a fundamental flaw in this study. Attendant anxiety may well have affected the judgements made, in itself leading to a higher rate of intervention.

There was no validation in a test set of patients.

Is this evidence about prognosis important? This is the next question to be tackled.

In relation to importance, two questions are relevant:

1. How probable are the outcomes over time?
2. How precise are the prognostic estimates?

Given the flaws of the study, I would question the validity and would not go on to determine the importance.

Two further questions then follow.

Were the study patients similar to your own, and will this evidence make a clinically important impact on your conclusions about what to offer or tell your patients? In this case, I would not change my practice on the basis of this study as its flaws render it non-valid. Perhaps the only change in practice I would make would be to be more careful that any bias regarding older women did not by itself increase the intervention rate.

Harm

Is this evidence about harm valid? Sackett et al (1997, p. 106) propose the following questions to assess the validity of studies to evaluate the possibility of harm:

1. Were there clearly defined groups of patients, similar in all-important ways other than exposure to the treatment or other cause?
2. Were treatment exposures and clinical outcomes measured the same ways in both groups (e.g. was the assessment of outcomes either objective (e.g. death) or blinded to exposure)?
3. Was the follow up of study patients complete and long enough?
4. Do the results satisfy some 'diagnostic tests for causation'?
   - Is it clear that the exposure preceded the onset of the outcome?
   - Is there a dose response gradient?
   - Is there positive evidence from a dechallenge rechallenge study?
   - Is the association consistent from study to study?
   - Does the association make biological sense?

This is a question of whether or not a treatment *caused* the harm experienced and thus, as Sackett et al tell us, 'benefits from what has been learned from classical epidemiology'. There are four possible designs for a study of the harmful effects of treatments. These are the randomized controlled trial, the cohort study, the case control study, or reports of one or two patients who have suffered from something that is unique and rare. Table 2.6 is a summary of the advantages and disadvantages of these approaches, as described by Sackett et al.

Let us look at the above questions with regard to a study to examine the effect of neonatal exposure to vitamin K on the risk of childhood cancer (Klebanoff et al 1993). The relationship between vitamin K and cancer

Table 2.6 Advantages and disadvantages of different kinds of harm study. (From Sackett et al (1997) with kind permission.)

Type of study	Advantages	Disadvantages
Randomized controlled trial	Randomization would make groups similar for all other features that would cause harm	For rare events, very large trials would be needed (once per thousand would need 3000 patients in order to be 95% certain of seeing at least one adverse reaction)
Cohort study	Next most powerful design	The groups of patients (cohorts) may not be identical in every respect. Other things apart from the treatment being evaluated such as severity of illness may affect outcome. Same problem of size applies
Case control studies	For rare or late complications of treatment, need to rely on studies in which those who already have the disease are assembled and compared with a group who do not have the disease	The problem of confounding (of prognosis with exposure) is worse with case control studies because it may be impossible to measure confounders in a case even if they are known
Case reports and case series	Reports of one or two patients who developed a complication while under treatment (e.g. phocomelia in children born to women who took thalidomide)	May be enough but usually point to the need for further studies

was examined in a nested case control study that used data from the Collaborative Perinatal Project, a multi-centre, prospective study of pregnancy, delivery and childhood that took place in the USA. Among 54 795 children born between 1959 and 1966, 48 cases of cancer were diagnosed after the first day of life and before the eighth birthday. Each case child was matched with randomly selected controls whose last study visit occurred at or after the age when the case child's cancer was diagnosed.

Were there clearly defined groups of patients, similar in all-important ways other than exposure to the treatment or other cause? The rarity of the disease in this case makes a randomized controlled trial impractical for answering the question of harm and makes the case control study the only practical design. Attempts were made to adjust for factors that might be associated with the development of childhood cancer (for example, race, sex, birth weight, maternal age, exposure to X-rays during pregnancy, and breast-feeding). Nevertheless, we cannot be confident that the groups were similar in every respect.

Were treatment exposures and clinical outcomes measured in the same ways in both groups (e.g. was the assessment of outcomes either objective, for example death, or blinded to exposure)? The question that follows concerns the examination of treatment exposures and outcomes. The report states that 'two investigators who were blinded to the child's vitamin K status examined all records of children with cancer. Definite cases of

cancer were required to have a histologically proved diagnosis of cancer, a clinical course including treatment consistent with the diagnosis or both' (Klebanoff et al 1993, p. 905).

Was the follow-up study of patients complete and long enough? There is no account of loss to follow-up, but the authors state that, afterwards, loss to follow-up was accounted for by life table methods. The study followed children up to 8 years of age.

Do the results satisfy some diagnostic tests for causation?

- *Is it clear that the exposure preceded the onset of the outcome?* It is as clear as can be that the exposure preceded the outcome. There was reclassification for children with cancer before their first birthday, and therefore with the possibility that the cancer started in pregnancy.
- *Is there a dose–response gradient?* No dose–response gradient was available, but babies whose mothers were given vitamin K in the intrapartum period were excluded. All babies received the intramuscular vitamin K. In addition, there was an analysis of effect according to the brand of vitamin K used. There was then reanalysis to exclude the children in whom the administration of vitamin K was uncertain.

Because this was part of a larger study not aimed primarily at the evaluation of the effect of vitamin K, it is particularly important to be sure that vitamin K was actually administered when it was recorded and that all vitamin K was recorded when given. Recording in this situation was probably more careful because this was part of a research study with special documentation that was checked for completeness. In addition, there was recording by an observer in the delivery room of any drugs administered.

- *Is there positive evidence from a dechallenge–rechallenge study?* The dechallenge–rechallenge question (seeing what happens if a drug is withdrawn or re-administered) is not appropriate to this drug.
- *Is the result consistent from study to study?* The answer to this is no. The authors comment on two earlier studies including an evaluation of the effect of the administration of oral vitamin K that found twice the expected risk of cancer during childhood with the administration of vitamin K.
- *Does the association make biological sense?* There is no biological link made explicit in this study, but the fact that the incidence of childhood cancer has not increased with the frequent administration of vitamin K at birth increases confidence in the findings of the study.

Are the valid results from this harm study important? Importance is evaluated against an estimation of the strength of the association between receiving the treatment and suffering the adverse effect. Strength here means the risk or odds of the adverse effect, with, as opposed to without, exposure to the treatment; the higher the risk or odds, the greater the strength and the more one should be impressed with it.

Different tactics are used for estimating the strength of the association for different studies. This is demonstrated in Table 2.7 (Sackett et al 1997, p. 147).

Using the data presented in the paper on vitamin K (Klebanoff et al 1993), the calculation is as shown in Table 2.8. In this case, there is no association demonstrated.

Can the study results be extrapolated to your patient? Given the situation in the USA, with such different demographic characteristics, I would extrapolate with caution. One factor that is pointed out by the authors as being different is that the vehicle for the vitamin K differs between the USA and the UK.

Therapy

If one wants to find out whether a treatment is likely to be of benefit, the most appropriate methodology to answer the question is a randomized controlled trial. There are so many factors that might influence the outcome of treatment that the only good way to control

Table 2.7 Different ways of calculating the strength of an association between a treatment and subsequent adverse outcomes. (Reproduced from Sackett et al 1997, with kind permission)

		Adverse outcome		Totals
		Present (Case)	Absent (Control)	
Exposed to the treatment	Yes (Cohort)	a	b	a+b
	No (Cohort)	c	d	c+d
Totals		a+c	b+d	a+b+c+d

In a randomized trial or cohort study: relative risk = RR = [a/(a+b)]/[c/(c+d)] In a case-control study: relative odds = RO = ad/bc

Table 2.8 Ways of calculating the strength of an association between treatment and subsequent adverse outcome

	Adverse Outcome	
	Present (Case)	Absent (Control)
Exposed to the treatment — Yes Cohort Vitamin K	33 a	171 b
	c	c
No Vitamin K Controls	15	69
	$\dfrac{33.69}{15.171}$	$\dfrac{2277}{2565} = 0.89$

for possible sources of bias is to allocate people randomly to different treatment conditions.

In this section, we will look at assessing the evidence from a single study. If several studies are available, the investigator should first look for a systematic review and use that as a starting point.

Before going on to assess the results of a study, one must first ask the following questions.

Are the results of this single study valid? The key questions to answer, following Sackett et al (1997, p. 92), are:

1. Was the assignment of patients to treatments randomised?
2. And was the randomisation list concealed?

3. Were patients and clinicians kept blind to which treatment was being received?
4. Aside from the experimental treatment, were the groups treated equally?
5. Were the groups similar at the start of the trial?

Studies of treatment or therapy compare outcomes in groups receiving the treatment with outcomes in groups either not receiving treatment or receiving an alternative treatment. It is essential that, at the outset, the groups being compared are as alike as possible. The only way to avoid bias when assigning people to groups is to make the assignments random. This does not guarantee that the groups will be identical, but it does ensure that any differences are caused by chance alone.

Say, for example, that you were looking for a treatment for pregnancy-induced nausea and had heard that acupuncture worked. You would want to make sure that your groups consisted of a mixture of women with different severities of the condition, different lifestyles and a different tolerance of the symptoms: An uneven distribution of these factors between groups is likely to exaggerate, counteract or even cancel the effects of the therapy. If such a distribution exaggerated the effects, this could lead to false positive results, and if it cancelled them, false negative conclusions could arise.

In addition, if the random allocation is concealed from clinicians, they will be unaware of the treatment that the patient is receiving and will not be able to distort the effect, either consciously or unconsciously.

You can match the number of patients who entered the trial with the number accounted for at its conclusion. Ideally, these should be the same: lost patients could have events that would change the conclusion. The authors suggest that to be sure of a trial's conclusion, its authors should be able to take all the patients who were lost along the way, assign them the worst case scenario and still be able to support the original conclusion. It would be unusual for a trial to withstand a worst case scenario if it lost more than 20% of its patients.

The correct form of analysis is intention-to-treat analysis, which means that patients are analysed in the groups to which they were assigned. Perhaps you have set up a randomized controlled trial of home birth, wanting to assess the effect of home birth on intervention rates. It might be that a number of women are transferred to hospital for failure to progress or some other problem. If you do not use intention-to-treat analysis, there will be a falsely low intervention rate in the home birth group. Such an analysis provides an even greater assurance that one can believe its results. It prevents both the reporting of the symptoms and their interpretation being affected by the woman's feelings about the treatment that she is receiving. It also prevents clinicians from adding co-interventions to one of the groups.

When patients and clinicians cannot be 'blinded', it is possible to have other 'blinded' clinicians come in to assess the medical records. You can look to see whether randomization was effective by looking to see whether the patients were similar at the start of the trial.

Are the results of this single preventive or therapeutic trial important? Sackett et al (1997) propose the calculation of a figure that is more meaningful to clinical practice: the number needed to treat (NNT). This is an important concept. If a valid study found, for example, that you needed to treat four people to have one respond to the treatment, this gives a clear indication of how many people you would need to treat and the chance of a response in the people you are caring for. The view of these numbers differs for the midwife and the childbearing woman. A midwife may want to know that for every four women she treats, one will respond to treatment. For the childbearing woman, the most useful presentation of these figures is that she has a 1 in 4 chance of responding to therapy.

Now, let us use the calculation in practice. One of the most troublesome aspects of pregnancy is nausea and vomiting, surveys indicating that nausea affects between 70% and 85% of women and vomiting approximately 50% (Jewell & Young 1998). One of the treatments for nausea and vomiting is a form of acupressure applied at the Neiguan point on the volar aspect of the wrist. Using the data from the Cochrane Library, let us work out how many women would need to be treated with acupressure to have one respond to treatment (the NNT).

Here is the calculation. Take the control event rate (CER; the events being the number of women who suffer from severe nausea and vomiting) and subtract the experimental event rate (EER) to calculate the absolute risk reduction (ARR). Then, to calculate NNT, divide 1 by the absolute risk reduction. The results from the table in the Cochrane Library on the effect of acupressure on the severity of nausea and vomiting show that 128 out of 259 women in the control group and 37 out of 145 women in the experimental group suffered from severe nausea and vomiting.

To work out the absolute risk reduction:

- divide 128 by 259
  $128/259 = 0.49$, or 49%
- then divide 37 by 145
  $37/145 = 0.25$, or 25%

- then subtract 25% from 49%
  49%–25% = 24%
- the absolute risk reduction is therefore 24%.

To calculate the number needed to treat:

- divide 1 by the absolute risk reduction, which we have already calculated to be 24% or 0.24
  1/24 = 4.1
- the NNT is thus 4.

The calculation is, therefore, as follows:
ARR = CER–EER
NNT = 1/ARR

Is this evidence from this systematic review valid?   If there are a number of randomized controlled trials (RCTs) of the treatment in which you are interested, it is better to look at a systematic review than to use individual studies. Sackett et al (1997, p. 97) propose the following questions to test the validity of a systematic review:

1. Is it an overview of RCTs of the treatment you are interested in?
2. Does it include a methods section that describes:
   a. Finding and including all the relevant trials?
   b. Assessing their individual validity?
3. Were the results consistent from study to study?

The first question asks whether you are sure that the treatment is the same as the one you are interested in and the others whether all the studies were carried out at the same, most powerful level of evidence.

For example, if a randomized controlled trial of vitamin K prophylaxis were available and you wanted to know whether oral vitamin K were effective, you would want to make sure that it was oral vitamin K that had been tested.

Some overviews combine randomized and non-randomized studies, and you should ensure that this was not the case.

Does it include a methods section that describes (a) finding and including all the relevant trials, and (b) assessing their individual validity? The most important point to remember is that carrying out a systematic review is just like carrying out research. In other words, it uses the same approach as research to avoid bias and should be reported like research. As in the assessment of research, look carefully at the methods section. You need to ensure that all-important 'data' in the case studies are included. This will include a description of how the studies were found, which were included and excluded, and why. Sackett et al (1997) describe the importance of having sought unpublished results and of hand-searching for reports. The methods section should also say how the validity of the study was judged.

Were the results consistent from study to study? Although we should not expect trials to show exactly the same degree of efficacy, it is reassuring if the results are not widely different.

Are the results of this systematic review important? Deciding whether or not a treatment is important depends on the size and potential benefits of the effects of the treatment you are interested in.

Translating the odds ratio to the NNT and NNH   Conversion to NNT was described earlier; because it is such a useful concept, let us remind ourselves what NNT is.

Sackett et al (1997, pp. 136–7) say that 'it represents the number of patients we would need to treat (NNT) with the experimental therapy in order to prevent one of them from developing the bad outcome. The formula is obviously the same for calculating NNH. The formula is applied to the data from the Cochrane Library systematic review on electronic fetal monitoring as in Box 2.4.

Box 2.4   Number needed to harm (NNH): caesarean section in association with electronic fetal monitoring

The following numbers are taken from the Cochrane review provided in this chapter.

Electronic fetal monitoring without pH estimation versus intermittent auscultation:

Experimental group
204/3509 = 0.058 (5.8%)

Control group
117/3418 = 0.034 (3.4%)

Then ARR =
   5.8%
   –3.4%
   2.4% (0.024)

NNH = 1/0.024 = 41.67
(where 0.024 is the absolute relative risk)

The following questions apply to whether or not you should apply these results to your patient (Sackett et al 1997, p. 167):

Do these results apply to your patient?

- Is your patient so different from those in the overview that its results can't help you?
- How great would the potential benefit of therapy actually be for your individual patient (e.g. what is the NNT)?
- Do your patients and you have a clear assessment of their values and preferences?
- Are they met by this regime and its consequences?

Assessing qualitative research

Qualitative research is important to all professionals in

the maternity services, but it is perhaps most important to midwives. Midwives hold the potential for strong and intimate relationships with childbearing women and their families as well as the potential for changing the experience of care and of pregnancy and birth.

Greenhalgh (1997, p. 151) describes clearly the limitations of quantitative research and the importance of qualitative research in 'seeking a deeper truth'. She quotes the aim of qualitative research as being 'to study things in their natural setting, attempting to make sense of, or interpret, phenomena in terms of the meanings that people bring to them', and that researchers use a 'holistic perspective which preserves the complexity of human behaviour (Denzin and Lincoln 1994)'.

There are a number of examples of sound qualitative research in the maternity services, drawing from the social science and anthropology backgrounds of a number of committed scholars, including Oakley and Kitzinger. Their work provides a mine of information regarding the perspectives of childbearing women using the maternity services and their experiences, in order to inform midwives who want to understand better and improve care.

Greenhalgh (1997, see pp. 155–61) suggests the following questions for assessing qualitative research. She is clear about the limits of such a checklist, and it should be used with caution. Qualitative research is by its very nature non-standard; this list of questions is taken from Greenhalgh to provide a structure. However, it is advisable to read Greenhalgh's chapter in full and to refer to the list of further reading at the end of that chapter.

Did the paper describe an important clinical problem examined through a clearly formulated question? As with quantitative research, the topic area needs to be clearly defined. The process is iterative so the question may emerge more clearly at the end of the project, although it should still be clearly stated.

Was a qualitative approach appropriate? It is most appropriate when the objective is to explore, interpret or obtain a deeper understanding of a particular issue.

How were the setting and subjects selected? The study should go beyond a convenience sample to a theoretical sample. Instead of taking an average view, the aim is to achieve an in-depth understanding of particular individuals, for example a group of Somali women receiving maternity care in west London.

What was the researcher's view, and has this been taken into account? It is important to recognize that there is no way of controlling for observer bias in qualitative research. It is thus important that the investigator's personal perspective is fully explained.

What methods did the researcher use for collecting data, and are these described in enough detail? The methods section is likely to be lengthy and discursive. You should ask the question. 'Have I been given enough information on methods?' There are no hard and fast rules.

What methods did the researcher use to analyse the data, and what quality control measures were implemented? The researcher must have found a systematic way of analysing the data. A number of methods are available, which include content analysis. A good paper will describe a method of quality control; in other words, it will not depend on just the interpretation of one person.

Are the results credible? Check to see whether qualitative researchers check actual data: the results should be independently and objectively verifiable. Are they sensible and believable, and do they matter in practice?

What conclusions were drawn, and were they justified by the results? Greenhalgh suggests using these three questions: how well does this analysis explain why people behave in the way they do, how comprehensive would this explanation be to a thoughtful participant in the setting, and how well does the explanation cohere with what we already know? (Mays & Pope 1996).

INTERPRETING A SYSTEMATIC REVIEW: AN EXAMPLE FROM THE COCHRANE LIBRARY

Systematic reviews should be your first port of call when looking for evidence. When carried out properly, a systematic review provides a 'gold standard' against which individual research reports and other sources of information may be judged. In this section, we will look in detail at one of the systematic reviews prepared by the Cochrane Collaboration. The particular review is 'Continuous electronic fetal heart monitoring during labor' (Thacker & Stroup, 1998), one of the regularly updated reviews published in the Cochrane Library. Because the review is regularly updated, you need to check the Cochrane Library periodically to see whether new data have been added that might have changed its results.

Continuous electronic monitoring during labour

Let us now turn to the complex question of fetal monitoring in labour and examine the analysis presented in the review by Thacker & Stroup (1998).

The first thing to notice about a systematic review is

that it is conducted and reported in the same way as any other research study: there are explicit objectives, a methods section describing how the data were collected, a results section and finally a discussion section. After a brief background discussion, Thacker & Stroup are explicit about their objective:

Objective. To compare the efficacy and safety of routine continuous electronic fetal monitoring of labor with intermittent auscultation, using the results of published randomized controlled trials.

They then go on to describe exactly what outcome measures they are going to use and, importantly, where they looked to find the studies that they were going to review. If there is a bias in how studies are selected for inclusion in the review, the results of the review will also be biased. In all Cochrane reviews, there is a description of the individual studies included in the review and a listing of the studies found but not included, along with the reasons for the studies not being included. In the case of continuous electronic fetal monitoring, 12 studies were found, but three had to be excluded (for example, because an auscultation group was not included). In total, the nine included studies reported on the results of 58 855 pregnancies.

The authors report on number of different outcome measures, but we will focus on three results: the effect of electronic fetal monitoring on.

1. the number of babies with 1-minute Apgar scores below 4;
2. the number of babies suffering neonatal seizures;
3. the number of women having caesarean deliveries.

It is important to separate the results of a review from the interpretation and discussion of those results. In the Thacker & Stroup review, the authors discuss the differences between studies in different countries, what happens when you look at only the large studies and so forth. While this is important detail, it is generally best to look at the figures and graphs themselves and to come to your own conclusions about what they mean before reading the author's conclusions.

The Cochrane reviews use a standard graph to display the results of the review. In most cases, this graph shows the risk (or odds) of an event in one group compared with the risk in the other group. For the outcome measures we are examining, the questions to be answered are:

- What is the risk of a 1-minute Apgar score below 4 in the group receiving electronic fetal monitoring compared with the risk in the group receiving intermittent auscultation?
- What is the risk of suffering a neonatal seizure in the group receiving electronic fetal monitoring compared with the risk of a seizure in the group receiving intermittent auscultation?
- What is the risk of the mother having a caesarean in the group receiving electronic fetal monitoring compared with the risk in the group receiving intermittent auscultation?

Point estimates

The method used to compare one risk with another is to form a ratio, that is, to divide one risk by the other. In the simplest situation, say that there were 10 seizures in one group and 20 in the other. We can compare the two numbers by dividing 10 by 20, in which case we get a ratio of 0.5 (as $10/20 = 0.5$). Similarly, if there were 8 seizures in the first group but only 4 in the second, we would divide 8 by 4, in which case we would get a ratio of 2 ($8/4 = 2$).

It should be obvious when using this method that, if both groups are the same (e.g. 10 seizures in each), the ratio will be 1 (e.g. $10/10 = 1$). Numbers greater than 1 indicate more 'outcomes' in the first group (e.g. $8/4 = 2$), while numbers less than 1 indicate more 'outcomes' in the second group (e.g. $4/8 = 0.5$).

In these examples, we are comparing single numbers, but the same principle applies when comparing risks. That is, if the risk is 1 in 4 ($1/4$) in one group, and 2 in 4 ($2/4$) in the other, we can divide $1/4$ by $2/4$, and get a single number – 0.5 – to express the result (as $1/4$ divided by $2/4 = 0.5$).

Using ratios, the results of each single study can be expressed as a single number. This number is called the point estimate of the effect. If we ignore all the other factors in any one study, this single number is the best estimate we have of the effects of the treatment. The point estimate is shown on the Cochrane review graphs as a square or diamond.

Once we have the results of each study expressed as a single number, we can combine these numbers statistically to get an overall estimate of the size of the effect. This process is known as meta-analysis.

Confidence intervals

The challenge when doing research is to tease out the effects of the treatment you are studying from all the other factors that might influence the outcomes in which you are interested. With respect to electronic fetal monitoring, the studies look at whether electronic fetal monitoring or intermittent auscultation was used. However, they gloss over questions such as how reliable was the equipment and how good were the midwives at interpreting traces and performing intermittent auscultation?

Random assignment to treatment and control groups is one method that researchers use to try to control for unknown factors that might influence outcomes, but the results of any one study are bound to be influenced by factors other than the independent variable. Even if a research study were repeated exactly, we would expect the results to be slightly different each time.

Although the point estimate is our best guess for the size of the effect of treatment, results are generally expressed in a range of values known as the confidence interval. This shows the range of results we would expect to find if we carried out the study over and over again. The 95% confidence interval, for example, means that 95 times out of 100, we would expect the results to be within that range. In the Metaview graphs, the confidence interval is the horizontal line.

Statistical significance

Results of meta-analyses are generally considered to be statistically significant if the confidence interval around the point estimate does not include 1.00, the line of no effect. A 95% confidence interval of 0.49–0.87, for example, does not include 1.00, and we would say that the results are statistically significant.

It is important to note that statistical significance is not the same as clinical significance, and there are considerations that must be borne in mind when interpreting statistical significance in the context of meta-analysis.

First, because the overall estimate of effect is an average of sorts, it is possible to get a 'significant' result when some studies show one thing and some show the complete opposite. This difference between studies is referred to as heterogeneity, meaning that the results of the different studies are not consistent. At a clinical level, there may be a good reason for the differences between studies. Perhaps the women have different histories, are from different socio-economic groups and so on. These differences should not be ignored when generalizing the results of the meta-analysis to the clinical situation. You are usually on safer ground when most of the studies show the same direction of effect.

The second consideration is that the ratio statistics show the *relative* difference between two groups, and the significance levels refer to the size of this relative difference. For example, if one group has an operative delivery rate of 20 in 100, and another has a rate of 10 in 100, this is a relative difference of 50% (10/20). The *absolute* difference between the groups is 10 in 100, or 10%, indicating that you have one fewer operation for every 10 people you see. Compare this case to one in which the difference in rate is 2 in 1000 compared with 1 in 1000. Here the relative difference is still 50% (i.e. 1/2), but the absolute difference is only 1 in 1000, indicating that you would have to see 1000 women to observe a difference of one operative delivery.

Interpreting the results

Apgar scores   The effect of electronic fetal monitoring with pH estimation versus intermittent auscultation on 1-minute Apgar scores under 4 is shown in Table 2.9. The results of five studies are shown. Note that the two smallest studies, the Copenhagen (1985) study and the Melbourne (1976) study, show the largest effects (i.e. the point estimates furthest from 1.0), but the confidence intervals are very large, indi-

Table 2.9   The effect of continuous electronic fetal monitoring versus intermittent auscultation on the 1-minute Apgar score. (Reproduced with kind permission from Update Software 1999.)

Review: Continuous electronic fetal monitoring
Comparison: Electronic monitoring with pH estimation versus intermittent auscultation.
Outcome: 1-min Apgar <4

Study	Expt n/N	Ctrl n/N	Relative Risk (95% CI Fixed)	Weight %	RR (95% CI Fixed)
Copenhagen 1985	5/485	7/493		5.8	0.73 [0.23,2.27]
Denver 1979	10/230	11/232		9.1	0.92 [0.40,2.12]
Dublin 1985	57/6530	62/6554		51.4	0.92 [0.65,1.32]
Melbourne 1976	4/175	6/175		5.0	0.67 [0.19,2.32]
Seattle 1987	38/122	35/124		28.8	1.10 [0.75,1.62]
Total (95% CI)	114/7542	121/7578		100.0	0.95 [0.75,1.21]
Chi-square 1.14 (df=4) Z=0.41					

.1   .2   1   5   10

Table 2.10 The effect of electronic monitoring with pH estimation versus intermittent auscultation on neonatal seizures. (Reproduced with kind permission from Update Software 1999.)

Review: Continuous electronic fetal monitoring
Comparison: Electronic monitoring with pH estimation versus intermittent auscultation.
Outcome: Neonatal seizures

Study	Expt n/N	Ctrl n/N	Relative Risk (95% CI Fixed)	Weight %	RR (95% CI Fixed)
neonatal seizures not receiving oxytocin					
xCopenhagen 198	0/485	0/493		0.0	Not Estimable
Denver 1979	0/230	2/232		4.8	0.20 [0.01,4.18]
Dublin 1985	8/6530	19/6554		36.6	0.42 [0.19,0.96]
Melbourne 1976	0/175	4/175		8.7	0.11 [0.01,2.05]
Seattle 1987	7/122	7/124		13.4	1.02 [0.37,2.81]
Subtotal (95% CI)	15/7542	32/7578		63.4	0.49 [0.27,0.88]
Chi-square 3.43 (df=3) Z=2.37					
neonatal seizures receiving oxytocin					
xCopenhagen 198	0/485	0/493		0.0	Not Estimable
Dublin 1985	4/6530	19/6554		36.6	0.21 [0.07,0.62]
Subtotal (95% CI)	4/7015	19/7047		36.6	0.21 [0.07,0.62]
Chi-square 0.00 (df=0) Z=2.83					
Total (95% CI)	19/14557	51/14625		100.0	0.39 [0.23,0.65]
Chi-square 5.60 (df=4) Z=3.63					

.1   .2   1   5   10

cating that the estimate of effect is not very reliable.

Overall, there were 114 cases of a low Apgar score out of 7542 deliveries in the group receiving electronic fetal monitoring, and 121 cases out of 7578 in the group receiving intermittent auscultation. The summary estimate of relative risk was 0.95, with a 95% confidence interval of 0.75–1.21, suggesting that the 'true' result could be anywhere in that range. As the point estimate is very close to 1.0 (the line of no effect), and the confidence interval clearly includes 1.0, it can be concluded that these studies showed no effect of electronic fetal monitoring on low Apgar scores at 1 minute.

Neonatal seizures The results of the studies looking at the effect of electronic fetal monitoring with pH estimation on neonatal seizures is shown in Table 2.10. The first thing to notice is how few seizures were observed. In the Copenhagen (1985) study, there were no seizures in either group, which means that the study does not allow us to calculate the relative effects of electronic fetal monitoring and auscultation. As a consequence, the study is ignored. Overall, however, the figures for the neonatal seizures in the group not receiving oxytocin indicate that there were statistically fewer seizures observed in the group receiving electronic fetal monitoring (15/7542) than in the group receiving intermittent auscultation (32/7578). The relative risk was 0.49 and the 95% confidence interval 0.27–0.88, which does not include 1.0, the line of no effect.

Caesarean sections The effect of electronic fetal monitoring without pH estimation on the incidence of caesarean deliveries is shown in Table 2.11. Notice that there are in this graph two subgroup analyses – caesarean deliveries with fetal indications and caesarean deliveries without fetal indications – followed by an overall analysis. In the group with fetal indications, there were clearly more caesarean deliveries in the groups receiving electronic fetal monitoring (88/1593) than in those receiving intermittent auscultation (30/1530), and the relative risk was 2.81 with a 95% confidence interval of 1.87–4.23.

The group without fetal indications is interesting because, in the largest study, the results are the opposite of those in the other studies: more caesareans were observed in the intermittent auscultation group. The subgroup summary, however, was consistent with that in the 'with fetal indications' subgroup, and the overall analysis shows a clear increase in the incidence of caesarean section in the groups receiving electronic fetal monitoring (relative risk = 1.69; 95% CI = 1.36–2.11).

Interpreting the meaning

A discussion of the results of this review might focus on the long-term significance of these outcomes, the lack of association between these measures and long-term morbidity, and the fact that the protective effect for an Apgar score below 4 at 1 minute was only found

Table 2.11 The effect of electronic monitoring without pH estimation versus intermittent auscultation on caesarean deliveries. (Reproduced with kind permission from Update Software 1999.)

Review: Continuous electronic fetal monitoring
Comparison: Electronic monitoring without pH estimation versus intermittent auscultation.
Outcome: Cesarean Deliveries

Study	Expt n/N	Ctrl n/N	Relative Risk (95% CI Fixed)	Weight %	RR (95% CI Fixed)
caesarean deliveries with fetal indications					
Athens 1993	40/746	16/682		14.0	2.29 [1.29,4.04]
Denver 1976	18/242	3/241		2.5	5.98 [1.78,20.02]
Denver 1979	16/230	1/232		0.8	16.14 [2.16,120.70]
Seattle 1987	10/122	7/124		5.8	1.45 [0.57,3.69]
Sheffield 1978	4/253	3/251		2.5	1.32 [0.30,5.85]
Subtotal (95% CI)	88/1593	30/1530		25.7	2.81 [1.87,4.23]
Chi-square 7.82 (df=4) Z=4.98					
caesarean deliveries without fetal indications					
Athens 1993	31/746	43/682		37.7	0.66 [0.42,1.03]
Denver 1976	22/242	13/241		10.9	1.69 [0.87,3.27]
Denver 1979	25/230	12/232		10.0	2.10 [1.08,4.08]
Melbourne 1981	18/445	10/482		8.1	1.95 [0.91,4.18]
Sheffield 1978	20/253	9/251		7.6	2.20 [1.02,4.75]
Subtotal (95% CI)	116/1916	87/1888		74.3	1.30 [1.00,1.70]
Chi-square 14.27 (df=4) Z=1.93					
Total (95% CI)	204/3509	117/3418		100.0	1.69 [1.36,2.11]
Chi-square 28.15 (df=9) Z=4.66					

.1   .2   1   5   10

in the US studies. It may be helpful to give the actual numbers as this provides a more realistic estimate of figures. The woman's decision will depend to a great extent on her feelings about the risk of caesarean and operative birth. It is important to note that the risk of caesarean section was greatest in low-risk pregnancies. The increase in rate of caesarean section associated with continuous electronic fetal monitoring may be even higher than this: although there is a large increase evident in the studies, the overall rate is not in fact as high as in many parts of the UK and other parts of the world. The largest study in this meta-analysis is from Dublin, where the rate of caesarean section is very low in comparison to many parts of the world.

There is another resource to help in giving information to the woman here – the MIDIRS informed choice leaflet (1999). It comes in two versions: the leaflet for professionals and the leaflet for women. Together, these provide an evidence-based resource that the woman can take away, read and consider.

Cochrane reviews take into account the main results of randomized controlled trials. The MIDIRS leaflets extract from different types of good evidence. They are carefully peer reviewed. The latest version of the leaflet on electronic fetal monitoring provides the following information to help midwives and women make decisions about the best way to monitor the heartbeat of the fetus in utero (MIDIRS/NHS Centre for Research and Dissemination 1999):

It remains unclear whether the addition of Fetal Blood Sampling (FBS) to Electronic Fetal Monitoring (EFM) reduces the false positive rate and unnecessary caesarean sections. Thacker et al's review (1997) does not support its perceived benefit. FBS has drawbacks e.g. discomfort for the woman, a skilled operator is required to do the procedure and it is a static measurement that often needs repeating to show a trend. Results are equivocal in relation to FBS's ability to identify actual fetal distress and it may be that with improved CTG interpretation skills, FBS will have a decreasing role in clinical practice (Clark and Paul 1985).

In one trial when EFM with ECG analysis is compared with EFM alone, the operative delivery rate for fetal distress was reduced but more research is needed to justify the adaptation of this technology into everyday practice (Westgate et al 1993, Mistry and Neilson 1998).

Also, EFM increases the caesarean section rate by 250% (Havercamp et al (1976) and (1979) and also Kelso et al (1978)). EFM reduces the rate of neonatal seizures but only on full term babies (Luthy et al 1987) undergoing a labour induced or augmented by oxytocin (MacDonald 1985).

CONCLUSION

Whereas a while ago, we might have felt pride in being all knowledgeable, that is no longer a realistic

It is important not to be intimidated by the mystique and sense of élitism that has surrounded research in midwifery for so long. We have presented a structured approach to assessing evidence. Just as you would use a structure in undertaking a clinical examination, this structure will help to make sure that you have not missed something important out. Do not be afraid to make judgements about whether or not the findings make sense on a basic level. Your everyday experience and the knowledge you gain from that experience give you an important basis for judging whether or not things simply make sense. Although you should be aware of the limitations of personal knowledge in making generalizations, it still gives you a more general sense of whether or not a piece of research is 'somehow just not right'.

Asking questions that arise from practice and being able to find, evaluate and implement the findings of research are crucial to ensuring that care is likely to be beneficial and to avoiding harm. However, we will often find that there is no strong evidence to help us to answer questions arising from practice. In that case, we need to learn to be honest about the sources used for answering questions and our uncertainty.

aim. The amount of knowledge at our disposal is so much that we can never know it all. The more laudable aim now is to know how to find out. This marks a fundamental change in the culture of midwifery practice and education.

REFERENCES

Cairns Library Oxford Teaching Materials on using Medline 1998 Widening or Narrowing your Search. Cairns Library, Oxford
CASP 1999 Evidence-based health care workbook and CDROM. Update Software, Oxford
Chalmers I, Enkin M E, Kierse M J N C 1989 Effective care in pregnancy and childbirth. Oxford University Press, Oxford
Clark S, Paul R 1985 Intrapartum fetal surveillance: the role of fetal scalp blood sampling. American Journal of Obstetrics and Gynecology 153: 717–20
Denzin N K, Lincoln Y S 1994 Handbook of qualitative research. Sage Publications, London
Gray J A Muir 1997 Evidence-based healthcare: how to make health policy and management decisions. Churchill Livingstone, Edinburgh
Greenhalgh T 1997 How to read a paper: the basics of evidence based medicine. BMJ Publishing Group, London
Harker L H, Thorpe K 1992 'The last egg in the basket'? Elderly primiparity – a review of findings. Birth 19 (1): 23–8
Haverkamp A D, Thompson H E, McFee J G et al 1976 The evaluation of continuous fetal heart rate monitoring in high-risk pregnancy. American Journal of Obstetrics and Gynecology 125(3): 309–20
Haverkamp A D, Orleans M, Langendoerfer S et al 1979 A controlled trial of the differential effects of intrapartum fetal monitoring. American Journal of Obstetrics and Gynecology 134(4): 399–532
Jewell D, Jones R, Kinmonth A-L 1995 Critical reading for primary care. Oxford University Press, Oxford
Jewell D, Young G 1998 Treatments for nausea and vomiting in early pregnancy. Cochrane Library, Issue 4. Update Software, Oxford
Kelso I M, Parsons R J, Lawrence G F et al 1978 An assessment of continuous fetal heart rate monitoring in labor: a randomized trial. American Journal of Obstetrics and Gynecology 131(5): 526–32
Klebanoff M A, Read J S, Mills J L, Shiono P H 1993 The risk of childhood cancer after neonatal exposure to vitamin K. New England Journal of Medicine 329(13): 905–8
Luthy D A, Shy K K, van Belle G et al 1987 A randomized trial of electronic fetal monitoring in preterm labor. Obstetrics and Gynecology 69(5): 687–95
MacDonald D, Grant A, Sheridan-Pereira M et al 1985 The Dublin randomized controlled trial of intrapartum fetal heart rate monitoring. American Journal of Obstetrics and Gynecology 152(5): 524–39
Mays N, Pope C 1996 Qualitative research in health care. BMJ Publishing Group, London
MIDIRS/NHS Centre for Research and Dissemination 1999 Informed choice for professionals: fetal heart rate monitoring in labour. Informed choice for women: fetal heart rate monitoring in labour. MIDIRS, Bristol
Mistry R, Neilson J 1998 Intrapartum fetal ECG plus heart rate recording. Cochrane Review, Issue 4, 1998–12–07. Update Software, Oxford
NHS Wales Health 1998 Evidence bulletins Wales: maternal and early child health protocols. NHS Wales, Cardiff
Olsen O 1997 Meta analysis of the safety of home birth. Birth 24: 4–13
Rosenthal A, Paterson-Brown S 1998 Is there an incremental

risk of obstetric intervention with increasing maternal age? British Journal of Obstetrics and Gynaecology 105: 1064–9.

Sackett D L, Richardson W S, Rosenberg W, Haynes B R 1997 Evidence-based medicine: how to practise and teach EBM. Churchill Livingstone, Edinburgh

Silverman W A 1980 Retrolental fibroplasia: a modern parable. Academic Press, London.

Strauss S, Badenoch D, Richardson Scott W, Rosenberge W, Sackett D L 1998 Practising evidence-based medicine. Tutor's manual, 3rd edn. Radcliffe Medical Press, Oxford

Thacker S, Stroup D 1998 Continuous electronic fetal heart monitoring during labor. Issue 1. Update Software, Oxford

Thacker S, Stroup D, Peterson H 1997 Continuous fetal heart monitoring during labour. Cochrane Library, Issue 4. Update Software, Oxford

University of Oxford 1998 Manual of Oxford workshop on teaching evidence-based medicine. University of Oxford, Oxford

Westgate J, Harris M, Curnow J S H, Green K R 1993 Plymouth randomized trial of cardiotocogram only vs waveform plus cardiotocogram from intrapartum monitoring in 2400 cases. American Journal of Obstetrics and Gynecology 169: 1151–60

USEFUL ADDRESS

MIDIRS
9 Elmdale Road
Clifton
Bristol BS8 1SL
Tel: 0800 581009
email: miders@dial.pipex.com
Website: http://www.miders.org

3

Making choices in childbirth

Deborah Harding

The birth culture of the 1990s provides a bewildering complexity of choices for the pregnant mother and her care-giver. Technology is entrenched in maternity care and continues to advance even as we discover and accept that some forms of technology, for example electronic fetal monitoring, do not enhance outcomes in normal births (Thacker et al 1995). Beliefs, attitudes, institutional policies, educational models and styles of practice all influence the decision-making and the decision-makers. A shared process between the client and the care-giver is emerging as the preferred paradigm shift in health care decision-making. Included in this process is the recognition of the right of the individual to participation and autonomy in making health care decisions.

This chapter concerns the decision-making process in maternity care and the centrality of the midwife–client relationship in supporting shared decision-making. A report of an exploratory study examines the midwife's perceptions of shared decision-making in practice.

HISTORICAL PERSPECTIVE

Throughout the ages, childbirth has traditionally involved a gathering of women. Friends, neighbours, relatives and midwives attended labouring women, surrounding them with support, caring and assistance, sharing their collective knowledge about birth (Kitzinger 1992), and it was the mother's choice who would be in attendance at the birth. She often looked to her contemporaries as well as to her midwife to help her decide what interventions might be useful or necessary when her labour was not proceeding easily. The decision-making was usually a collective undertaking, the final decision being approved by the group of women in attendance (Kitzinger 1992). The focus was centred on the birthing woman and her needs. She could trust her community to safeguard and respect her autonomy and her choices.

By the start of the 20th century, women had less and less input into how their maternity care would be managed (Wertz & Wertz 1979, Leavitt 1987, Mason 1988). The invention of forceps and the interest of the medical profession in obstetrics had firmly established the male presence in childbirth. Childbirth practices changed: medical practitioners replaced midwives, women moved from their homes into hospitals to deliver, and the use of technology and surgical interventions became commonplace. The decision-making process changed from a woman-led, community-supported, inclusive discussion to a professional-led, patriarchal, 'scientific', exclusive determination.

Medical knowledge increased, the medical monopoly in obstetrics strengthened, and as physicians became more confident and familiar with the procedures currently in use, their desire for autonomy in decision-making became paramount. According to Leavitt (1987, p. 244):

Physicians told one another to eschew the advice of all other participants – birthing women, husbands, friends, clergy: to delimit the debate solely on the issue of medical safety; to remove their patients to hospitals, where medical considerations could be paramount; and to establish science as the primary focus.

Physicians promoted themselves as the experts laying claim to the decision-making authority (Leavitt 1987).

Dr George McKelway summed it up thus: 'It would hardly seem necessary for me to emphasize the fact that the obstetrician alone must be the judge of what is to be done' (McKelway 1892, cited in Leavitt 1987, p. 244). Physicians also deemed themselves to be the only ones who could take into account, without bias, the interests of both mother and fetus. Many physicians began consciously to withhold information from women, believing them incapable of making rational or objective decisions (Leavitt 1987). It was the beginning of the medical profession appointing itself as the advocate for the fetus (Duden 1993) and the consolidation of the primary care-giver, now the physician, having control of decision-making.

Until the 1960s, the physician's claim to decision-making authority in obstetrics was unchallenged. Societal mores and childbirth practices supported this paradigm until the inception of the women's health movement and childbirth education classes promoted women's awareness of their right to information, choices and self-determination (Faulder 1985, Clement 1987). Women began to seek alternatives in maternity care, and in many countries, the re-emergence of midwifery care played an important part in women reclaiming childbirth.

DECISION-MAKING RELATIONSHIPS

Over the past 30 years, the public, especially childbearing women, have indicated that they want a stronger voice in the decisions regarding their health care (Newby 1990). Some health care providers have responded to this expressed need for change, but evidence suggests that the pace of change toward increased patient autonomy and participation is slow. Many of the traditional hierarchical relationships are still functioning alongside emerging relationships of increased patient/client participation (Faulder 1985, Greenfield et al 1985). Taylor (1985) notes that while obstetricians have been slow to respond to this change, 'midwives have responded wonderfully well to changed circumstances' (p. 38).

Paternalism

Historically, absolute paternalism was considered to be the appropriate professional etiquette in medicine. Paternalistic physicians listen to the patient and answer questions but see their responsibility as making decisions based on their expertise and guiding the patient to an understanding of them (McKinstry 1992). Christie & Hoffmaster (1986, p. 56) state, '[at] the heart of medical paternalism is the usurpation of the decision making from a patient by a person who thinks he knows better than the patient does what is in the patient's best interest'. Women, particularly, were socialized to regard the power of the expert in health care as absolute (Oakley, 1980). The following quote illustrates the inherent belief in paternalistic decision-making that has been prevalent in health care over the years.

Wise women choose their doctors and trust them. The wisest ask the fewest questions. The terrible patients are nervous women with long memories, who question much where answers are difficult. The nervous woman should be made to comprehend at the outset that the physician means to have his way unhampered by the subtle distinctions with which bedridden women are apt to trouble those who most desire to help them (S. Weir Mitchell 1888, cited in Wertz & Wertz 1979).

The layperson was thus distanced from the information needed to participate effectively in decision-making, and a hierarchical relationship between physician and patient became entrenched in health care (Fisher 1986). The asymmetry in such a relationship is supported by the physician's control of the information and his or her power to determine clinical treatment. This 'gate-keeping' is what Starr (1982) calls 'cultural authority' and is legitimized by the belief that physicians will only make decisions based on scientific knowledge, medical expertise and their professional commitment to act in the patient's best interests (Haug & Levin 1983, Fisher 1986). Paterson (1966, cited in Siegler & Osmond 1973) has labelled this power an 'aesculapian authority' (after Aesculapius, the God of medicine in ancient Roman mythology), which is used to manage and control patients in the 'sick role'. Kalisch (1975 p. 22) explains, 'This awesome authority, which rules out any patient participation in the decision-making process, stems from a three-pronged power base; the physicians expertise, the patient's faith in him, and the belief that he has almost mystical powers'.

In this paradigm of the physician as primary decision-maker, acquiesence by the patient is expected, and a dependency role is reinforced. Should a patient decide to reject a decision or make choices about how care or treatment will be administered, he or she is labelled as non-compliant. Non-compliance has been recognized as 'an assertion of individual autonomy' (Haug & Levin 1983). If non-compliance is used as an indicator of acceptance of this paternalistic model of decision-making, the reported estimates that 33–50% of patients are non-compliant suggest that this paradigm is not effective and does not find favour with a large proportion of the population (Blackwell 1992, Donovan & Blake 1992, Wright 1993). Even though the evidence informs us that 33–50% of the population do not comply with medical advice, pregnant women choosing alternative courses of action are regarded and treated differently.

The growing specialty of fetal medicine, supported by prenatal diagnostics, has separated the mother and the fetus from what was once considered an integral unit of what Rothman (1982) calls a 'conflicting dyad'. The 'conflict' has been created by physicians who have appointed themselves as advocates for the fetus (Arney 1982, Oakley & Houd 1990, Duden 1993) and in recent years have asserted their authority by using the judicial system to obtain compliance with their decisions regarding care and treatment (Maier 1992, Warren 1992). The attitude that prevails with this separation of the mother's and the baby's interests reduces decision-making to an unacceptable choice of extremes: either the safe delivery of the baby or a positive birth experience (Goer 1995). As Goer (1995, p. 356) states 'they frame the issue in such a way that the woman cannot answer, "I want both".' A coercive element manifests when women are admonished for questioning care-giver's decisions and are accused of being selfish and putting their babies at risk (Francis 1985).

Central to the discussion of paternalism in medicine is the context of the 'sick role'. Komrad (1983) maintains that 'all illness represents a state of diminished autonomy' (p. 41), encompassing vulnerability, dependency and an involuntary loss of freedoms that invite the physician to act paternalistically. Whereas many of the current maternity practices and obstetric care appear not to question the appropriateness of applying the 'sick role' to pregnancy and birth, the consumer and midwifery movements view childbirth as a normal, healthy, physiological process.

Proponents of paternalism question the ability of patients or family to make rational, objective and educated decisions regarding medical treatment (Scholmann 1992). Physicians, particularly specialists, consider that they have specialized knowledge central to medical decision-making and that fully to discuss diagnosis or treatment options can be problematic, time-consuming and potentially very stressful, not only for the patient and family, but also for the practitioner (Zanner & Bliton 1991). Indeed, some physicians affirm their paternalistic stance and medical orientation towards childbirth, questioning women's entitlement to participate in planning their care. Jaiyesimi & Ballard (1992, p. 170) point out that 'in no other profession does the client dictate the management approach to the professional, and in no medical specialty other than obstetrics does the patient present the practitioner with a management option'.

Green et al (1990) reported that some professionals argue that women who are *allowed* (emphasis added) to participate in obstetric decision-making may become anxious, confused or panicky, and may experience negative consequences such as an inability to relax or a feeling of being overburdened with the responsibility. The findings of the study did not support this hypothesis, and in fact women felt empowered by receiving information and more in control of their birth processes, which led to a happier postpartum period.

Shapiro et al (1983) found that women generally fail to obtain all the information they want during obstetric care; however, 'patients leave the encounter essentially satisfied with the interaction and apparently unaware their interests have been set aside' (p. 145). Kirkham (1989) also found that whereas midwives stressed the importance of informing the woman at all times, the actual quality and amount of information that women received was inconsistent and usually less than the midwife's perception. Currently, paternalism remains the primary approach to medical decision-making, and decisions are often presented to the patient as a *fait accompli*, i.e. as the designated course of treatment (Buchanan 1983, Thomasma 1983, Taylor et al 1989). Information-giving and receiving remains problematic because of the paternalistic attitudes, the presumption that the expert's advice will be accepted and the socialization of the pregnant woman as a 'patient'. Many health care-givers claim the intention to involve the patient, but entrenched practices and the realities of the health care system often stop this happening.

Patient autonomy

Patient autonomy is an ethical principle that recognizes the right of a patient to self-determination and encompasses freedom of action and freedom of choice (Dworkin 1982, Komrad 1983). Autonomy in health care presupposes the ability and capacity of a patient to make choices, manage his or her own affairs and assume responsibility for his or her own life (Christie & Hofmaster 1986). Although there is an agreement in the literature for increased patient autonomy, there are concerns and criticisms raised about its workability in practice (Komrad 1983, Thomasma 1983, Christie & Hoffmaster 1986). According to Thomasma (1983, p. 245), the patient autonomy model does not address the impact that illness has on 'personal integrity'. Christie & Hoffmaster (1986) agree, pointing out the emotional, vulnerable and compromised physical state that accompanies illness or disease. This view implies that a patient's ability to make decisions while coping with the effects of illness is also compromised. However, the midwifery philosophy that recognizes pregnancy as a state of health and childbirth as a normal physiological process does not support this view, instead recognizing women as competent decision-makers in their social and health context.

McKinstry (1992) questions why medical decisions should be considered differently from other difficult life decisions. He suggests that 'doctors may be able to claim superior technical knowledge, but they must realize that their ethical or moral skills cannot be considered better than those of the patient' (p. 342). Although there may be a disparity of knowledge and health care information between practitioners and patients, how the information is presented can influence the decision-making process. A study by Kerrigan et al (1993) found that a combination of oral and written information improved patient comprehension, allowing for the incorporation of patient preferences in the decision-making process.

A primary role in decision-making in health care is not a familiar one for most women. A study by Sjogren & Uddenberg (1988) on the decision-making process surrounding prenatal diagnostic procedures found that although women felt autonomous in choosing the procedures, they also found it difficult to refuse them once they had been offered.

King (1991) raises the point that decisional autonomy may be affected by the institutional environment. Institutional policies do not often take into account the preferences, needs and experiences of both the practitioner and the patient (Mander 1993), and also have the potential to create a conflict between the practitioner and the client. Women sometimes create a choice for themselves in regard to hospital policies by consciously avoiding them. They leave it until the last possible moment to go to hospital and leave as soon after the birth as they can arrange.

Taylor (1985) reminds us of the many obstetric treatments that have been discarded over the years, as well as some present forms of management that are also being reconsidered; he notes that it is unreasonable to expect consumers to continue to accept 'blanket prohibitions or advice'. Taylor's position in favour of patient autonomy is clear: 'While a normal physiological process exists, the individual preferences of the mother must be allowed to overrule other considerations – such as convenience.' He further clarifies, 'In abnormal situations she still has the right to make her own decisions' (p. 38). Applebaum (1984, cited in Bastion 1990, p. 344) proposes that the resolution lies in cooperation: 'Demands for patient autonomy, just like the corresponding demands for physician dominance in decision-making … reflect the failure of each side to recognize that neither can act independently of the other'.

Shared decision-making

The focus on 'woman-centered' midwifery care has encouraged a 'partnership' between women and midwives and a collaborative style in decision-making. The process of shared decision-making is predicated on the notion of active patient (client) participation. A substantial body of literature supports the desire of patients to be actively involved in their decision-making and indicates that this participation may improve health outcomes (Greenfield et al 1985, Morris & Royle 1988, England & Evans 1992). Conversely, other studies show that patients do not always welcome this more active role, participating only as 'reluctant collaborators' (Waterworth & Luker 1990, Biley 1992). Strull et al (1984) reported that 53% of patients wanted to be involved in the decision-making, while 63% preferred the clinician to be the decision-maker. These findings may or may not be representative of healthy, pregnant women accessing maternity care.

Patient participation often requires active intervention, support and guidance by health care providers (Greenfield et al 1985, England & Evans 1992). It is well documented that patients desire more information but that they are not very proactive in obtaining it (Haug & Lavin 1983, Shapiro et al 1983, Street 1991). The nature of the support provided to midwifery clients may affect their level of comfort with and confidence in decision-making. Studies have shown that receiving information, feeling in control and having input into their care are important to childbearing women and are factors in long-term satisfaction and subsequent emotional well-being (Green et al 1990, Simkin 1991). The Winterton report (House of Commons Health Committee 1992) identified that women wish to be:

full participants in their own pregnancies and empowered to make genuinely informed decisions about their own care. Everything else issues naturally from this. Women want choice; in the overwhelming majority of cases there is no medical argument against this; and so the maternity services should be designed to give it to them.

The Expert Maternity Group, in their 1993 report (Department of Health 1993), noted that women should be encouraged to be closely involved in the planning of their care and that the decisions made should address the unique needs of the individual (p. 5). The report also indicated that a woman's right to choose her place of birth and her primary care-giver should be respected and that any plans for the birth should be flexible and open to change. Schain (1980) notes that a 'shared responsibility' model of decision-making requires the promotion of personalism rather than paternalism.

THE EMERGING MIDWIFERY MODEL OF CARE

Midwifery care has been undergoing a transformation and renewal in many parts of the world over the past 20 years. Some supporters and midwives view this resurgence as a collective movement, women reclaiming birth being linked with midwives reclaiming their profession (Farnsworth 1994). Women and midwives together have created an emerging model of midwifery practice based on a philosophy that understands pregnancy as a state of health, childbirth as a normal physiological process, and midwives and women as equal partners (Newby 1990, Donley 1993). This midwifery philosophy recognizes childbirth as a profound event taking place in the social context of a woman's life, and midwifery practice as encompassing the social, emotional, cultural, spiritual, physical and psychological aspects of the woman's childbearing experience. The philosophy also envisions the midwife as an autonomous primary care-giver.

The fundamental principles of this model are:

- continuity of care and care-giver
- informed choice
- shared decision-making
- choice of birth place

and are provided in the context of collaborative relationships within the health care system. These principles underlie a new direction of working in partnership with women (Donley 1993, College of Midwives of British Columbia 1995). As Guilliland (1993, p. 785) explains, 'Partnership utilizes the collective knowledge and wisdom of the midwife and the specific self knowledge and wisdom of the woman and her family'.

The definition of the midwife as a primary care-giver is an important distinction that recognizes a midwife's expertise and skills. The importance of autonomous practice relates directly to a midwife's ability to respect, promote and facilitate women's choices regarding their care. As a primary care-giver, the midwife is well situated in a community base providing midwifery care in all settings – hospital, home and birth centres – according to the woman's choice. This model of midwifery practice is compatible with the International Definition of a Midwife and is supported by the 1986 World Health Organization Report on Health Promotion and Birth (Wagner 1994).

The premise of this model is to integrate all the important and unique aspects of midwifery practice into an holistic system of care. Women have expressed their difficulties with the fragmentation that now exists in many systems of maternity health care. Some of the problems in these systems far outweigh the positive aspects and overwhelm the efforts of midwives to provide high-quality care. The promotion of this particular model of midwifery care does not imply that other forms of midwifery practice are inadequate. Instead, it suggests that the midwifery profession is responding to women's expressed needs and preferences for more individualized, personalized forms of care.

INFORMED CHOICE VERSUS INFORMED CONSENT

The model of midwifery practice discussed above includes informed choice as a fundamental principle and the cornerstone of a shared decision-making process. In order actively to participate in their care and make appropriate decisions, clients need to be able to access relevant information. The ethical concept of informed consent was initiated in the late 1950s and came into widespread use in the 1970s, primarily as a remedy for the lack of power that consumers were experiencing in the delivery of their health care.

Informed consent is designed to inform health care consumers of all the risks and benefits of a particular treatment and of possible treatment alternatives in order to protect them against unwanted medical treatment and to make possible their active participation in the decision-making process (American College of Obstetricians and Gynecologists 1993, Donohue 1993, Rachlis & Kushner 1994). As Faulder (1985, p. 128) states:

Giving our informed consent to medical treatment is the ultimate expression of the responsibility each one of us has for our own person ... Our bodies belong to us. They are who we are.

Weil (1993) states that the true purpose of informed consent is to enhance the autonomy of the patient. However, in practice, the process is often reduced to a 'perfunctory permission-granting activity' aimed primarily at meeting a policy or a legal requirement (Lidz et al 1988, Pinch & Spielman 1990, p. 715). Thompson (1982) addresses this discrepancy, noting that there are no mechanisms in place to ensure that informed consent is obtained in a manner that fulfills its mandate. Thus, information may be presented in a manner that is misleading, manipulative, inadequate, framed to reflect a care-giver's preference or introduced at a time that is not conducive to making carefully considered decisions (e.g. the night before scheduled surgery). Consent is often obtained by co-optation, women are treated as part of the team, and decisions are presented as a joint venture, for example 'We need to do a non-stress test or we want to have a healthy baby don't we?' Faulder (1985, p. 33) states that 'the elements of *choice* and *voluntariness* are essential to the concept of consent' and reminds us that 'choice implies ... at least one alternative to the action proposed – that of saying no'. For informed choice or informed consent to be employed in an ethical manner, the client needs to be fully aware of the options available and to feel that her choice will be 'unhampered by any hint of coercion' (Faulder, 1985, p. 33) or threats such as a withdrawal of services.

There is evidence to show that people will make different decisions depending on how the information is presented to them (Tversky & Kahneman 1981, Redelmeier et al 1993). The public in many instances assumes that it has to give its consent once it has entered the health care system and that the only option available is the one presented to it. People do not realize that they actually do have a choice: they can consent or refuse, or in some instances reach a compromise (Jones

1994). Although informed consent is a vehicle for increased client autonomy and participation, it remains, considering how it is generally employed in clinical practice, limited as an aid to shared decision-making.

Informed choice has been described as an expression of respect for the autonomy of the client and respect for her right to self-determination regarding reproductive choices. Informed choice requires complete, relevant objective information provided in the context of a non-authoritarian, collaborative relationship and the active involvement of the client (Van Wagner 1991, Farnsworth & Saxell 1994). It also requires a commitment from the practitioner and a belief that (Gibson 1991, p. 357):

individuals have the ability to make decisions and act on their own behalf, although they may need information and help to do so. Individuals have competencies that are present or possible, both internal and external. They often know what changes have to be made and can direct their own destinies.

As with informed consent, the application of informed choice in clinical practice varies considerably and is not yet widely understood. Some practitioners and clients view informed choice as being necessary only when a situation or complication dictates the need to make a particular decision, for example induction for post dates or transfer from home to hospital for a prolonged labour. Many of the 'routine' tests and procedures in pregnancy are viewed as not falling within the scope of informed choice; it is taken for granted that they will be automatically carried out. Maternity care is still characterized by technology, protocols and procedures that have not been adequately scientifically evaluated before being put into widespread use (Wagner 1994). Pregnant women have for so long been conditioned to accept 'routine' procedures that it does not occur to them that they may have a choice. Similarly, it does not occur to many practitioners that they should be offering women a choice.

Ultrasound scanning is a case in point. This technology very quickly became routinely and often repeatedly performed during pregnancy, and its widespread dissemination preceded proper evaluation (Wagner 1994). Although concerns about routine ultrasound scanning have been expressed for over 10 years, the procedure is now an entrenched part of pregnancy care and is rarely questioned by either client or practitioner. Despite evidence to the contrary, the medical profession in British Columbia, for example, has recently come out with the recommendation for a routine scan for all pregnant women at 18 weeks.

The World Health Organization (1984):

strongly endorses the principle of informed choice with regard to technology use. The health care providers have the moral responsibility; fully to inform the public about what is known and not known about ultrasound scanning during pregnancy; and fully to inform each woman prior to an ultrasound examination as to the clinical indication for ultrasound, its hoped for benefit, its potential risk, and alternative available, if any.

In this and other similar matters in maternity care, it is doubtful whether this counsel for informed choice is widely followed in practice.

Midwives, practising within the context of woman-centred care, should view the concept of informed choice as the precursor to all decisions within the course of care, starting with the choice of primary care provider and place of birth. If the woman is viewed as the primary decision-maker and the midwife as a resource person, midwifery care takes on a different form. Care becomes personal and individualized, the midwife as partner fulfills the role of 'the skilled companion' (Page, 1995), and the woman is empowered throughout the childbearing experience. According to Gibson (1991, p. 359), 'empowerment is a social process of recognizing, promoting and enhancing people's abilities to meet their own needs, solve their own problems and mobilize the necessary resources in order to feel in control of their lives'.

The philosophy of midwifery care previously discussed contains an expectation that midwives will actively encourage women's participation and promote decision-making as a shared responsibility. Transforming this expectation into clinical practice is empowerment. When empowerment is valued as a fundamental principle of shared decision-making, 'it is an enabling factor that assists women and midwives to achieve the unique and personal childbearing goals that have been identified as being so significant in their lives (Simkin 1991).

Informed choice, informed consent and informed decision-making are all similar and sometimes interchangeable terms for a concept that is being recognized as an essential part of health care today. There may be differences in the interpretation, but the basic premise needs to be the same:

- Clients should be invited and encouraged to participate in the decision-making involved in their health care.
- Clients need complete and relevant and objective information.
- This information should be provided at the appropriate time in an appropriate manner.
- The choices, risks and benefits need to be clearly

outlined, and the decision of the client will be respected even if it runs counter to professional advice (Rachlis & Kushner 1994).

SHARED DECISION-MAKING IN MIDWIFERY PRACTICE

Shared decision-making has been recognized as a desirable change in health care relationships, and women have expressed their wish to have a voice in the planning of their childbearing care. The adaptations inherent in this paradigm shift will incorporate changes in these relationships, particularly with regard to the balance of power: the acknowledgement of the woman as primary decision-maker and an appreciation of the multifaceted nature of decision-making. As Box 3.1 illustrates, there are many factors that will influence a woman's and a midwife's decision-making process. A shared decision-making process is based on the axiom that a woman's care needs to be considered in the social and cultural context of her life.

Box 3.1 Sources of input and factors influencing decision making.	
Woman	**Midwife**
Partner	Model of practice
Family/friends	Values/beliefs
Values/beliefs	Education/training
Midwife	Experience
Education	Woman's birth plan
Physician	Professional guidelines
Previous birth experience	Physician relationships
Cultural beliefs	Theoretical frameworks
Social context	Colleagues
Availability of options	Ability to support options

Midwives' experience of shared decision-making in midwifery practice

The concept of shared decision-making and the woman as the primary decision-maker will be new to many practitioners. Some midwives may say that it is too simplistic and question its feasibility in practice. Others will express shared decision-making as a fundamental premise of their practice. The report below of a small exploratory study will explore how midwives experience and implement shared decision-making in midwifery practice. The study utilized a semi-structured interview format to facilitate the sharing of information and experience. The interviews were guided by a schedule of open-ended questions to allow for individual variation, expression and spontaneous digression, which often enhance the research interaction (Reinharz 1992, Roter & Frankel 1992).

At the time the study was conducted, midwifery services were not an integrated part of the health care system in British Columbia. The model of midwifery practised at this time (one outside the usual regulatory processes) had developed out of the expressed demands of the women seeking midwifery care. It was a model based on continuity of care and care-giver, the majority of care being provided in a community setting. The study included midwives from a hospital-based programme, which, constrained by institutional policies and employment contracts, was unable to provide continuity of care-giver or choice of birth place. In 1993, the Ministry of Health, after 15 years of lobbying, recognized midwifery as a designated health care profession, and its incorporation into the health care system began. The hospital practice has adapted to a community-based model following the registration of midwives.

A total of 15 midwives participated in the study, 10 of whom were practising in a community setting providing the full scope of midwifery care (antepartum, intrapartum and postpartum) in a continuity of care framework. Their clients predominately chose home births. Five midwives were practising in a hospital-based programme, also providing the full scope of midwifery care and hospital births under the supervision of GPs. The midwives' length of time in practice ranged from 2 to 20 years, and the number of primary care clients from 60 to over 400.

The interviews were audiotaped and transcribed verbatim, the transcripts being returned to the participants for clarification and feedback. The data were analysed, referring to the objectives of the study. From the findings, there emerged three areas for discussion: the importance of the midwife–client relationship; strategies in decision-making conflicts; and the notion that the midwife's paradigm of shared decision-making defines midwifery practice.

The importance of the midwife–client relationship

The midwives were asked whether the relationships they had with their clients had a bearing on the decision-making process. Most midwives considered the midwife–client relationship to be the foundation of a shared decision-making process. This relationship, based on trust, respect and commitment, facilitates communication and enhances care. The midwives stressed the importance of listening to women and valuing what they had to say. Many described how the

relationship enhanced care. Knowing the woman enabled midwives to assess the degree of assistance, support and encouragement she might need to participate fully in the decision-making process. The relationship built with the client throughout the pregnancy informed the midwives of what was important for that woman, her wishes, her hopes and fears, all of which guided the decision-making process.

Most of the midwives felt that their relationship with their clients established trust, and trust was crucial for both midwife and client:

They need to feel they can trust you … you really need to have a trusting relationship beforehand, they need to understand where you're coming from and you absolutely need to understand where they're coming from. (Midwife M4)

As one midwife expressed, the need is for the parents:

to trust me as a midwife for the decisions I make on their behalf

and for the midwife:

to trust the parents, that they have enough knowledge and are making their decisions from a knowledgeable base, not just an emotional one. (M13)

Another midwife (M13) stated that 'trust is the cornerstone'. It is not a blind 'I'll do whatever you think best' trust, one that is encouraged by paternalism and expected by authoritarianism, but a trust based on mutual respect and confidence. This trust enables the midwife to speak for the woman if necessary and enables the woman to have confidence that the midwife knows what is important to her and will act accordingly (Page 1990).

Continuity of care and care-giver was mentioned as an essential ingredient for the midwife–client relationship as it can take several visits for a mutual relationship to develop. Midwives who had worked in the hospital setting reported that it was very different giving care to women they had never met before and that it was difficult to establish the same degree of understanding and communication. One community midwife was unwilling to accept clients late in the pregnancy, having run into difficulties in the past.

Having a relationship was seen as facilitating communication, which enabled midwives to give and receive input. The interface between each woman's and each midwife's communication style was felt to have an effect on informed choice. Again it was mentioned that this getting to know one another:

took time, effort, a lot of honesty and a kind of humility. You need to be able to have people disagree with you and be able to talk about it. (M4)

Several midwives expressed how they felt women had a lot of knowledge within themselves and how, in the context of a trusting relationship, midwives could help women to get in touch with their inner resources. Midwives trusted that women knew what was best for them and their babies. Therefore, it was important for midwives to listen to women. For some midwives practising in the community, it provided reassurance:

listening to the Mum, really, really closely, is my safety net in a home birth practice because I feel there is a subconscious level where she knows what she needs. (M5)

The midwife–client relationship contains reciprocal caring. It is a complementary dynamic: the caring promotes the relationship and the relationship promotes the caring. As Ann Oakley (1993, p. 77) states, caring is a fundamental necessity rather than being a soft option and is as important as technical knowledge or science.

The midwife–client relationship models the shared decision-making process. The midwife and client are partners, they share information, they consider each other's opinion and they trust each other to make intelligent decisions. Thus, the relationship creates and maintains accountability.

Informed choice

The midwife's paradigm of shared decision-making has several component parts: the midwife–client relationship based on trust, respect and caring; the principles and implementation of informed choice; and the commitment to the midwifery model of care. The midwives often used the terms '*shared decision-making*' and '*informed choice*' interchangeably. However, as the findings were analysed, a distinction emerged. Shared decision-making is a broader concept than informed choice and is more indicative of what actually occurs in practice.

The midwives interviewed perceived shared decision-making to be an integral part of the midwifery model and assumed the responsibility to introduce and implement informed choice as part of their midwifery care. Midwives shared how they saw themselves as facilitators and educators because many women are not used to participating in decision-making and taking responsibility in their health care:

We have to face a whole cultural change as far as women feeling it is their right to make decisions. (M11)

Most midwives introduced the concept of shared decision-making, in some way, at the initial visit. In outlining their care, midwives usually presented a partnership concept, explaining their expectation of an equal, collaborative relationship and the woman's active participation in decision-making. Midwives felt that they had an important role to play in encouraging women to take responsibility in their health care decisions and expected it would be ongoing in the pregnancy. They felt that one of the reasons clients chose midwifery care was because clients wanted to know all the options and to receive support in making their decisions:

I find a lot of time is spent helping the woman understand that the decisions are hers and it's constantly being reiterated in different ways. (M11)

Midwives described informed choice primarily as information-giving, helping clients to understand the information and identifying their choices. Informed choice was presented in various ways. One midwife gave clients a handout that described their rights to have all the relevant information about any particular issue and included the midwife's expectations regarding the clients' responsibility to educate themselves. Another felt it important to disclose her qualifications and experience in order to enable clients to make an informed decision in their choice of midwife. Community midwives would discuss in detail all the pertinent information regarding home birth to ensure that their clients were clearly making an informed choice regarding place of birth.

All midwives emphasized the importance of complete and honest disclosure. They saw themselves as responsible for providing all the relevant information to clients and helping them to understand it. The midwives felt it was incumbent on them to be conversant with the latest research. Their role was to present all the options, including the option of not doing anything, and to explain the implications of choosing any particular option. As one midwife remarked:

If you don't know what your choices are then you don't have any. (M14)

Over half the midwives openly expressed the difficulty of presenting information in an impartial manner without inserting subtle cues to reinforce their opinions and beliefs. Several were conscious of their preferences in certain situations and the need to work hard at not emphasizing certain information or options. As Ann Oakley (1993, p. 187) notes, 'It means giving them information about their situation rather than stories about what other people would like their situation to be'.

Most midwives felt a responsibility honestly to identify their biases to their clients and made it clear that their own beliefs would not affect their support of the client's decision. They were prepared to state their preferences if asked, and in many instances midwives clearly identified to their clients that they had:

a strong bias … so I'll just let you know that right now. I'll try and present you with the pro's and con's that I'm aware of but I do have a bias and aside from that I respect whatever decision you make. (M15)

One midwife felt that the specifics of the situation influenced how she presented information. For example:

if it's something that's critical and life threatening, I'll give the options and weight the plus's and minus's, and if it's not as critical I don't usually weight it, I just give the information and help them make the [decision]. (M12)

The midwives were cognizant of the influence that they could have and did have over their clients:

We tend to still push them one way or another and that we need to keep thinking about it. You always need to be aware of what you are doing. (M4)

One midwife acknowledged consciously directing her client's choices, in her view, toward safe care. Oakley & Houd (1990) noted that, at times, midwives felt their expertise should overrule a client's wishes.

Recognizing that midwives do have direct power over women giving birth (Oakley & Houd 1990), the midwives expressed the need to have an ongoing awareness of how the decision-making process was made manifest in their practice and a need to review the decisions and the process on a regular basis. It is evident that the midwives are aware of the complexities involved in a woman's birth process and that decision-making is linked to power and control, respect and trust. One midwife described a learning experience with a client who wanted to birth out in the woods, far away from all amenities. By exploring what was behind the decision the midwife discovered:

What she really wanted was just the power to make decisions and [to] feel she was making the decisions … she needed to know she was supported and wouldn't be abandoned. She just wanted to do it on her own and us to be witnesses to that power. (M9)

In reaching that understanding, the midwife was able to provide the right physical, emotional and psychological environment for that woman to birth safely, with the power and dignity that she desired.

The midwives in the study were asked how they learned to use informed choice in their practice. All of them answered that it was something they learned experientially. Most of them expressed how it had evolved from their personal and political beliefs, including their beliefs regarding women's rights, their beliefs as feminists and their belief that the birth belongs to the woman and her family. Many of

the midwives had developed their commitment to informed choice from witnessing births in which women's power was completely taken away and by watching how women are completely taken for granted and expected to conform within the health care system. Some midwives learned from watching and networking with more experienced midwives. One midwife related how communications courses and midwifery conferences had enhanced her awareness and skills in using this concept. No midwives answered that shared decision-making or informed choice was something that they learned as part of their training. Two midwives indicated that the model of practice they encountered during their training was one in which women were expected to do what the midwife told them (Scotland) and that women were like children who needed gentle, firm guidance (England). A midwife whose training included an apprenticeship with an experienced midwife reported that her teacher stressed the parents' rights to make choices, although this was not at that time called informed choice.

The primary decision-maker

The midwives were asked to describe their understanding of the woman as the primary decision-maker. One midwife suggested that it implied respect – respect for women's voices, for their abilities to make appropriate decisions for themselves and their babies, and for birth as a major life event:

It means just that, we recognize the woman as the primary decision maker. This is her experience, this is her rite of passage. I am there to provide what I can in the way of assistance, but this is something she does, not that I do. She gives birth, I don't deliver her baby. (M14)

As part of investigating how decision-making manifests in practice, midwives were asked what proportion of clients wished to be primary decision-makers and what proportion preferred the midwife to take a more directive role. Estimates from midwives ranged from 10% to 25% for women wishing a primary role and 0% to 15% for women wanting direction. Two midwives had noticed that the client often looked to the midwife for direction when she was experiencing pressure from family members or physicians to make certain decisions. Overall, the midwives identified that the majority of women preferred to work collaboratively.

This range of preferences reflects the necessity for an individualized approach to practice. As one midwife discussed, some clients have highly specific needs and expectations, one of her clients expressing hers thus:

I came to the midwives so that I could feel safe and be told exactly what to do all the time. I don't want all this natural childbirth. I don't want all these choices. I want you to tell me what's best. (M4)

Which is a choice in itself. Midwives reported that clients asked many questions; they wanted information; they wanted their midwives to give their opinions, especially for situations requiring medical expertise; and they wanted affirmations for the decisions they had made. Midwives were asked whether they had noticed any specific periods or circumstances in which clients wished to hand over the decision-making to their caregiver. Labour, especially a long, difficult one, was cited as the most common time. In times of intense stress, midwives felt that clients looked to them for guidance and support; this might include trusting the midwife to make the decision for them:

I guess the relationship and rapport we had and the sense of trust was such that the woman chose to go along with what I felt was the safest thing at that time for her and the baby. (M8)

Emergencies were also cited as a time when clients not only wanted to hand over decision-making, but also expected to. As several midwives expressed:

As a professional midwife I'm supposed to be able to advise them to take them to a good outcome. That's why they hired me. (M1)

Some midwives noticed, as the pregnancy progressed, an increase in women's confidence and a readiness to take more responsibility in decision-making. Each woman had individual needs, and the midwifery care needed to be tailored to meet them.

Several midwives noted a difference between clients who chose home birth and those who wanted to birth in the hospital with labour support. They commented that clients choosing hospital birth were generally more accepting of turning over the decision-making and responsibility for what happened to them, handing over their power more easily. They explained that, as hospital policies are implemented, the woman begins to feel that she is losing control and will sometimes give up her autonomy, saying, 'You make the decisions, I don't care any more'.

Decision-making conflicts

Decision-making conflicts were explored with all the participating midwives. They were asked what they did when clients chose not to follow their advice or recommendations. The initial response of most midwives was that it depended on the nature of the situation and that such situations were quite uncommon. One community midwife stated that she had clear guidelines on how she handled complications and required autonomy in making clinical decisions. If clients did not agree with this approach or were unhappy with her decisions or prescribed management, she suggested the option of finding another midwife.

The dividing line between different courses of action seemed to be whether safety was an issue. Most midwives felt reasonably comfortable with clients refusing ultrasound examinations, glucose tolerance tests or non-stress tests, for example. They noted that clients mostly rejected routine protocols or hospital policies, and in many instances midwives found themselves acting as a buffer between these policies, the physician and the client. If a more critical issue arose, one that might affect the short- or long-term well-being of the mother and baby, most midwives felt that further communication was paramount:

You need to communicate further with them to see if you can find out what their beliefs are, what their feelings are, why they're choosing a particular course of action. (M3)

Several midwives commented that people do not usually make unhealthy choices so a conflict of this nature indicated a need to evaluate the situation. They felt that it was important to determine whether the client had all the relevant information, to assess whether she understood that information and to decide whether she had any misinformation or fears that were influencing her decision. The midwives felt quite committed to spending as much time as it took to help their clients to understand the situation and make a wise decision. Several midwives expressed that they would go to colleagues for consultation and support.

Most midwives reiterated supporting the philosophy of a woman's right to make her own decisions; however, some community midwives felt that they might, in extreme situations, have to withdraw their care:

I'm very flexible except in life or death situations. (M1)

However, in these instances, they would provide referrals to other midwives or physicians. Most midwives identified that they would not abandon care; however, they felt that, in some instances, they needed to take a strong stand:

I'm not convinced that some people don't kind of blackmail you a little bit. (M15)

The midwives felt the situations were very individual and needed individual consideration. Most of them identified that clients were usually receptive to their explanations, especially when (the midwife's) lack of experience was a factor:

I find that when I state my limitations to my clients they're very respectful most of the time, because that's part of the collaborative effort too. (M15)

Seven midwives had not encountered any major conflict situations or had had to deal with only minor issues. Seven other midwives had been in conflict situations and most of the problems had been resolved, to everyone's satisfaction, prior to the birth. Some midwives reported that clients occasionally just did not return for further care.

An ethical dilemma

Decision-making conflict was a very topical issue. Six months previously, one of the midwives had attended a woman having her fourth baby, which was in a frank breech position at term. The woman was insistent on having her baby at home. Her other choices were to have an elective caesarean section in the community hospital or to leave her family and travel to a larger centre where she could access a physician and a hospital that would allow her to attempt a vaginal breech delivery. The midwife, who had been in community practice for almost 20 years, had minimal experience with breech deliveries. She tried to give her clients as much information as possible:

This [breech] was the kind of thing where informed choice is a big issue ... making them look at all aspects, all sides of it. What if the baby does get stuck? I shared everything with her, the only way I could be totally accountable was to share everything. (M10)

The midwife offered all possible options: exercises, acupuncture and external cephalic version. The midwife was even able to elicit support from a community physician (experienced in breech deliveries), who agreed to assist them in a vaginal birth if they showed up at the hospital very late in labour, although it was against hospital policy. In the end, the mother decided to give birth at home:

For her [the mother] it was not to disturb God's perfect work and that was what was true for her, that was her belief system. She prayed about it. Who am I to question that? It's pretty hard to argue with maternal instincts and unswerving faith, religious faith. It's real hard to argue with those. (M10)

The midwife described how she examined her options, her motives and her responsibilities, not only to her clients, but also to herself, her colleagues and the emerging midwifery profession in British Columbia. In the end, she said:

I would go back to thine own self be true. Like, midwife is with woman, it's not with the doctors, or with the politics, it's with the woman.

The birth took place at home with the midwife in attendance, the arms were extended (which had not been identified on the ultrasound), and the baby died during the birth. Several of the community midwives mentioned this birth during our interviews. They described how it had provoked much soul-searching, much discussion and much compassion for the midwife involved. They acknowledged how difficult it would be to refuse care to the woman given the midwifery philosophy and code of ethics, and how hard it would be to provide care given her limited experience with breech deliveries and the political climate. This birth was a valuable learning experience for the midwifery community. They learned that these dilemmas do occur and that midwives may have to face up to where they stand on the moral, ethical and professional issues. They also learned that the professional association stood behind their philosophy and code of ethics: the midwife was supported in her decision. The midwife advised that the family is moving through their grieving process and that the mother is at peace with her decision.

Strategies for resolving conflicts

According to the midwives interviewed, decision-making conflicts are not common in midwifery care. The midwife–client relationship, the non-interventional style of practice and the commitment to informed choice lend themselves to harmony rather than conflict. Most discord arises over routine procedures where the refusals are least likely to compromise the mother or baby. Many difficulties are related to providing a midwifery model of care within the context of a medical establishment.

The midwives described a unique approach to resolving conflicts. Their first inclination was to examine the process surrounding the decision-making. They questioned their practice instead of judging their clients. Did the clients need more information? Did they understand the implications? Was there another issue that needed to be talked through? The midwives' awareness of the potential to misuse their power in these situations was unique and respectful. The bottom line seemed to be that midwives have a responsibility to respect and support their clients' decisions; after all, it is the mother who is giving birth.

Summary

All the midwives felt that shared decision-making and informed choice in the context of a collaborative relationship were an essential part of midwifery practice.

Although the midwives had learned, through their own philosophy and experience, to incorporate shared decision-making and informed choice in their practice, they felt it was something that should be included in midwifery training.

Most midwives viewed informed choice as a process that promoted women's participation in decision-making. They also acknowledged it was a challenge to address their own particular biases and to recognize where and how they influenced women during their care.

Prenatal preparation and discussion avoided most decision-making conflicts and enabled both midwife and client to feel secure. Difficult dilemmas sometimes arise when clients do not agree with the midwife's recommendations, but in general midwives felt that these situations could be resolved with good communication and creative solutions.

Many midwives feel the midwife–client relationship is at the heart of shared decision-making. Their relationships with their clients foster mutual trust, respect and commitment, enabling midwives to practise in an environment that may be unsupportive or even openly hostile. Recognizing the contribution that a woman's inner knowledge about herself and her pregnancy can bring to the decision-making process draws another dimension into the midwife–client communications and adds to the midwifery knowledge in relation to this women's care. Midwives can view these relationships as an opportunity to increase the choices for all by reinforcing for women the power and importance of their own voices.

The midwives also demonstrated that they make a concerted effort to promote shared decision-making on an individual basis. This enables women to become aware of their own capacities and provides an opportunity for them to exercise their personal power in their childbearing. The process synergistically empowers both the woman and the midwife. Shared decision-making reflects the equal, collaborative nature of the midwife–client relationship wherein the professional context and the specific expertise of the midwife can be situated as a resource rather than a directing factor. As long as midwives remain aware of the potential for asymmetry in their relationships with clients, this partnership model of practice will go a long way to help women to reclaim their central role in childbearing.

IMPLICATIONS FOR THE FUTURE OF MIDWIFERY

As hierarchical and paternalistic decision-making structures lose credibility across Western cultures, more care-fully nuanced collaborative processes are emerging for the purpose of safeguarding mutual respect, which in turn expands collective knowledge.

Given the profound influence of the midwife–client relationship on the efficacy of shared decision-making in childbirth, we can anticipate certain disciplines, skill sets and areas of knowledge that midwives require now and in the future. Midwives will need to be equipped to clarify at the outset of their relationship with their clients what each party to the relationship needs and expects from the other and what will happen should a conflict arise. It will presumably be their particular responsibility to assimilate knowledge from professional sources and to communicate that knowledge in ways that support their clients' participation in decision-making. Midwives will also need to be sufficiently self-aware to name the implications of divergent contexts and accountabilities, to identify their biases, to distinguish facts from opinions and to deal creatively with the ambiguity of differences. Midwifery practice in our time requires preparation for ethical discernment and wisdom in relationships, as well as skills for clinical judgement.

CONCLUSION

'Giving birth to a child is a transformative experience for women ... and a rite of passage' (Bergum 1989). Recognizing and honouring the significance of the childbearing experience compels midwives to facilitate the discovery and implementation of the woman's choices. Situating the midwife–client relationship in the context of a partnership is the foundation of a different approach to maternity care, one that values women's voices and their power, and has confidence in their abilities to make wise choices that will enable them to give birth to their babies safely.

Pointers for practice

- The woman should be the primary decision-maker and the midwife the resource person and facilitator.
- The relationship should be one of partnership.
- The midwife–woman relationship is fundamental to this model of decision-making.
- Midwives have an important part to play in encouraging women to take responsibility for their health care decisions.
- Midwives should be conversant with latest research.
- Midwives should be aware of their own biases.

REFERENCES

American College of Obstetricians and Gynecologists 1993 Ethical dimensions of informed consent. Women's Health Issues 3(1): 1–10

Arney W R 1982 Power and the profession of obstetrics. University of Chicago Press, Chicago

Bastion H 1990 Obstetrics and litigation: a consumer perspective. Medical Journal of Australia 153(6): 340–5

Bergum V 1989 Woman to mother. Bergin & Garvey, Massachusetts

Biley F C 1992 Some determinants that effect patient participation in decision-making about nursing care. Journal of Advanced Nursing 17: 414–21

Blackwell B 1992 Compliance. Psychotherapeutics and Psychosomatics 58: 161–9

Buchanan A E 1983 Medical paternalism. In Satorius R (ed.) Paternalism. University of Minnesota, Minneapolis

Christie R J, Hoffmaster C B 1986 Ethical issues in family medicine. Oxford University Press, Oxford

Clement C 1987 Women and health: from passive to active. Health Promotion 25(4): 5–8

College of Midwives 1997 Philosophy of care. In College of Midwives Registrants Handbook. College of Midwives, Vancouver

Department of Health (1993) Changing Childbirth. Part 1. Report of the Expert Maternity Group. HMSO, London

Donley J 1993 Independent midwifery. Proceedings of the International Confederation of Midwives 23rd International Congress, 9–14 May, Vancouver, Canada

Donohue M 1993 Maternal–fetal health: ethical issues. Association of Women's Health, Obstetric, and Neonatal Nurses. Clinical Issues in Perinatal and Women's Health Nursing 4(4): 561–9

Donovan J L, Blake D R 1992 Patient non-compliance: deviance or reasoned decision-making? Social Science and Medicine 34(5): 507–13

Duden B (1993) Disembodying women. Harvard University Press, London

Dworkin G 1982 Appendix F: Autonomy and informed consent. In: Making health care decisions. The ethical and legal implications of informed consent in the patient–practitioner relationship, vol. 3: Appendices studies on the foundations of informed consent. President's Commission for the Study of Ethical Problems in Medicine and Biomedical and Behavioural Research. US Government Printing Office, Washington, DC

England S L, Evans J 1992 Patients' choices and perceptions after an invitation to participate in treatment decisions. Social Science and Medicine 34(11): 1217–25

Farnsworth D 1994 Midwifery rising: the politics of midwifery in British Columbia and New Zealand. Unpublished paper, Master's degree programme, Thames Valley University

Farnsworth D R, Saxell L 1994 Midwives and women in partnership: informed choice. Aspiring Midwife (4): 16–17

Faulder C 1985 Whose body is it? Virago, London

Fisher S 1986 In the patient's best interests: women and the politics of medical decisions. Rutgers, University Press, New Jersey

Francis H H 1985 Obstetrics: a consumer orientated service? The case against. Maternal and Child Health (March): 68–72

Gibson C 1991 A concept analysis of empowerment. Journal of Advanced Nursing 16: 354–61

Green J M, Coupland V A, Kitzinger J V 1990 Expectations, experiences, and psychological outcomes of childbirth: a prospective study of 825 women. Birth 17(1): 15–24

Greenfield S, Kaplan S, Ware J E 1985 Expanding patient involvement in care. Annals of Internal Medicine 102(4): 520–8

Goer H 1995 Obstetric myths versus research realities. Bergin & Garvey, Connecticut

Guilliland K 1993 Professionalism versus partnership: midwives and women hear the heartbeat of the future. Proceedings of the International Confederation of Midwives 23rd International Congress, 9–14 May, Vancouver, Canada.

Haug M, Lavin B 1983 Consumerism in medicine. Sage, London

House of Commons Health Committee 1992 Second report on maternity services (Winterton report). HMSO, London

Jaiyesimi R A, Ballard R M 1992 The birth plan – patient demands without responsibility. Maternal and Child Health (June): 166–70

Jones S 1994 Ethics in midwifery. Mosby, London.

Kalisch B J 1975 Of half gods and mortals: Aesculapian authority. Nursing Outlook 23(1): 22–8

Kerrigan D D, Thevasagayam R S, Woods T O et al 1993 Who's afraid of informed consent? British Medical Journal 306: 298–300

King N M 1991 Maternal–fetal conflicts: ethical and legal implications for nurse-midwives. Journal of Nurse-Midwifery 36: 361–5

Kirkham M 1989 Midwives and information-giving during labour. In Robinson S, Thomson A (eds) Midwives, research and childbirth, Vol. 1. Chapman & Hall, London

Kitzinger S 1992 Ourselves as mothers. Bantam, London

Komrad M S 1983 A defence of medical paternalism: maximising patients' autonomy. Journal of Medical Ethics 9: 38–44

Leavitt J 1987 The growth of medical authority: technology and morals in turn-of-the-century obstetrics. Medical Anthropology Quarterly 1: 230–55

Lidz C W, Applebaum P S, Meisel A 1988 Two models of implementing informed consent. Archives of Internal Medicine 148: 1385–9

McKinstry B 1992 Paternalism and the doctor–patient relationship in general practice. British Journal of General Practice 42: 340–2

Maier K 1992 Forced cesarean section as reproductive control and violence: feminist social work perspective on the 'Baby R' case. Unpublished Masters thesis, Department of Women's Studies, Simon Fraser University, Canada

Mander R 1993 Autonomy in midwifery and maternity care. Midwives Chronicle and Nursing Notes (October): 369–74

Mason J 1988 Midwifery in Canada. In: Kitzinger S (ed.) The midwife challenge. Pandora, London

Morris J, Royle G T 1988 Offering patients a choice of surgery for early breast cancer: a reduction in anxiety and depression in patients and their husbands. Social Science and Medicine 26: 583–5

Newby L 1990 The politics of women's health. Journal of the Australian College of Midwives 2(4): 7–14

Oakley A 1980 Women confined: towards a sociology of childbirth. Martin Robertson, Oxford

Oakley A 1993 Essays on women, medicine and health. Edinburgh University Press, Edinburgh

Oakley A, Houd S 1990 Helpers in childbirth: midwifery today. World Health Organization, Regional Office for Europe. Hemisphere, London

Page L 1990 A question of trust. AIMS Quarterly Journal 3(3): 9

Page L 1995 (ed.) Effective group practice in midwifery. Blackwell Science, London

Pinch W J, Spielman M L 1990 The parents' perspective: ethical decision-making in neonatal intensive care. Journal of Advanced Nursing 15: 712–19

Rachlis M, Kushner C 1994 Strong medicine. Harper Collins, Toronto

Redelmeier D A, Rozin P, Kahneman D 1993 Understanding patient's decisions: cognitive and emotional perspectives. Journal of the American Medical Association 270(1): 72–6

Reinharz S 1992 Feminist methods in social research. Oxford University Press, Oxford

Roter D, Frankel R 1992 Quantitative and qualitative approaches to the evaluation of the medical dialogue. Social Science and Medicine 34(10): 1097–103

Rothman B K 1982 In labour: women and power in the birthplace. WW Norton, New York

Schain W S 1980 Patient's rights in decision making: the case for personalism versus paternalism in health care. Cancer 46(suppl.) 1034–41

Scholman P 1992 Ethical considerations of the aggressive care of very low birthweight infants. Neonatal Network 11: 31–6

Shapiro M C, Najman J M, Chang A, Keeping J D, Morrison J, Western J S 1983 Information control and the exercise of power in the obstetrical encounter. Social Science and Medicine 17(3): 139–46

Siegler M, Osmond H 1973 Aesculapian authority. Hastings Center Studies 1(2): 41–52

Simkin P 1991 Just another day in a woman's life? Women's long term perceptions of their first birth experience. Birth 18(4): 203–10

Sjogren B, Uddenberg N 1988 Decision making during the prenatal diagnostic procedure. A questionaire and interview study of 211 women participating in prenatal diagnosis. Prenatal Diagnosis 8: 263–73

Starr P 1982 The social transformation of American medicine. Basic Books, New York

Street R 1991 Information-giving in medical consultations: the influence of patients' communicative styles and personal characteristics. Social Science and Medicine 32(5): 541–8

Strull W M, Lo B, Charles G 1984 Do patients want to participate in medical decision making? Journal of the American Medical Association 252(21): 2990–4

Taylor R W 1985 Obstetrics: a consumer oriented service? The case in favour. Maternal and Child Health (February): 37–38

Taylor S G, Pickens J M, Geden E A 1989 Interactional styles of nurse practitioners and physicians regarding patient decision making. Nursing Research 38(1): 50–5

Thacker S B, Stroup D F, Peterson H B 1995 Efficacy and safety of intrapartum electronic fetal monitoring: an update. Obstetrics and Gynaecology 86: 613–20

Thomasma D C 1983 Beyond medical paternalism and patient autonomy: a model of physician conscience for the physician–patient relationship. Annals of Internal Medicine 98: 243–8

Thompson W C 1982 Appendix H: psychological issues in informed consent in the patient–practitioner relationship. Volume Three: Appendices studies on the foundations of informed consent. Presidents Commission for the Study of Ethical Problems in Medical and Biomedical Behavioural Research. US Government Printing Office, Washington DC

Tversky A, Kahneman D 1981 The framing of decisions and the psychology of choice. Science 211(30): 453–8

Wagner M 1994 Pursuing the birth machine. Ace Graphics, Camperdown, New South Wales

Wagner V Van 1991 With women: community midwifery in Ontario. Unpublished Master's thesis, Department of Environmental Studies, York University, Ontario, Canada

Warren M A 1992 The moral significance of birth. In: Holmes H B, Purdy L M (eds) Feminist perspectives in medical ethics. Indiana University Press, Indianapolis

Waterworth S, Luker K A 1990 Reluctant collaborators: do patients want to be involved in decisions concerning care? Journal of Advanced Nursing 15: 971–6

Weil W B 1993 Commentary: Ethical issues of informed consent. Women's Health Issues 3(1): 1–10

Wertz D C, Wertz R W 1979 Lying-in. A history of childbirth in America. Free Press, New York

World Health Organization 1984 Diagnostic ultrasound in pregnancy: WHO view on routine screening. Lancet ii: 361

Wright E C 1993 Compliance – or how many aunts has Matilda? Lancet 342 (October 9): 909–13

Zanner R M, Bliton M J 1991 Decisions in the NICU: the moral authority of parents. Children's Health Care Quarterly 20(1): 19–25

4

Risk: theoretical or actual

Lee Saxell

Very little research has been carried out to investigate the perceptions that pregnant women have of being labelled as 'high-risk' and the subsequent impact of this on the pregnancy, birth and postpartum period. This chapter begins by reviewing the literature on the purpose and efficacy of risk-screening and scoring systems. The 'high-risk' label has become an integral part of the language of childbirth and is one with which most pregnant women are familiar. The label is intended to direct attention and provide specialized care to women at risk of poor perinatal outcome. Although risk-screening is a widely accepted concept throughout the obstetric literature, opinions on the validity of scoring systems for determining high-risk vary widely, and their efficacy has yet to be determined (Alexander & Keirse 1989, Hall, 1994). Oakley (1992a) asserts that risk-scoring systems are used to control women, ostensibly in the interests of their own health and that of their babies, while Sapolsky (1990) infers that people's fears about risks can be used to maintain control by the institutions that have the power to define and categorize these risks.

Although many interventions in obstetrics are appropriate and have led to improved perinatal outcome, no intervention is free of risk. The assignment of a high-risk status to a woman's pregnancy may lead to what has been described as a 'cascade effect' of intervention of dubious benefit and potential harm (Brody & Thompson 1981). These potentially unnecessary interventions may allocate scarce resources to a group of women who do not need them. In addition, the label of high risk can create stress and anxiety in a pregnant woman, which can cause a diminished sense of competence and a loss of confidence in her ability to give birth safely (Chalmers 1982).

Medicine has had the power to define what is normal in childbirth, so that any deviation from this standard is viewed as 'abnormal' and justifies the further surveillance of pregnant women (Arney 1982). The range of normal has shifted drastically throughout the 20th century as new tests, procedures and technology redefine it. Rothman (1982) observed that conditions of pregnancy and childbirth that would have been considered normal or marginal in the past are now being labelled high risk. In contrast, that which is presently considered 'high risk' may, at a later date, turn out to be within the 'normal' range (Overall 1989). The lack of precision in risk identification tools means there is no factual 'scientific' basis for denying women choice regarding their care or for insisting that all women give birth in an institutional setting.

With respect to maternal death, childbirth has never been safer in the developed world; paradoxically, the concept of risk to the *fetus* has expanded to unprecedented levels (Queniart 1992). Growing interest in 'fetal well-being' has resulted in far more public discourse on the dangers of pregnancy. Although overall risks to the fetus depend on a multitude of different factors, the public focus has shifted to maternal behaviour and lifestyle. Recent legal developments threaten pregnant women's privacy and autonomy by using control measures in court 'whenever [a woman's] behaviour is seen to be detrimental to the fetus she carries' (Rodgers 1989, p. 174). The identification of the fetus as having a risk distinct from that of the mother has enormous implications for the future of risk assessment in pregnancy and childbirth.

This chapter also includes a small study, carried out in British Columbia, Canada, that is exploratory in nature and intended to probe the meaning that women and midwives place on risk and the label of 'high risk'. In interviews, some of the following questions were asked. What does the term high-risk mean to you? Who has the right to define what is high risk? Do you believe that women have the right to refuse treatment and control where they will give birth, if they have been labelled as high risk? Do you believe that identifying a woman as high risk could change her perception of the pregnancy and adversely affect the outcome? Although this study is limited in its scope with selected participants, it suggests that there is a need to incorporate women's perceptions of health and risk into the development of midwifery guidelines for practice. Furthermore, any risk-screening systems should remain flexible in order to foster greater choice to women regarding their care and place of birth.

THE PURPOSE AND EFFICACY OF RISK-SCORING SYSTEMS

Uncertainty is a permanent part of life and life's beginnings. It is also at the heart of the definition of risk. (Hall 1994, p. 1239)

Since antiquity, it has been recognized that some pregnancies have a poorer outcome than others. Hippocrates recognized the difference between those risk factors present at the time of pregnancy and those developing during pregnancy (James & Stirrat 1988). Early in the 20th century, obstetric textbooks began containing lists of risks associated with poor outcome during pregnancy and childbirth (Stander 1936). Clinicians have long identified risk factors in pregnancy, but formalized risk-scoring systems did not become common until the 1960s, when computerized databanks became available. Dozens of scoring systems have been developed, some widely in use, others having been abandoned (Alexander & Keirse 1989).

The primary *purpose* of a risk-scoring system is to 'permit classification of individual women into different categories, for which actions can then be planned' (Enkin et al 1994, p. 7). The *goal* of risk assessment from a public health perspective is to understand the rate of occurrence of a condition in a given population and calculate the risk that other population groups have of developing the same condition (Handwerker 1994). The definition of a pregnancy 'at risk' is one in which the likelihood of an adverse outcome for the mother or her baby is greater than that for the general population (James & Stirrat 1988). However, there are questions of whether risk-scoring systems can be generalized from one population to another, if '... many of the values we measure are probably only surrogates for the true etiologic variable' (Spasoff & McDowell, quoted in Hayes 1992, p. 406). According to Murphy (1994, p. 67), 'most risk factors, even if they are strongly associated with outcomes in populations, do not predict adverse outcomes very well for individuals.'

Risk-scoring involves allocating a number to each adverse factor and combining them to achieve an overall score. These cumulative scores are then assigned a category of risk from low to high, although they often display unequal weighting of risk factors and fail to address how to account for compounding risk factors (Lilford & Chard 1983, Lazarus 1990). For example, in a risk-scoring system developed by Hobel (1978), a maternal age of 35 years or more has the same weight as acute pyelonephritis, habitual abortion, rhesus sensitization and excessive drug use. Furthermore, there is little consensus on what the appropriate risk factors are, much less on how to weigh them (Alexander & Keirse 1989). Hall (1994) observes that 'there is no evidence that a woman with a risk factor of 9 is three times more likely to have a problem than a woman whose score is 3'.

It would appear that a formal risk-scoring tool would be more accurate than the rather subjective process of clinical impressions. However, risk factors are only statistically *associated* with the outcome being scored for and are not the *cause* of the adverse outcome. Since certainty is rare, risk can only be defined in terms of the *probability* that the risk factor will lead to a poor outcome (Murphy 1994). Therefore, removing or correcting the risk factor does not eliminate the possibility of an adverse outcome. Lilford & Chard (1983) have argued that risk-scoring systems do not make a precise prediction of the chances of an adverse outcome and therefore cannot be used in formal decision analysis. In order for risk assessments to be effective, the 'poor outcomes' for which a woman is at risk must be clearly specified, otherwise 'the outcome measures are so prone to bias that the scoring system can easily become no more than a self-fulfilling prophecy' (Alexander & Keirse 1989, p. 347).

To the expectant woman, the label of 'high risk' is only beneficial when something can be done to decrease or eliminate the risk factor. It is not useful to predict a poor outcome if it is too late in the pregnancy to positively influence the outcome predicted (Enkin et al 1994). While some antepartum problems can be prevented and corrected, Hall (1994, p. 1241) asserts that, when this occurs, 'the risk score should be reduced, but typically risk scores are never deflated'. Unfortunately, risk assessment tools only refer the woman and her baby up the ladder of risk and rarely down, even if the factors that caused her to be labelled as high risk have disappeared (Handwerker 1994, Perkins 1994). Also, as pregnancy risk is dynamic and complex in nature, a screening test applied even at serial points during pregnancy can never effectively assess the dynamic character of pregnancy (Wall, 1988).

HOW WELL DO RISK-SCORING SYSTEMS WORK?

Scoring systems will perform better in assessing the risk if they are implemented late in pregnancy or if they allow for readjustment during pregnancy. This leads to the paradox that the most precise risk prediction is made at a time when there is little or no further need for it, whereas the potentially more useful early identification of risk is relatively imprecise. (Enkin et al 1994)

Opinions on the efficacy of scoring systems vary widely. Fortney & Whitehorne (1982, p. 501) comment 'that unreasonable demands are made of high-risk indices … no index can satisfy all requirements'. A US Institute of Medicine (1982) report evaluating 33 published risk assessment methods concluded that the methods varied widely, were not successful in identifying women most at risk and frequently incorrectly

identified women as high risk. The conclusion was that risk assessment tools were not appropriate for predicting risk in individuals, and the authors recommended that clinical judgement be used in determining treatment for individual women, risk tools being only a 'useful adjunct' (p. 52). Alexander & Keirse (1989, p. 350) noted that, with formal risk-scoring, 'women may be assigned to the high-risk group because of rigid definitions of the risk markers, whereas a capable clinician could have assessed the situation more sensitively thanks to implicit clinical judgment'.

According to Perkins (1994, p. 24), more than 20 risk assessment instruments have been developed in the USA, while in Canada, there are currently at least 12 risk-scoring systems reported in use, with varying degrees of compliance and success (Hall 1994). Although it has been well established that low socioeconomic status is associated with increased perinatal risk (see, for example, Osofsky & Kendall 1973, Lazarus 1990, Handwerker 1994), only 2 out of the 12 scoring systems make provision for any social factors. In addition, seven do not include either smoking or alcohol use as predictors of risk (Hall 1994).

Perkins (1994, p. 24) found that, in 1973, 'the application of one well-known [risk assessment] instrument led to the inference that 60% to 90% of the patients at every obstetric service in San Diego were high-risk'. Wall (1988) estimates that the high-risk label is assigned to between 16% and 55% of all pregnant women, with an average of about 30%. The consequences of false negative results (high-risk women being classified as low risk) may result in increased mortality or morbidity for the mother or baby. Conversely, the consequences of a false positive result (low-risk women being classified as high risk) may subject a woman to unnecessary and potentially harmful interventions (Murphy 1994). Fortney & Whitehorne (1982) estimate that the number of false positives can be as high as 96%, while Mohide and Grant (1989, p. 78) suggest that 'there is a relatively large number of false positives for each true positive and the balance of benefits and risks may actually swing to a net hazard'. According to Wall (1988, p. 155), 'seventy percent or more of adverse perinatal outcomes appear to be unpredictable by existing assessment methods'. Indeed, the system of Hobel et al (1973) predicted poor outcomes in only one-third of women thought to be high risk.

Even the presence of many risk factors is no guarantee that a bad outcome will occur. The combination of poor specificity (a test with many false positives) and the low prevalence of most adverse outcomes creates a low predictive value for positive test results. The appearance of benefit, however, reinforces the perceived value of risk screening and timely intervention and makes it difficult to question whether assessment and intervention programs are beneficial or not. (Murphy 1994)

DEVELOPING 'HOLISTIC' RISK-SCREENING SYSTEMS

By their nature, standardized measurement systems are antithetical to assessments based upon the intuition and experience of primary health care providers. (Hayes 1991)

As early as 1950, numerous studies have demonstrated that psychological and/or social factors play a role in pregnancy outcome and that interventions in these areas can decrease the incidence of problems (Katchner 1950, Kapp et al 1963, McDonald 1968, Nuckolls et al 1972, Gorsuch & Key 1974, Crandon 1979, Laukaran & van den Berg 1980, Chalmers 1982, Oakley 1992a). In 1983, Grimes et al developed a holistic, phenomenological approach to risk-screening to test for accuracy against a more traditional medical approach. As well as her medical and obstetric history, consideration was given to a woman's nutritional status, life and relationship stress, behavioural patterns, coping styles, beliefs and attitudes about childbirth, and energy levels in relation to strength. The authors concluded, 'this alternative method of risk assessment is more successful than traditional medical methodology' (p. 27).

Smilkstein et al (1984) developed and applied a 'biopsychosocial' model of risk-screening to 93 pregnant women and compared the results with those of a control group screened using only biomedical risk factors. They found that while biomedical risk factors alone were not substantially related to complications, psychosocial risk was related to both delivery and postpartum complications. Family function and biomedical risk also reliably predicted complications. The authors suggest that an interaction of biomedical and psychosocial risk screening 'will offer significant improvement in identifying women who may experience pregnancy complications' (p. 315).

In a study carried out in the USA by Marshall (1989), midwives providing care in a free-standing birth centre developed their own assessment tool for screening potentially acceptable clients and compared it with Hobel's (1978, p. 7) scoring system. They found that neither tool performed well when applied to a sample of 699 women, inferring that 'to date there is no instrument that can improve on provider judgment'.

Social support (support systems) have been related to fewer complications of labour and delivery, including shorter labour, fewer caesarean sections (Sosa et al 1980, Oakley 1992a) and lower rates of postpartum depression (Aaronson 1989). A survey in Canada of 125 family physicians (Carroll et al 1994) found that while 90% believed that identifying psychosocial risk factors in pregnancy was 'very important', the frequency of inquiry about these problems (abuse in the relationship, alcohol or drug use, etc.) was much lower. This is confirmed by two other studies estimating that 10% of women appear to be abused (Swanson 1984), while physicians identify only 1 in 10 of these (Mehta & Dandrea 1988). Support systems should be carefully evaluated during pregnancy, and appropriate referrals should be made to ensure that women have the support they need.

Although much is written about the 'midwifery model of care', midwives have not, to date, clearly defined what constitutes this model. While midwifery care is fairly uniform in the Netherlands, the model of midwifery care practised in the USA varies widely, with great dissension among practising midwives about how the model 'should' be practised. In the UK, Canada and New Zealand, midwifery is redefining itself into a new model of care intent on blending the art and science of midwifery. Midwives should aim future research at identifying the 'midwifery model of care' and its outcomes, both qualitative and quantitative, in order to offer women a better informed choice about the care they are choosing.

PERCEPTIONS OF RISK AND RISK DISCOURSE

The literature on risk acceptance and risk perception in the health domain tends not to account for the influence of the sociocapculture contexts within which risk perception takes place and the political uses to which risk discourse is put. (Lupton 1993, p. 427)

According to Douglas (1990), the word 'risk' was once a neutral term referring to the probability of an event occurring and could refer to either a positive or negative outcome. The author suggests that the word 'risk' has changed its meaning in contemporary society. Any risk is now negative: it has come to mean danger, while 'high-risk means a lot of danger' (p. 3).

While medical practitioners ascribe risk factors to the population at large via a seemingly objective, scientific realm, women experience pregnancy as part of their social world (Oakley 1992a). In the context of a woman's life, she has her own standards by which she evaluates risk, and it is often a concept with multiple meanings that is ideologically loaded (Lupton 1993, p. 425). Even though notions of risk are presented as well defined by the medical profession, differing cultural and moral beliefs result in conflicting percep-tions. Women's understanding of risk may reflect their values, education and social class, which brings multi-ple interpretations of risk that are embedded in their everyday lives (Rapp 1988). Health care providers' understanding of risk reflects their specialized knowl-edge and training as well as their personal values and experiences (Handwerker 1994). Lupton (1993) argues that research methods into risk perception ignore respondents' belief systems regarding their health. Nickerson (1990) notes that this narrow approach to the study of risk perception misses the impact of different cultural factors and belief systems upon behaviour.

Perceptions of risk among different care-givers reflect how levels of risk are defined and how women will fit into each category. Hall (1994) found that, out of 12 risk assessment guides, only three defined a category of pregnancy that is at 'no predictable risk'. Obstetricians often discredit the very existence of low risk, explaining that a 'low-risk pregnancy is not definable, except in retrospect' (Wilson & Schifrin 1980, p. 655). In contrast, midwives generally perceive pregnancy and childbirth as a normal, physiological event, one which the majority of women can complete with few or no complications or interventions. Queniart (1992) states that the medical interventions of testing, screening and technology have created a 'risk factor ideology', shifting women's perceptions and experiences of pregnancy from a natural to a risky process, and focusing society on the risks associated with pregnancy while ignoring its essentially normal nature.

According to Riessman & Nathanson (1986, p. 267):

subjective judgments in medical decision-making give the practitioner a great deal of freedom in the interpretation of physical signs as indicators of risk, especially in situations that are ambiguous.

These judgements are influenced by the metaphor of the body as a machine, stripped of its social and cul-tural context, which continues to dominate medical practice and both 'underlies and accounts for our will-ingness to apply technology to birth and to intervene in the process' (Martin 1989, p. 54).

For most pregnant women, whose medical knowl-edge is limited, it becomes virtually impossible to con-test the medical evaluations of their pregnancy and progress in labour. In addition, women's status as a minority group and the authority of the medical pro-fession make it difficult for women to assert their rights and offer their own interpretations of their health (Treichler 1990). This reinforces the unequal power relationship that women experience with the medical profession (Kuipers 1989).

Many risk-screening systems have determined which women will receive care from which provider and, in some settings, which women are candidates for home birth. According to Oakley (1992a), there are no risk-assessment systems that include an evaluation of risk by the women themselves, even though women's own perspectives on their health often conflict with medi-cine's view of women's bodies. Yet, if a woman is labelled high risk, she may be left without decision-making autonomy over who her care providers will be, where she will give birth and what interventions will take place.

Michaelson (1988) noted that, in obstetrics, risk factors are usually presented to women in negative terms, which describe the worst possible (and least likely) outcomes. Most pregnant women depend on their care providers' advice; however, their decision-making will depend on how the information is pre-sented. According to Hayes (1992, p. 404):

Language is context dependent – the meaning of words derive from the settings and circumstances in which they are used and shaped by the power relationships involved in their use.

Rapp (1988) found that physicians often slant informa-tion about risks that appeal to their patients' fears and anxieties, in order to secure compliance. If a woman's behaviour or the course of her labour does not con-form to the pattern of normalcy defined by medicine, the tendency has been to view her as deviant or deficient. If she is classified as high risk, medicine assumes that she will 'cooperate' (i.e. accept medical authority) since she has requested medical services. There are women who refuse the interventions that accompany their diagnosis of 'at risk', but their opin-ions are generally not requested or respected, and they are assumed to be misguided. It is not considered that the risk-screening system itself could be at fault. 'Thus, reasons why individual women fail to take action to reduce their risk may be, in part, because they are act-ing on a concept of risk that is qualitatively different from clinical risk as discussed in a prenatal setting (Handwerker 1994, p. 670). These differing interpreta-tions of risk affect pregnant women's ability to 'com-ply' with medical advice in the face of diagnosed risks (Nickerson 1990).

In the USA, McClain (1983) studied the risk percep-tions of pregnant women regarding childbirth and its medical management, and whether risk/benefit accounting played a role in their choice of birth setting and care provider. Women choosing home birth with a lay midwife, an alternative birth centre in hospital with a nurse-midwife, and birth in a private hospital with a private obstetrician were included in the study.

McClain found that all of the women, regardless of choice of birth place or provider:

discount the risks and magnify the benefits of the chosen birth service, and exaggerate the risks and minimize the advantages of the rejected services. (p. 1857)

She refers to the women as 'bolstering' their choices: enhancing the appeal and building up the benefits of their choice while emphasizing the risks of the other alternatives.

A study undertaken by Handwerker (1994) found that, for health practitioners, risk assessment is a highly subjective process and the weighing of certain risk factors can be more idiosyncratic than scientific. She observed the tendency of health practitioners to designate Asians, Caucasians and Hispanics as 'low risk' and black women as 'high-risk'. One Caucasian practitioner inconsistently labelled two women from different ethnic backgrounds who shared the same risk factor. While she considered a pregnant black woman with a poor diet to be high risk, she did not label as high risk a pregnant Asian woman who also had a poor diet. She attributed the Asian woman's poor diet to cultural differences. Douglas (1990) observed that, despite our sophisticated understanding underlying conceptions of disease, we still seek explanations based on behaviour, ethnicity or social stereotypes.

A study carried out by Hurst and Summey (1984) in the USA found that women from lower socio-economic classes tended to score as higher risk on various risk indices than did middle-class women. However, it was middle-class women who received more of the procedures developed for 'high-risk' pregnancies, such as caesarean sections. In their research on nulliparous pregnancy in women over the age of 35, it is interesting to note that both Neuhoff et al (1989) and Roberts et al (1994) found that the rate of caesarean section was higher among private patients than among clinic patients. Gordon et al (1991) noted an increase in the rate of caesarean section for primiparous women over 35 as income increased from less than $20 000 to more than $30 000. This supports Hurst and Summey's (1984) suggestion that risk assessment and the use of medical technology appear to hinge on social factors as well as 'scientific' assessment.

The news media plays an integral role in the public perception of health risk. Media coverage can set the agenda for risk discourse in the public arena (Lupton 1993). Russell (1993) discusses how, during the 1970s, consumer groups pushing for natural childbirth received widespread media coverage. However, by placing the topic of childbirth within the public domain, an ever-growing list of pregnancy 'don'ts' has also appeared (p. 192). If women are relying upon the media for information and advice regarding their pregnancies, they can be left feeling panicked and confused (Lebow & Arkin 1993). The media is interested in attracting a large audience and tends to overdramatize or oversimplify information regarding risks. Peterson & Sims (1993) assert that members of the media need to understand basic epidemiological methods and terms, while researchers need to communicate their findings more clearly.

More research is needed into how risk is communicated to women by physicians, midwives, government and the media. Whose judgement is to be considered in evaluating the acceptability of the risk? What level of certainty about the risk is required before it is communicated? What are the rules of evidence that should guide standards of practice and policy decisions? In order for women to accept responsibility for the decisions they make, they must be made fully aware of the limitations of the information/data and the risks versus benefits on which they are basing their decisions.

RISK IDENTIFICATION AND SOCIAL CONTROL

This new medical intrusion in the lives of women may be diffuse, but it is certainly insidious, legitimating its interventions and its discourse not only in the name of science, as it has up to now, but in the name of the fetus itself. (Queniart 1992, p. 163)

What women *wanted* was viewed in the 1920s and 30s as an important force shaping maternity care. After the 1950s, women's wishes came to be seen as a 'luxury' and incompatible with the medical determination of risk (Oakley 1984). Obstetricians began to dominate higher levels of policy-making, control the introduction of new procedures and define who was at risk. Riessman & Nathanson (1986) argue that the development of the concept of risk was essential to the maintenance of birth as a medical problem and that obstetrics extended its boundary over clearly pathological birth by expanding the concept of risk to include births that were *potentially* pathological (Ehrenreich & English 1973). In 1985, the 17th edition of *Williams' Obstetrics* added to 'high risk' and 'low risk' the new category of 'growing risk', broadening the definition of what constitutes risk (Queniart 1992). Arney (1982, p. 26) states that 'the concepts of "normal" and "abnormal" took on a new relationship to one another. No longer was there a clear demarcation between the two; a gray area had been created that was capable of taking on added dimensionality.'

In *Discipline and Punish*, Focault (1979) describes a

panopticon, a structure of power that has the capacity for constant and total surveillance, which effects a new form of control based on behaviour that is self-regulated through the fear of observation. Arney (1982) relates the panopticon to obstetrics, in which women are subjected to constant and total visibility, and in which technologies and monitoring allow obstetrics to extend into every aspect of women's pregnancies. Power and control are magnified by making risk factors more 'known' through multiple monitoring schemes; 'risk-scores thus became a vehicle for expanding the scope of surveillance to all aspects of a woman's life' (p. 143).

Douglas & Wildavsky (1982) contend that the selection of risk is a social process: the risks selected may be of little or no danger, but they are culturally identified as important. For women, childbirth has never been safer, and Arney (1982, p. 137) believes that obstetricians have now become fetal advocates, drastically altering the orientation of obstetrics. The fetus is becoming increasingly more autonomous and is gradually being perceived as the primary patient (Maier, 1992). Duden (1993) discusses how 'seeing' the fetus with ultrasound and the publication of Nilsson's (1965) photographs of the fetus in utero have changed the public's perception of pregnancy and allowed physicians, friends, family members, judges and strangers the freedom to judge and condemn women for their 'risky' behaviour. Society has now shifted its gaze to the fetus, and the resulting social control over pregnant women is legitimated in the name of fetal protection (Rodgers 1989). As prenatal testing and other medical interventions become more routinized and therefore accepted as a 'normal' part of care, expectations about women's behaviour will expand. It becomes very difficult for women to refuse testing and interventions when they are presented as being 'for the good of the baby' (Gregg 1993).

In recent years, physicians have asserted their control over the definition of risk by using the judicial system to apprehend the baby in utero if the mother is not complying with medical advice. A woman's right to refuse medical treatment and surgery has been overruled by the courts in North America (Rodgers 1989). However, Nelkin (1989) argues that these definitions of risk tend to apportion blame upon stigmatized minorities. This is supported by the findings of Kolder et al (1987), who reported an alarming increase in attempts to prosecute what essentially constitute poor pregnant women, primarily from ethnic minorities, for failing to follow medical advice. It is noteworthy that Maier (1992) found, in cases of court-ordered caesarean sections sought to protect the baby from the mother's non-compliance, that women who *did not* undergo surgery delivered safely with no adverse outcome.

Medicine and society are now defining what constitutes *risky behaviour* (Gregg 1993). When risk is believed to be internally imposed because of a lack of self-control or willpower, blame is placed on the 'lifestyle choices' made by the individual. Yet there has never been a clear demarcation between socially produced risks (poverty, illiteracy, abuse issues, drug addiction and lack of housing) and biologically produced risks (genetic traits, age and blood type). When socially produced risks are identified, pregnancy surveillance is increased and women are cautioned to avoid harming the baby. Interventions in the root causes of the risk are rarely carried out; they include more money, educational programmes, better and safe housing, addiction treatment and counselling (Oakley 1992a). A new trend that views pregnant women and their unborn babies in an antagonistic relationship raises serious questions about 'pregnant women's right to privacy and autonomy … through direct pressures and explicit social sanctions regarding their choices' (Gregg 1993, p. 67). This alarming violation of women's reproductive freedom and the assessment of the fetus as having a risk distinct from the mother's health have enormous implications for the future of risk assessment in obstetrics.

COMMUNICATING RISK

What are the ethics of assessing all women to identify hypothetical risk factors (that may or may not predict disease with accuracy) in order to prescribe interventions (which may be of dubious value and possible harm) in the hopes of preventing an outcome (that will never happen to most of those subjected to this process)? (Murphy 1994, p. 68)

In order to facilitate informed decision-making, women require their midwives to provide information that is objective, evidence based and unswayed by emotion and ideologies. They must also be fully informed of the risks *as we know them to be* without slanting or biasing the information.

Women learn to make decisions long before they come to the midwife's office. These decisions take place in contexts – contexts of feeling and of prior experience and learning. They learn to make decisions that 'feel right' to them (Bursztajn et al 1990). Women do not define risk solely as the number of deaths or injuries but as how well they can control their exposure and whether they have assumed the risk voluntarily (Radford 1997). There is virtually no human activity that can be completely free from risk, and it is up to the individual to decide what constitutes an acceptable risk. Despite the anxiety that risk-taking can induce, successful risk-taking can induce a feeling of euphoria, with a sense of power to reinvent every-day life.

For medicine, risk is a statistical artefact, while for the woman, risk is a subjective experience. All risk cal-culations involve the juggling of personal understand-ing about not just the danger, but also experience (Gabe 1995). Risk can take on a different content and meaning depending on whether the language being used to describe it is epidemiological, clinical or lay. While the epidemiologist quotes the number of deaths per 1000 that occur with a given complication, the clin-ical risk is expressed in comments such as 'I have seen 10 babies die...'.

Women who know someone who has had a stillbirth are much more aware of that hazard than those who do not. For professionals, those who have dealt with a serious complication are subsequently more likely to see the risk of that complication as being higher than it actually is. Kaufert & O'Neil (1993) found, when talk-ing with health professionals, that their fear of child-birth was related to concerns about competence and being able to cope in an emergency. The burden of responsibility is enormous, and the experience of the last case can inordinately affect judgement. In labour, care decisions can be influenced by fear of litigation, the common response often being overinvestigation or overtreatment, subjecting labouring women to treat-ment regimens based on hospital policies rather than an individualized care plan.

Even in situations where the diagnosis is certain, the appropriate treatment may be far from certain (Harvey 1996). However, when women express a desire to deviate from the recommended standard of care (such as home birth), risk discourse often moves into the emotional realm, the clinician conjuring up images of past obstetric disasters. In the case of home birth, how far does the hysteria surrounding it reflect a balanced view of the risk inherent in all areas of modern life?

The individualization of risk has legitimated the routine use of invasive techniques such as the aug-mentation of uterine activity and drug administration in pregnancy and childbirth, all potentially hazardous. When labour is not progressing 'normally', an assumption is made that women are at risk because of the pending failure of their bodies. A large number of interventions are begun for 'failure to progress in labour,' which incorporates the lack of progressive dilatation of the cervix and maternal exhaustion. Lane (1995, p. 63) argues that this term merely describes an existing state:

They are not reasons, but states of being. These states of being may seem legitimate reasons for medical intervention, but they do not provide a causal explanation.

Contextual factors, including positive and negative social exchanges and emotional responses to physical surroundings, are rarely examined or considered in the causal framework. However, these contextual fac-tors may be the primary determinants of risk precipi-tating medical intervention.

Lupton (1993) observed that the discourse of risk is weighted toward disaster and anxiety rather than peace of mind. Oakley (1993) writes about the connec-tion between peace of mind and a competent cervix, and emotional confidence and a coordinated uterus. Every aspect of human experience influences health in some way, and when a midwife promotes a woman's self-confidence, intuition, trust in her body and ability to give birth, these may well be the primary deter-minants for avoiding medical intervention.

REDUCING RISK IN MIDWIFERY PRACTICE

In recent years major changes in the nature of the risks associated with pregnancy have occurred, however, and in the way those risks are perceived. Is it time to change the very concept of risk? (Enkin 1994)

According to McDonnell (1997) midwives should employ a 'risk management' approach to improve care and reduce liability. In the group practice where I am a partner, there are five midwives working in partner-ships of two, providing care and sharing call on a 50/50 basis (1 week on, 1 week off). The fifth midwife 'floats' through the practice, providing locum care for 10 months of the year while each midwife takes 2.5 months' vacation per year. Women alternate ante-natal visits between the two midwives sharing her care. The group meets weekly for clinical rounds, where we discuss antenatal problems and birth outcomes, with a focus on how our care could be improved. With the two other midwifery practices in our community, we meet monthly and are developing guidelines to practice and protocols that reflect our philosophy and model of care. We strive to improve our care and reduce risk by:

- having the 'locum' for vacations as an ongoing part of our practice, someone we all know and trust;
- providing continuity of care with no more than two midwives caring for one woman; this has the added benefit of preventing burn-out;
- having a weekly chart review and frank discussion of outcomes;

- having regular drills in emergency skills, for example resuscitation and shoulder dystocia;
- developing protocols that reflect our philosophy of care, that are grounded in evidence-based practice and that include information on complementary therapies, these protocols being made available to our clients;
- following protocols developed by our professional college clearly delineating our responsibility to consult and transfer care;
- embracing an informed choice approach to care, in which the woman has control over her body and her birth, and is the ultimate authority in decision-making;
- carefully documenting any discussions of procedures and interventions, with verbal or written confirmation from the woman when she decides to decline or accept treatment; documentation on the client's chart should indicate the topics discussed; each point discussed may be initialled and dated following discussion;
- providing a prompt and truthful explanation to our clients when things go wrong, with a commitment to provide them with ongoing information and support.

FACILITATING INFORMED DECISION-MAKING

Informed consent conceptually promotes the transfer of knowledge and power to the recipient of services, further equalizing the relationship between midwife and pregnant woman. (Spindel & Suarez 1995)

According to Mann and Albers (1997), there are two basic moral principles underlining the theory of informed consent:

1. *Beneficence*: promoting the well-being of the client and doing no harm.
2. *Respect for autonomy*: honouring individual views, choices and values, resulting in patient self-determination.

The ethical and legal imperatives of informed consent require a full discussion of all procedures and interventions, the benefits and risks of each, and the expected results with or without the proposed treatment. In general, it is agreed that any person has the right to refuse medical treatment and that treatment cannot be carried out without informed consent.

Hayes (1992) proposes that the 'notion of risk as wager' – assessing both losses and gains – would seem a more appropriate conception of risk in relation to 'risk-taking'. A discussion of the positive and negative aspects of interventions provides women with the opportunity to play an active role in evaluating risk and its significance to them, thereby grappling exclusive power to determine risk away from the 'expert'. It is the midwife's responsibility to provide women with a basis for making an informed decision while at the same time stressing the importance of personal responsibility and the free agency of the individual. Four aspects are important here.

First, discussion in pregnancy should take place on all topics requiring decision-making, for example maternal serum screening, ultrasound examination, amniocentesis, induction for post-dates and external cephalic version. In our practice, we have files for clients to sign out that include papers providing a simple explanation of the problem or procedure as well as papers on the latest research on the topic. The client takes the package home to read in between visits. If a woman's baby is presenting in a breech position, she takes home the file on 'Turning a breech baby', which includes information on homeopathic remedies, massage, the slant board, acupuncture and playing music. If the baby remains breech and the woman is nearing term, she is given the file 'External cephalic version', which outlines the procedure and includes its pros and cons.

Second, at the following prenatal visit, the client asks questions regarding the information in the file. When presenting evidence to the woman, account must be taken of medical uncertainty. The woman also needs to be know whether her decision deviates from the community 'standard of care' (care provided by the majority of obstetrical care-givers) so that she can prepare to stand behind her choices. In our practice, we recently had a client who was screened out from a home birth in her first pregnancy for pregnancy-induced hypertension. The subsequent intervention in hospital (antihypertensive drugs, fetal monitoring, etc.) was very traumatic for both her and her partner and, she felt intuitively, ultimately unnecessary. In this pregnancy, the woman again developed pregnancy-induced hypertension and claimed control over how it would be managed. She extensively researched the condition and planned a home water birth in which *she* would decide whether her blood pressure required hospitalization based on the length of labour and the information provided to her. She had a 6-hour labour using relaxation and visualization to control her blood pressure and had an empowering, healing home birth. In the event of a transfer to hospital, she had prepared a birth plan, which communicated that she was well informed of the risks surrounding her choices and accepted responsibility for taking them.

Third, the woman's own perception of risk should be explored by the midwife and taken into consideration when assisting her in decision-making. For example, a woman planning a home birth in our practice had a close friend whose baby had died from meconium aspiration syndrome following a home birth. After reviewing all the information available on meconium aspiration syndrome, the woman and her partner decided that, if any meconium were present, they would prefer to transfer to hospital to complete the birth.

Fourth, decision-making during labour is problematic because of the presence of contractions and pain. Information overload can occur, which has been shown to decrease the quality of choice and increase the variability of the response (Mann & Albers 1997). The recollection of information regarding procedures and interventions is greater when prenatal discussion has taken place. For many procedures, consent or refusal can be obtained prior to labour, which is always, of course, subject to change. For example, a woman may specify that she does not want to be offered pain medication or that she would prefer an epidural in the event of a caesarean section.

According to Giddens (1990), we are living in a period in which the judgements of experts are constantly open to scrutiny or 'chronically contested', and are either accepted or rejected by lay people on the basis of pragmatic calculations about the risks involved. Lane (1995, p. 53) refers to this as 'the now voluble level of reaction against the cult of the expert in diverse professional spheres'. Douglas (1990) believes that when the larger question of risk is evaluated, the debate moves away from the specific question 'How much risk is acceptable to you?' to the more general question 'What kind of society do you want?' The question concerns who has the power to define risk and to insist that their view should prevail over those of others.

WOMEN'S AND MIDWIVES' PERCEPTIONS OF RISK

This study explores the perceptions that midwives and women in their care have about childbearing risks and the labelling of women as high risk. The study was carried out in Vancouver, British Columbia, Canada in 1994. At this time in British Columbia, there were no provisions in the health care system for the practice of midwifery. However, midwives had been practising outside the regulated system for two decades, largely carrying out home births, with a few midwives providing care in hospital under a physician's supervision. On 1 January 1998, midwives became registered

in British Columbia and now provide care within the system in both the home and hospital. Midwives became the first non-physicians with independent hospital-admitting privileges and are fully funded within the health care system.

The limitations of the study were recognized at the outset. The volume of data generated from the interviews limited the study participants to a total of 20. The findings are limited in that all of the respondents were white, well educated, middle class and shared an alternative philosophy of care that is not necessarily shared by most women. Because of the illegal status of midwifery in British Columbia at the time of these interviews, fewer than 1% of women sought out midwifery care (Burtch 1994). Therefore, the women in this study represent an exceptional minority. In addition, the midwives were all known to be *radicals* by care providers within the health care system, and their views are also of the minority.

A semi-structured interview with open-ended questions was chosen as the most appropriate for this exploratory research and for hearing the respondents' opinions in their own words (Palys 1989). One criticism of the interview process is that data are being collected retrospectively, relying on memory for detail that may not be accurate or reliable (Kirby & McKenna 1989). However, the information sought in this study was about individual perceptions and therefore required a process of reflection rather than recollection of specific events.

Two groups of participants were interviewed. The first group comprised 10 currently practising midwives; the second group numbered 10 nulliparous women over 35, who were clients of the midwives in the study. Lather (1986) discusses the importance of validating findings by recycling them back through the respondents. The transcribed interviews were mailed out to all the participants for feedback, correction and clarification, as well as providing an opportunity to add additional comments. This proved to be worthwhile. The comments and additions added much to the original transcripts, and the respondents appreciated being able further to articulate some of their ideas.

Although this study does shed some light on the research question, these findings cannot be generalized to other populations of women or midwives, and more representative studies are warranted. According to Oakley (1992b, p. 8), 'the best research is that which breeds more'. The expansion of this research into a larger, more representative sample of women is necessary to explore concepts of risk and their influence on outcomes. However, this study reinforces the need to value and listen to women's experiences. At the same time, social, emotional and other factors that place women at risk need to be studied more systematically, involving not only expert knowledge, but also the lived experiences of the women concerned.

The women

Ten nulliparous women, all 35 years or older at the time of giving birth, were chosen by interval sampling from a list of 29. All of the women had received primary care from a midwife during the pregnancy, labour and postpartum period. They had all given birth 38 months prior to the date of the interview; five women planned to give birth at home and five planned to give birth in the hospital.

During the interview, women were asked how they felt about risk assignment and risk-labelling. For example, if they had experienced being labelled as high risk, how did that make them feel? Women were asked what the term 'high risk' meant to them, most remarking that they felt this was a difficult question to answer. They expressed that it was the most thought-provoking question in the interview, and it generated the most discussion. More than half of the women perceived the term to mean that complications could develop or that the baby might not be healthy. Half of the women mentioned knowing on an intuitive level that neither they nor their babies were at risk. One woman described it as a 'gut feeling' that everything was all right, while another explained, 'In my heart of hearts, I really didn't think that I was at risk.'

Two women perceived it to mean 'that somebody's in danger and that it's life that's at risk'. For them, the term 'high risk' took on a much more serious meaning than one simply indicating that complications could develop. As one woman explains: '[High risk means] that the baby's going to die! Actually, I though, oh my God! High-risk! I'm going to lose the baby tonight. Yeah, it scared the hell out of me.'

One woman, a nurse, thought that the term was an invitation for more medical intervention:

To me, it is a negative term. That's the first thing, as soon as I hear high-risk – it's negative. And it means you need to be alerted to more intervention. Needing more medical support, more medical intervening. It just kind of puts a label on someone. By saying the word 'risk' we're making a lot of definitions that make people act, and make the medical system put on one thousand million tests.

One woman expressed her anger at being labelled as high risk and believed it to be a negative bias toward women and ageing:

They're huge, I mean those two little tiny four-letter words but they're HUGE in your mind when you are first pregnant Yeah. I wasn't high-risk. High-risk in whose definition of risk? And certainly not because of my age. That appears to me to be a blatant prejudice, from looking at the other side.

Another woman described the loss of control and sense of powerlessness that she felt when she was labelled high-risk antenatally:

I think it kind of leads people to believe that they need more help and they can't help themselves as much. It takes some of the control out of decision making because you've already been labeled something … and you have to leave it up to your so-called experts to decide. And if they want to they'll let you help in the decision making, but because they are the experts, they'll have the final word. That's what that term does to women who are labeled high risk. It takes their power and control away.

Most of the woman characterized the 'risk' as belonging to the baby. Generally, they did not view themselves as being at risk: 'In terms of risk to me, it would be so very very rare that it would be fatal … so that became very minor to me. I think that the focus became the risk to the child.'

However, one woman described how she herself felt at risk when, after a long labour, she had an epidural:

Once I'd gotten the epidural, my expectations of what I was perceiving as the nice normal vaginal birth, those dreams were … starting to fade and I had to recalculate the whole situation. I remember often thinking about the baby's welfare in the pregnancy. But not so much in labour, I kind of pushed that aside. It was kind of my own sense of survival I felt.

All of the women in the study had the experience of being labelled as high risk either during their pregnancies or in labour. Most women felt angry or resentful that a label was being placed on them that could drastically alter their care. Several women described their frustration when dealing with their physicians' opinions or approach to their choices:

My family doctor that I had originally, when I discussed home birth with her absolutely forbade it! She said it was just a horrible idea and pointed out to me – especially at my age! She had no business sharing her opinion in the manner she did; she is certainly entitled to her opinion and can voice that to me in an atmosphere of concern. But to say to me I would not support you, in essence, I forbid you to do that. She didn't scare me at all by telling me … that my age would make it risky. I've never gone back to her since.'

Three women developed risk factors during the pregnancy and/or birth. One woman, whose blood pressure went up in pregnancy, describes her feelings of being treated as high risk:

I remember feeling threatened that I was being almost told that I was a bad girl for working too hard and that was one of the reasons my blood pressure was up. No one was taking into consideration my personality and what is good for me. I remember feeling actually quite angry about it ... being told what to do. So I withdrew and I didn't do the things they told me to do; like a child I'm gonna show them! I almost felt like our options were disappearing. They were controlling my options.

Another woman was diagnosed near term as having a small-for-dates baby. Shortly after being induced, the baby experienced fetal distress and the client underwent an emergency caesarean section. The baby was fine at birth but was diagnosed with a congenital heart defect shortly afterward. The mother gives this account:

When I went in for the ultrasound and they told me how they estimated a 4 pound 13 ounce baby ... it was nerve wracking because I instinctually knew something was wrong ... the baby had to come out. My partner, who was resistant to that, 'these god-damned physicians – just when *they* wanna do it!' Then once it all came down and he [the baby] was diagnosed, it was a really wonderful thing because we all ended up being grateful that it was caught and that they were as professional as they were. They looked after him.

All of the women in the study believed that they were low risk and planned to have a natural, spontaneous birth (half of the women had spontaneous vaginal births, two had caesarean sections, and three had instrumental deliveries). The women were asked whether their perception of risk had changed since the birth of their child. All of the women indicated that their perception of risk *did not* change, half seeing themselves as being even lower risk than they were for the first birth: 'I would be lower risk in that my body knows what to do.' All of the women who had undergone caesarean sections or instrumental deliveries *did not* perceive that their low-risk status changed. One woman who agreed to a caesarean section for fetal distress (although the baby was not in distress when born) said:

I still feel that, even though I had a cesarean section I didn't feel that I had enough information to properly assess whether my babe was at risk ... and I acquiesced to a c-section. As far as my own risk, I was right in feeling that I wasn't high risk, because I have a healthy, bright active child. And I'm fine. So, no, I don't think my ideas of what risk meant have changed, they were validated in a way.

Even if they had experienced serious complications during the pregnancy and/or birth, women remained adamant that their risk status did not change to high-risk because of it. One woman, who had experienced a difficult forceps delivery and whose baby had serious medical problems postpartum, said the following:

They seem far fewer! I mean, even in the discussion when you talk about high-risk I'm thinking, what was all the fuss about? What was the risk? What are they? And I'd have to go back and think. There really weren't that many of them.

Another woman whose baby died in utero at term and proceeded to give birth at home was planning her next birth at home with a midwife. She described what she perceived to be the risks she faced:

I'm really solid in the fact that there's other factors that enter in besides your age. I'm confident and I'm ready and I still have that little bit of fear nagging at me, what if. I mean life is like that, it could happen again ... life is a chance. That's a risk, right? Just getting pregnant is a risk! [laughter] Talking about risk!! When you've had your heart broken you almost want to protect it. I guess it must be okay because I'm doing it [trying to get pregnant].

The women were asked whether they consciously avoided risk-labelling and what, if anything, they did to keep risk factors from developing during the pregnancy and birth. Why they had chosen alternative care for their pregnancy and birth, especially given that midwifery was not part of the health care system in British Columbia at this time. Was it to avoid being labelled as high risk?

Almost all the women in the study chose midwifery care because they viewed having a midwife as an opportunity to have more holistic care. As one woman said, 'It wasn't just looking after my state of health or looking after the medical problems that were happening, it was looking after me!' Another woman described how she had hired a midwife in order to have a home birth: 'I did not realize all the other benefits came with midwifery.' Women emphasized that it was the type of care a midwife had to offer that they were seeking. They had already rejected the label of high risk and anticipated that the midwife would agree with them. Several women believed that midwives 'give the woman power': 'It had to do with empowering me as a woman and as a person, and so the decision to have midwifery care had nothing to do actually with my age.' Another woman, an actress, explains:

I wanted a midwife. She was magnificent! She was sort of like the director of my play, in that she told me what to expect and what was coming so it didn't scare me. She reminded me to relax between each contraction, that a whole different thing was going to happen. I could ask her questions. She knows who I am. She knows all my secrets.

Two women indicated that they had hired a midwife to protect them from interference from the medical profession:

The midwives were between me and the medical profession. I [felt] that the birth would stay in my hands. That I would retain my rights as the mother, as the person who was doing it! I've always thought that anybody that did midwifery as a profession was a very special person and I wanted that to be part of my life.

Although all the women believed that a midwife

would not emphasize risks unnecessarily, only one woman said she went to a midwife to avoid being labelled high risk because of her age:

I had already decided before I was even pregnant that I would have a midwife. She was a very good mediator between what the medical system wished to do and what I wished to do. So yes, in a sense, because of my age I did choose a midwife, in order to lessen the interventions if possible.

In order to stay healthy during the pregnancy and prevent risk factors developing, all the women in the study agreed that a healthy mind and attitude were as important as a healthy body. Most women mentioned the same regime: eating well, exercising, no drugs, smoking or alcohol, and in general leading what one woman described as 'a balanced lifestyle'. Asked whether they believed that attitudes, anxiety and emotional health could have an impact on pregnancy and birth, women answered adamantly that they believed it *did* influence outcome. One woman replied, 'I think your attitude is going to direct your care.' Another woman went as far as to say, 'If you perceive you're going to have a risk you will have a risk. And if you don't you never will.' Almost all of the women believed that a positive attitude and emotional well-being were integral to achieving a healthy, uncomplicated pregnancy. Even in the face of complications, women tried to think positively, talk to the baby and stay as relaxed as possible. One woman described the role she felt anxiety could play thus:

Hospitals frighten me, hospitals make me anxious. So if my anxiety can contribute to longer labour, stronger contractions, more difficulty in birth, ... if anxiety can contribute to that, and I'm anxious being in a hospital, then I'm setting myself up.

The majority of women agreed that a mind–body connection was an integral part of avoiding risk factors. However, one woman was sceptical about whether this was indeed true:

I think the feminist in me wants to believe that but I also know that women have babies in the middle of wars. Healthy, beautiful babies in the middle of the most horrendous circumstances. So a part of me believes that pregnancy is a thing unto itself, that it is about a third force, its not about the woman and her particular circumstances. My child was other than who I was. And she was going to come out one way or another. It was another force, it was another soul speaking.

Most women tried to avoid conflict and stress. One woman explained: 'I like to be peaceful. I like to not put myself in stressful situations that I think could upset the baby.' Another woman described trusting in herself: 'I kept telling myself to listen to my body, to

trust it and know that it was strong. The mind and body together, that things were going well and just to keep that in mind.'

The midwives

A list of 16 midwives currently practising in the lower mainland of British Columbia was generated, and the first 10 midwives on this list who agreed to be interviewed were selected. Five midwives primarily practised in hospital, and five primarily attended home births. All were licensed to practise midwifery in another jurisdiction and were current members of the Midwives Association of British Columbia.

The interview explored midwives' perceptions of 'risk' and how it effects the care they provide to women. Midwives were asked what the term 'high risk' meant to them, as well as what rights a woman has over the choices available regarding her care and place of birth. Should she be able to continue making her own choices if the midwife believes that her pregnancy has become high risk? What is the midwife's obligation to the woman who refuses to follow her advice on risk prevention, treatment or screening? Many of the midwives found these questions very hard to answer. With regard to the meaning of the term 'high risk', one midwife replied, 'That's a loaded question. I don't really know.' Many of the midwives mentioned that they did not like the term 'high risk'. The majority of the midwives felt that high risk implied that the woman had a medical disorder:

First of all, I hate the term. So I'd like to scrap the term. But if you wanted to define high-risk I'd look at somebody who had some medical condition that would actually place the pregnancy in a risky situation. Like someone with heart disease, cancer, cystic fibrosis, those kinds of things I consider at high-risk.

One midwife felt that labelling women as high risk was a way of establishing medicine's authority over birth:

I think the whole classification of risk has been a way to establish and entrench the medical establishments hold on birth and I think they truly believe in it – which is the sad part – and even sadder is that women then believe them.

Most of the midwives mentioned that they felt the term was grossly overused – 'I think that a lot of things we label high-risk are not' – while another mentioned '*and then* she's been classified high-risk and it ain't necessarily so'. Several midwives characterized the term 'high risk' as having 'a very large gray area'.

One midwife suggested that there should be three categories of 'high risk' for example low, medium and high, in order to identify the severity of the problem.

One midwife considered a woman as high risk when there 'is somebody I can't handle and I need to refer her out of midwifery care'. Another felt that the label of high risk could not be applied to a woman unless she agreed to it:

High-risk is a relative term, because I may see one part of risk meaning something to me, but more important is what the client sees as risks. Things can change in terms of their health or fetal health which then force people to make decisions as to what they're going to do with the information. If you follow this path there may be risk. If you don't follow this path there may not. But whose decision is it? It's not me as the caregiver; it's them as the family.

If risk factors did develop during the pregnancy, all of the midwives felt that women should have the right to accept or refuse treatment and still 'have every right to choose her place of birth'. One midwife remarked, 'I might disagree with her strongly, but what can you do? You can't put a gun to people's heads!' Another midwife said:

The decision lies with the mother and her family. It's not my decision whether someone has a hospital birth or a home birth. I can only say, ... in your case it might be better if, then I'd have to tell them that the 'better if' is my idea, not necessarily their idea of 'better if'. I have no right to make that decision for them.

However, several of the midwives expressed that this right to choose was a very difficult issue in clinical practice. All but three of the respondents felt that the midwife should have the right to refuse care if she 'did not feel competent or confident to deal with the problem' presenting. One midwife said, 'I'd have to ask her to find another caregiver, because I feel it's very irresponsible to take on something that you don't think you have the skills to do.' Another said, 'She might have the right to choose, but I wouldn't do a breech birth at home no matter what age she was!' The following quote explains one midwife's dilemma:

I think that there need to be guidelines around place of birth, based on what good research shows us is the safest environment for a mother in certain situations. I would like to feel that I would have the right to say no in an environment that I really didn't feel comfortable in. But given that ... feel there should also be choice of place of birth for women.

The remaining midwives felt very strongly that midwives should not be able to refuse a woman care in any circumstances. 'We have an ethical responsibility to attend her. Who are we to question this woman's decision?' One of these midwives also believed that 'any woman making an informed choice chooses responsibly for herself and her baby'. Another felt it was imperative that the midwife always supported the woman's choice because of the threat that 'fetal rights' has placed on her personal autonomy:

I feel personally very strongly, as a woman, that it's her body. What I see more and more that really disturbs me is that a lot of decisions have been made based on the fetus ... 'fetal rights'. What's right for the mum is right the babe, and when a woman's making that decision, I have to support her in that decision.

One midwife expressed concern about how we would balance the woman's right to choose against the midwife's right to refuse care if she did not feel competent to provide it: 'It's a bit of a quandary for me actually, how that will be reconciled when we're legal.'

Another objective was to investigate whether midwives believed that labelling a woman as high risk could actually effect the outcome of her pregnancy and birth. Did they believe that it was important to avoid labelling the woman as high risk? What did they do, if anything to promote normalcy and help women to prevent risk factors developing?

When midwives were asked whether they believed that labelling a woman as high risk could affect the outcome of the pregnancy and/or birth, they unanimously answered 'yes' in the most emphatic terms used during the whole interview process: 'Definitely', 'Absolutely, absolutely', 'I think so very firmly.' One midwife exclaimed, 'I've always said that when doctors go looking hard enough for complications, that women will often end up producing some for them.' She added:

I think that's true about risk labelling in general. I think it sets up a situation in which women begin to doubt their abilities to be healthy, to grow a healthy baby, to have a normal, healthy birth.

Another midwife felt that the emphasis on complications in pregnancy eroded a woman's self-confidence:

I think that when women have a picture of illness given to them at the start of a pregnancy, ... then it can effect the way their pregnancy progresses because they see themselves in an illness model. It takes away from their own sense of health and empowerment so that they themselves may begin to manifest a picture of illness. They lose their own confidence.

Several midwives felt that a woman's perception of risk could affect the outcome of the birth. One midwife offered an example:

If you're very nervous about a situation, that can definitely effect your blood pressure. That's been proven. When women go into doctor's offices and they are tense, they have higher blood pressures.

One midwife, whose practice was based in the hospital, included nurses as other care-givers who could affect the outcome of the birth:

The power of the mind and the power of suggestion are very strong. I feel strongly that the nurse's view and her subsequent care will greatly effect the way a woman's labour goes.

When asked what they did during the pregnancy to promote normalcy and avoid risk-labelling, almost all of the midwives agreed that education and information-sharing were the most important tools. One midwife advised: 'Giving them knowledge and the tools to pass through the pregnancy and birth as easily as possible.' Another believed it was important to be 'involving [the woman] in all her care. Giving her all the information that she would need.' Many midwives talked about the need to re-educate women about birth and 'continually emphasize the normalcy of pregnancy':

I think people get so much psychological pollution around how scary birth is and how something's definitely going to go wrong. In this culture, it's the role of the midwife to re-frame that for them. Women get filled with so much fear and negativity around birth. To really support women about their own intuitive powers; encourage them when they have a good, instinctual positive thought. So that they feel some of their own power. That I don't want to be their expert either.

All of the midwives believed it was very important to avoid risk-labelling a woman and to be careful with language and terminology. One midwife explains how important this can be to the birth experience:

I think you have to be very, very careful what words you choose when you're talking to anyone and simply calling someone high-risk. Even if you have a good outcome in terms of healthy baby and a healthy mum, you usually don't have a healthy birth experience. I spend most of my practice trying to get people out of fear, more than anything else.

DEVELOPING A RISK PREVENTION AND ASSESSMENT MODEL FOR MIDWIFERY PRACTICE

Is a unified theory so compelling that it brings about its own existence or does it need a creator? (Hawking 1989)

Strategies for the future include a vision of care for all childbearing women in which care is continuous, personalized and non-authoritarian, responding to a woman's physical, social, emotional and cultural needs (Page 1993). Care is thus built on a model of cooperation between women and their health care providers, women being encouraged to participate and make choices regarding their care (Guililland 1990, Donley 1993). In essence, what is needed is to reconstruct the biomedical model of care, to redefine what knowing about health really is.

Benston (1986) proposes a 'science *for* the people', in which professionals develop socially responsible applications of their expertise and make this expertise available where it is most needed. Obstetric care providers need to address their marked disagreement on what constitutes effective care, what the objectives of care are and what are the best means of achieving effective care. According to Enkin et al (1989, p. 15), 'there is no place for rivalry or competition, optimal care can only occur when both caregivers recognize their complementary roles'. Careful consideration must be given to the reliability and validity of research evidence in order to establish a rational basis for selecting the studies most likely to cause no harm and enhance the care we provide. This would allow for a model of care based on the evidence of effective care rather than on ideologies or individual opinions. Also, pervasive class, race and gender inequities must be addressed to ensure that care is available, accessible and affordable to all women who require it (Lazarus 1990, Handwerker 1994).

Benston (1986) proposes a second model, 'science *with* the people', in which professionals and the lay public combine their expertise to create a synthesis of knowledge. This cooperation would assist in the reduction of the hierarchical imbalance between expert and lay knowledge. This strategy could bring together medicine, midwifery and the lay public, which would create a more democratic process for determining what constitutes effective care as well as how health care resources are allocated.

Benston's (1986) third approach, 'science *by* the people', provides lay people with the resources to learn more about the areas of technical expertise that affect their everyday lives. Morgan (1993) believes that when women are given balanced information and time to reflect on it, they can do a remarkably good job of deciding what problems are important and of systematically addressing decisions concerning risks. Benston's theory argues that only by removing the connection between expert knowledge and power would we open up a dialogue with women and minorities. Obstetrics has been dominated by the medical model of knowledge, and physicians are believed to be the main experts on women's health (Queniart, 1992). This change would require discarding the social role of 'expert' and acknowledging women's expertise about their bodies and health care needs. Alexander & Keirse (1989, p. 382) suggest that 'research to investigate women's feelings about risk assignments and the way in which it does or does not change their perception of pregnancy and childbirth may be of benefit to both the receivers and providers of care'. Women have not been included in defining health, and Benston's model would allow them to reclaim the ability to define the meaning and experience of childbirth. A model of care could be developed that is more responsive to women's social, emotional and economic needs, one that requires less intervention and technology in childbirth and redirects health care dollars to provide an integrated range of support services for pregnant women and their families.

Midwifery, in many countries including Canada, has come to represent a counter-movement that seeks to reclaim childbirth for women (Burtch 1994). This model of midwifery care reconceptualizes 'risk' by rejecting risk-markers as categorical and applying a more holistic approach to risk-screening that is continuous and assesses the whole person (Gaskin 1978, Davis 1987). To these midwives, the pregnant body is not simply a machine but instead a complexity of mind, body, feelings and emotions, all impacting on the well-being of the fetus. According to Scheper-Hughes & Lock (1987), a great ferment and restlessness is taking place, with the appearance of alternative medical care. Health is being viewed in a more holistic way in which the mind–body connection is seen as valid. Cassell (1986) points out there is hardly a patient today who is unaware that the mind has a powerful effect on the body, both in sickness and in health. Midwives need clearly to define this holistic model of risk screening so that we can move towards a better understanding with our medical colleagues: 'The goal is difference without opposition' (Oakley 1993, p. 342).

Midwifery, in partnership with women, must develop and clearly define its own model or framework for

> **Pointers for practice**
>
> - The label of high risk is intended to direct attention and provide specialized care for particular women or groups of women. It may, however, be used by institutions to control women.
> - Clinical judgement should be used in determining treatment for individual women, risk tools being a useful adjunct.
> - Pregnant women depend on care-givers' advice. Their decision-making will be influenced by how the information is presented.
> - It is up to the individual to decide what constitutes an acceptable risk.
> - Risk assessment tools and strategies lack precision and are of poor predictive value.
> - Non-medical risk factors such as poverty are often ignored.

risk assessment, based on principles that are holistic in scope and incorporate what midwives refer to as a *midwifery philosophy* of care.

According to Enkin & Chalmers (1982, p. 285):

the effects of warmth and kindness on measurable outcomes of pregnancy may be difficult to demonstrate, but these qualities are simply good in themselves. Many things that really count cannot be counted.

Although they may be difficult to count, perhaps the involvement of women in defining risk would see the inclusion of the effects of warmth and kindness more often.

REFERENCES

Aaronson L S 1989 Perceived and received support: effects on health and behavior during pregnancy. Nursing Research 38(1): 4–9

Alexander S, Keirse M J N C 1989 Formal risk scoring during pregnancy. In: Chalmers I, Enkin M, Keirse M J N C. Effective care in pregnancy and childbirth, vol. 1. Oxford University Press, Oxford

Arney W R 1982 Power and the profession of obstetrics. University of Chicago Press, Chicago

Benston M L 1986 Questioning authority: feminism and scientific experts. Resources for Feminist Research 15: 71–2

Brody H, Thompson J R 1981 The maximin strategy in modern obstetrics. Journal of Family Practice 12: 977–86

Bursztajn H J, Feinbloom R I, Hamm R M, Brodsky A 1990 Medical choices, medical chances: how patients, families, and physicians can cope with uncertainty, 2nd edn. Routledge/Chapman & Hall, New York

Burtch B 1994 Trials of labour: the re-emergence of midwifery in Canada. McGill Queen's University Press, Montreal

Carroll J C, Reid A J, Biringer A, Wilson L M, Midmer D K

(1994) Psychosocial risk factors during pregnancy: what do family physicians ask about? Canadian Family Physician 40: 1280–9

Cassell E 1986 The rise and fall and rise and fall of new views of disease. Daedalus 115: 19–42

Chalmers B 1982 Psychological aspects of pregnancy: some thoughts for the eighties. Social Science and Medicine 6: 323–31

Chalmers I, Enkin M, Keirse M J N C (eds) 1989 Effective care in pregnancy and childbirth. Oxford University Press, Oxford

Crandon A J 1979 Maternal anxiety and obstetric complications. Journal of Psychosomatic Research 23: 109–11

Davis E 1987 A guide to midwifery: heart and hands, 2nd edn. John Muir Publications, New Mexico

Donley J (1993) Independent midwifery. In: Proceedings of the International Confederation of Midwives 23rd International Congress of Midwives, May, Vancouver, Canada

Douglas M 1990 Risk as a forensic resource. Daedalus 119: 1–16

Douglas M, Wildavsky A 1982 Risk and culture. Basil Blackwell, Oxford

Duden B 1993 Disembodying women: perspectives on pregnancy and the unborn. Harvard University Press, Cambridge

Ehrenreich B, English D 1973 Witches, midwives and nurses: a history of women healers. Feminist Press, New York

Enkin M 1994 Risk in pregnancy: the reality, the perception, and the concept. Birth 21(3): 131–4

Enkin M, Chalmers I (eds) 1982 Effectiveness and satisfaction in antenatal care. Spastics International Medical Publications, London

Enkin M, Keirse M J N C, Chalmers I (eds) 1989 A guide to effective care in pregnancy and childbirth, Oxford University Press, Oxford

Fortney J, Whitehorne A M 1982 The development of an index of high risk pregnancy. American Journal of Obstetrics and Gynecology 143: 501–8

Foucault M 1979 Discipline and punish: the birth of the prison. Random House/Vintage Books, New York

Gabe J (ed.) 1995 Medicine, health and risk: sociological approaches. Blackwell Publications, Oxford

Gaskin I M 1978 Spiritual midwifery. Book Publishing Company, Summertown, Tennessee

Giddens A 1990 The consequences of modernity. Polity Press, Cambridge

Gordon D, Milberg J, Daling J, Hickok D 1991 Advanced maternal age as a risk factor for caesarean section. Obstetrics and Gynecology 77(4): 493–7

Gorsuch R L, Key M K 1974 Abnormalities of pregnancy as a function of anxiety and life stress. Psychosomatic Medicine 36: 352–62

Gregg R 1993 'Choice' as a double-edged sword: information, guilt and mother-blaming in a high-tech age. Women and Health 20(3): 53–73

Grimes L, Mehl L, McRae J, Peterson G 1983 Phenomenological risk screening for childbirth: successful prospective differentiation of risk for medically low risk mothers. Journal of Nurse Midwifery 28: 27–30

Guililland K 1990 Women and midwives: a partnership in progress. Proceedings of the International Confederation of Midwives 21st International Congress of Midwives, October, Kobe, Japan

Hall P F 1994 Editorial: Rethinking risk. Canadian Family Physician 40: 1239–44

Handwerker L 1994 Medical risk: implicating poor pregnant women. Social Science and Medicine 38(5): 66–75

Harvey J 1996 Achieving the indeterminate: accomplishing degrees of certainty in life and death situations. Editorial Board of Sociological Review. Blackwell Publishers, Oxford

Hawking S 1989 A brief history of time. Bantam Books, New York

Hayes M V 1991 The risk approach: unassailable logic? Social Science and Medicine 33(1): 55–70

Hayes M V 1992 On the epistemology of risk: language, logic and social science. Social Science and Medicine 35(4): 401–7

Hobel C J 1978 Risk assessment in perinatal medicine. Clinical Obstetrics and Gynecology 21(2): 287–95

Hobel C J, Hyvarinen M A, Okada D M, Oh W 1973 Prenatal and intrapartum high-risk screening: prediction of the high-risk neonate. American Journal of Obstetrics and Gynecology 117: 1–9

Hurst M, Summey P S 1984 Childbirth and social class: the case of caesarean delivery. Social Science and Medicine 18: 621–63

Institute of Medicine and National Research Council (1982) Research issues in the assessment of birth settings. National Academy Press, Washington

James D K, Stirrat G M (eds) 1988 Pregnancy and risk: the basis for rational management. John Wiley & Sons, New York

Kapp F T, Hornstein S, Graham V T 1963 Some psychological factors in prolonged labor due to inefficient uterine action. Comparative Psychiatry 4: 9–13

Katchner F D 1950 A study of the emotional reactions during labor. American Journal of Obstetrics and Gynecology 60: 19–29

Kaufert P A, O'Neil J 1993 Analysis of a dialogue on risks in childbirth: clinicians, epidemiologists, and Inuit women. In: Lindenbaum S, Lock M (eds) Knowledge, power and practice: the anthropology of medicine and everyday life. University of California Press, Los Angeles

Kirby S, McKenna K 1989 Experience, research, social change: methods from the margins. Bantam Books, Toronto

Kolder V, Gallagher J, Parsons M 1987 Court-ordered obstetrical interventions. New England Journal of Medicine 316(19): 1192–6

Kuipers J C 1989 'Medical discourse' in anthropological context: views of language and power. Medical Anthropology Quarterly 3(2): 99–123

Lane K 1995 The medical model of the body as a site of risk: a case study of childbirth. In: Gabe J (ed.) Medicine, health and risk: sociological approaches. Blackwell Publications, Oxford

Lather P 1986 Issues of validity in openly ideological research: between a rock and a soft place. Interchange 17(4): 63–84

Laukaran V H, van den Berg B J 1980 The relationship of maternal attitude to pregnancy outcomes and obstetric complications. American Journal of Obstetrics and Gynecology 136: 374–9

Lazarus E S 1990 Falling through the cracks: contradictions and barriers to care in a prenatal clinic. Medical Anthropology Quarterly 12: 269–87

Lebow M, Arkin E B 1993 Women's health and the mass media: the reporting of risk. Women's Health International 3(4): 181–90

Lilford R J, Chard T 1983 Problems and pitfalls of risk assessment in antenatal care. British Journal of Obstetrics and Gynaecology 90: 507–10

Lupton D 1993 Risk as moral danger: the social and political functions of risk discourse in public health. International Health Surveys 23(3): 425–35

McClain C S 1983 Perceived risk and choice of childbirth service. Social Science and Medicine 17(23): 1857–65

McDonald R L 1968 The role of emotional factors in obstetric complications: a review. Psychosomatic Medicine 30(2): 222–37

McDonnell R 1997 Risk management in pregnancy. MIDIRS Midwifery Digest 7(3): 291–4

Maier K E 1992 Forced cesarean section as reproductive control and violence: a feminist social work perspective on the 'Baby R' case. Unpublished Master's thesis, Women's Studies, Simon Fraser University, Canada

Mann O H, Albers L L 1997 Informed consent for epidural analgesia in labour. Journal of Nurse Midwifery 42(5): 389–92

Marshall V A 1989 A comparison of two obstetric risk assessment tools. Journal of Nurse Midwifery 34(1): 3–7

Martin E 1989 The woman in the body: a cultural analysis of reproduction. Open University Press, Milton Keynes

Mehta P, Dandrea L A 1988 The battered woman. American Family Physican 37(1): 193–9

Michaelson K L 1988 Introduction: A brief history and contemporary issues. In: Michaelson K L (ed.) Childbirth in America: anthropological perspectives. Bergin & Garvey, Boston

Mohide P, Grant A 1989 Evaluating diagnosis and screening during pregnancy and childbirth. In: Chalmers I, Enkin M, Keirse M J N C (eds) Effective care in pregnancy and childbirth, vol. 1. Oxford University Press, Oxford

Morgan M G 1993 Risk analysis and management. Scientific American 269(1): 32–41

Murphy P A 1994 Editorial: Risk, risk assessment and risk labels. Journal of Nurse Midwifery 39(2): 67–9

Nelkin D 1989 Communicating technological risk: social construction of risk perception. Annual Review of Public Health 10: 95–113

Neuhoff D, Burke M S, Porreco R P 1989 Caesarean birth for failed progress in labor. Obstetrics and Gynecology 73: 915–20

Nickerson C A E 1990 The attitude/behaviour discrepancy as a methodological artifact: comment on 'Sexually active adolescents and condoms'. American Journal of Public Health 80: 117–19

Nilsson L 1965 A child is born – the drama of life before birth. Dell Publishing, New York

Nuckolls K, Cassel J, Kaplan B 1972 Psychosocial assets, life crisis and the prognosis of pregnancy. American Journal of Epidemiology 95(5): 431–41

Oakley A 1984 The captured womb: a history of the medical care of pregnant women. Basil Blackwell, Oxford

Oakley A 1992a Social support and motherhood: the natural history of a research project. Blackwell Publishers, Oxford

Oakley A 1992b Commentary: The best research is that which breeds more. Birth 19(1): 8–9

Oakley A 1993 Women, health and knowledge: travel through and beyond foreign parts. Health Care for Women International 14: 327–44

Osofsky H J, Kendall N 1973 Poverty as a criterion of risk. Clinical Obstetrics and Gynecology 18: 103–9

Overall C (ed.) 1989 The future of human reproduction. Women's Press, Toronto

Page L 1993 Midwives hear the heartbeat of the future. In: Proceedings of the International Confederation of Midwives 23rd International Congress of Midwives, Vancouver, Canada

Palys T S 1989 Research questions: quantitative and qualitative perspectives. Simon Fraser University, Vancouver

Perkins B B 1994 Intensity, stratification, and risk in perinatal care: redefining problems and restructuring levels. Women and Health 21(1): 17–31

Peterson H S, Sims A M 1993 Epidemiologic studies and the media: the challenge of communicating women's health risks. Women's Health International 3(3): 198–203

Queniart A 1992 Risky business: medical definitions of pregnancy. In: Currie D H, Raoul V (eds) Anatomy of gender: women's struggle for the body. Canada: Carleton University Press, Ontario

Radford T 1997 Juggling life's comical odds. Guardian, 5 December, p. 21

Rapp R 1988 Chromosomes and communication: the discourse of genetic counseling. Medical Anthropology Quarterly 2(2): 143–57

Riessman C K, Nathanson C A 1986 The management of reproduction: social construction of risk and responsibility. In: Aiken L H, Mechanic D (eds) Applications of social science: to clinical medicine and health policy. Rutgers University Press, New Jersey

Roberts C, Algert C S, March L M 1994 Delayed childbearing: are there any risks? Medical Journal of Australia 160: 539–44

Rodgers S 1989 Pregnancy as justification for loss of juridical autonomy In: Overall C (ed.) The future of human reproduction. Women's Press, Toronto

Rothman B 1982 In labor: women and power in the birthplace. WW Norton, New York

Russell C 1993 Hype, hysteria, and women's health risks: the role of the media. Women's Health International 3(4): 191–7

Sapolsky R A 1990 The politics of risk. Daedalus 119: 83–96

Scheper-Hughes N, Lock M M 1987 The mindful body: a prolegomenon to future work in medical anthropology. Medical Anthropology Quarterly 1(1): 6–41

Smilkstein G, Helsper-Lucas A, Ashworth C, Montano D, Pagel M (1984) Predictions of pregnancy complications: an application of the biopsychosocial model. Social Science and Medicine 18(4): 315–21

Sosa R, Kennell J, Klaus M, Robertson S, Urrutia J 1980 The effect of a supportive companion on perinatal problems, length of labor, and mother–infant interaction. New England Journal of Medicine 33: 597–600

Spindel P G, Suarez S H 1995 Informed consent and home birth. Journal of Nurse Midwifery 40(6): 541–54

Stander H J 1936 Williams' Obstetrics, 7th edn. D Appleton-Century, New York

Swanson R W 1984 Battered wife syndrome. Canadian Medical Association Journal 130: 709–12

Treichler P A 1990 Feminism, medicine, and the meaning of childbirth. In: Jacobus M, Keller E F, Shuttleworth S (eds) Body/politics: women and the discourse of science. Routledge, New York

Wall E M 1988 Assessing obstetric risk: a review of obstetric risk-scoring systems. Journal of Family Practice 27(2): 43–5

Wilson R W, Schifrin B S 1980 Is any pregnancy low risk? Obstetrics and Gynecology 55(5): 653–6

5

Keeping birth normal

Lesley Ann Page

WHAT DOES 'NORMAL' MEAN?

Midwives are the only professionals who specialize in the overall care of childbearing women and their babies when there are no complications, in what is usually called 'normal' pregnancy and birth. It is generally accepted that midwives are required to refer to a doctor if complications arise, yet less attention is paid to the need for midwives to confirm the normal and to be able to support, protect and encourage healthy birth and the avoidance of unnecessary interventions. There has never been a greater need for midwives to protect and support normal processes. The operative delivery rate is rising in many parts of the industrialized world, and it is even suggested that women should have the choice of elective caesarean birth (Patterson-Brown 1998). Birth through an abdominal incision is fast becoming a 'normal event', although the safety of this approach is debatable (Amu et al 1998). If this trend is to be controlled, the enhancement of 'normal' pregnancy and birth is more important than ever, and midwives are the professionals in the best position to do this.

But what is 'normal'? The words 'normal' and 'natural' are simply 'constructs' that are affected by the culture in which we live and practise, and hold a number of meanings. If we define the normal as the average and consider a number of services with a high epidural rate, we would think of a birth that is induced and in which the majority of women would have an epidural as being 'normal'. In fact, it is in many maternity services extremely difficult to protect normal birth, if we consider normal birth to be birth without any medical intervention. The understanding of what is normal is altered by a number of deeply entrenched regimens, many of which have not been adequately evaluated, for example the active management of labour (Thornton & Lilford 1994). This active management includes a number of factors, such as the arbitrary establishment of strict time limits to labour and the frequent use of oxytocin augmentation, that are highly invasive interventions. Perhaps the worst aspect of this active management is that it has been translated into practice in countries other than Ireland, without the most important aspect of the package as O'Driscoll et al (1984) conceived it, the constant presence of 'the nurse'.

Might we then define the 'normal' as natural birth? Even here, we run into difficulties because the society and culture in which birth takes place affect what is considered to be natural. Local customs and values all affect the behaviour and expectations surrounding birth as well as the outcomes of birth. Perhaps by saying that we believe in natural birth, we mean that nature should be allowed to take its course. Surely not: nature can be cruel as well as kind. The definition of normal then is clearly difficult because intervention will at times be necessary. The question becomes one of when do we interfere with nature, and at what point do we use intervention?

The definition of normal is so problematic that I have found it simpler to be guided by two simple principles:

- Intervention should only be used if there are clear evidence-based clinical indicators and clear evidence that the intervention is more likely to do good than harm in the particular situation (see Chapter 1 for an example of the use of this principle in practice), or if a woman asks for it.
- The provision of adequate support, which includes providing enough and appropriate information to women, is fundamental to avoiding unnecessary intervention in pregnancy and birth.

At present the 'rules' of the UK, and of most other countries, that govern midwifery practice usually require that midwives should be able to refer or call medical help when there is what the United Kingdom Central Council for Nursing, Midwifery and Health Visiting (UKCC; 1998) refers to as 'a deviation from the norm'. Of course, it is important to know when medical assistance is required. However, the identification of a deviation from the norm presents great difficulties in modern-day care, where the definition of 'normal' is so restricted by current practices. For example, a second stage of more than 1 hour is in many places viewed as abnormal, and it is considered to be 'normal' for all women to have a cervical dilatation of at least 1 cm per hour in active labour.

I would rather see the first rule of midwifery being the need to 'confirm the absence of any real, evidence-based indicators for intervention' and the second as the need 'to refer to a medical colleague when there is an evidence-based indicator for medical intervention'. For example, if it is considered that a doctor should be involved in the care of women who are over 40 years old, there should be good evidence that there is a higher probability of poor outcome. As always, apparently simple principles are not easy to put into practice, particularly in services where it is 'normal' to induce labour, to augment labour and to use continuous electronic monitoring.

Below, I will focus on some practical ways of supporting what I will refer to as 'the normal' in the context of labour and birth. This choice is intentional. First, labor and birth is a critical point in the pregnancy, a time at which the actions and decisions of the midwife are likely to have profound effects. The decisions that the midwife makes at this time, and her approach to the woman in her care, may make a difference not only between life and death, good health and severe disability, but also in the emotional well-being of the woman and her family. They will affect the mother, baby and family in a number of ways for years to come. Memories of good and poor care tend to be profound, and memories of birth are in themselves an important outcome. This is not intended to downplay the importance of midwifery care in the antenatal and postnatal period, and this is discussed in other chapters. However, the birth of a baby is like no other event in human life. As Simkin (1992, p. 64) reminds us:

The birth of a child, especially a first child, represents a landmark event in the lives of all involved. For the mother particularly, childbirth has a profound physical, mental, emotional and social effect. No other event involves pain, emotional stress, vulnerability, possible physical injury or death, and permanent role change, and includes responsibility for a dependent, helpless human being. Moreover, it generally all takes place within a single day. It is not surprising that women tend to remember their first birth experiences vividly and with deep emotion.

The acute and critical nature of labour and birth call for an integration of a number of skills in the midwife, many of which are practical physical and interpersonal in nature.

In this chapter, I will do two things: indicate the importance of the practical aspects of midwifery by an example drawn from one area of midwifery, and draw on some important evidence to show how midwives might 'keep birth normal'. Other chapters emphasize the critical analysis of evidence, clinical decision-making, the importance of relationships and some of the science that is the foundation of midwifery. However, the practical work that is the focus of this chapter emphasizes that hands and heart as well as head are important to midwifery practice. The work of midwifery is, by its very nature, very practical. The practical aspects taken as an example in this chapter are concerned with supporting women so that they may give birth to their children without unnecessary interference (Fig. 5.1). I will focus on four discrete areas:

- helping women to cope with the pain of labour to avoid epidural anaesthesia wherever possible;
- there being a constant presence in labour;
- helping women move as they wish in labour;
- using intermittent auscultation rather than continuous electronic fetal monitoring when there are no complications in labour.

The reviews of the evidence to be used as a platform for indicating how birth might be kept normal are available to every midwife. These include the MIDIRS 'Informed choice' leaflets (MIDIRS 1996a–1996d) and reviews from the Cochrane Library. In particular, this evidence indicates that continuous electronic fetal monitoring and the use of epidural anaesthesia are associated with a higher rate of operative delivery, and that a constant presence in labour is associated with a lower rate of the use of analgesia in labour and of operative delivery.

This evidence, then, indicates that it is possible that three things may help in keeping birth normal:

- the use of intermittent auscultation rather than continuous electronic monitoring;
- helping women to cope with the pain of labour so that they are less likely to require analgesia, particularly epidural anaesthesia;
- the constant presence of a midwife or trained person in labour.

The text will also draw on my own experience of what I have found helpful in supporting women during childbirth.

HELPING WOMEN TO COPE WITH THE PAIN OF LABOUR

Whether or not it is right to discourage women from using analgesia is a frequent topic of debate. Certainly,

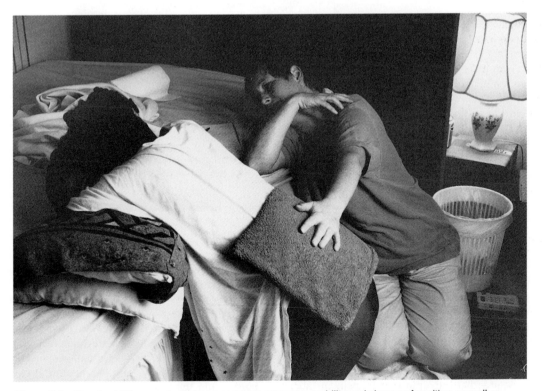

Figure 5.1 Keeping birth normal requires a constant presence, mobility and change of position, as well as comforting touch. These pictures illustrate this approach. Immersion in water, as well as providing pain relief, helps the women to adopt comfortable positions more easily and creates tranquility and privacy. (Reproduced with kind permission from Marcia-May.)

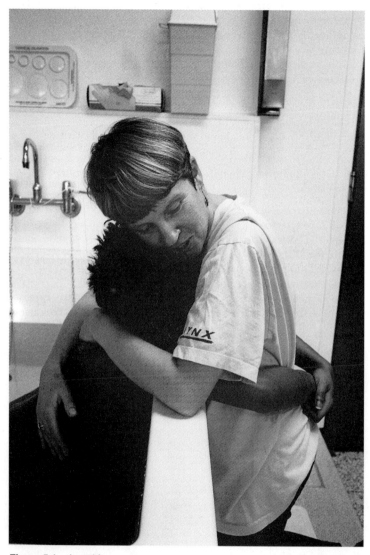

Figure 5.1   (cont'd)

many of the anaesthetists I work with think that complete pain relief is an end in itself and that to avoid it is old fashioned. Given the potential complications of many of the methods of analgesia, and for the potential of a positive birth experience without invasive methods of pain relief when adequate support is provided, the topic is of fundamental concern.

As the use of epidural analgesia becomes more common, it seems that our approach to pain in labour changes. The belief that the normal pain of childbirth is something to be erased at all costs deserves scrutiny. As Leap (1997) says, 'The allure of pain relief in labour is almost irresistible in a society that sees the relief of pain as a major benefit of modern living.'

Leap describes what she calls the menu approach to pain relief – the provision of a list of options. In her interviews of 10 midwives who had developed a rationale for not routinely offering pain relief to women in labour, she describes consistent responses. These include the importance of differentiating between the normal and the abnormal pain of childbirth, and the idea that most women can cope with the pain of labour aided by the body's endogenous opiates, which are stimulated by pain. The purpose of pain includes the transition to motherhood empowering the woman through a sense of achievement. Pain is also seen as being of benefit in triggering the neurohormonal cascades that keep birth normal.

I recently listened to a series of lectures by a very experienced midwife from Holland. Coming as she did from a country where home birth is common and the level of intervention very low compared with that of most of the industrialized world, her view of pain in labour was enlightening and considerably altered my own views. Smulders also believes that the pain of labour is necessary for the release of hormones that stimulate labour and progress in birth and is, as such, to be welcomed. She describes the importance of midwives being able to differentiate between normal and abnormal pain in labour (Smulders 1999).

The MIDIRS 'Informed choice' leaflet (1996c, pp. 3–5) gives the following information on the research evidence on epidurals:

The research evidence relating to epidurals is far from adequate, although the overall safety of the technique has been well demonstrated. The controlled studies, which have looked at outcomes for mother and baby, have involved quite small numbers of women. Many other studies have been concerned only with variations of the drug requirements.

Effectiveness
The majority of women, about 93%, find their epidural to be of great benefit in terms of pain relief. About 6%–8% find their epidural to be of little or no use. Women's satisfaction with epidural is correspondingly high: 88% of those women who gained effective pain relief would request an epidural in a subsequent pregnancy.

There are a number of adverse effects and complications associated with the technique. These include:

- A threefold increase in the use of oxytocin during labour and a significant increase in the length of the second stage of labour
- A threefold increase in the instrumental delivery rate. Allowing the epidural to wear off in second stage of labour is effective in promoting spontaneous delivery but the reappearance of pain may not be acceptable to women. It may not be necessary when low dose combinations of drugs are used. Encouraging early pushing (i.e. as soon as full dilatation is reached) results in a higher rate of delivery by rotational forceps. Delaying pushing until the vertex is visible at the introitus does not appear to be detrimental to the fetus.
- The evidence from randomised controlled trials suggests that epidurals are associated with a doubling of the caesarean rate for dystocia
- The loss of pain from the uterus is accompanied by some loss of normal sensation in the lower part of the body. The block of motor nerves results in reduced mobility. Except in the case of mobile epidurals, this will confine the woman to bed and may result in difficulties with pushing in the second stage of labour. Some women feel that the loss of mobility and sensation with an epidural is unacceptable

- Loss of sensation to the bladder may lead to the need for catheterisation
- Epidurals can cause hypotension. Ephedrine is needed for up to 2% of women having an epidural
- Epidurals can cause a rise in the maternal temperature
- When opiates are used women may experience varying degrees of itching of the skin
- Potentially life-threatening complications occur in 1 in 4000 cases. Death associated with epidural anaesthesia is very rare
- 80% of women where the epidural has been associated with dural tap will develop a headache
- Serious neurological damage associated with epidural is extremely rare (4–18 per 10 000 women)
- Several studies have demonstrated the association between epidurals and new backache. Most of this evidence has not been able to demonstrate a convincing cause and association.

Effect on the newborn
- There are no consistent differences in the condition of the babies at birth following epidural anaesthesia or non-epidural analgesia as measured by Apgar scores and cord blood gases. Detailed neurobehavioural studies demonstrated dose-related effects on newborn tone and behaviour, but there is little information on whether these effects were clinically significant. In a 5-year follow up of one randomised study, no behavioural differences between the groups of children were detected.

A later meta-analysis in the Cochrane Library confirms the information in the MIDIRS 'Informed choice' leaflet. It concludes that further long-term follow-up studies of both mother and baby are required (Howell 1997).

Women should be supported in such a way that they are less likely to need analgesia, particularly the more invasive methods such as epidural or combined spinal epidural, if we are to reduce the rates of operative delivery.

Rather than use the title 'analgesia for labour', I have intentionally used the phrase 'helping women to cope with the pain of labour'. This is for the following reasons. All the studies that have evaluated the provision of some form of extra support for women in labour have resulted in a lower use of analgesia and are often associated with higher satisfaction (Green et al 1998). Moreover, complete pain relief is not necessarily associated with greater satisfaction (Morgan 1982) but is linked to the extent to which a woman feels in control of her experience (Green et al 1988, Simkin 1992). Indeed, women who have coped with the pain of labour without interventions such as epidural analgesia may feel proud of their achievement if they feel that decisions have been within their control. Thus, it seems that rather than asking the question 'Should all women be offered analgesia for labour?', we should be focusing instead on the provision of adequate support.

This is not to say that we should deny women analgesia if they need it. There are a number of women who, even if they receive appropriate support, will still need analgesia in labour, and if they are denied it, they may be traumatized by the experience of labour and birth. During my 5 years as Director of a large maternity service, I saw a large majority of the women who complained about their care and of severe personal distress following birth. In a number of these situations, good pain relief was asked for and denied. Decisions are individual. It is best to have full discussions about pain relief and possible complications before labour starts. If possible, this should be between the woman and the care-givers who are likely to be with her in labour (Royal College of Obstetricians and Gynaecologists 1995).

Women will sometimes decide in the antenatal period that they wish to avoid analgesia or epidural anaesthesia; then, during labour, they change their minds. If the midwife knows the woman ahead of time, and feels that the woman she is caring for may regret it afterwards if she changes her mind about pain relief in labour, she may want to encourage her to try to cope without it. This particularly applies if events in labour are right (not too prolonged, etc.). This is one of the trickiest areas of judgement for midwives in labour care. It involves a careful balance of supporting and encouraging the woman to manage without an epidural and knowing when the decision should be changed. In the evaluation of One-to-One midwifery, (see Chapter 6), there was a significant reduction in the rate of uptake of combined spinal epidurals in the One-to-One group. However, women in the One-to-One group generally felt satisfied with their pain relief, and more found the experience of birth positive. More in the One-to-One group than in the control group said that birth was 'hard work but wonderful' (McCourt & Page 1996). The test of an appropriate avoidance of epidural anaesthesia is whether or not the woman feels supported and that she is involved in decision-making. Certainly, epidurals should not be denied when they are really needed.

Alternatives to analgesia and epidural anaesthesia

There are a number of alternatives to conventional medical analgesics. However, it is important to remember that tension and fear are a part of the cycle of pain, and everything possible should be done to reduce these. This includes giving adequate information, both before and during labour, as well as the factors mentioned above. These alternatives work in a number of different ways:

- masking the pain by the use of alternative sensations (e.g. heat and cold, perhaps a hot water bottle) or deep massage (e.g. hard pressure to or massage of the sacral area during contractions);
- soothing the pain and helping the woman to adopt different positions with ease (e.g. by using water in a shower, bath or birthing pool);
- affecting nerve pathways (e.g. transcutaneous nerve stimulation; TENS);
- acting as a diversion.

The use of massage

There are a number of ways in which massage may be used. Although many of these have not been systematically evaluated, one can assess them on individual women by simply asking whether one can try something and then asking whether it is helping! The woman's partner may have learned some massage techniques in prenatal classes, and supporting the partner in this important activity is likely to be very helpful.

A number of different approaches may help individual women. These include:

- light efflourage of the abdomen during contractions, the finger tips tracing a figure of eight (this was the method taught in La maze classes in the 1980s);
- deep massage of the sacral area or applying pressure with the heels of the hands during contractions;
- firm massage of the hands, feet or shoulders using some type of oil.

The golden rule is to watch the woman and to check with her that what is being done is helpful. Many women simply want to be left to close their eyes and turn inwards during a contraction and may not want to be touched at all.

I used always to massage the perineum during the second stage of labour. After my own pregnancy, when I found any touching of my perineal area terribly painful, I started to wonder about its efficacy and increasingly felt that the procedure seemed very intrusive. However, I still sometimes apply a hot cloth to the perineum if there is a lot of pain in this area during the second stage.

The use of water

With the exception of home birth, the issue that has

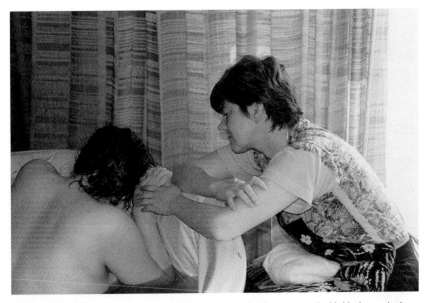

Figure 5.2   A pool allows the woman to move easily. (Reproduced with kind permission from Uwe Kitzinger.)

created the most controversy over the past decade has been the use of immersion in water for labour and birth (Figs 5.2 and 5.3). Wagner (1996, p. 4) says that this is because 'you can't attend a waterbirth and keep your sophisticated cool and dignity'. He makes the point that water helps the women but 'sure doesn't help the birth attendant'. There are, of course, a number of considerations for the birth attendant, including protection of the back.

When using a birthing pool, I have found the following approach the most practical:

- Do not attempt to get into the pool but use a seat on the side, which means you do not have to lean over.
- Use a waterproof Doppler device (sonicaid) or cover the transducer with a condom or plastic bag for listening to the fetal heart.
- Measure the temperature of the water with a floating thermometer. It is generally recommended that the pool is at body temperature, although in an observational study of a series of 1000 low-risk births using immersion in water where the mother chose the temperature of the water, no complications were reported (Muscat 1996).
- When in the hospital, involve the infection control department in ensuring that filling and emptying devices avoid contamination and agree a protocol for sterilization.

Approaches to management of the birth differ. If there is a good sense of rapport with the woman and she is able to follow verbal advice regarding bearing down during the second stage of labour, it will probably not be necessary to use any hands on the perineum or crowning head. The mother should be helped to take her baby out of the water soon after birth. Some midwives keep the woman in water for the third stage, while some feel better about having the woman get out. Discuss the woman's preference for this ahead of time; it is, however, quite possible that she will change her mind.

More detailed advice and information regarding the use of a birthing pool is contained in the proceedings of the First International Waterbirth Conference (Beech 1996).

Like many other procedures that require further evaluation, including such procedures as the use of epidurals, the outcomes of immersion in water should be carefully audited. The Cochrane Library (Nikodem 1999) indicates the following:

Comparisons of immersion versus no immersion before labour or during the second stage of labour are not available yet. Only three trials reported on immersion versus no immersion during labour; two of the trials had only a small number of participants. Many of the outcomes only reflect the results of one trial.

The benefits and risks of the use of water immersion during labour has shown no significant differences on maternal, fetal or neonatal outcomes. No significant adverse effects have been detected.

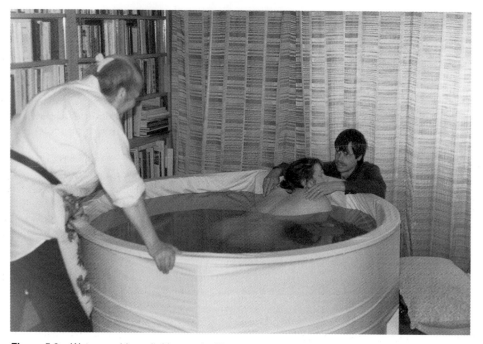

Figure 5.3   Water provides relief from pain. (Reproduced with kind permission from Uwe Kitzinger.)

One important effect of using a birthing pool is the calm it creates. The addition of a pool to the room changes the atmosphere completely, and staff seem to be deterred from coming in and out of the room at will – maybe because they are worried about confronting a naked woman.

If a birthing pool is not available, a bath or a shower is often helpful. The major advantage of the birthing pool over these is that, if it is deep enough, it helps the woman to move around freely.

Creating a positive atmosphere and arranging furniture

One of the basic ways of reducing anxiety and tension, and of helping women to cope with the pain of labour, may be by intentionally creating a calm, positive, welcoming atmosphere. Over the past decade, I have talked with many midwives in many parts of the world. What many of them, particularly those who work in large hospitals, have told me is that the delivery suite or labour ward is a place that evokes anxiety in them. I have also found that when community midwives are rotated into the delivery suite to upgrade their skills, they find it a frightening experience. In contrast, the atmosphere of a home birth is usually very different. Home is home; a sense of home is per-sonal and can *never* be created in an institution or birth centre, although such a centre certainly can, and should be, more homely (Fig. 5.4). Home is a place in which the woman is in her own surroundings, supported by chosen people and loved ones, in which it is far easier to get comfortable. Usually, only one or two professionals are in attendance.

It is far harder to create a positive calm atmosphere in a hospital. This is possibly because of the combined effect of having so many people in one area, people who are often overworked and rushed, constantly dealing with such a critical event, constantly looking after women in severe pain, so that anxiety spreads from one person to another. It is also difficult with conventional patterns of staffing to have long enough to care for one mother and baby at a time, adding to the sense of frustration and crisis. The area is often more like an intensive care unit than a place where babies are brought into the world.

It is important to think consciously about the atmosphere in which you practise because it is likely to affect you and other staff, who will in turn affect the women they are caring for. The atmosphere will also have a direct effect on the woman herself. A midwife working in a delivery suite permanently may be in a position to do something to make the atmosphere calmer, for example setting up strategies for staff support, getting

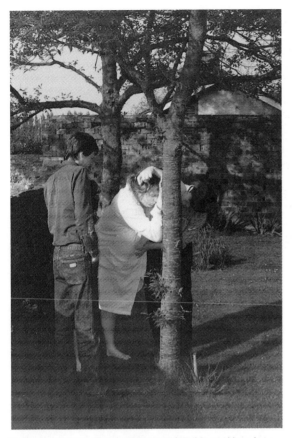

Figure 5.4 It is easier to adopt comfortable positions in home-like settings. (Reproduced with kind permission from Uwe Kitzinger.)

all the staff (both midwives and doctors) to talk together and finding time for debriefing sessions.

Even if the atmosphere as a whole cannot be altered, midwives can do something about the room or rooms in which they work and about protecting themselves from the atmosphere if it is unsupportive. They can be aware of their feelings and reactions, and carry out deep breathing when they go into or return to a room. Concentrating on the woman (or women) for whom they are caring at that moment will consciously keep them calm. It is also important not to have numerous strangers wandering in and out of the room when the woman is in labour. She should feel that she is in a protected environment where she is able to focus on herself and put all her energy into coping with labour.

One of my most vivid memories when I gave birth to my son David was the worry that staff other than those who were caring for me would come into the room, leaving me highly embarrassed. Looking back, it seems strange that I was not worried about safety, but I think we, as midwives, tend to underestimate the intimacy of the situation and how important it is for the woman to have privacy. Go out of the room to talk to doctors and colleagues about the woman's progress if that is expected; invite them in to meet the woman at an early stage, at an appropriate time and in a pre-arranged way if you think you may need to make a referral or require advice.

Despite the efforts of many midwives over recent years, many delivery rooms are still very ugly places. The bed is often dominant (and uncomfortable!) and right in the centre of the room. Altering the position of furniture will encourage women to move about. Put the bed against the wall and make a space that invites the woman to move and walk around, also leaving room for 'props' to support her in adopting different positions. Such props may include people, beanbags, rocking chairs, over-bed tables and the end of the bed itself. In one hospital in Iceland, I saw a padded swing, high enough for the woman to lean on and rock herself during contractions; it was very popular. If a delivery suite has not had the 'Laura Ashley treatment' given to a number of hospitals, turning down the lighting may help in creating a more aesthetic and calm atmosphere. Despite all this, it must be remembered that it is probably the people working in the suite who will make most difference in the long run.

In the 1980s, there was a noticeable change in many delivery suites in response to the work of Leboyer. Some of the impact of his work seems to have been lost and forgotten now, but it is worth reconsideration. Leboyer wrote of how traumatic it could be for the baby to be born. He proposed that there should be silence for the birth of the baby, the cord should not be clamped and cut until pulsation had stopped, and the baby should have skin-to-skin contact on the mother's abdomen after birth. He also proposed that the baby should be massaged and given a bath after birth in order to adjust to a totally new environment (Leboyer 1975). The silent, darkened delivery room makes sense for the baby, but also makes sense for the woman in labour, who will be given the chance to draw in on herself, and her own resources, for the challenge of labour and birth. The idea of the calm, quiet, darkened room is very different from that of the hospital hustle and bustle that is often observed.

Presence, comfort and encouragement

One of the most important and effective things we can do in labour is to ensure that women have constant support. Such support has been shown not only to provide a woman with emotional back-up, so that she is happier and more likely to be relaxed, but also to have a strong positive effect on the physiology and outcomes of labour (MIDIRS 1996a). In recognizing the importance of this constant attendance in labour, *Changing Childbirth* (Department of Health 1993) recommended that:

The aims of the service should be for every woman to have a midwife with her throughout her labour, if she wishes. If possible the same midwife should stay with the woman throughout.

A range of people in addition to the woman's partner – family members, friends, trained lay people (doulas), student midwives and midwives – can provide this birth support (MIDIRS 1996a).

A constant presence

Staying in the room is not enough as it is easy to be present without really *being* present. It is important to be able to give all one's attention to the woman. In most hospital systems, there is a major deterrent to attending properly and being 'with' the woman in labour, even when staffing is adequate. This deterrent is the paperwork, which is often irrationally organized, documentation being repeated in a number of places and requiring much duplication. Yet recording progress and decisions made and actions taken is crucial to good care. If possible records should be made 'midwife friendly'. If this cannot be done, the midwife should be aware that keeping records may take her concentration away from the woman and her supporters, and should try to combat this. Everything possible should be done to organize midwifery so as to allow this one-to-one presence in labour and birth.

Hodnett (1995) undertook a systematic review of 10 randomized controlled trials that included over 10 000 women. She found that, despite the different countries and conditions covered by the study, 'there was a remarkable consistency in the description of the experimental intervention across all trials. In all instances the intervention included continuous presence, at least during active labour. Eight trials also included mention of comforting touch and words of praise and encouragement.'

Hodnett also reported:

a considerable consistency in the results of the trials, even when they are separated into 'accompanied' and 'unaccompanied'. This is despite the disparities in obstetrical routines, hospital conditions, and obstetrical risk status of the participants, the differences in policies about the presence of significant others, and the differences in the professional qualifications of the women who provided the support.

Regardless of whether or not a support person of the woman's own choosing could be present, the continuous presence of a trained support person who had no prior social bond with the labouring woman reduced (MIDIRS 1996a, p. 3; see also Hodnett 1995):

● the likelihood of medication for pain relief
● duration of labour
● operative vaginal delivery
● A 5-minute Apgar score of < 7

In settings which did not permit the presence of significant others the presence of a trained support person also

● Reduced the likelihood of caesarean delivery

All four trials, which looked at women's preferences, found that continuous support in labour is associated with:

● Labour being better than expected
● A more positive overall experience for the woman

Individual trials found that continuous support in labour is associated with:

● Less perineal trauma
● Women more likely to be breastfeeding at six weeks
● Less depression at six weeks
● Less difficulty in mothering
● Fewer unsatisfactory relationships between midwife and father

There were no negative outcomes associated with support in labour.

All this research took place in hospitals and focused on support given by women, with or without the baby's father also being present. The most beneficial effect was found to be when a woman who had some experience of supporting other women in labour provided the constant support. In many countries, this might be the midwife.

A constant presence is easier to ensure when there is an effective 'continuity of care' scheme in operation in which a midwife will follow a woman into labour. In the One-to-One practice, over 90% of women receiving One-to-One care received constant attendance in labour compared with 50% of those in the conventional service. Nor did this service cost any more than the provision of conventional care (McCourt & Page 1996).

Alternatively, an extra two midwives may be needed for a service possessing a typical pattern of staffing with typical UK levels and 4000 deliveries annually (MIDIRS 1996a). It should, however, be recognized that there are other difficulties in providing this constant support with a traditional staffing pattern. This traditional staffing pattern requires midwives to be permanently affiliated to the delivery suite for a period of time, and it may well be difficult to provide this constant support in this situation. 'Labour support is so intense and demanding that no one can do it

40 hours a week' (Simkin 1992). As far as I know, no evaluation of the effect of permanent placement on a labour ward with respect to the potential for burn-out has been undertaken; the results would certainly be interesting.

Words of praise, comfort, encouragement and reassurance

It would be wrong to reduce the way in which we may use words of encouragement and support to a technique. As in most communication, the importance is in listening to and attending to the individual needs and preferences of the woman and her partner, as well as in responding to those individual needs. Robertson (1997), in her excellent book on supporting women in labour, calls it tuning in to women. This is far more than listening to what the woman is saying: it is also watching and sensing.

Sometimes, when I have a good rapport with a woman, it helps at difficult times, for example the transition to the second stage of labour, to stand still for a moment and try to imagine how the woman is feeling. I can remember one time that was particularly difficult because I had been torn between the care of a number of women. I was looking after a first-time mother I had never met before who really wanted to avoid analgesia. She had been making good progress, but then I was called into another room, and when I got back she was in the second stage, distressed and apparently not making the progress I had expected. I stood quietly for a moment trying to imagine what she was feeling. I suspected that she was finding the contractions so painful that she was frightened to follow her urge to push. She seemed to be poised at that moment when there is no turning back and the pain has to be endured, when it hurts not to push and it hurts as much if you do. I simply touched her hand and said, 'I wonder if you are frightened to push because you are in so much pain; I know it is painful, but there is no turning back, you have to go on.' At that point, she looked at her husband, took a deep breath and started to bear down with contractions, spontaneously following her own urges. She wrote me later saying how this had helped. Soon she had given birth to her baby and she and her husband were ecstatic, pleased too that she had managed the birth without analgesia.

Words of praise, comfort and reassurance will vary from midwife to midwife, and different women need different approaches. These may include giving information about progress in a positive rather than a negative way, telling a woman that she and her baby are doing well, and, if there are concerns, letting the woman know in a way that is not frightening. Asking for permission before undertaking any procedure and talking through decisions in an appropriate way is crucial. It is also important to know when to be quiet. The midwife should attend to the signals emanating from the woman and her support partner(s), and respond to them.

I try to talk in a kind of shorthand, and I am often also silent. These are the kind of phrase I might use: 'You are doing well', 'You are breathing well', 'This contraction will soon be over', 'I can see some of the baby's head', 'Would you like to feel your baby's head?', 'Would it help you to relax more if I rubbed your shoulders?' Even when I have not met the woman before labour starts, I always find myself developing a kind of tenderness mixed with great respect for the woman I am looking after, so much so that I often want to use terms of endearment, although I do not in case it is viewed as patronizing.

Once, when I worked with a very experienced midwife, a senior midwife in a delivery suite, I noticed that she smiled – really beamed – at the woman and her partner whenever she talked to the couple she was with. There was such a lot in that smile. It was not false, and it seemed to say so many things: everything is fine, there is nothing to worry about, we will soon see your baby, and I am enjoying what I am doing.

All of this is far easier if you have met the woman before and have some kind of working relationship with her. This helps too in sorting out some important decisions beforehand, particularly in knowing how the woman feels about using analgesia and electronic fetal monitoring. Then, during labour, such discussions can be in the shorthand that is possible between two people who know and understand each other (see Chapter 1).

Comforting through touch, massage and physical support

In describing the differences in the purposes of touching that they encountered in past and present literature, Hedstrom & Newton (1986) reported that the only purpose for touching common to both times was touching for pain relief. They said that, although there was still much to be learned about the effects of human touching, the studies that they reviewed indicated that the effect could be profound.

In her chapter 'Authoritative touch in childbirth', Kitzinger (1977) reminds us that, within Western culture, great stress is placed on verbal communication, while the unspoken elements in discourse tend to be trivialized and ignored. Yet touch is an important element in the interaction of human bodies. In an account of the way in which touch has been used in childbirth through different times and across different cultures, Kitzinger makes a classification of different types of touch: blessing touch, comfort touch, physically supportive touch, diagnostic touch, manipulative touch, restraining touch and punitive touch. Much of birth now occurs inside a hospital setting, thus taking the woman away from the potential for a more natural circle of family friends and supporters who may, in their own surroundings, be more likely to use physical contact and touch in a spontaneous way. In addition, the ritual of medicalized birth, particularly where there is a reliance on technology for enhancing and monitoring labour, may restrict and alter the way in which we use touch to comfort, support and encourage women through labour. This is especially so because staff in hospitals tend to be rushed and overworked, and may have no prior bond or relationship with the women in labour for whom they are caring. The potential power of touch is thus restricted, or touch is more likely to be used to control rather than to help.

When touch is used with the intention of comforting and supporting, and when it is sensitive to the woman's needs and reaction, experience teaches that it is extremely powerful. I vividly remember a story told by a woman doctor at a conference in Canada: the story of her own labour and the birth of her own baby. She told of the point in her labour when she felt she could not go on, so her midwife encouraged her to have a shower. When she got out of the shower, she described how her midwife brushed her hair with such tenderness that it gave her the power and will to continue. Touch used for physical support may be close contact, cradling of the woman for comfort and to help her to maintain her posture or position, or providing a neck or shoulders to lean on. Touch may be slight, perhaps a touch of the hand or forehead, or massage that may be either gentle or firm. In Western society, where touch is restricted by culture, massage may be an acceptable form of touch and be considered less invasive and more acceptable. While the touch of massage may be an effective form of pain relief in itself, a light touch may simply be a way of saying, 'I am here with you, you are not alone'. It is the direct contact of one with another, the support of and contact with another person who cares about you as an individual, that is crucial at such a time.

While touch may be comforting and supportive, it is true, as Kitzinger (1997) says, that it may also be used to restrain and punish, and may cause pain. I have often seen a woman's arms restrained as she reached out to hold her baby at birth – because they would 'contaminate the sterile field'. Also, touch during contractions and vaginal examinations may be very painful. Touch may also be invasive, particularly in childbirth. Consider the vaginal examination, often performed by staff whom the woman has never met before, to whom she has barely had an introduction, and sometimes without full consent. In everyday life, such touch would be seen as one of the worst forms of assault. In labour, it is extremely painful. Touch should be a response to the woman's needs rather than a routine or protocol to be followed, otherwise it can be, as Kitzinger comments, irritating and painful.

MOBILITY AND POSITIONS FOR LABOUR AND BIRTH

Most women being cared for in hospital will stay in bed during labour. In England and Wales, 74% of women adopt a semi-recumbent position (MIDIRS 1996b). This is to a great extent because of the frequent use of continuous electronic fetal monitoring, which fundamentally restrains and alters the experience of labour. Yet the freedom to move and to adopt different positions is an important way of helping women to cope with the pain of labour and may aid progress.

The research

The MIDIRS 'Informed choice' leaflet on positions in labour and delivery (1996b) comments that research into the effect of maternal position in labour on outcome has not been thorough. Many of the trials conducted on the first stage are methodologically poor, and most of the second-stage trials have focused only on the use of birth chairs (MIDIRS 1996b, pp. 3–4).

The limited evidence available suggests that women being upright in the first stage of labour results in:

- less severe pain
- less need for epidural anaesthesia and for narcotics
- lower rate of loss of beat-to-beat variability in the fetal heart rate
- reduced length of the first stage of labour

No measurable effects were detected on:

- rate of assisted delivery
- rate of caesarean delivery
- fetal or neonatal outcomes

The second stage
In 13 of the 17 randomised controlled trials which assess the effects of position on the second stage of labour, women sat on something: in three studies they were propped up in bed, in one they sat on a cushion, and in nine they used a rigid chair or stool. Thus, the findings may reflect the use of a birth

chair rather than the position per se. Systematic review of these trials shows that being upright in second stage results in:

- less discomfort
- less intolerable pain
- a shorter second stage of labour
- bearing down being less difficult
- fewer assisted and caesarean births
- fewer perineal and vaginal tears
- more labial tears
- more women with a blood loss over 500 mls (in women using birth chairs or stools)
- fewer postpartum wound infections.

Helping women to choose appropriate positions and move freely

The MIDIRS leaflet (1996b) comments that while 87% of units claim that women are 'allowed' to adopt whatever position they choose, the great majority of women spend all their labour either recumbent or semi-recumbent.

This may be because of the strong cultural norm of lying down for labour and birth. In this situation, the midwife needs positively to encourage and support women in adopting different positions and moving freely. Encouragement is given by suggestions, the use of props, creating enough space and active encouragement; the key is assessing what is best for the individual woman and her circumstances. However, encouraging women to move about, and to adopt the most comfortable positions, should not be taken to extremes. A number of women will want and need some rest during labour, often when in advanced labour, so rest and activity should be kept in balance. The woman should never lie flat on her back because of the danger of aortocaval compression and compromised uterine blood flow.

Such changes of position may integrate the use of water. I once looked after a very petite woman (5 ft; 1.53 m), who spent most of her labour curled up in the bottom of a shower cubicle with warm water playing on her back. When she got close to second stage, she got out and moved around. She gave birth to a baby that was well over 10 lb (4.5 kg) over an intact perineum.

Kitzinger (1997) describes the 'birth dance' that women do when they are left to their own devices and encouraged to move. Rocking, hip circling and adjustments of position may help to relieve pain and aid the progress of the baby through the birth canal.

USING INTERMITTENT AUSCULTATION IN LABOUR

We listen to the fetal heart in labour to screen for hypoxia in the fetus. This can be done by electronic fetal monitoring (either periodic or continuous) or intermittent auscultation. The evidence indicates that the use of intermittent auscultation in labour is associated with a higher rate of non-operative delivery and that the outcome for the baby is not generally compromised. We should be aware, when deciding how to monitor the baby's heart beat in labour, that the method chosen may affect not only the normal vaginal delivery rate, but also the nature of the birth and the experience. In addition, we should remember that the most effective monitor is the constant presence of a competent and attentive midwife who can interpret the data relating to fetal health. These data include an assessment of the fetal heart rate, using either intermittent auscultation or electronic fetal monitoring. The use of continuous electronic fetal monitoring in labour makes the experience more like that of an intensive care unit experience, limits mobility in the woman and may deflect attention from the labouring woman to the monitor. Belts, transducers and pressure gauges are extremely uncomfortable and need constant reapplication with movement of the mother or the baby.

Moreover, the accuracy of fetal monitoring in screening for fetal distress is questionable. Interpretation of the cardiotocograph (CTG) is often flawed. Electronic fetal monitoring has a low specificity. Not only is it associated with a high number of false positives, but there are also a number of false negatives (i.e. the diagnosis of fetal distress when there is none and the failure to detect distress when there is). For years, there has been an effort to improve the reliability of interpretation of CTGs through education, yet the problems remain. Moreover, electronic fetal monitoring is a screening tool that is more likely to be accurate in high-risk pregnancies. Thus, the routine use of electronic fetal monitoring in low-risk pregnancies increases the problems that this technique has caused. This is because, in low-risk pregnancies where there is a low prevalence of true fetal distress, the false positive rate will be higher (see Chapter 1).

Although policies in a number of countries, including the UK, the USA and Canada, have supported the use of intermittent auscultation for normal labour, the rate of routine use of electronic fetal monitoring remains high. Such monitoring is associated with a higher rate of operative delivery, including caesarean section.

The MIDIRS 'Informed choice' leaflet on fetal heart rate monitoring in labour (1996d, p. 4) includes the following information on electronic fetal monitoring (EFM), summarized from the best evidence:

When compared with intermittent auscultation:

- EFM, even when combined with fetal blood sampling (FBS), has not been shown to reduce perinatal mortality
- EFM, even when combined with FBS, has not been shown to reduce the incidence of cerebral palsy. Indeed, what evidence we have indicates a slight increase in cerebral palsy among infants who have been monitored
- EFM alone increases the caesarean section rate by about 160%. When used with FBS the rate of caesarean section increases by 30%
- EFM reduces the rate of neonatal seizures. However, those babies suffering neonatal seizures did not have any long-term problems, suggesting that the type of seizures prevented were not those which presage cerebral palsy.
- EFM increases the operative vaginal delivery rate by 30%
- There is no evidence of any benefit arising from the use of EFM in relation to the number of babies with low or very low Apgar scores or admissions to SCBU.

A more recent review and meta-analysis of fetal monitoring in labour indicates similar findings: no difference in Apgar score between groups receiving electronic fetal monitoring and intermittent ausculta-

tion, a slight increase in the rate of seizure in association with intermittent auscultation, and a higher incidence of operative delivery in association with electronic fetal monitoring (Thacker and Stroup, 1998; see also Chapter 2).

Based on a scientific study of the best available evidence, the Royal College of Obstetricians and Gynaecologists scientific study group on intrapartum fetal surveillance proposed the following guidelines (1993, pp. 390–1):

Auscultation is the method of choice for women at the normal end of the continuum of fetal risk. A Doppler device should be used in order to identify the fetal heart and distinguish the characteristic heart valve movements from the soufflé of blood flow in a vessel, which may be maternal.

The standard of intermittent auscultation evaluated by randomized controlled trial is as follows: auscultation for one complete minute beginning immediately after the end of a contraction, repeated every 15 minutes during first stage and while not pushing in the second stage, and after every maternal effort while pushing. All values should be recorded.

If the auscultated heart gives cause for concern then a

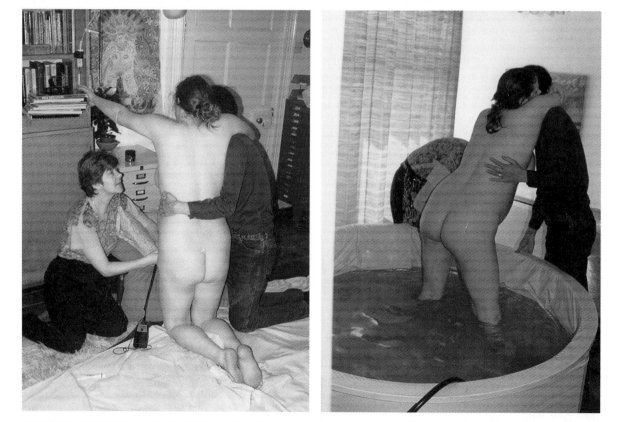

Figure 5.5   A Sonicaid enables the fetal heart to be heard when the woman adopts different positions. (Reproduced with kind permission from Uwe Kitzinger.)

continuous reading of the fetal heart rate should be obtained using an electronic fetal monitor (EFM). Blood sampling will be appropriate if the EFM record also causes concern.

Indications for EFM:
EFM should be used whenever there is an increased risk of hypoxaemia/acidaemia developing during labour.

A reduction or absence of liquor before labour and the appearance of meconium are indications for continuous FHR monitoring during labour.

Neilson (1993) recommends electronic fetal monitoring for *thick* meconium. It is difficult, however, to know why midwives continue to use the technique so frequently. It may in part be because they have lost the skill of intermittent auscultation. In encouraging the use of intermittent auscultation in any unit, it may help to undergo some retraining and to agree some protocols, based on the Royal College of Obstetricians and Gynaecologists' or other appropriate guidelines.

The following hints may help:

- If the woman has no objection to its use, a Doppler device (Sonicaid) will aid in listening to the fetal heart while the woman adopts different positions for labour and birth (Figs 5.5 and 5.6).
- During your first assessment of the women in labour, palpate carefully to determine the place where the heart will be heard (over the baby's shoulder and on the same side as the back).
- Auscultate the fetal heart while the woman is recumbent (but not flat on her back) so that you know where to find it when the woman is mobile and in different positions.
- I usually count during a contraction as well as afterwards, listening for any accelerations, which are indicative of an intact central nervous system and good fetal health.
- Use the knowledge you have gained from the interpretation of CTGs in interpreting the fetal heart rate.
- Record all values carefully.

(For further reading, see Page 1993.)

One of the advantages of intermittent auscultation is that it encourages a regular direct contact between midwife and mother through touch and words. It provides an opportunity for the midwife to give feedback to the labouring woman and to think about what she is assessing. It is also a point at which to use encouragement and support, for example 'Your baby sounds fine'.

In contrast, using a monitor for continuous electronic monitoring allows the midwife to be absent. I recently visited a large delivery suite where the CTGs from individual rooms were relayed onto one central bank of monitors, presumably to allow surveillance

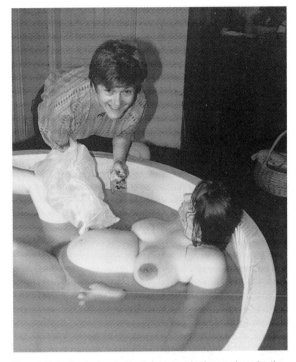

Figure 5.6 Listening to the fetal heart in the pool: a plastic bag protects the Sonicaid from the water. (Reproduced with kind permission from Uwe Kitzinger.)

from outside the individual rooms. It gave the impression of a modern-day nightmare.

However, for the times when electronic fetal monitoring is needed, it is important that midwives and doctors work together to standardize interpretation and for the continuation of professional development. It is also important that technology should be up to date and in working order and with all parts (especially belts, etc.) present. Importantly, the CTG should be interpreted regularly and a note made on the trace of the interpretation. It is vital to ensure that the attention of all who enter and stay in the room is on the woman rather than the screen.

I have suggested that, unless there is a clear indication or it is the wish of the woman, midwives should help the childbearing woman to avoid the use of continuous electronic fetal monitoring in labour and analgesia in labour. It is important that the woman is given good information ahead of labour so that she may consider her choices carefully. Any preferences she has should be recorded clearly in the medical records or on a birth plan. Aids such as the MIDIRS 'Informed choice' leaflets (1996a–1996d) will help a great deal in providing clear evidence-based information to women.

Pointers for practice

- An important function of the midwife is to confirm the normal and to support and protect physiological processes and healthy outcomes.
- The use of intermittent auscultation to monitor the fetal heart rate is associated with a lower operative delivery rate.
- Current guidelines recommend that intermittent auscultation should be used for labours at the normal end of the continuum.
- The use of epidural anaesthesia is associated with an increase in the operative delivery rate and needs a further evaluation of long-term outcomes for both mother and baby.
- Effective support is associated with a decrease in the need for analgesia, including epidural anaesthesia.
- Midwives should stay with women in labour and use words of praise and encouragement, as well as comforting touch.

CONCLUSION

In this chapter, I have not attempted to give a compre-

hensive overview of all aspects of care for labour and birth, nor have I examined clinical decision-making, which is in itself an important aspect of keeping birth 'normal' (see, however, the discussion in Chapter 1). Instead, I have chosen to suggest ways to help women to cope with the pain of labour without resorting to epidural anaesthesia, and have advised monitoring the fetal heart by intermittent auscultation, to increase the woman's likelihood of a non-operative vaginal birth. I have presented a summary of strong evidence indicating that the midwife's most important action for the mother and baby is to stay with them during labour. The approach to support in labour that I have described requires an integration of a constant presence, personal sensitivity and a calm atmosphere. It will be made much more likely if there is a good continuity-of-care scheme in place. I hope that this chapter has given at least a limited indication of some of the practical ways in which midwives may help women to 'keep birth normal'.

REFERENCES

Amu O, Rajendran S, Bolaji I 1998 Maternal choice alone should not determine method of delivery. British Medical Journal 317: 463–5

Beech B 1996 Water birth unplugged: proceedings of the first water birth conference. Books for Midwives Press, Cheshire

Department of Health 1993 Changing childbirth. Part 1. Report of the Expert Maternity Group (Cumberlege report). HMSO, London

Green J, Coupland B A, Kitzinger J 1988 Great expectations: a prospective study of women's expectations and experiences of childbirth. Child Care and Development Group, Cambridge

Green J, Curtis P, Price H, Renfrew M 1998 Continuing to care: the organization of midwifery services in the UK: a structured review of the evidence. Books for Midwives Press, Cheshire

Hedstrom L, Newton N 1986 Touch in labor: a comparison of cultures and eras. Birth 13(3): 181–6

Hodnett E D 1995 Support from caregivers during childbirth. Cochrane Database of Systematic Reviews, Issue 2. Update Software, Oxford

Howell C J 1997 Epidural vs non epidural analgesia in labour. In: Neilson J P, Crowther C A, Hodnett E D, Hofmeyr G J (eds) Pregnancy and childbirth module of the Cochrane Database of Systematic Reviews, updated 02 December 1997). Available in the Cochrane Library (database on disk and CDROM). Cochrane Collaboration, Issue 1. Update Software, Oxford

Kitzinger S 1997 Authoritative touch in childbirth. In: Davis-Floyd R E, Sargent C F (eds) Childbirth and authoritative knowledge: cross cultural perspectives. University of California Press, London

Leap N 1997 Birthwrite: being with women in pain – do midwives need to rethink their role? British Journal of Midwifery 3(5): 263

Leboyer F 1975 Birth without violence. Alfred A Knopf, New York

McCourt C, Page L 1996 Report on the evaluation of one-to-one midwifery. Thames Valley University, London

MIDIRS and NHS Centre for Reviews and Dissemination 1996a Informed choice for professionals: support in labour. MIDIRS, Bristol

MIDIRS and NHS Centre for Reviews and Dissemination 1996b Informed choice for professionals: positions in labour and delivery. MIDIRS, Bristol

MIDIRS and NHS Centre for Reviews and Dissemination 1996c Informed choice for professionals: epidurals for pain relief in labour. MIDIRS, Bristol

MIDIRS and NHS Centre for Reviews and Dissemination 1996d Informed choice for professionals: fetal heart rate monitoring in labour. MIDIRS, Bristol

Morgan B, Bulpitt C J, Clifton P, Lewis P J 1982 Analgesia and satisfaction in childbirth (the Queen Charlotte's 1,000 mother survey). Lancet ii: 808–10

Muscat J 1996 A thousand water births: selection criteria and outcome. In: Beech B (ed.) Water birth unplugged. Books for Midwives Press, Chestire

Neilson J 1993 Cardiotocography during labour: unsatisfactory technique but nothing better yet. British Medical Journal 306: 347–8

Nikodem V C 1999 Immersion in water during pregnancy labour and birth. Cochrane Review. Cochrane Library, Issue 1, Update Software, Oxford.

O'Driscoll K, Foley M, MacDonald D 1984 Active management of labour as an alternative to caesarean for dystocia. American Journal of Obstetrics and Gynecology 63: 485–90

Page L 1993 How and who should be monitored: the midwife's view. In: Ward M, Spencer J (eds) Intrapartum fetal surveillance in labour. RCOG, London

Patterson-Brown S 1998 Controversies in management. Should doctors perform an elective caesarean section on request? Yes, as long as the woman is fully informed. British Medical Journal 317: 462–3

Royal College of Obstetricians and Gynaecologists 1993 Recommendations on intra partum fetal surveillance In: Ward M, Spencer J (eds) Intrapartum fetal surveillance in labour. RCOG, London

Royal College of Obstetricians and Gynaecologists, Joint Working Group of the RCOG and RCM 1995 Communication standards obstetrics. RCOG, London

Robertson A 1997 The midwife companion: the art of support during birth. Ace Graphics, Sydney

Simkin P 1992 Just another day in a woman's life? Part II: Nature and consistency of women's long term memories of their first birth experiences. Birth 19(2): 64–81

Smulders B 1999 Future birth conferences. Ace Graphics, Australia

Thacker S B, Stroup D F 1998 Continuous electronic fetal heart monitoring during labor. Cochrane Library, Issue 4. Update Software, Oxford

Thornton J G, Lilford R J 1994 Active management of labour: current knowledge and research issues. British Medical Journal 309: 366–9

United Kingdom Central Council for Nursing, Midwifery and Health Visiting 1998 Midwives rules and code of practice. UKCC, London

Wagner M 1996 Birth in the 21st century: where are we going? In: Beech B (ed.) Water birth unplugged. Books for Midwives Press, Cheshire

6

Providing one-to-one practice and enjoying it

Lesley Ann Page   Pauline Cooke
Patricia Percival

For the childbearing woman, there is a world of difference between having a known and trusted midwife who is with her through the whole of pregnancy, birth and the early weeks of newborn life, and being in the care of strangers, no matter how kind. For midwives also, there is a world of difference between being with childbearing women through the entire journey of pregnancy and birth, and providing random and fragmented care to a number of different women. There is a mutual satisfaction in this relationship of being truly with the childbearing woman, which, as Sharpe, a midwife lecturer practitioner from McMaster University Ontario, Canada, comments 'supports and nourishes the caregiver as well as the woman' (personal communication 1997).

Campbell (1984), in his description of skilled companionship, says that companionship means being with rather than doing to. This implies a sense of personal involvement even with 'unpopular and difficult people'. This idea of companionship is particularly apt for midwives, who are with women as they journey through pregnancy and birth – an important and challenging journey or rite of passage. It is a journey during which physical and psychological growth and development, and growing love for the baby, help the woman and her partner to adapt to the new roles and challenges of mothering and fathering the child. Being with the woman and helping her to discover her own strengths, while offering skilled companionship, is crucial to this journey of adaptation, an adaptation in role to what are the most important and probably the most exacting responsibilities of adult life. Being able to accompany her on all parts of this journey, that is, caring for her during all the phases of pregnancy, labour, birth and the postnatal period, is important in terms of 'being with', rather than 'doing to'.

In recent decades in many countries, the dominant pattern of care has been fragmented and hospital based. This fragmentation has limited both the ability of midwives to follow women through the system of care, and the extent of their personal involvement with individual women. In this chapter, we propose a change to the conventional organization of practice, which will allow midwives to follow individual women through the entire system of care, including labour and birth. The movement away from fragmented structures in which midwives staff wards, departments or communities rather than care for individual women, requires both different organizations of practice and different approaches to practice. We believe that it should be the right of every childbearing woman to receive this care. We also believe that it is the right of every midwife to be able to practise in this way, and that this form of practice will, if managed appropriately, provide greater satisfaction to midwives.

In this chapter, we review some of the changes and policies that have supported midwives in the provision of continuous care. However, our main aim is to provide practical advice on how to set up, and practise within, systems that enable One-to-One relationships between childbearing women and midwives. The systems we propose should also enable professional autonomy and professional growth for midwives. Importantly, we present them as systems that undoubtedly call for commitment but which are potentially the most enjoyable form of midwifery practice available.

BEING WITH THE WOMAN: ORGANIZING FOR CONTINUOUS SENSITIVE CARE

Continuous sensitive care means responding knowledgeably and sensitively to the individual needs of women and their families. The provision of woman-centred care requires a particular organization of practice such as One-to-One care. We will describe One-to-One midwifery in more detail later in the chapter. The practice should allow what has come to be called 'continuity of carer'. In everyday language, this means enabling midwives to organize their practice so that they may form a continuing working relationship with women in their care. It means enabling midwives to work with women through the whole of pregnancy, birth and the early weeks of newborn life, so that they may get to know each other and form a relationship that is based on trust between the two. This relationship, of trust and mutual respect, is fundamental to midwifery. Such a relationship – the working friendship – goes beyond like and dislike, and is a strong foundation for the sensitivity and effective use of skills and knowledge that are crucial to midwifery.

One-to-One midwifery practice enables individual midwives to provide most of the hands-on care, to lead care and to be with individual women in their care whenever possible for labour and birth. It is important, and possible, when planning different organizations, to be aware of the personal needs of midwives for adequate time off from practice and support for effective practice.

We view a change in the pattern of practice to allow continuity of carer as a necessary but not sufficient measure to develop woman-centred care. New patterns of practice are necessary to provide constant support in labour, to provide information at the right time and in the right place and to respond to women's individual needs. However, sensitive care also requires of midwives skills and positive attitudes. In particular, it demands personal sensitivity, clinical competence, skills and knowledge. Continuous care is the most likely form of care to enable sensitive scientific practice.

Place of care

The most extreme opposites in terms of place of care and birth are home versus acute care hospital. Although it may seem like a contradiction in terms, many of the alternative birth centres have tried to create a more home-like environment in a hospital setting, as for example, in home-from-home units (MacVicar et al 1993) and hospital-attached birth centres. There are also a number of free-standing birth centres that are not attached to any hospital. In Britain, a number of small, community-based or GP unit maternity centres have survived. These seem to have detracted from the need to set up alternative birth centres, which are more common in Australia and the USA. In Australia from the 1970s onward, the number of birth centres has increased to 24 in 1997 (Waldenstrom & Lawson 1997). Although a major impetus was consumer demand, a federal grant of A$6.4 million to fund alternative birthing services assisted the setting-up of such centres. Regardless of the number of birth centres, at present fewer than 3% of women giving birth do so in such settings. Moreover, equitable access may be limited by a number of factors not related to consumer choice. For example, women deemed to be 'too old' or 'not low risk' may be denied access even when the birth centre is attached to a maternity hospital. Furthermore, geographic factors may mitigate against some women being able to access such care. Lecky-Thompson (1995) argued that the increasing number of birth centres has actually led to a disintegration in the consumer voice calling for change: they allow women a choice, but this choice is limited by a number of factors.

The place of care is likely to be the most important determinant of the way in which a midwife practises and may be a strong influence on the outcome of birth (see Chapter 1). Despite all the alternatives created, it should be remembered that home birth still offers the best opportunity for enhancing the experience and clinical outcome of birth for those women without complications who wish to give birth at home. Oakley (1997) commented on the fact that the majority of women who give birth at home find the experience enjoyable, whereas, despite efforts for many years to 'humanize' hospital birth, it never quite seems to work (see Chapter 1). Institutions, by their very nature, will always have a tendency to depersonalize care. It requires constant attention to ensure that each woman and her family are cared for as individuals, particularly in large institutions.

Clarifying the concepts

Any institution, whether it be a small birthing centre or a large hospital, is unlikely to provide exactly what a home birth can offer. However, in most of the industrialized world, hospital birth has become the norm. It is important, therefore, to push back the boundaries of practice to provide the most individual, sensitive and safest care possible when women choose to give birth in a hospital setting. Nowadays, hospitals are regarded as the safest place to give birth, yet there are a number of potential dangers of hospital birth, which need to be considered carefully and counteracted (see, for example, Audit Commission 1998). These include:

- the tendency to leave women unattended in labour;
- fragmented care;
- the frequent routine use of medical interventions such as acceleration of labour and induction of labour;
- the frequent routine use of electronic fetal monitoring.

New organizations of midwifery, such as the Know Your Midwife practice and One-to-One midwifery practice, were developed for a number of reasons, including to provide more individual care that is responsive to the needs of the individual woman and her family, and to challenge the increasingly surgical approach to birth. When women receive most of their care from one named lead professional, it usually enhances their experience of pregnancy, birth and care, and increases their confidence in mothering (McCourt & Page 1996) (see Chapters 11 and 12). There has been

less success in reducing the frequency of medical and surgical interventions in birth apart from the performance of episiotomy and the need for pain relief in labour (Green et al 1998).

For nearly two decades, there have been attempts by hospitals to provide what has come to be known as 'woman-centred care', that is, care which is intended primarily to meet the individual needs of the woman and her family rather than meeting the needs of the institution. Many of these changes have been successful, but many have not. Confusion seems to surround the ideas or concepts that underlie these changes, and unless they are clearly defined, understood and agreed, no organizational change can succeed.

There are a number of key concepts in the move to more woman-centred structures of care, and it is necessary to be clear about what is meant when we use words to describe these concepts or ideas. Such conceptual clarification is important for a number of reasons. First, effective organizational change requires that the purpose is clear, and such clarity of purpose requires that everyone involved be speaking the same language. Second, these abstract concepts can be different, and have very different effects, when they are applied in practice.

Below we offer some definitions of the most important concepts.

Continuity of care or continuity of carer?

In most industrialized countries, with the exception of a few such as the Netherlands and now New Zealand and Canada, the majority of midwives practise within an institutional setting. Where this is the case, the development of systems of care that allow midwives to work in a continuous relationship with women and their families, over most of the process of maternity, requires a dramatic shift in the way in which these institutions function. In fact, midwives have become so used to what is an industrial model of care that continuity of care is seen as the alternative rather than being fundamental to midwifery. Practice has been influenced by a society in which factory organizations have affected many forms of work and life. Thus, the most common model of midwifery care over recent decades has been an assembly line approach, the woman progressing along the line at different points in her pregnancy. Industrial society also brought about a clearer separation of personal and professional life than had been known before, Midwives were once part of the communities where they practised; now their lives and work are quite separate. Changes in the organization of practice, such as the development of

One-to-One midwifery, often create an easy integration and balancing of personal and professional life.

It is possibly because there is such a strong norm towards these industrial models of practice that the creation of continuity of carer across whole services has been quite difficult. In addition, the development of alternatives such as team midwifery, group practice or One-to-One midwifery creates a number of practical organizational challenges and requires a huge change in attitudes. It may be these practical difficulties which have led to the continued debate on and controversy over continuity of care and what it means. Some have claimed that women want continuity of care (consistency of policy and approach from a team of care-givers) rather than continuity of carer (the majority of care coming from a named individual midwife supported by a small number of other midwives).

The development of systems of care that allow midwives to work in relationship with women and allow midwives to practise autonomously were influenced by the Know Your Midwife project (Flint et al 1989), a title that is explicit about the relationship between midwife and woman. Later, team midwifery was set up in a number of places. These teams sometimes moved away from the fundamental idea of having a small number of midwives looking after individual women, to much larger teams that were often hospital based. Later, in order to move on from a whole variety of forms of care subsumed under the name of team midwifery, the term 'midwifery group practice' was developed. This implies smaller groups of midwives caring for individual women, and those midwives 'carried a caseload' (Page 1995a). Later, a distinction was made between carrying a team caseload (a team of midwives looking after individual women) and carrying a personal caseload (in which an individual midwife takes the responsibility for the care of individual women) but with the support of other midwives in the group.

In Australia, women can access continuity of carer within birth centres, for home births and in some mainstream hospital settings (Rowley et al 1995, Rowley 1998). Midwives within a birth centre setting may work within a small team or group, with either a team or personal caseload, and are usually employed by the birth centre or attached hospital. Those independent midwives working within a home birth setting may work alone, or closely with one or two colleagues, to provide continuity of carer and are in most cases employed by the pregnant woman.

Although progress has been slower than in the UK, a number of exciting and innovative programmes have been set up during the late 1980s and 90s within Australian mainstream hospital settings to provide continuity of carer. Published reports of these programmes include those of Rowley et al (1995) Kenny et al (1994), Aiken (1997), Gumley et al (1997) and Waldenstrom (1996). A number of other programmes are also being planned or have recently commenced throughout Australia. Such programmes are largely the result of the efforts of midwives committed to improving maternity care for women.

Shared care

This term usually implies care that is shared between the consultant medical team and the GP or family doctor. It has become the dominant form of care in most of the industrialized world. In Britain, this has usually meant that the woman is seen by a number of different people. The GP team will often consist of a community midwife and one or more GPs, and the consultant team will consist of a number of doctors of different ranks, any of whom might see the woman. This system of shared care was intended to give all women access to and assessment by a specialist; in general, however, it has led to highly fragmented care. Even when the woman has full hospital care, she may be seen by a number of different people. In Australia and many other parts of the world, the role of the midwife may be very limited during the antenatal period in some shared care teams. During labour, a midwife provides care, but in many situations, the obstetrician or GP will attend the birth. Similarly, a midwife provides postnatal care, but a doctor also visits the woman in hospital. As well as being the recipients of fragmented and duplicated care, women may also be the recipients of a greater number of obstetric interventions. For example, Australia has one of the highest rates of obstetric intervention in the developed world (Day et al 1997).

Continuity of care

This term implies a shared philosophy and approaches to care. It is not enough in itself to satisfy the needs of women for a continuing *relationship* with a midwife.

Named midwife

The named midwife is the primary midwife, who is responsible for planning care together with the woman and her family, and ensuring that care is of a high standard. The named midwife should be accessible to the women in her care for the majority of time and provides most of the direct hands-on care. The named midwife may well work with the support of a number of other midwives in her practice. In Britain, all women, whether low or high risk, receive midwifery care, so the named midwife may or may not be the lead professional.

Lead professional

The named midwife may be the lead professional for women with low-risk pregnancies. The lead professional is legally responsible and accountable to the woman and her family, and to the institution in which care is provided, for the provision of effective and appropriate care. The lead professional may be a doctor or a midwife. It is important that the lead professional provides most of the hands-on care and is involved, together with the woman, in making decisions about place of birth and treatment.

Midwifery-led care

This encompasses a system in which midwives are accountable for and take responsibility for the care of a number of low-risk women. It may also imply an explicit midwifery philosophy and midwifery protocols or guidelines that reflect the need to support physiological processes. This does not mean that the woman never sees a doctor as cross-referral may often be needed.

Alternative birthing centre

Birth or birthing centres offer a physical environment that is conducive to physiological birth or normal birth. They are usually explicitly family centred and put a particular philosophy into practice. They may be privately funded and are often small enough for a sharing of values and ways of working among all staff. They may also be small enough for families to get to know all staff very easily, although they may not seek to achieve continuity of care. Birth centres may be free standing, that is, away from hospital, or be part of a hospital setting, either in the grounds or in the hospital building itself.

Home-from-home

The first home-from-home unit was developed in Leicester in the 1980s. The unit is usually a part of the labour and delivery area but is furnished in a more homely way. It is a place for the care of women with low-risk pregnancies who will be transferred to conventional care if complications arise (MacVicar et al 1993).

Choice and control

The Winterton report (House of Commons 1992) highlighted the need for women to have choice, continuity and control in the birth of their babies. Simply speaking, choice and control imply that women should have a choice of where they give birth, who should look after them and the kind of treatment they should receive. To a great extent, the idea of giving childbearing women choice and control has become rhetoric. This is a simple idea that is a shorthand for a number of important principles that may have a profound outcome on the short- and long-term health and welfare of the individuals and families concerned.

Perhaps the best short description of giving women control is given in the report of the Expert Maternity Group (Department of Health 1993; see also Chapter 3):

The woman must be the focus of maternity care. She should be able to feel that she is in control of what is happening to her and able to make decisions about her care, based on her needs, having discussed matters fully with the professionals involved.

Skilled companion

The term 'skilled companion' is taken from the book *Moderated Love* by Campbell (1984). He originally formulated the concept to describe the relationship between a nurse and a patient, and used the imagery of a journey in which companionship arises from a chance meeting and is terminated when the joint purpose that keeps the companions together no longer applies (p. 49). Four features of this relationship are outlined:

1. Companionship involves a bodily presence and necessitates sensitivity.
2. Companionship includes the notion of helping another to move onward on the journey with encouragement and hope.
3. Companionship means 'being with' rather than just 'doing to' in the sense of personal involvement, even with 'unpopular' and 'difficult' people.
4. Companionship involves a limited commitment that is for the duration of the journey, recognizing that both companions have their own lives to lead.

Caseload practice

In caseload practice, the midwife 'carries a caseload'; in other words, she is responsible for, and provides most of the care for, a number of women and their families through the whole process of pregnancy, labour and birth, and during the early weeks after the baby's birth. It implies following the woman through the system rather than staffing wards and departments or communities.

It is important to emphasize the term 'practice'. Implicit in this term is the sense of midwives organizing their own practice in the way in which a group of doctors might, in other words being responsible for cover and setting and monitoring standards (National Childbirth Trust 1995).

One-to-One midwifery practice

One-to-One midwifery practice integrates a high degree of continuity in which a named midwife provides most of the care for a number of women and their families, and acts as lead professional (midwifery-led care) when a woman has a low-risk pregnancy. The One-to-One midwife will also care for 'high-risk' women, for whom she will be the named midwife and work together with the responsible doctor. It is more than a structural organization, however. The term 'One-to-One' is meant to imply creating the potential for the development of the special relationship that is possible between the woman and her midwife, a supportive organization in which the midwife may practise and fully develop her skills. One-to-One midwives are organized in small group practices and 'carry a caseload'. They are generally responsible for women in a limited locality, which makes the practice more effective. They usually relate to a small number of family doctors' practices in order to enhance appropriate referral and communication between professionals.

Midwives take on a 'personal' caseload; that is, they are named midwife for individual women and provide most of the care for those women. If the named midwife is off duty, her partner, who has met and knows the women in the named midwife's practice, is on call. This is different from a 'team caseload', in which a team of six or more midwives takes the on-call for a number of women whom they may or may not have met. Being on call for known women seems to be easier than being on call for unknown women.

The initial One-to-One midwifery programme in London was set up in 1993 to put the principles of the *Changing Childbirth* report (Department of Health 1993) into practice in one maternity service. This was the first time that such a service had been implemented within the NHS, although One-to-One midwifery practice is very similar to the way in which independent midwives practise and are organized. Since then, the scheme has been replicated in a number of other maternity services, including Shrewsbury and Leicester.

It was intended as a change to both the structure and the culture of care. Twenty midwives were organized into partnerships. These partners form three group practices, providing total care for 40 women from each midwife. The named midwife provides most of the care for individual women, but the partner gets to know the women and covers when the named midwife is unavailable. A high level of continuity has been achieved. There are a number of important elements to this scheme:

- a shift of most care to the community;
- a high level of continuity;
- midwives carrying a personal caseload rather than being on call for a number of women they do not know;
- professional autonomy and flexibility, so that midwives may be in control of, organize and prioritize their own work;
- the combination of responsibility for a personal caseload combined with partner and group support.

The evaluation of One-to-One midwifery indicated a reduction in some important interventions in association with One-to-One care as well as showing that it cost no more than conventional care. There were more positive responses from women receiving One-to-One care than from women in the control group (McCourt & Page 1996, Page 1996, Piercey et al 1996, Page et al 1997, Beake et al 1998, McCourt et al 1998).

The continuum of care

Many of these ideas can be usefully viewed on a continuum, particular forms or models of care representing a particular place on the continuum (Fig. 6.1).

FROM STAFFING THE SERVICE TO CARING FOR INDIVIDUAL WOMEN AND THEIR FAMILIES

Moving policy into practice

In most parts of the industrialized world, the shift from structures where midwives worked as obstetric nurses, for the most part staffing wards and departments in hospitals, to systems in which the midwife 'worked with women where and when wanted', started about the early 1980s. Where midwives staff the service, they may be permanently allocated to one area, for example the delivery suite or the community, or they may rotate around the various areas. Such an approach centres on the needs of the institution rather than the needs of individual women. It is likely, as

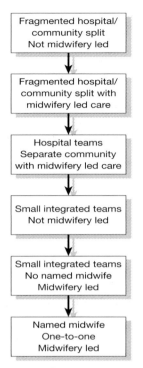

Fig. 6.1   The continuum of care.

Brodie (1997) notes, to lead to an allegiance to the institution rather than the woman. The shift to woman-centred care has helped to transcend the barriers that hospital work and a rigid shift system represented: it has offered the opportunity to profoundly change practice for both childbearing women and midwives. Although independent and lay midwives in many parts of the world, particularly Britain, Canada and the USA, had continued to provide such women-centred rather than institutionally centred care, this was confined to small numbers of women.

What is significant to the shift in emphasis that started in a very practical way in the 1980s is that it sought to reach the women who were part of the mainstream maternity service. For example, the Grace Hospital Low Risk Midwifery Project in Vancouver (Weatherston 1985) and the Know Your Midwife project (Flint et al 1989) both provided care for a small number of women and families who were attending hospital for their care. Both involved four midwives getting to know and caring for a small number of women and families, and both projects were based on a high degree of continuity of carer. Moreover, the midwives in both projects saw them as prototypes of systems that they wished to see developed for all women.

A substantial change has occurred in the majority of maternity services in Britain and in some maternity services in other parts of the world. This change has, however, usually been confined to a portion of the service rather than involving a change to the service overall. The extent of the change is also quite variable, from large teams that are hospital based to One-to-One midwifery practices. In Britain, between 1987 and 1990, over 100 maternity services had set up some form of team midwifery (Wraight et al 1993). The emphasis in Britain has been in transforming the hospital service and in moving a substantial amount of care to the community. This has been made possible because, in the main, maternity services have always been integrated between the hospital and the community.

Other parts of the world, including some provinces of Canada and New Zealand, have established midwifery as a primary care service and put midwives on a par with medical practitioners, giving women the right to choose between doctor- or midwifery-led care.

Policy changes

To a large extent, the policy changes that occurred in Britain followed changes that had already started in a practical way. Nonetheless, the importance and significance of these policy changes should not be underestimated. Putting policy into practice, especially with such fundamental change, is never easy. However, having policy backing makes such change easier than it would be without such backing. Importantly, the creation of government policy that pronounced the values of giving women control in the birth of their babies, of having midwives practise their skills fully and of the importance of a known and trusted carer to women and their families signified a shift in the mainstream of thought.

Earlier government policy documents had emphasized the importance of continuity of care to women but had still accepted the dogma of the importance of inadequately evaluated technology such as fetal monitoring. Even despite a movement to increasing continuity of care, shared care was promoted as an ideal form of practice with little apparent awareness that this was a contradiction in terms (Maternity Services Advisory Committee 1982, Department of Health Maternity Services 1992).

The Winterton report (House of Commons 1992) marked a watershed in thinking in Britain. It is a detailed piece of work, with a number of recommendations. It is also a broad report dealing with a number of social as well as health care issues that affect women's and children's health. This was the first report to question what had amounted to a faith in the indiscriminate use of technology such as electronic fetal heart rate monitoring.

The Cumberlege report (Department of Health 1993) was the English government's response to the Winterton report. *Changing Childbirth* set an agenda for change in the maternity services in England and became policy for the maternity services in 1993 (NHSE). In many ways, *Changing Childbirth* reflected Winterton, but it was focused on the provision of the maternity services. It set specific targets and indicators of success for the providers and commissioners of maternity care. The recommendations of the report were based on three fundamental principles of care (Department of Health 1993, p. 18):

The woman must be the focus of maternity care. She should be able to feel that she is in control of what is happening to her and able to make decisions about her care, based on her needs, having discussed matters fully with the professionals involved.

Maternity services must be readily and easily accessible to all. They should be sensitive to the needs of the local population and based primarily in the community.

Women should be involved in the monitoring and planning of maternity services to ensure that they are responsive to the needs of a changing society. In addition care should be effective and resources used efficiently.

The following indicators of success give an indication of the nature of the practical changes proposed.

Within 5 years

1. All women should be entitled to carry their own case notes.

2. Every woman should know one midwife who ensures the continuity of her midwifery care – the named midwife.

3. At least 30% of women should have the midwife as the named professional.

4. Every woman should know the lead professional who has a key role in the planning and provision of care.

5. At least 75% of women should know the person who cares for them during their delivery.

6. Midwives should have direct access to some beds in all maternity units.

7. At least 30% of women delivered in a maternity unit should be admitted under the management of the midwife.

8. The total number of antenatal visits for women with uncomplicated pregnancies should have been reviewed in the light of the available evidence and the Royal College of Obstetricians and Gynaecologists' guidelines.

9. All front-line ambulances should have a para-

medic able to support the midwife who needs to transfer a woman to the hospital in an emergency.

10. All women should have access to information about the services available in their locality.

Health Authorities and National Health Service Trusts were given 5 years in which to implement Changing Childbirth Services (National Health Service Executive 1994). This Changing Childbirth policy has been endorsed by the subsequent government and by other policy documents (Department of Health 1997, 1998).

The strength of these British reports was the specific timeframe given in which to implement changes. In Australia, during the late 1980s and 90s, a number of maternity care reviews were conducted, which resulted in specific recommendations. However, in many cases, these recommendations lacked specific timeframes for their implementation as well as adequate indicators to measure success (Ministerial Task Force on Obstetrical Services in New South Wales 1989; Ministerial Review of Birthing Services in Victoria 1990; Ministerial Task Force WA 1990, Select Committee on Intervention in Childbirth 1995, National Health and Medical Research Council 1996).

Evaluation of innovations

The majority of maternity services in Britain have now piloted either continuity of care schemes or midwifery-led services. Many of these have not been evaluated (Wraight et al 1993, Green et al 1998). Although this is a real lost opportunity, it is not surprising: midwives have had few resources or support to evaluate such innovations. Moreover, the work was politically sensitive and often accomplished against great difficulties. It was extremely hard to obtain funding for such projects, and experience indicates that there always has been, and continues to be, cynicism about such innovations. In addition, the evaluation of such innovations is technically difficult. Neither is the randomized controlled trial, the dominant methodology in the health services, the most appropriate or practical form of evaluation.

However, a number of evaluations have been undertaken (Green et al 1998). As yet, there is no complete and comprehensive systematic review of all the evidence. Such a review will require an integration of qualitative research with quantitative research if it is to be useful. A limited 'structured' review of a number of studies is available, but a number of the important evaluations are excluded, and there is no account of qualitative research in this review. The conclusion that 'the evidence does not suggest a need for the enormous efforts of service reorganisation which are need-ed to ensure that a woman is cared for in labour by a midwife that she knows' is questionable and goes beyond the evidence cited (Green et al 1998, p. 138).

THE KNOWN AND TRUSTED MIDWIFE

Why is continuity of carer important, and how is it best provided?

The issue of whether or not continuity of carer is important to women and acceptable to midwives has been, as well as the basis of welcome change, the major divisive issue in midwifery in much of the industrial-ized world over the past decade. It may be divisive because the provision of continuity of carer brings about truly fundamental change, a change that alters the experience of pregnancy and birth for women in a profound way. Similarly, it profoundly alters the meaning, experience and expectations of midwifery for midwives. In general, it alters the allegiance of the mid-wife from being primarily to the institution, to being with the woman (Brodie 1997). Such a profound change tends to affect individuals and organizations deeply, on a number of levels and in a number of ways, and may provoke great support but also great hostility.

The most difficult aspect of continuity of carer to organize is that for labour and birth. This also seems to be the most contentious issue among the critics. Some argue that existing evidence does not support the view that women want continuity of care in labour (Green et al 1998). However, in this case, qualitative research (for example, Rutter 1996, Proctor 1997, McCourt et al 1998), which may better answer the question of what it is that women value about continuity of care for labour and birth, has been ignored.

In general, quantitative research is too limited to identify any links between continuity of carer and par-ticular outcomes, or indeed whether or not a known midwife in labour is important to women. The imple-mentation of continuity of carer brings about the intro-duction of a whole package of care. Indeed, that is the very purpose of these schemes: to change the structure so that other aims, such as constant support in labour, the provision of better information and more sensitive care, may be accomplished. These other factors are sometimes seen by researchers as confounding vari-ables rather than part of the change. Evaluating a new model of care that entails a different approach does not lend itself to the manipulation of different variables to see what is associated with what, an approach that has been suggested for future research (Green et al 1998).

Where evidence does exist, fundamental problems often arise in interpreting the importance of a known carer in labour. It is common sense that having a known carer in labour will not be important if that carer is unskilled or insensitive, yet a number of stud-ies continue to rank women's wants in a way indicat-ing that a known carer in labour is less important than other things. Indeed, Green et al (1998) conclude that 'What probably matters most is that she [the child-bearing woman] should feel that they are competent and that they care – about her.' Of course, any woman having to choose between a known carer, and kind-ness, skill and enough information, would choose the latter. In life, the aim is to provide a known midwife who is also sensitive, knowledgeable and kind. Green et al overlook the problem of caring for the individual woman when the system mitigates against this.

The most difficult issue of all in establishing the importance of a known carer for labour and birth arises from the difficulty of adequately evaluating women's responses to care. Measures of satisfaction are rarely adequate in establishing any answers to such ques-tions. As we commented in the evaluation of One-to-One practice (McCourt et al 1998, p. 79):

satisfaction surveys are fraught with difficulties, from defining or deconstructing, the concept of satisfaction to deciding how questions should be asked. On the whole, responses to consumer surveys tend to be neutralised by the use of broad satisfaction measures.

More open-ended data, such as those gained from open-ended responses or from interviews, may be con-sistent with more concrete responses but may reveal greater differences in perception between groups (McCourt et al 1998). These more open, less structured responses may also explain what it is about continuity that women appreciate.

There are a number of fundamental problems in establishing whether or not new forms of care, such as the provision of a known midwife in labour, are of importance to women. The most important of these is the tendency for women to be satisfied with what they expect, that is, what is must be best (Porter & Macintyre 1984). Moreover, many women feel immense obligation to the staff who have cared for them and relief at having a live baby; these feelings may be expressed in broad terms as satisfaction with the service even when the women have experienced great distress (McCourt et al 1998).

Continuity and knowing one's carers were the most common themes across both groups in the evaluation of One-to-One midwifery practice. Women in the One-to-One group said that this was something they want-ed to keep and advocated extending the service to other areas, while women in the control group high-lighted this as an aspect needing change or improve-ment (McCourt & Page 1996). In general, the evidence from this study was overwhelmingly that women pre-fer continuity of care and carer where it is possible (McCourt & Page 1996).

We are now, with the availability of more open-ended qualitative research, beginning to understand what it is that women appreciate about continuity. It is important to understand that it is valuable in its own right. As one woman, comparing her experience with a previous birth, commented (Garcia et al 1998, p. 60):

My first delivery was with a selection of different midwives and students who came and went as they pleased which I found very distressing and upsetting. My most recent delivery was totally different. So much different – it was wonderful to have a midwife I had met before and who stayed with me the whole time – I just wish this had been the case the first time as I am sure that it wouldn't have been so horrendous or distressing if this had been the case.

A structure that allows continuity of care-giver also allows the development of a special relationship, one that is something like friendship but not exactly that (Wilkins 1995, Sharpe, personal communication 1997). In the One-to-One project, women reported feeling closer to a midwife than other health professionals, and this was likely to be their named midwife (McCourt & Page 1996).

Women who value this special relationship and the availability of a known trusted midwife emphasize the confidence, support and reassurance that knowing one's midwife provides (McCourt & Page 1996). This finding was supported by comments made by women in Garcia's study; as one woman commented: 'It was wonderful knowing them [a team of midwives]. It gave me a lot more confidence in my care' (Garcia et al 1998, p. 58).

Continuity of care-giver may also improve the amount of information given to women and the way in which it is provided. This was an issue raised by nearly all women in the qualitative evaluation of One-to-One care. Control group women were far more likely to mention information or communication as a problem, and of the ethnic minority women in the control group, only one was happy about the level of informa-tion received (McCourt & Page 1996)

Naturally, women do not want continuity enhanced in one area of care to the detriment of continuity in another. In the Audit Commission study (1998), 23 women commented voluntarily on continuity of care in the antenatal period, although there were no ques-tions related to this in the survey. Quite a few of these comments about continuity referred to the difficulties of having to explain things to different members of staff, as well as to women's worries that clinical care might not be as good when many care-givers were involved (Garcia et al 1998). The One-to-One evalua-tion found that although most women in both groups wanted to see their main carer for antenatal care, this applied more in the study group (86.3% versus 49.3%).

Those women who have had the experience of being cared for in labour by a known midwife tend to rate this as being more important (McCourt & Page 1996, Green et al 1998). Continuity in labour is important for a number of reasons. First, it allows a constant pres-ence in labour, a factor important to both mother and baby (Hodnett 1998). In the One-to-One study, we found that the majority of One-to-One women had constant support in labour compared with just over half the control group. Women value continuity for a number of reasons. When asked in the antenatal period, 'would you prefer your main carer to attend the birth' few women in either group said that they would rather not know the person (7 controls versus 1 One-to-One woman). A large majority (84%) of One-to-One women said, 'yes very much'. The views of control group women were fairly widely spread. Although their most frequent response was that they did not mind whether this person was available (27.5%), this was closely followed by 'yes very much' (26.9%). Both mothers who knew and those who did not know about the One-to-One service expressed the belief that labour and delivery would have been much easier if they had known the midwife beforehand. Rutter (1996), who undertook an independent analysis of open-ended responses, confirmed this finding.

Proctor (1997), in her study of perceptions of quality in the maternity services, also describes a consistent theme from her antenatal interviews of the importance of familiarity with the midwife. They wanted, she comments, to feel that they would know, or even rec-ognize, the person who would care for them in labour. She comments that, during the process of labour, the significance of continuity of carer seemed to increase in importance from the early hours to during the actu-al delivery. Interestingly, in the same study, midwives' comments on the perceived importance of continuity for the mother were divided (Proctor 1997).

Morrison et al (1999), in a phenomenological study of families who gave birth at home, found that a consistent theme was the midwife knowing the person in labour and a person knowing them and what they wanted. Coyle (1998) undertook a qualitative study of 17 women who gave birth in a birth centre but had previously given birth in a hospital, reporting that women emphasized the importance of cumulative interactions and the opportunity to develop an ongoing relationship with the midwife. These cumulative interactions resulted in:

- women being comfortable with carers and at ease; and
- women being known by carers.

In both of the above, it was particularly important in labour that the midwife knew them, what they wanted, how they might act, their fears and so on.

Despite these problems, data that point to the importance of continuity of carer and explain why it is important to women do exist. In addition, some work is ongoing; for example, a further analysis of open-ended and interview and focus group responses from women receiving One-to-One care is in process.

In Allen et al's (1997) study, the majority of women who had experienced the presence of their named midwife at delivery said that it mattered a lot. In general, they valued the enormous rapport that had been built up and the trust that had been established. Although, in general, the demand for continuity of care is greater from women who know that they can expect it, many other women also express a desire for greater continuity. For example, women receiving One-to-One care had higher levels of continuity of care-giver and midwife-led care than those in conventional care. Both groups of women expressed a desire for continuity of care-giver and midwife-led care, and wanted this in a community setting, although this was more pronounced in the study group. Nevertheless, a number of women in the control group who were not offered such care expressed a desire for change in this direction (McCourt et al 1998).

An ethnographic study was undertaken by Walsh, which involved women cared for by midwives in the Bumps (Birth under midwife) scheme in Leicester. This scheme was set up to replicate One-to-One midwifery practice. From his interviews of 10 women who had experienced the care, Walsh described a significant positive impact on women's experience of childbirth. The relationship that evolved between women and their midwives was highly valued by women. Walsh describes this relationship as being of overriding significance and differing when compared with earlier childbirth experiences. Birth under the Bumps' system led to an experience that was described in the interviews in terms of friendship with the midwife, a known midwife for intrapartum care and expressions of delight and gratitude. Walsh described the reflections of care, which were given as 'I was' statements, and characteristics were described using the midwives' names. In contrast, previous experiences of

birth were a 'powerful negative experience of maternity care in a hospital context and critical, depersonalised "S/he was" and "they were" statements about caregivers' (Walsh 1998, p. 49). These depersonalized statements perhaps reflect the depersonalization of the care experienced. Walsh mentions the possible bias of his sample because the majority of women in his study had given birth at home (Walsh 1998). However, his report reflects the experience of other women receiving such highly personal midwifery care in the One-to-One system: that it is as likely to be the relationship of care as the setting that leads to such responses.

Labour is a critical time for the woman, but it should be remembered that the postnatal period may also be a distressing time, and supportive care is crucial in the postpartum period. As Garcia et al (1998) comment, lack of continuity at this time may lead to conflicting advice, something that many parents find very difficult.

It is naturally important, as Green et al (1998) note, that expectations of continuity are not raised without the probability of their being fulfilled. This is likely to lead to increased disappointment. It is particularly important, therefore, to develop a system allowing continuity through the whole period and all trimesters of pregnancy, that is unlikely to fail the woman. In this respect, the One-to-One project was particularly successful (McCourt & Page 1996).

Why is continuity important to midwives, and how is such practice best organized?

The commitment of many of the midwives who implemented continuity of carer schemes has come from the direct experience of providing a personal and continuous service to individual women through pregnancy, birth and the weeks thereafter. It is an experience that may transform approaches and attitudes to practice (see, for example, Bissett 1995, Couves 1995, Minns 1995, Page 1995b, Farmer & Chipperfield 1996, Brodie 1997).

Common themes

Many midwives who practise in continuity of care schemes apply to do so because of extreme dissatisfaction with the conventional service and because they feel their role to be limited by it. Once in a continuity of care scheme, they usually express a reluctance to return to the conventional service. Midwives commonly express intense satisfaction when providing continuity of care. One of the most important aspects of this satisfaction seems to be the possibility of special relationships with women in their care, a finding confirmed by Sandall (1997). This is often referred to as a friendship (Wilkins 1995, James 1997, Walsh 1998, Sharpe, personal communication 1997). Other commonly encountered themes are the flexibility and autonomy enabled by such schemes, the intense learning that this form of practice provides and encourages, and the ability to identify and meet women's real needs.

The familiar way of practice for the majority of midwives practising in the industrialized world is primarily hospital based. Midwives, in general, work shifts and do not follow women through the system. When we work in our own familiar systems, there is a tendency to take familiar ways and routines for granted. Looking outside to a completely different way of practice often casts a different light on the things that are taken for granted. In countries such as Britain, private practice or independent midwifery still exists, although in very small numbers. In Canada, where midwifery has only recently been regulated in a number of provinces, midwives worked outside the formal health care system in a private practice arrangement. Now, in the provinces that have started to regulate midwifery, midwifery remains community based with a requirement for the provision of continuity of carer. In New Zealand, which has undertaken radical reforms of midwifery and the provision of maternity services, there is a regulatory and professional recognition and acceptance of the underlying principle of partnership in the definition of midwifery, and midwifery is community based (Guilliland & Pairman 1995). These models of practice offer an insight into a different way of practising as a midwife.

Changing Childbirth (Department of Health 1993) was based on an understanding of the importance of the relationship between the woman and her midwife, and the power of the establishment of trust between the two. Similarly, Guilliland & Pairman (1995) are explicit about the woman–midwife relationship, which they define as a partnership in which there is a sharing between the woman and the midwife involving trust, shared control and responsibility, and shared meaning through mutual understanding.

Institutional needs or long-established precedents have not hampered the development of these innovative practices established in Canada and New Zealand. They are united by a number of principles of care, the most fundamental of which is the importance of the relationship between the childbearing woman and the midwife. In her PhD thesis, James (1997) explores the nature of the midwifery relationship in great depth.

Her study was conducted in Alberta, among 'lay midwives' and the women they cared for. Such a situation allows for the emergence of a form of practice characterized by close relationships between childbearing women and their midwives. Sharpe, in her 'thoughts about continuity of care' (personal communication 1997) describes a situation in a province where midwifery is now regulated and is part of the health care system. The midwives in Ontario are reimbursed directly by the Medicare system and provide a primary care service. The provision of continuity of care is a requirement of midwifery practice. Guilliland & Pairman have described the midwifery partnership that is integral to practice in New Zealand (1995).

Pairman (1998) undertook an in-depth study of both the nature and understanding of the relationship between midwives and women during pregnancy, labour and birth in New Zealand. She found that both the midwife and the woman contribute equally to the relationship and value what each brings to it. The 'real' continuity that was offered by the midwives in this study, being available and getting to know women over time, allowed this relationship to develop and seemed to be of mutual benefit to both women and midwives. 'Friendship' and 'partnership' are terms used by both the women and the midwives in this study. The midwife–woman relationship is one of equal status and shared power and control. What is striking in the accounts of the relationship in this study is the sense of attention to the experience as well as the physical outcome of birth, and the thoughtful attention to shared decision-making (see also Chapter 3).

These new (or perhaps renewed) patterns of practice have one fundamental aspect in common – the relationship between the childbearing woman and her midwife, and the development of a relationship of trust, is paramount. James' (1997) thesis, based on a study that used hermeneutic phenomenology as a method of investigation, unfolds and illuminates the experience of 'being with woman as midwife'. The thesis provides a way of understanding the potential of such relationships, relationships that go far beyond any idea of relationship as simply transactional, to a depth of mutuality and understanding that transforms midwifery. James describes the midwifery relationship as a special friendship that is usually terminated once the relationship is over. This 'attention to this woman in all her relations', which James describes, is truly woman-centred care. It is mutual in a number of respects, including the way in which it allows pregnancy and birth to transform both woman and midwife.

Sharpe also highlights the need to attend and to give attention to the individual woman. Like James (1997), Sharpe (personal communication 1997) emphasizes getting to know the woman over time and the difference between this and our ordinary understanding of friendship. This relationship goes beyond liking or disliking. Like Walsh (1998), who describes the challenge to traditional professional roles that is represented by personal midwifery practice, James reminds us that in most professional relationships, there is not usually a blending of the personal and the professional roles. Both Sharpe and James advocate this blending of roles. Perhaps the crux of this woman–midwife relationship is its mutual concern with the pregnancy and birth of this baby and this mother, and the shared intention of the best experience possible on their journey. This epitomizes the differences, described clearly by Brodie (1997), between loyalty to the institution and loyalty to individual women when we think about 'staffing women' rather than 'staffing wards'.

The relationship between the woman and her midwife is, in most of these situations, one in which both the woman and the midwife bring particular expertise and knowledge into the relationship. The woman holds her own personal knowledge of what is best for her and her situation; the midwife brings accumulated knowledge and expertise in childbirth. There is a theoretical basis to midwifery practice, but in this equal sharing of relationship, it is important that, as James (1997, p. 95) comments, 'we find new ways so that the authority of the theory does not become the central focus of our being together'. In this relationship, then, the woman and her needs determine what happens. Kitzinger (1991, p. 76) describes the role of the midwife as a professional who relates to the woman with mutual respect, warmth and openness:

A good midwife loves women. She does not dominate, direct, or even instruct. Except on the rare occasion when she needs to take decisive action to avert danger, she follows rather than leads. She is the midwife to all the dreams and hopes surrounding the coming to being of that child, and to the process of maturing and growth that is involved for both parents.

PRACTICAL ASPECTS OF PROVIDING PERSONAL, CONTINUOUS CARE

We draw on the experience of practising in the One-to-One midwifery scheme because it is a system that provides a high level of continuity. In addition, it shares many of the features of other leading edge practices in British Columbia and Ontario, Canada, and some practices in New Zealand.

Developing the relationship: being with the woman

One-to-One midwifery practice was developed explicitly to change both the structure and culture of care. It is intended to allow midwives to develop a relationship with women, a relationship that enables midwives to be skilled companions to women on their journey through pregnancy and birth. Lifting the barriers of inflexible shift systems, and allocations to one area of a service, allows the midwife to work with women in this way. However, the change demands a careful consideration on the part of the midwife of how she will develop appropriate relationships that are sensitive and supportive without developing undue dependency. It is possible in such a situation to go overboard. Midwives who practise in this way sometimes become overprotective or have unrealistic expectations of what they can achieve. For example, it may not be possible to get long-term problems of housing or substance abuse sorted out in such a short time. One-to-One midwives, who serve a deprived area (including one of the most deprived in the UK), discovered that they had to outline boundaries and define their role as midwives. Some midwives found themselves acting as friends, general supporters, counsellors and social workers. It has been reported that educating women in their role helps to overcome these problems (Farmer & Chipperfield 1996, McCourt & Page 1996). There is also the potential to meet one's own needs to be needed through such work, setting up a relationship of dependency that is helpful to neither the childbearing woman nor the midwife.

The concept of skilled companionship has been described by a number of midwives (Smith 1991, Cooke & Bewley 1995, Page 1995a). However, this concept has been criticized by others. Leap (1996) argues that rather than acting as companions, midwives should facilitate friendship and support among the woman's community through networking at antenatal and postnatal groups. Leap (1997) further highlights the potential of creating mutual dependency in continuity schemes if too much emphasis is placed on exclusive special relationships between women and midwives. Although Leap acknowledges the emergence of friendships, and indeed their importance in engaging in joint efforts to improve maternity services, she suggests that they should not be the *focus* of care provision.

This theme of dependency is one highlighted in the literature on continuity. Allen et al (1997) found some evidence of it in their study of three midwifery group practices. Downe (1997) warns of the 'culture of dependency' that may result with intense involvement with women, and Sandall (1996) writes of the 'dependency relationship', which may grow from a trusting relationship between woman and midwife. However, it is becoming evident that developing meaningful relationships with women is a protective factor against burn-out (Sandall 1997), while a lack of such relationships may lead to frustration, stress and disillusionment. Clearly, for effect, there needs to be a balance. While continuity of carer may provide intense satisfaction for both woman and midwife, it is also important that the midwife establishes parameters for her practice and relationship with her client, enabling the woman to build a sense of personal control over her own pregnancy.

How to provide personal and continuous care

The provision of continuity of carer means having individual midwives planning midwifery care together with individual women and their families, and providing most of the care, including, whenever possible, care during labour and birth. There are a number of ways of organizing such a system while keeping the principles intact.

In One-to-One midwifery practice, one named midwife coordinates and provides most of the care for 40 women per year on her personal caseload. Midwives are loosely affiliated to GP practices for the purpose of selecting women for One-to-One care and ensuring that the majority of the caseload is within a small geographical area. Midwives are encouraged to plan well ahead and to accept women on to their caseload according to the expected date of birth. Planning for four births per month, apart from when time is taken for annual leave, will produce an annual caseload of about 40 births. Women with low-risk pregnancies will usually receive midwife-led care, and most of their antenatal care will take place in their own homes. Women with high-risk pregnancies will receive obstetrician-led care, the obstetrician providing a point of referral and decision-making alongside the named midwife.

The named midwife works with a partner who shares the antenatal care and provides care when the named midwife is unavailable. This ensures the presence of a known midwife if the woman goes into labour when the named midwife is not on call. In practice, 92% of women were attended by a known midwife in labour between November 1996 and October 1997, 75% of them by the named midwife and 17% by the midwife's partner. Postnatally, the named midwife will again provide the majority of care, visiting according to the woman's need until transfer to the health visitor.

How to avoid burn-out

Observing the principles and key themes of Sandall's (1997) work, we will describe how One-to-One midwives manage their personal and professional lives, successfully integrating them and avoiding stress and burn-out.

Occupational autonomy. Moving from the security of a shift system with rostered days off, usually known weeks in advance, to providing 24-hour cover is not easy and is a source of concern to midwives moving into caseload practice (Farmer & Chipperfield 1996). However, the advantage of working flexibly means that midwives are only 'at work' when either clients or colleagues need them. Antenatal and postnatal visits are planned effectively so that midwives maximize the use of their time and do not travel long distances unnecessarily. Time off is organized within the partnership so that only one midwife is on call at night or over weekends. The only time that rotas are drawn up is over Christmas and New Year, when usually only two or three members of the group practice work, and time off with family and friends can be ensured with a first, second and third on-call system in place. Annual leave is planned well in advance, with, ideally, only two members of the group practice away at any one time.

Being the lead professional for women with low-risk pregnancies and decision-making in partnership with women adds to the sense of occupational autonomy. The responsibility and accountability are clearly attractive to One-to-One midwives and contribute to their own sense of control (Stevens 1996). Twenty-four hour referral to an on-call registrar at the two units where One-to-One works provides support in situations of clinical uncertainty.

Developing meaningful relationships with women. Many One-to-One midwives moved into caseload midwifery because of frustration with the traditional, fragmented system of practice. The opportunity to develop meaningful relationships with women and their families in order to respond more specifically and effectively to their needs is a major source of satisfaction. As Farmer & Chipperfield (1996, p. 20) write, 'it is simply much easier and more satisfying to look after someone you know'. The potential for creating dependency was highlighted in the early days of the scheme when enthusiastic midwives virtually promised women the earth! A psychologist provided a valuable session on developing professional parameters for practice. Practically, the midwives focus on three areas:

1. describing their role as midwives at the initial booking interview;

2. educating women in how, why and when they might best contact their midwife;

3. ensuring that the women receive some antenatal care from the named midwife's partner.

We have found, in keeping with Sandall's research (1997), that continuity of carer is as important to midwives as it is to women. Campbell's (1984) concept of 'reciprocity' within the relationship between client and professional helper may be pertinent. The notion that both parties experience mutual benefit within the professional relationship is evident from our work.

Social support. In the One-to-One programme, both peer support at work and emotional and social support at home have been significant in reducing stress and preventing burn-out. It was important to the first midwives selected to practise within the One-to-One scheme that they could choose their partners and then form themselves into group practices of six or eight midwives. Working predominantly in the community is potentially isolating, and the support of the midwife partner and wider group practice has been essential. Weekly group practice meetings are held to discuss issues, solve problems, plan ahead and get an overall picture of current workload. When problems have arisen with dissatisfaction, the root has often been a failure to communicate with the rest of the group in terms of either giving or receiving support.

Peer review, described in detail by Cooke & Bewley (1995), has also been a means of expressing support, usually in terms of a midwife's action or decision. To know that one's colleagues would have made a similar decision in an uncertain situation, or to be challenged constructively and helped to see a different way, can be enormously supportive.

Monthly whole practice meetings and regular away-days provide 'time out' for One-to-One midwives to meet each other. Social occasions such as birthday celebrations, leaving parties or preparing for the annual hospital Christmas review have been important to many of the midwives and provide a focus for fun and relaxation.

Emotional and social support from family and friends and having a life outside work are also important. Planning holidays well in advance has enabled midwives to pursue their own interests, which have included white water rafting in Colorado and cycling around Thailand!

Managerial support is important; it should be facilitative rather than directive. Midwives should have an infrastructure of support for referrals and clerical work. In Britain, the research of Stapleton et al (1998) in relation to the supervision of midwives has included an in-depth account of the culture of midwifery. This culture has not been a supportive one. The authors explain this culture with reference to the work of Freire (1972), who described a cycle of oppression in which those who have been oppressed continue to oppress each other. They describe what is called 'horizontal violence', a form of institutional bullying that they see as part of the culture of midwifery. Certainly, in many situations where there has been a new project set up, midwives working in these innovative areas have not always felt supported by their colleagues. Those setting up and those working within the innovations may suffer what Brodie also calls horizontal violence (1997).

In setting up new projects, it is important to attend to the culture of practice as a whole, making it more positive and supporting and paying attention to all midwives in the service rather than only those taking the innovation forward. However, boundaries and frameworks of expectation are required, so that it is clear that destruction of the innovation by rumours and innuendo will not be sanctioned.

Time management

Midwives moving into One-to-One practice benefit from thinking about, or training in, time management skills. In the hospital system, although midwives may need good time management skills at work, they do not have to manage 24-hour time periods in the same way. This is partly because work is contained by the working day and going off duty provides a clear physical break between professional and personal life. In One-to-One practice, a number of priorities and commitments may easily spread over 24 hours if they are allowed to, but with good management, a caseload of 40 births a year can be managed in an average week of 37.5 hours (McCourt 1998).

Flexibility and the ability of an individual midwife to manage her own time are crucial to allow for both the provision of care that meets the woman's needs, and the midwife's ability to balance personal and professional life. This latter factor is crucial to a profession that consists mainly of women. To provide such flexibility, it is important that set commitments are kept to a minimum. Midwives working in this way should never be expected to staff wards. With a caseload of 40, the daily work of a midwife will consist of a number of antenatal and postnatal visits. If a labouring woman calls her, it is relatively easy for her to cancel such visits or have her partner undertake them.

In Britain, the development of the One-to-One

practice has led to much discussion about how much on call is best for midwives. With a partnership model, although the midwife may be 'available' to women for half the time, call-outs will be relatively rare. In One-to-One practice, one midwife and her partner are on call for eight births per month, compared with team midwifery where, with a team caseload of 240 births per year, team midwives are on call for 20 births per month. In addition, communications are simpler, and it is not as complicated to ensure that the woman knows both of the midwives. If, however, a 'team' of six undertakes to do a 1 in 6 rota, the midwife is far more likely to be called out on her night on call, is more likely to have a number of women in labour at once and has a higher chance of being called for women she does not know well or even at all. The approach described by Saxell in Chapter 4, of taking 1 week on and 1 week off, makes a great deal of sense. The One-to-One midwives arrange their availability time to suit themselves. They carry out their visits from home and do not need to visit the hospital first. Arranging visits at mutually convenient times with women in their practice means that they can sleep later and work later, or take their children to school or the nursery before starting work.

Time management skills are important to modern-day life whichever walk of life we are in. We found that a time management workshop given 6 months after the One-to-One project had started helped the One-to-One midwives enormously. The flexibility offered by caseload practice requires that midwives pace themselves. If it is probable that midwives will be called out at night, they should try to have an easier day. This is difficult when midwives have been used to going to work and working flat out on a shift.

Two tools that are crucial to midwives in caseload practice are a mobile telephone or pager, and a good diary system. Setting priorities, making lists and keeping addresses and telephone numbers together is essential.

The future

It was recommended that the One-to-One service be

Pointers for practice

- Women appreciate having a known and trusted midwife who is available to them for all periods of maternity care, especially for labour and birth. Continuity is also satisfying to midwives.
- This is best provided by a named midwife who works with a partner, giving her time off.
- As well as changing the structure of care, attention should be paid to the development of skills, personal sensitivity and an adequate knowledge base.
- One-to-One continuity is possible throughout the whole of maternity care, even when the named midwife takes time off.
- Attention should be paid to a structure that works for midwives as well as for women.

---

extended under continuing evaluation. At present, there are plans to extend caseload practice, which includes the most successful aspects of One-to-One and other continuity of care schemes, to other adjacent health services.

CONCLUSION

We have described some of the changes in policy and practice that have occurred in the development of systems that provide continuity of care-giver in many parts of the world. We have also, drawing from many years of experience in setting up such schemes and practising within them, offered some practical advice. Readers may wish to refer to the references below for more detailed advice. In setting up such systems, it is important to remember that the creation of a new structure may be necessary but not sufficient in developing more sensitive and scientific care. The development of an adequate knowledge base, and clinical, personal and intellectual skills, is also crucial to putting science and sensitivity into practice.

REFERENCES

Aiken N 1997 Team midwifery: a challenge for Australian midwives. Australian College of Midwives Conference Proceedings, 10th Biennial National Conference. ACMI, Melbourne, Australia

Allen I, Bourke Dowling S, Williams S 1997 A leading role for midwives? Evaluation of midwifery group practice development projects. Policy Studies Institute, London

Audit Commission 1998 First class delivery: improving maternity services in England and Wales. Audit Commission, Abingdon

Beake S, McCourt C, Page L 1998 The use of clinical audit in evaluating maternity services reform: a critical reflection. Journal of Clinical Evaluation in Clinical Practice 4(1): 75–83

Bissett S 1995 One-to-One midwifery: a personal experience. British Journal of Midwifery 3(3): 142–61

Brodie P 1997 Being with women: the experiences of Australian team midwives. Degree of Masters of Nursing Thesis, University of Technology, Sydney

Campbell A V 1984 Moderated love: a theology of professional care. SPCK, London

Cooke P, Bewley C 1995 Developing scholarship in practice. In: Page L (ed.) Effective group practice in midwifery: working with women. Blackwell Science, Oxford

Couves J 1995 Working in practice. In Page L (ed.) Effective group practice in midwifery: working with women. Blackwell Science, Oxford

Coyle K 1998 Women's perceptions of birth centre care: a qualitative approach. Unpublished thesis, Edith Cowan University, Perth, Western Australia

Day P, Lancaster P, Huan G J 1997 Australia's mothers and babies. AIHW National Statistics Unit, Sydney

Department of Health 1982 Maternity care in action. HMSO, London

Department of Health 1993 Changing childbirth. Report of the Expert Maternity Group (Cumberlege report). HMSO, London

Department of Health 1997 Pregnant women should have more choice. Press Release by Baroness Jay

Department of Health 1998 Midwifery: delivering our future. Report by the Standing Nursing and Midwifery Advisory Committee. Department of Health, London

Department of Health Maternity Services 1992 Government response to the second report from the Health Committee Session 1991–92. HMSO, London

Downe S 1997 The less we do, the more we give. British Journal of Midwifery 5(1): 43

Farmer E, Chipperfield C 1996 One-to-One midwifery: problems and solutions. Modern Midwife (Apr): 19–21

Flint C, Poulengeris P, Grant A 1989 The 'Know your midwife' scheme – a randomised trial of continuity of care by a team of midwives. Midwifery 5: 11–16

Freire P 1972 The pedagogy of the oppressed. Penguin, Harmondsworth

Garcia J, Redshaw M, Fitzsimmons B, Keene J 1998 First class delivery: a national survey of woman's views on maternity care. Audit Commission, London

Green J M, Curtis P, Price, H, Renfrew M J 1998 Continuing to care. The organization of midwifery services in the UK: a structured review of the evidence. Books for Midwives Press, Hale

Guilliland K, Pairman K 1995 The midwifery partnership: a model for practice. Victoria University of Wellington, New Zealand

Gumley S, Haines H, Holland J (1997) Midwife care project: a partnership between Wngaratta District Base Hospital and Ovens and King Community Health Service. ACMI Conference Proceedings, 10th Biennial National Conference. ACMI, Melbourne, Australia.

Hodnett E D 1998 Continuity of caregivers during pregnancy and childbirth. Cochrane Review. Cochrane Library, Issue 3. Update Software, Oxford

House of Commons 1992 Second report on the maternity services by the Health Services Select Committee (Winterton report). HMSO, London

James S G 1997 With woman: the nature of the midwifery relation. Doctor of Philosophy thesis, University of Alberta, Edmonton

Kenny P, Brodie P, Eckermann S, Hall J 1994 Westmead Hospital team midwifery project evaluation. Final Report. Westmead Hospital, Sydney

Kitzinger K 1991 Homebirth: the essential guide to giving birth outside of the hospital. Macmillan, Canada

Leap N 1996 Caseload practice: a recipe for burn-out? British Journal of Midwifery 4(6): 329–30

Leap N 1997 Caseload practice that works. MIDIRS Midwifery Digest 7(4): 416–18

Lecky-Thompson M 1995 Independent midwifery in Australia. In: Murphy Black T (ed.) Issues in midwifery. Churchill Livingstone, Edinburgh

McCourt C 1998 Working patterns of caseload midwives: a diary analysis. British Journal of Midwifery 6(9): 580–5

McCourt C, Page L 1996 Report on the evaluation of One-to-One midwifery. Thames Valley University, London

McCourt C, Page L, Hewison J, Vail A 1998 Evaluation of One-to-One midwifery: women's responses to care. Birth 25(2): 73–80

MacVicar J, Dobbie G, Owen-Johnstone L, Jagger C, Hopkins M, Kennedy J 1993 Simulated home delivery in hospital: a randomised controlled trial. British Journal of Obstetrics and Gynaecology 100: 316–23

Maternity Services Advisory Committee 1982 First report on maternity care in action. Part 1: Antenatal care. HMSO, London

Ministerial Review of Birthing Services in Victoria 1990 Having a baby in Victoria. Department of Health, Victoria, Australia

Ministerial Task Force WA 1990 Report of the Ministerial Task Force to review obstetric, neonatal and gynaecological services in Western Australia 1990. Health Department, Perth, Western Australia

Ministerial Task Force on Obstetrical Services in New South Wales 1989 Maternity services in New South Wales. NSW Department of Health, Sydney

Minns H 1995 Teaching in practice. In: Page L (ed). Effective group practice in midwifery: working with women. Blackwell Science, Oxford

Morrison S, Percival P, Haucky Y, McMurray A 1999 Birthing at home: the resolution of expectations. Midwifery 15: 32–39

National Childbirth Trust 1995 Midwife caseloads. National Childbirth Trust, London

National Health and Medical Research Council 1996 Options for effective care in childbirth final report. Australian Government Printing Service, Canberra

National Health Service Executive 1994 Women centred maternity services. Executive Letter Department of Health, London (94)9

Oakley A 1997 Women's responses. In: Chamberlain G, Wraight A, Crowley P (eds) Home births: the report of the 1994 confidential enquiry by the National Birthday Trust. Partheron, Carnforth

Page L 1995a Effective group practice in midwifery: working with women. Blackwell Science, Oxford

Page L 1995b Putting principles into practice. In: Page L (ed.) Effective group practice in midwifery: working with women. Blackwell Science, Oxford

Page L A 1996 16th Dame Rosalind Paget memorial lecture: reclaiming midwifery. Midwives Chronicle 109(1304): 248–53

Page L A, McCourt C, Cooke P 1997 One-to-One midwifery. New Generation 20: 2–3

Pairman S 1998 The midwifery partnership: an exploration of the midwife/woman relationship. MA thesis, Victoria University of Wellington, New Zealand

Piercey J, Wilson D, Chapman P 1996 Evaluation of One-to-One Midwifery practice. York Health Economic Consortium and Centre for Midwifery Practice, University of York

Proctor S R 1997 Perceptions of quality in maternity services. Doctoral thesis, University of Bradford, Yorkshire

Porter M, Macintyre S 1984 What is, must be best: a research note on conservative or deferential responses to antenatal care provision. Social Science and Medicine 19(11): 1197–200

Rowley M J 1998 Evaluation of team midwifery care in pregnancy and childbirth: a randomised controlled trial. Doctor of Philosophy thesis, University of Newcastle, New South Wales

Rowley M, Hensley M, Brinstead M, Wlodarczyk J 1995 Continuity of care by a midwife team versus routine care during pregnancy and birth: a randomised trial. Medical Journal of Australia 163: 289–93

Rutter D 1996 An analysis of the open-ended questionnaire responses. In: McCourt C, Page L (eds) Report on the evaluation of One-to-One midwifery. Thames Valley University and Hammersmith Hospitals NHS Trust, London

Sandall J 1996 Moving towards caseload practice: what evidence do we have? British Journal of Midwifery 4(12): 620–1

Sandall J 1997 Midwives' burnout and continuity of care. British Journal of Midwifery 5(2): 106–11

Select Committee on Intervention in Childbirth (1995) Report on intervention in childbirth. State Law Publisher, Perth

Smith A 1991 Newborn optimism. Nursing Times 87(16): 56–9

Stapleton H, Duerden J, Kirkham M 1998 Evaluation of the impact of the supervision of midwives on professional practice and the quality of midwifery care. English National Board for Nursing, Midwifery and Health Visiting/United Kingdom Central Council for Nursing, Midwifery and Health Visiting, London

Stevens 1996 Cavalry strangers: what a changing childbirth service means to obstetricians. MSc dissertation, London Guildhall University

Waldenstrom U 1996 Midwives in current debate and in the future. Australian College of Midwives Incorporated Journal (Mar): 3–9

Waldenstrom U, Lawson J 1997 Birth centre practices in Australia. Unpublished report. Royal Women's Hospital, Melbourne

Walsh D 1998 An ethnographic study of women's experience of partnership caseload midwifery practice (the BUMPS scheme). Masters dissertation, Leicester Royal Infirmary NHS Trust, Leicester

Weatherston L 1985 Midwifery in the hospital: a team approach to perinatal care. Dimensions in Health Service 62(4): 15–16, 22

Weatherston L A, Carty E, Rice A, Tier T 1985 Hospital based midwifery: meeting the needs of childbearing women. Canadian Nurse 81: 35–7

Wilkins R 1995 Sociological aspects of the mother/community midwife relationship. PhD thesis, University of Surrey

Wraight A, Ball J, Seccombe I, Stock J 1993 Mapping team midwifery: a report to the Department of Health. IMS Report Series 242. Institute of Manpower Studies, Brighton

7

A public health view of the maternity services

Jean Chapple

This chapter looks at the common aims of personal and public health services, how health needs to achieve better outcomes for pregnant women are assessed for a community and how an evidence-based policy of care can help to improve the health of mothers, babies and families.

ACHIEVING BETTER OUTCOMES OF MATERNITY SERVICES: THE ROLE OF PUBLIC HEALTH

What is public health?

Public health is the science and art of preventing disease, prolonging life and promoting health through the organized efforts of society (Acheson 1988). Public health specialists differ from the nurses, midwives and doctors involved in clinical medicine in that their 'patients' are whole communities rather than the individuals who make up that community. This creates a potential tension between those making health policy decisions that affect society as a whole and those who have day-to-day contact with individuals and who need the resources to deliver that clinical care.

In general, what is good for the individual is also good for society, but this is not inevitably the case. Every parent contemplating immunization for their child wants vaccination for every other child but their own in order to provide herd immunity. This would mean that their own child would not come into contact with the disease and would be protected without encountering any of the extremely small but individually important risks of immunization. This argument is not sustainable for the country as a whole: living in a democratic community means compromise. We have to follow rules and forego some individual choices to live in harmony with others. Imagine the chaos if we did not follow laws to drive on a given side of the road or to dispose of rubbish in a hygienic manner. Similar rules must apply if we are to have a publicly funded health service. We cannot all have every diagnostic test or treatment that we might desire or the health service bank will run dry at an even faster rate than it already does; diagnosing and treating one person might mean that no resources are left to diagnose and treat another. We often face similar decisions in our home budgets – having to choose between a new suite of furniture or a holiday, or to compromise by opting for having both but selecting the cheapest options available. These are opportunity costs, the opportunity for one doctor to treat one person being affected by the decisions made by another. Dr Paul may be robbing Dr Peter of his chance to treat the patient sitting in front of him (Mooney 1992).

Setting priorities through health needs assessment

As health service resources are finite, tough decisions are needed on what services should be provided and for which members of the community. Care in publicly funded health care systems is rarely rationed (given as a fixed allowance to restrict supply) but is prioritized or ranked in order of preference. Public health specialists help in this process through needs assessment to ensure that resources are targeted to those who need them most. Some specific groups, such as people who are mentally ill, the elderly and those with learning disabilities, will lose out in a system in which the person or service that shouts loudest gets most. In an ideal world, public health would cover more than just health services – it would also cover the health impact of plans formulated by other parts of government, for example those dealing with housing, social policy on benefits and environmental issues such as new roads and air pollution.

Health needs assessment is not an exact science but studies:

- how common any given condition is and its impact on the health of the affected individual and the population;
- changes in disease patterns, for example the re-emergence of old diseases such as tuberculosis and the development of new ones such as HIV and AIDS;
- the development of new health care interventions, new drugs and new techniques in terms of *effectiveness* (does it change the natural history of the disease?; Cochrane 1972) and *efficiency* (is it used in a way which produces the best results for the total population?) as judged by scientifically rigorous studies – *evidence-based medicine*;

- the effects of national initiatives to improve quality of care, such as *Changing Childbirth* (Department of Health 1993)
- what the public expects from the health care services for which it pays through taxes.

The chief tool of public health and needs assessment is *epidemiology*.

What is epidemiology and what does it have to offer midwives?

Epidemiology is the study of the distribution and determinants of disease: who gets what disease, where they live, and when and why they get it. There is a need to put an individual patient in the context of the community of which he or she is a member. For example, we know through population-based studies that a woman with insulin-dependent diabetes has five times the risk of losing her baby than does her neighbour without this disease (Casson et al 1997, Hawthorne et al 1997). We therefore focus attention on this individual before and during pregnancy – even if she appears well and has no social or other disadvantages – because, in general, women like her have a higher risk of having a baby with a congenital malformation and macrosomia. Midwives can use epidemiology to tell them which members of their local community are at higher risk of a complication of pregnancy and thus need more monitoring and support.

Populations with problems: what is risk?

We never say that there is a risk we may win the lottery but that we think we have a chance of winning (Silman 1997). This implies that the term 'risk' adds a negative emotive element to the *probability* or *likelihood* of an event happening. This element is also subjective: the risk of any event may be viewed and expressed in a very different light by different people (Calman & Royston 1997). Contraceptive pill scares in the media produce the common phenomenon of a woman rushing to her doctor and appearing surprised that the doctor is far more concerned about the risk of thrombosis from her smoking habit – which she refuses to contemplate giving up – than about changing her pill.

There is also a conflict here between a population and a personal health approach. Epidemiological studies can supply accurate figures on the probability or chance of having a baby with an abnormality on which to base informed consent, but if you are one of the small percentage of high-risk patients in a total population of a thousand, that is 100% of you. It is the value judgements linked to this probability by clinicians and their patients that may cause conflict and concern.

IDENTIFYING PEOPLE WITH PROBLEMS IN THE POPULATION

Methods

There are three methods of identifying high risk populations:

1. needs assessment to identify high risk groups with features that predispose them to problems within a population
2. case finding to identify high risk individuals within a population attending for health care
3. screening to identify high risk individuals within a population invited for screening

Needs assessment can identify the characteristics of the local population and alert both those buying care and those providing it to specific services that are needed. Anonymous HIV testing in neonates (which acts as a proxy for maternal HIV infection) has identified that, in London, there are populations in whom the prevalence (the proportion of people in the population with HIV at any given time) is 1 in 150 pregnant women. Services to encourage all women to be screened for HIV, to look after mothers and to minimize the transmission to their babies are needed in these districts. In other parts of the UK, prevalence assessed through neonatal screening is so low that screening for HIV is targeted at women with a known high-risk lifestyle, such as those injecting drugs (Nicoll et al 1998).

Case-finding involves clinicians looking for illness or its predictors whenever a patient presents to them for another reason, seen, for example, in checking blood pressure when a woman comes to a clinic for a cervical smear. Case-finding is usually carried out at the same place where definitive diagnosis and therapy are offered (for example, in a primary care setting), so there are few problems linking those identified as high risk to a source of care (Sackett et al 1991).

Antenatal care usually involves case-finding as midwives check for a range of social and clinical complications, ranging from evidence of domestic violence (Mezey & Bewley 1997) to signs of pregnancy hypertension, at each visit. Formal counselling or permission to case-find is not usually sought as most women and their carers accept that this is a normal part of pregnancy care, although midwives take care to explain what they are doing and why. Ultrasound scanning is a very non-specific type of case-finding; a woman may be informed that the scan is to confirm her dates, but the ultrasonographer may then measure the nuchal skinfold thickness as a 'routine' part of the scanning process to assess the risk of Down syndrome without formal or informed consent.

Screening involves inviting the public to undergo screening tests to separate them into groups with higher and lower probabilities of disease. Those with a high probability of disease will be offered a diagnostic test. Specific screening programmes are set within pregnancy care, for example offering testing for Down syndrome through serum screening, or screening for rhesus status. These screening programmes usually involve some form of pretest counselling and are formalized, with protocols and literature for women to take away and discuss with their partners.

Needs assessment and case-finding: which groups of women develop which pregnancy complications and when?

Some women are at risk even before they conceive. The number of deaths resulting from lethal congenital malformations is falling because of prenatal diagnosis with termination of the affected pregnancies. Some families are aware that they carry genes for severe genetic disease and seek advice before pregnancy.

Random errors in the division of the egg can lead to fetal chromosomal abnormalities or multiple pregnancy, both of which are more common in older mothers. Some trisomies, such as trisomy 18 (Edwards' syndrome) and trisomy 13 (Patau syndrome), are rapidly lethal, often in the middle or third trimester, but others, for example trisomy 21 (Down syndrome), may produce a viable fetus if there is no major structural abnormality such as a congenital heart defect.

Multiple births are exposed to many hazards and are becoming more common with the increasing use of infertility treatment. Multiple placentation and increased nutritional demands made by two or more fetuses can result in fetal growth retardation. In monozygous twins, cords can become entangled in a single amniotic sac, competition for placental tissues may occur, or one twin may transfuse blood into the other, resulting in a marked size difference between them or the death of one twin. The rate of premature delivery is also very high, especially in higher-order births.

Fetal anomaly scanning may reveal structural abnormalities such as spina bifida in women who do not have a family history of the problem and enable a fall in perinatal mortality because of their detection (Saari-Kemppainen et al 1990). However, routine scanning has not been shown to reduce mortality from and improve outcome in any other cause (Bucher & Schmidt 1993, Ewigman et al 1993).

Some maternal infections, such as rubella and toxoplasmosis, may be transmitted vertically from mother to child and cause severe malformation. Although the birth prevalence of severe malformation and death caused by these may be falling, it remains to be seen whether public health programmes to immunize children against rubella, to prevent the spread of toxoplasmosis through personal and food hygiene (Royal College of Obstetricians and Gynaecologists 1992) and to prevent neural tube defects by a periconceptional increase in maternal folic acid intake (MRC Vitamin Study Research Group 1991, Czeizel & Dudas 1992, Czeizel 1993) will actually result in the primary prevention of malformation.

Environmental factors acting in pregnancy

External environment

There are many well-recognized teratogens and other fetal toxins that may cause the deaths of a very few fetuses in developed countries. These include viral infections such as fetal rubella, cytomegalovirus and toxoplasmosis, which may cause minimal symptoms in a pregnant woman if caught during pregnancy but can seriously damage a fetus, especially in the first trimester. Other organisms, such as *Listeria*, *Salmonella* and Parvovirus (fifth disease) can cause death through prematurity with or without intrauterine or neonatal infection.

Altitude plays a part in producing low birth weight: about 30% of babies born in Colorado above 10 000 m were of low birth weight in Lubchencho's classic (1963) study on birth weight distribution for gestational age, compared with 7% in the UK today. This may be an important factor for fetal health in some countries.

Exposure to occupational or environmental hazards such as radiation or lead can contribute to perinatal mortality, but the literature is unclear on the risk, mainly because the numbers of births considered are generally too small to achieve sufficient statistical power to assess risk (Rosenberg et al 1987, Savitz et al 1989). A retrospective case control study of over 1000 perinatal deaths in Leicester between 1976 and 1982 showed that leather-workers were at increased risk of perinatal death, particularly from congenital malformation and macerated stillbirth, compared with other manual workers in the same class (Clarke & Mason 1985).

The effect of occupational hazards on perinatal mortality may also be mediated through an increased risk of prematurity or low birth weight, both of which have a major influence on the risk of a baby dying. One study has shown a dose-related association between blood lead and risk of preterm delivery (McMichael et al 1986). In a large study in Scotland between 1981 and 1984 (Sanjose et al 1991), the risk of preterm delivery and low birth weight was shown to be over 50% higher in the children of women who worked with electrical, metal or leather goods than in other female manual workers and was more frequent in the children of mothers and fathers employed in manual rather than non-manual jobs. Women in jobs for which high physical exertion is needed have a higher rate of preterm and low birth weight delivery (Homer et al 1990).

In utero environment

The effects on the fetus of maternal smoking have been intensively studied since the 1950s. The actual contribution made by maternal smoking to the risk of perinatal death is not direct but appears to depend on the presence of other adverse factors as smoking reduces fetal growth rate and therefore adds to other detrimental influences. However, its importance is shown by the estimate that, in England and Wales in 1984, 18% of instances of low birth weight were attributable to maternal smoking (Simpson & Armand Smith 1986). Women who stop smoking by the third trimester are not at increased risk of a low birth weight baby compared with non-smokers, but women who begin smoking during the second or third trimester have a risk of a low birth weight baby similar to that of women who have smoked throughout their pregnancy. The risk in the third trimester is also dose related: the more cigarettes smoked, the higher the risk of a small baby (Liberman et al 1994).

The role of undernutrition and specific dietary constituents is still uncertain (Naismith 1981) but will also vary with the underlying health of the mother. A study carried out in London showed that mothers of low birth weight babies are not randomly distributed among mothers at all nutritional levels but are concentrated among mothers of poor nutritional status (Wynn et al 1991). This study also found that vitamin and mineral supplementation in the last two trimesters of pregnancy had no significant effect on birth dimensions; thus diet may have its maximum effect during ovulatory maturation and early embryonic development (Doyle et al 1990).

Maternal nutrition may have an even more longlasting effect. There is currently much debate about the Barker programming hypothesis – that it is earlier rather than later adverse circumstances that have the major impact on diseases seen later in life. The hypothesis is that a programming stimulus or insult (such as a drug or hormone) during certain critical periods of development have a lasting or lifelong effect on the structure or function of organs, tissues and body functions. Work initially done on the midwifery records of a cohort of males born in Hertfordshire from 1911 onwards who were followed up many years later suggests that cardiovascular and chronic lung disease in adult life may have important causes in fetal and early life, such as poor maternal nutrition (Barker 1992).

Which babies are at risk?

Birth weight is the best predictor of perinatal mortality. In England and Wales in 1990, 59% of perinatal deaths occurred in the 6.5% of babies who weighed less than 2500 g at birth, and 36% of perinatal deaths occurred in the 0.9% of babies who weighed less than 1500 g at birth.

Most of the factors contributing to perinatal death do so by influencing fetal growth rate, gestational age or both. The size of any baby is influenced by genetic factors (including the presence of congenital malformation, and parental height and weight), birth order and ethnic group (Thomson 1983). These are all closely associated with socio-economic status, as is the risk of exposure to environmental health hazards, for example those at work, and personal health behaviour, such as smoking. All of these factors produce very robust birth weight distributions that change only slowly with time. There has been virtually no change in the birth weight distribution in England and Wales between 1983 and 1996. The fall in mortality over these years is the result not of a decrease in the proportion of low birth weight babies but of improved survival rates, especially in low and very low birth weight babies. However, there is much debate over whether there are limits to the gestational age and birth weight below which aggressive resuscitation and active treatment should not be instituted as there is considerable short- and long-term morbidity in survivors (Walker & Patel 1987, Allen et al 1993). The cut-off in improved survival appears to be at 25 weeks gestation and 750 g birth weight (Hack & Fanaroff 1989).

Growth-retarded babies are at higher risk of perinatal mortality. A study in Sweden showed that growth-retarded babies had four times the perinatal mortality rate of the general population, even after deaths resulting from congenital malformation were excluded (Wennergren et al 1988). In Ontario, preterm growth-retarded babies had a perinatal mortality rate of 180 per 1000 (Fitzhardinge & Inwood 1989), and in Baltimore, 86% of perinatal deaths occurred in growth-retarded babies (Callan & Witter 1990).

Intrauterine growth retardation is also associated with an increased risk of perinatal death, not only through its link with low birth weight, but because of an increased association with major congenital abnormalities. Studies report a birth prevalence of 4.6–11% (Butler 1974, Wennergren et al 1988) in small-for-gestational-age infants and 31.6% in small-for-gestational-age infants under 1500 g birth weight (Drillien 1974).

Social factors causing problems

Most social factors act through causing prematurity and/or growth retardation.

Hellier (1977) showed that almost a quarter of the reduction in perinatal mortality rate that occurred in England and Wales between 1953 and 1978 was explained by the demographic changes in maternal age, parity and social class that had occurred. These included:

- more women bearing children at a safer age;
- improvements in the standard of living, with relative poverty becoming more of a problem than absolute poverty (Kawachi & Kennedy 1997);
- a decrease in the number of mothers of very large families;
- a general rise in the standard of nutrition and stature of women;
- more widespread use of contraception;
- the legalization of abortion following the 1967 Act.

'Elderly' primiparae and women with more than four previous births are often seen as high-risk patients. The data on which this perception is based are collected through national record systems that produce cross-sectional data at one point in time, as birth registration records in the UK cannot be linked. Cross-sectional studies look at all subjects at the same point in time. Such studies of pregnancy loss show a U-shaped curve for the distribution of perinatal mortality rate and parity, the death rate being high for first births, dipping to a lower level for first births and women under 20 years of age, and rising for fourth and subsequent births and for women aged over 35. Analysis in this way gives an erroneous view of the risks, as reproductive compensation may apply to women who have previously lost babies. Women who lose babies usually go on to have further pregnancies in order to achieve the size of family they want. They are at high risk because of the previous poor outcome and are therefore of higher parity and, of necessity, older. Longitudinal studies follow the same women over a period of time by linking each episode of health care. They show that fetal mortality for each pregnancy goes down as the mother's parity increases (Billewicz 1973, Roman et al 1978, Bakketeig & Hoffman 1979, 1981). For babies of the same mother, the risk of each baby dying seems to fall steadily with each pregnancy, but children from families that end up large are all at higher risk of perinatal death regardless of their birth order compared with children from small families. Higher age and parity in subsequent pregnancies may be the result of poor pregnancy outcome rather than its cause.

Longitudinal studies can also examine the effects of birth interval: a close spacing of pregnancy may contribute to an increased risk of perinatal death, and there is also a tendency for repeated perinatal death with the same mothers.

There is still great disparity between perinatal mortality rates in different social classes in Britain, although the increasing proportion of babies born to unmarried women – now over one-third – has meant that illegitimate babies are now less disadvantaged at birth than they once were.

Women from ethnic minority groups appear to have a higher risk of perinatal death than do indigenous mothers. A minor part of this may be the result of a difference in birth weight distribution, but the incidence of malformation may be very different. The increased incidence of lethal congenital malformations in British Pakistanis made a large contribution to a perinatal mortality rate of 18 per 1000 in 1984 for this group compared with 12 per 1000 in other ethnic groups – a 50% excess (Balarajan & Botting 1989, Chitty & Winter 1989). The access to and use of maternity services may also affect outcome (Clarke et al 1988).

Finding problems by screening

Screening is a service that detects the predisposition for a particular disease or its early, treatable stages in people who are generally considered to be disease free when the screen is carried out. Public health specialists evaluate how well screening tests perform in picking up individuals who will develop disease.

Screening can be carried out by specific questions or by tests using blood samples or ultrasound. For example, the questions 'How old are you?' and 'What ethnic group do you belong to?' are both screening tests to determine a subgroup who are at higher risk of having a baby with a problem than the general population: trisomy 21 in the case of maternal age, and sickle cell anaemia, thalassaemia or Tay–Sachs disease in the case of ethnic group. We treat questions as part of case-finding and as of little importance. We certainly do not counsel people before we ask their age, and may not warn that we are measuring nuchal skinfold when we perform a dating scan, and a woman needs to make a definite move to opt out of this type of screening. However, we should reflect on why the offer of a blood test to estimate the risk of Down syndrome triggers long sessions explaining the condition and the screening process, and relies on the woman opting in and giving verbal informed consent. It is important that counselling or questioning is non-directive – enabling rather than prescriptive – and does not involve carers in putting their own views forward, although with the best will in the world, body language and intonation of voice can betray one's own thoughts (Hollingsworth 1994).

A screening test is not usually in itself diagnostic; it detects a subgroup of those tested who are at higher risk of having the disease or disorder than the original population screened. This subgroup needs further investigation with a diagnostic test that is usually more time-consuming, invasive and expensive than the screening test.

Screening programmes

Prenatal screening is a two-edged sword that can do good and harm, often at the same time to the same person (Abramsky 1994). To maximize benefit and minimize detriment, screening should not be introduced because a screening test has just been devised, but should be part of a planned and evaluated programme that is:

- cost-effective, with the costs of screening weighed against the benefits gained from the programme and the opportunity of using the money for other projects that are foregone;
- planned, with an agreed policy on who to screen;
- preceded by a campaign of education of both professionals and those who are being offered screening;
- offering good, sympathetic, non-directive counselling;
- monitored to see that it is, and continues to be, effective;
- continuous rather than one-off;
- providing treatment services for those who are missed by screening or do not take up the offer of screening, prenatal diagnosis or therapeutic abortion for whatever reason.

Any screening programme must be preceded by good diagnostic and treatment facilities. It is no good offering a neonatal hearing screening service if there is a 6-month wait for an audiology appointment to diagnose the child and to fit hearing aids.

Some sort of cost–benefit evaluation is needed for all screening programmes, together with surveys on what those who are most affected by the results – the parents – think of what is offered to them.

What infrastructure is needed for a screening programme?

Without a functioning infrastructure in place, any genetic screening programme is likely to cause more problems than it alleviates and run into disrepute. Any screening programme needs (Modell 1990):

- a programme of information and education for health professionals and the target population;
- a system for collecting samples from a cohort of the population and delivering them to the laboratory where the tests will be conducted, or a system for imaging, such as ultrasound;
- a network of diagnostic laboratories and ultrasound departments with a quality control system;
- an information storage and retrieval system;
- a system for notifying results to those tested and their medical advisors and for storing the results in their medical records;
- an information and counselling service for the target population;
- an adequate number of expert centres for counselling couples at risk and providing prenatal diagnosis;
- a system of monitoring the service.

What is an ideal disease to screen for?

There are many sets of criteria by which to judge whether a screening programme is likely to bring benefits to those screened (Thorner & Remein 1961, McKeown 1968, Wilson & Jungner 1968, Cochrane & Holland 1971, Cuckle & Wald 1984).

In summary, screening programmes work well if the disease they are intended to pick up is:

- well defined;
- of known natural history;
- an important health problem for the individual and for the community as it is severe, common or both;
- of known incidence and prevalence;
- preventable by acceptable methods.

Case study: toxoplasmosis screening in the UK and France

The parasite *Toxoplasma gondii* can cause fetal infection, which may result in severe and lasting neurological damage in the baby, when the mother contracts the infection for the first time in pregnancy. The disease in the mother is usually symptomless, and not all infections in pregnancy produce disability in the baby. Screening programmes on maternal blood have been running in France and Austria for some time. An initial test is carried out at booking, and if the mother has not had a previous *Toxoplasma* infection, the tests are repeated monthly to ensure that any new infection is detected and treated in utero or a termination of pregnancy is offered if necessary. About 20–25% of French women need repeated testing (*Lancet* 1990).

In Britain, about 25 new cases of congenital toxoplasmosis in 680 000 births are reported each year to the British Paediatric Surveillance Unit. This is about half the expected number estimated from data on acute toxoplasma infection in pregnancy and transmission rates (*Lancet* 1990). Only 20% of women tested in London had previously contracted a toxoplasmosis infection (Fleck 1969), so a screening programme in the UK would need to test 680 000 women at the start of their pregnancy and subsequently 80% (or 540 000 pregnant women) in each month of their pregnancy to produce the chance of detecting 25–50 cases each year.

The expense of this means that it is highly unlikely that *Toxoplasma* screening will be introduced in Britain. This is in spite of vigorous lobbying by well-informed and highly motivated pressure groups of families who have discovered that their child has been damaged by a potentially detectable and treatable disease. The cost per case discovered, however beneficial to the individual family concerned, is simply too high. Greater benefit to the community as a whole may result in spending the same amount of money on other forms of more cost-beneficial health care. Health education on minimizing the risks of contracting toxoplasmosis during pregnancy through food hygiene in preparing raw meat and in avoiding cat faeces is a more cost-effective way of reducing the incidence (Royal College of Obstetricians and Gynaecologists 1992).

Case study: 'normality' – what messages do we give by screening?

There are now numerous ways of screening for Down syndrome: asking for maternal age, fetal nuchal translucency measurement with ultrasonography and the use of a variety of biochemical markers from maternal blood in combination with maternal age. None of these programmes picks up all cases of trisomy 21, and all produce false positive results that cause untold worry and may lead to the loss of a pregnancy after an invasive diagnostic test. Counselling about these tests takes considerable time and effort.

Smoking overall produces more ill-health in women and babies than any genetic disorder; however, we do not routinely offer clinical screening for smoking but instead rely on self-reporting. Why do clinicians and the general public pay so much attention to the Down screening programme but pay less attention to, and use fewer resources on, other more important health messages?

What messages are we giving to women by these programmes? Do women think that people with trisomy 21 have such a poor quality of life that clinicians are determined on a 'search and destroy policy' by inventing more and more tests? As the birth prevalence of the disorder decreases with increased testing, fewer lay people and professional staff will come into contact with families who have a member with trisomy 21. There is a high risk that continued emphasis on screening for the most common chromosomal disorder in liveborn babies will present a skewed public view of its effects and a stigmatization of families and people with the syndrome.

Amniocentesis will pick up chromosomal variations other than trisomy 21, but parents are often not forewarned that this may happen. Some (trisomy 13 and trisomy 18) are lethal, but many, such as a sex chromosome trisomy, an apparently balanced structural rearrangement or a mosaicism, are not. These are often reported as chromosomal abnormalities rather than variations. What messages does this give to parents and clinicians?

It is difficult to give a prognosis with respect to the physical or intellectual effect of many of these variations. Many perceptions are based on data that are collected in a way which is biased. Males with XXY chromosomes (Klinefelter syndrome) are found in approximately 1 in 1000 male births. Not long ago, the traditional textbook description of a Klinefelter syndrome was of a mentally retarded male, lacking in male secondary characteristics and with breast enlargement – an alarming prospect for future parents. This picture resulted from a bias in selection, since originally only those boys with the most severe physical manifestations had their chromosomes analysed. Long-term prospective and population studies suggest that many people with Klinefelter syndrome look and act 'normally' and may not be found to have the syndrome until karyotyping is carried out as part of investigations for infertility (Robinson et al 1992, Abramsky & Chapple 1997).

What are the characteristics of an ideal screening test?

The screening test must:

- be simple, safe and acceptable;
- be valid, that is, both sensitive and specific, with a high predictive value;
- be repeatable;
- be relatively inexpensive;
- have a distribution of test values in affected and unaffected individuals that is known, a sufficiently small extent of overlap and a suitable, defined, cut-off level.

As screening tests are applied to people who are regarded as being fit and well in an attempt to stop future ill-health, it is vital that the tests are acceptable and do not cause iatrogenic disease. Acceptability varies according to culture and perceived seriousness of the disorder. It is accepted in Western countries that women should not mind having a vaginal examination with a speculum in order for a cervical smear to be taken because it is perceived that the screening procedure will have a significant effect on mortality from cervical cancer.

In any screening programme, it is inevitable that certain individuals will be subjected to what is later proved to be unnecessary worry and that some will be falsely reassured, thus being even more devastated by the birth of a child with a congenital malformation. The evaluation of screening programmes is therefore essential if individuals in society are to have access to appropriate technology that, overall, does more good than harm.

Case study: screening for trisomy 21

Screening programmes based on offering amniocentesis to older mothers (37 years old or more) subject about 5% of pregnancies in Britain to amniocentesis and pick up about one-third of fetuses with trisomy 21 (Down syndrome). Newer techniques, using markers found in maternal blood, have been shown to pick up nearly half of all cases for the same amniocentesis rate (Wald et al, 1992). However, to keep to the same 5% amniocentesis rate, older mothers will have to forego their absolute right to a diagnostic test and will only have an amniocentesis if indicated by the blood test, which misses a few cases.

The aim of needs assessment, case finding and

screening programmes is to target resources at women who will benefit most from them. This is done with the aim of improving the outcome of pregnancy for the woman, her child and her family. How can we measure whether we are achieving this aim?

Measuring better outcomes of maternity services

Modern technology gives us countless methods of investigating and treating health and disease. However, many of the procedures carried out by health professionals are ineffective and do not produce a better state of health for those individuals who have sought clinical help (Enkin et al 1989). In a tax-funded health care system such as the NHS, it is inevitable that interest focuses on funding good results, or outcomes, of health care rather than on emphasizing the processes (such as the number of operations or other procedures).

Health is not merely the absence of disease and infirmity but a state of complete physical, mental and social well-being (World Health Organization 1992), and should be a universal human right (Saracci 1997). Better health outcomes will therefore also include social aspects of pregnancy and childbirth, but these may be difficult to measure. For example, a good outcome is for every women to be satisfied with the support she has received during pregnancy, delivery and the postpartum period, and to feel that she and her baby have been at the centre of care. Some tools to measure this are available (Mason 1989, Lamping & Rowe 1996, Audit Commission 1997). In small surveys, a response rate of about 70% can be expected with postal questionnaires, but there will be a bias in those who respond: women with visual problems or learning disabilities, or who do not speak English, will find it difficult to give their views. It is also difficult to look at changes in behaviour as a result of care; a good outcome would be for smokers to reduce or give up smoking during pregnancy and afterwards, but monitoring this is difficult if it relies on self-assessment (Walsh et al 1996) and intrusive if it requires urinary testing for cotinine, a byproduct of nicotine. Some physical problems after childbirth, such as urinary or faecal incontinence, are also important but are often hidden by women. Many of these outcome measures are not included in routinely collected data systems but would need special surveys to monitor them. It is therefore unsurprising to see that the chief measure of outcome used in the past has been death, an event that has to be registered in the UK by law, as does birth, so figures are readily available.

Looking at death as an outcome

One of the earliest outcome measures used in the NHS was perinatal mortality. This measure was first proposed in an article published in 1948 (Peller 1948), which suggested combining stillbirth and first-week death rates as the time trends for early neonatal deaths were more like those for stillbirths than other death rates in infancy.

Staff working in maternity services have a long history of investigating deaths through confidential enquiries, a form of external clinical audit (Shaw 1980). In such studies, each death is reviewed individually by a group of clinicians from different disciplines concerned in maternity care, and 'avoidable', 'adverse' or 'notable' factors that may have contributed to the death are ascertained. The identification of less than optimal resources and practice can be fed back anonymously to all clinicians to make them rethink how they provide maternity care.

From 1928 onwards, the main concern of obstetricians was maternal rather than perinatal death, as the maternal mortality rate was 4.4 deaths per 1000 total births, or 3000 mothers dying each year in England and Wales. This led to a national confidential enquiry into maternal deaths. The persisting difference in the rates of death of babies between countries and between regions in England and Wales in the 1970s led to interest in applying the methodology of confidential enquiries to perinatal deaths, although as there were then 10 perinatal deaths for each maternal death, the task was much greater (Chalmers 1979, Chalmers & McIlwaine 1980). Several regions (Northern, South East Thames, Wessex and Mersey; Mersey Region Working Party on Perinatal Mortality 1982) started enquiries at this time.

Defining perinatal mortality

Different countries have different methods of collecting data on perinatal death as well as different definitions. This section deals with the situation in England and Wales. Greater detail can be found in volume 1 of *Birth Counts* (Macfarlane & Mugford 1984).

The perinatal mortality rate per 1000 births is calculated using the equation:

$$\frac{(\text{Stillbirths} + \text{deaths at 0--6 days after live birth}) \times 1000}{\text{Live births} + \text{stillbirths}}$$

Definitions of live births and stillbirths, and hence perinatal mortality, vary with national policy and time. A stillborn baby in the UK must be registered with the local Registrar of Births and Deaths and is currently defined (under section 41 of the Births and

Deaths Registration Act 1953) as a child issuing forth from its mother after the 24th completed week of pregnancy that did not at any time after being completely expelled from its mother breathe or show any other signs of life. This definition came into force on 1 October 1992; prior to this, the cut-off gestational age was 28 weeks. This change in definition will increase the perinatal mortality rate, as babies dying between 25 and 28 weeks will now be included in the figures, although the Office of National Statistics will continue to supply figures based on both definitions for some time. Stillborn babies are defined by the time at which they were born rather than the gestation at which they died, so a papyraceous twin who has died months before its sibling is born should be registered as a stillbirth.

All liveborn babies must also be registered. A liveborn baby is a child who breathes or shows signs of life after complete expulsion from its mother, regardless of length of gestation. This categorization varies greatly from one country to another as there are different legal definitions excluding live births below defined lower limits of gestational age or birth weight. Laws relating to the timing of registration may also affect whether the child is certified as live or stillborn (Macfarlane & Mugford 1984).

In addition, individual judgement plays a part in the certification of perinatal deaths (Keirse 1984) and judgements about viability (Fenton et al 1990). Some fetuses are born so early that they are not viable but may still show visible signs of life for a few minutes. The current abortion law in England, Wales and Scotland allows the termination of pregnancy for severe fetal malformation at any gestational age. If the termination is carried out after 24 weeks gestation and the fetus is dead at birth, it should officially be registered as a stillbirth, and the legal forms relating to termination of pregnancy must also be completed. If feticide is not carried out prior to delivery, such a fetus may be liveborn and die after delivery, and this should again be registered as a live birth and subsequent death, with official disposal of the body and with completed termination documentation. However, it is not unknown for clinicians to be influenced by perceptions of how the parents will feel about official form-filling and about financial considerations with regard to maternity benefit and the cost of burial. This is understandable – the legal cut-off points are artificial and parental grief is unchanged by the stage of pregnancy at which a baby is lost – but technically illegal.

A full national Confidential Enquiry into Stillbirths and Deaths in Infancy (CESDI) was instituted in England, Wales and Northern Ireland from 1 January 1993. Slightly contrary to its name, CESDI covers all deaths from the 20th week of pregnancy to the end of the first year of life. For the first year, a confidential assessment was undertaken by local regional multidisciplinary panels of obstetricians, paediatricians, midwives, GPs, pathologists and others of all babies over 2500 g birth weight with no severe congenital malformation who died from a perinatal cause during labour or the first week of life. The type of case assessed will change according to an agreed programme. Annual reports for CESDI highlight factors contributing to death (Department of Health 1994, 1997). It is hoped that timely feedback will make clinicians aware of possible problems and how to avoid them.

Are perinatal mortality rates a good outcome measure of maternity and neonatal care?

There are several factors that make the continued use of perinatal mortality rates as a measure of the effectiveness of maternity and neonatal care increasingly unsafe.

Perinatal rates include only deaths in the first week of life. Many babies who would previously have died within this period are now, thanks to improved paediatric care, surviving beyond the first week but still die before they are a month old. There is a strong case for including late neonatal deaths in analyses of deaths occurring round the time of delivery to prevent the postponement of death artificially lowering perinatal rates.

The place of delivery of premature babies of less than 28 weeks' gestation (on the delivery suite or on a gynaecology ward) may affect their classification and hence figures for perinatal mortality (Fenton et al 1990). The onus of judgement regarding viability and classification is often placed on relatively junior staff. There is a theoretical possibility that there may be pressure on clinical staff to regard a fetus as non-registrable if the clinical performance of their unit is judged on its crude perinatal rate alone.

Crude comparisons of perinatal mortality, by either hospital or district of residence, can be highly misleading because of the problems caused by statistics involving very small numbers in numerator data and large denominators: are the figures the result of random variation? Increasingly small numbers and rates of deaths have led the Office of National Statistics to publish rates for combined 3-year periods, with 95% and 99% confidence limits to give some idea of the reliability of the crude figures.

Low and very low birth weight are such strong determinants of perinatal survival that any maternity hospital with a neonatal unit, especially one that takes tertiary referrals, will have a high crude perinatal rate simply because of the types of cases for which it cares. Evaluating its services on this basis is akin to castigating a geriatric hospital because of its high number of deaths – units looking after high-risk patients have high death rates. Some effort should be made to adjust perinatal rates for case mix and referral patterns to produce a meaningful result (Clarke et al 1993). Calculating birth weight-specific perinatal rates may help, although the number at individual hospitals will again be very small. Even when this is done, it is difficult to compare the effectiveness of hospital units using perinatal mortality rates because of the increasingly small subset of perinatal deaths that are amenable to medical intervention (Field et al 1988).

Other outcome or risk assessment scores may be much more useful. A reliable assessment of neonatal care is impossible without correcting for major risk factors, particularly initial disease severity (Tarnow-Modi et al 1990). One robust method of assessing initial neonatal risk that is more predictive of outcome than birth weight alone is the clinical risk index for babies score (International Neonatal Network 1993). This includes birth weight, gestational age, congenital malformation, maximum base excess in the first 12 hours, and minimum and maximum appropriate fraction of inspired oxygen in the first 12 hours. On the obstetric side, Buekens (1990) describes six outcome measures influenced by the process of care and its quality: maternal and perinatal mortality, postpartum haemorrhage, the sequelae of obstructed labour, the Apgar score and very early neonatal seizures.

While all perinatal deaths are tragic and should not be dismissed lightly, there is concern that death may be preferable to severe long-term impairment and anxiety about the quality of life for some very small babies who would have become part of the perinatal mortali-

---

Pointers for practice

- Public health specialists have as their patients whole communities.
- Epidemiology (the study of the distribution and determinants of disease) is the chief tool of public health.
- A number of environmental factors, both external and acting in utero, may affect pregnancy.
- The risk of exposure to environmental hazards is associated with socio-economic status.
- Birth weight is the best predictor of perinatal mortality.
- The factors that influence birth size are closely associated with socio-economic status.
- Screening detects the predisposition towards a particular disease at its early treatable stages in people who are generally considered to be disease free when the screen is carried out; a screening test is not usually in itself diagnostic.
- In any screening programme, certain individuals will be prone to unnecessary worry and some falsely reassured. An evaluation of the screening programme is essential to ensure that it does more good than harm.
- Perinatal mortality rates are not in themselves a good outcome measure of maternity and neonatal care.

---

ty statistics had modern technology not been used to save them. It is important that, in the future, as much attention is paid to morbidity arising in the antenatal and perinatal period as has been paid to perinatal mortality in the past. This will require better information systems to collect data on each pregnancy as a routine part of care. It is also important that data from child health information systems can be linked to details of the pregnancy that produced that child to provide long-term follow-up. Midwives have a vital part to play in collecting reliable and clinically relevant information to link the health of the mother to the outcome for the baby.

REFERENCES

Abramsky L 1994 In: Prenatal diagnosis – the human side. Abramsky L, Chapple J (eds). Chapman & Hall, London

Abramsky L, Chapple J 1997 47,XXY (Klinefelter syndrome) and 47,XYY: estimated rates and indication for postnatal diagnosis with implications for prenatal counselling. Prenatal Diagnosis 14(4): 363–8

Acheson D 1988 Public health in England – the report of the committee of enquiry into the future development of the public health function. London HO Cm 289. HMSO, London

Allen M C, Donohoe P K, Dusman A E 1993 The limit of viability – neonatal outcome of infants born at 22 to 25 weeks' gestation. New England Journal of Medicine 329: 1597–1601

Audit Commission (1997) First class delivery: improving maternity services in England and Wales. Audit Commission, London

Bakketeig L S, Hoffman H J 1979 Perinatal mortality by birth order within cohorts based on sibship size. British Medical Journal 2: 693–6

Bakketeig L S, Hoffman H J 1981 Epidemiology of preterm birth. In: Elder M G, Hendricks C H (eds) Results from a longitudinal study of births in Norway in preterm labour. Butterworths International Medical Reviews. Butterworth, London

Balarajan R, Botting B 1989 Perinatal mortality in England and Wales: variations by mother's country of birth (1982–1985). Health Trends 21: 79–84

Barker D J P 1992 Fetal and infant origins of adult disease. BMJ Publishing, London

Billewicz W Z 1973 Some implications of self selection for pregnancy. British Journal of Preventive and Social Medicine 27: 49–52

Bucher H C, Schmidt J G 1993 Does routine ultrasound scanning improve outcome in pregnancy? Meta-analysis of various outcome measures. British Medical Journal 307: 13–17

Buekens P 1990 Outcome measures of obstetrical and perinatal care. Quality Assurance in Health Care 2: 253–62

Butler N R 1974 Late postnatal consequences of fetal malnutrition. Current Concepts in Nutrition 2: 173–8

Callan N A, Witter F R 1990 Intrauterine growth retardation: characteristics, risk factors and gestational age. International Journal of Obstetrics and Gynaecology 33: 215–20

Calman K C, Royston G H D 1997 Risk language and dialects. British Medical Journal 315: 939–42

Casson I F, Clarke C A, Howard C V et al 1997 Outcomes of pregnancy in insulin dependent diabetic women: results of a five year population cohort study. British Medical Journal 315: 275–8

Chalmers I 1979 Desirability and feasibility of a 4th National Perinatal Survey: report submitted to the Children's and Reproductive Research Liaison Group's Research Division of the DHSS. National Perinatal Epidemiology Unit, Oxford

Chalmers I, McIlwaine G (eds) 1980 Perinatal audit and surveillance. Proceedings of the 8th study group. Royal College of Obstetricians, London

Chitty L S, Winter R M 1989 Perinatal mortality in different ethnic groups. Archives of Disease in Childhood 64: 1036–41

Clarke M, Mason E S 1985 Leatherwork: a possible hazard to reproduction. British Medical Journal 290: 1235–7

Clarke M, Clayton D G, Mason E S, MacVicar J 1988 Asian mothers' risk factors for perinatal death – the same or different? A ten year review of Leicestershire perinatal deaths. British Medical Journal 297: 384–7

Clarke M, Mason E S, MacVicar J, Clayton D G 1993 Evaluating perinatal mortality rates: effects of referral and case mix. British Medical Journal 306: 824–7

Cochrane A L 1972 Effectiveness and efficiency – random reflections on health services. Nuffield Provincial Hospitals Trust, London

Cochrane A L, Holland W W 1971 Validation of screening procedures. British Medical Bulletin 27: 3

Cuckle H S, Wald N J 1984 Principles of screening. In: Wald N J (ed.) Antenatal and neonatal screening. Oxford University Press, Oxford

Czeizel A E 1993 Prevention of congenital abnormalities by periconceptional multivitamin supplementation. British Medical Journal 306: 1645–8

Czeizel A E, Dudas I 1992 Prevention of the first occurrence of neural tube defects by periconceptional vitamin supplementation. New England Journal of Medicine 327: 1832–5

Department of Health 1993 Changing childbirth. Report of the Expert Maternity Group (Cumberlege report). HMSO, London

Department of Health 1994 Annual report for Confidential Enquiry into Stillbirths and Deaths in Infancy for 1 January–31 December 1993. Department of Health, London

Department of Health 1997 Annual report for Confidential Enquiry into Stillbirths and Deaths in Infancy for 1 January–31 December 1996. Department of Health, London

Doyle W, Crawford M, Wynn A, Wynn S 1990 The association between maternal diet and birth dimensions. Journal of Nutritional Medicine 1: 9–17

Drillien C M 1974 Prenatal and perinatal factors in etiology and outcome of low birth weight. Clinics in Perinatalogy 1: 197–211

Enkin M, Keirse J N C, Chalmers I 1989 A guide to effective care in pregnancy and childbirth. Oxford University Press, Oxford

Ewigman B G, Crane J P, Frigoletto F D, Lefevre M L, Bain R P, McNellis D 1993 Effect of ultrasound screening on perinatal outcome. New England Journal of Medicine 329: 821–7

Fenton A C, Field D J, Mason E, Clarke M 1990 Attitudes to viability of preterm infants and their affect on figures for perinatal mortality. British Medical Journal 300: 434–6

Field D J, Smith H, Mason E, Milner A D 1988 Is perinatal mortality a good indicator of perinatal care? Paediatric and Perinatal Epidemiology 2: 213–19

Fitzhardinge P M, Inwood S 1989 Long term growth in small for date children. Acta Paediatrica Scandinavica 349: 27–33

Fleck D G 1969 Toxoplasmosis. Public Health 83: 131–5

Hack M H, Fanaroff A A 1989 Outcomes of extremely low birth weight infants between 1982 and 1988. New England Journal of Medicine 321: 1642–7

Hawthorne G, Robson S, Ryall E A, Sen D, Roberts S H, Ward Platt M P 1997 Prospective population based survey of outcome of pregnancy in diabetic women: results of the Northern Diabetic Pregnancy Audit. British Medical Journal 315: 279–81

Hellier J 1977 Perinatal mortality 1950 and 1973 Population Trends 10: 13–15

Hollingsworth J 1994 The sonographer's dilemma. In: Abramsky L, Chapple J (eds) Prenatal diagnosis – the human side. Chapman & Hall, London

Homer C J, Beresford S A, James S A, Siegel E, Wilcox S 1990 Work-related physical exertion and risk of preterm low birth weight delivery. Paediatric and Perinatal Epidemiology 4(2): 161–74

International Neonatal Network 1993 The CRIB (clinical risk index for babies) score: a tool for assessing initial neonatal risk and comparing performance for neonatal intensive care units. Lancet 342: 193–8

Kawachi I, Kennedy B P (1997) Health and social cohesion: why care about income inequality? British Medical Journal 314: 1037–40

Keirse M J N C 1984 Perinatal mortality rates do not contain what they purport to contain. Lancet i: 1166–9

Lamping D L, Rowe P 1996 Survey of women's experience of maternity services (short form): user's manual for purchasers and providers. Health Services Research Unit, London School of Hygiene and Tropical Medicine

Lancet 1990 Antenatal screening for toxoplasmosis in the United Kingdom. Lancet ii: 346–7 (editorial)

Liberman E, Gremy I, Lang J M, Cohen A P 1994 Low birthweight at term and the timing of fetal exposure to maternal smoking. American Journal of Public Health 84(7): 1127–31

Lubchenco L O, Hansman C, Dressler M, Boyd E 1963 Intrauterine growth as estimated from liveborn birthweight data at 24 to 42 weeks of gestation. Pediatrics 32: 793–800

Macfarlane A, Mugford M 1984 Birth counts: statistics of pregnancy and chilbirth. National Perinatal Epidemiology Unit, OPCS/HMSO, London

McKeown T 1968 Validation of screening procedures. In: Screening in medical care. Reviewing the evidence. Nuffield Provincial Hospital Trust/Oxford University Press, Oxford

McMichael A J, Vimpani G V, Robertson E F, Baghurst P A, Clark P D 1986 The Port Pirie cohort study: maternal blood lead and pregnancy outcome. Journal of Epidemiology and Community Health 40: 18–25

Mason V 1989 Women's experience of maternity care – a survey manual. HMSO, London

Mersey Region Working Party on Perinatal Mortality 1982 Confidential inquiry into perinatal deaths in the Mersey region. Lancet i: 491–4

Mezey G C, Bewley S 1997 Domestic violence and pregnancy. British Journal of Obstetrics and Gynaecology 104: 528–31

Modell B 1990 Cystic fibrosis screening and community genetics. Journal of Medical Genetics 27: 475–9

Mooney G 1992 Economics, medicine and health care, 2nd edn. Harvester Wheatsheaf, England

MRC Vitamin Study Research Group 1991 Prevention of neural tube defects: results of the Medical Research Council Vitamin Study. Lancet 338: 131–7

Naismith D J 1981 Diet during pregnancy – a rationale for prescription. In: Dobbing J (ed.) Maternal nutrition in pregnancy. Eating for two? Academic Press, London

Nicoll A, McGarrigle C, Brady A R et al 1998 Epidemiology and detection of HIV-1 among pregnant women in the United Kingdom: results from a national surveillance 1988–96. British Medical Journal 316: 253–8

Northern, South East Thames, Wessex and Mersey. Mersey Region Working Party on Perinatal Mortality 1982

Peller S 1948 Mortality past and future. Population Studies 1: 405–6

Robinson A, Bender B G, Linden M G 1992 Prognosis of prenatally diagnosed children with sex chromosome aneuploidy. American Journal of Medical Genetics 44: 365–8

Roman E, Doyle P, Beral V, Alberman E, Pharoah P 1978 Fetal loss, gravidity and pregnancy order. Early Human Development 2: 131–8

Rosenberg M J, Feldblum P J, Marshall E G 1987 Occupational influences on reproduction: a review of the recent literature. Journal of Occupational Medicine 29: 584–91

Royal College of Obstetricians and Gynaecologists, Multidisciplinary Working Group 1992 Prenatal screening for toxoplasmosis in the United Kingdom. Royal College of Obstetricians and Gynaecologists, London

Saari-Kemppainen A, Karjalainen O, Ylostalo P,

Heinonen O P 1990 Ultrasound screening and perinatal mortality: controlled trial of systematic one-stage screening in pregnancy. Lancet 336: 387–91

Sackett D L, Haynes R B, Guyatt G H, Tugwell P 1991 Clinical epidemiology – a basic science for clinical medicine, 2nd edn. Little, Brown, Boston

Sanjose S, Roman E, Beral V 1991 Low birthweight and preterm delivery, Scotland, 1981–1984: effect of parents' occupation. Lancet 338: 428–31

Saracci R 1997 The World Health Organisation needs to reconsider its definition of health. British Medical Journal 314: 1409–10

Savitz D A, Whelan E A, Kleckner R C 1989 Effect of parents' occupational exposures on risk of stillbirths, preterm delivery, and small for gestational age infants. American Journal of Epidemiology 129: 1201–18

Shaw C D 1980 Aspects of audit. British Medical Journal 1: 1256

Silman R 1997 The social and ethical issues of risk assessment. In: Grudzinskas J G, Ward R H T (eds) Screening for Down syndrome in the first trimester. RCOG, London

Simpson R J, Armand Smith N G 1986 Maternal smoking and low birthweight: implications for antenatal care. Journal of Epidemiology and Community Helath 40: 223–7

Tarnow-Modi W, Ogston S, Wilkinson A R et al 1990 Predicting death from initial disease severity in very low birthweight infants: a method for comparing the performance of neonatal units. British Medical Journal 300: 1611–14

Thomson A M 1983 Fetal growth and size at birth. In: Barron S L, Thomson A M (eds) Obstetrical epidemiology. Academic Press, London

Thorner R M, Remein Q R 1961 Principles and procedures in the evaluation of screening for disease. Public Health Monograph No. 67. US Department of Health Education and Welfare. Public Health Service Publication No. 846. US Department of Health and Human Services, Public Health Service, National Institutes of Health, Besthesda

Wald N J, Kennard A, Densem J W et al 1992 Antenatal maternal serum screening for Down's syndrome: results of a demonstration project. British Medical Journal 305: 391–4

Walker E M, Patel N B 1987 Mortality and morbidity in infants born between 20 and 28 weeks gestation. British Journal of Obstetrics and Gynaecology 94: 670–4

Walsh R A, Redman S, Adamson L 1996 The accuracy of self report of smoking status in pregnant women. Addictive Behaviours 21: 675–9

Wennergren M, Wennergren G, Vilbergsson G 1988 Obstetric characteristics and neonatal performance in a four-year small for gestational age population. Obstetrics and Gynecology 72: 615–20

Wilson J M C, Jungner G 1968 Principles and practice of screening for disease. Public Health Papers No. 34. WHO, Geneva

World Health Organization 1992 Basic document, 39th edn. WHO, Geneva

Wynn A, Crawford M, Doyle W, Wynn S 1991 Nutrition of women in anticipation of pregnancy. Nutrition and Health 7: 69–88

8

Exploring new worlds of midwifery

*Jane Sandall   Patricia Percival
Trudy Stevens*

This chapter has three aims. The first is that the reader will be able to think about where research questions come from and be aware of the research process. Second, it should be realized different questions require different research methods to answer them. Third, it is hoped that readers will reflect on the politics of research, the process of producing research knowledge and how that knowledge is used.

WHY DO RESEARCH?

Very little work has examined the development of midwifery research and research policy. Robinson & Thomson review the current state of play (1989, 1991, 1994, 1996), and Wilkins (1993) provides a critique of midwifery research from a sociological perspective. Traynor & Rafferty (1997) and Sandall (1996) have also discussed the place of nursing and midwifery research in the UK research and development strategy. The reasons for the difficulties that midwife researchers encounter in getting their findings valued and implemented by the midwifery profession are discussed by Hicks (1992, 1995).

To develop new midwifery knowledge?

Midwives have become involved in research more recently than other occupations, and there is a view that its professional status is legitimized by the movement of midwifery training into higher education and by an involvement in research. It has also been suggested that midwifery needs to develop a body of knowledge to underpin practice (Bryar 1995).

To improve the experience of childbirth for women and to give women a voice?

Some research has been inspired by a commitment towards giving women a voice and using their perspectives and experiences to inform a feminist political agenda. Much of this work has been carried out not by midwives but by social scientists (Macintyre 1977, Cartwright 1979, Green et al 1990). It has highlighted the competing views of women and doctors (Graham & Oakley 1981), and placed women's experiences of reproduction into a wider theoretical framework examining the impact of patriarchy on women in society (Oakley 1980). Other researchers have focused on the needs of women from various ethnic groups (Baxter 1996).

To change practice and make sure that care is effective?

Individual midwives have often embarked on research because of their unhappiness with current practice. They have been motivated by a desire to demonstrate that a different way of doing things has a better outcome. Such research uses scientific principles to challenge the supremacy of clinical experience. Initiated by medical epidemiologists (Chalmers & Richards 1977) and using the randomized controlled trial to evaluate effectiveness, epidemiologists have uncovered the iatrogenic consequences arising from obstetric technologies (Chalmers et al 1989, Neilson et al 1997). Midwives have been involved in this movement from an early stage, and midwives collaborating with epidemiologists have examined the effectiveness of midwifery practices such as perineal suturing, and nipple preparation for breastfeeding (Sleep 1991, Alexander 1996).

To examine the role of health professionals and the organization of care?

In general, this research has been conducted by social scientists using social research methods such as surveys, interviews and observation. For example, Robinson et al's (1983) research investigated the imbalance in professional power and made recommendations for future midwifery training. The findings highlighted the medical domination of maternity care and the constrained role of the midwife, particularly in specialist units. Subsequent research focused on the provision of less medicalized, woman-centred midwifery care (Green et al 1986) and the impact of midwifery policies on practice (Garcia & Garforth 1991). The difficulties of shedding the professional perspective when carrying out ethnographic research in this area have been raised by Hunt & Symons (1995) and will be addressed later in the chapter.

A second strand of the research into occupational roles has examined the organization of care and the implementation of new developments (Davies & Evans 1991). Research into the organization of care proliferated following *Changing Childbirth* (Department of Health 1993a). Studies have looked at team and caseload midwifery (Wraight et al 1993, McCourt and Page 1996, Allen et al 1997), but most of this work has been descriptive and has had a strong evaluative component, which has resulted in the undertheorization of broader issues.

Very little research has explored in a reflective sense the experiences of midwives as workers. Lewis (1991) examined those of male midwives and Sandall (1997) the health of midwives who were working mothers. Workforce issues, for example career paths (Robinson & Owen 1994) and the impact of the organization of care on the midwifery workforce (Stock & Wraight 1993) have been explored by social scientists. Midwifery teachers have focused on the experiences of students (Mander 1994). Again, such research needs explicitly to address the ethics of those in a position of power conducting research within their own institution.

To examine the process of midwifery care?

This stream of midwifery research has been concerned with the components of 'sensitive midwifery' and has usually been conducted by midwives, tending to focus on the primacy of the midwife–woman relationship. Examples include communication (Kirkham 1987) and continuity of care (Flint et al 1989). More recent midwifery research has tended to be dominated by a concern with continuity of care rather than broader issues. The examination of the effectiveness of the psychosocial aspects of care has mainly been undertaken by medical sociologists drawing on a broader theoretical framework of similar work in other areas of health care, for example Oakley et al's (1996) work looking at the effect of social support in pregnancy.

As historical research?

There has been a stream of historical study into midwifery, usually undertaken by historians and sociologists. A wide range of research has examined the historical aspects of midwifery in Britain and abroad (e.g. Donnison 1988, Marland & Rafferty 1997). Other work has viewed midwifery history from a critical perspective: Heagerty (1997) and Hannam (1996), for example, have examined the role of the Midwives Institute, while Witz (1992), Leap & Hunter (1993) and Sandall (1996) have looked at the development of midwifery as a profession and the relationship between gender and social class. Yet other research (Oakley 1984, Williams 1997) has looked more broadly at women's experiences of motherhood and maternity care during the 20th century.

As part of a course requirement or job?

Many midwives are now being asked to undertake small-scale projects as part of their job. As in any other area of midwifery practice, midwives should be trained and competent to do the work. Thus, midwives who are asked to do research should make sure that they have training and adequate supervision for the project. Other midwives have to carry out research as a requirement for a higher degree. It is important to remember that the reason for this involvement is that it is considered to be part of the educational and personal development of that particular midwife. Such midwives are often tempted into taking on large and complex research projects at work, which should really be the remit of midwives who have professional research training and experience.

WHERE DO OUR QUESTIONS COME FROM?

Research should be driven by curiosity, and at the start of all research lie the questions that arise daily through our work. Not all of these may be suitable so they will need to be reframed as research questions, a good one being important, interesting and answerable. For example, how would midwifery policy and practice and women's experiences of care be changed if the research questions were answered?

Deciding what and how topics get researched is also a political question. Those who set the research agenda and who define the research questions to be addressed hold a powerful position, and there is a danger that what gets researched is driven by the interests of powerful professional groups and the policy agenda. As a result, issues that are more important to users and to the improvement of health in a broader sense get neglected. This could lead to reluctance on the part of government to fund research that might yield uncomfortable evidence questioning or challenging policy (Pollit et al 1990).

At an individual level, questions come from listening to women, observing and reflecting on practice, our own experiences, reading the paper, watching television, reading journals, talking to colleagues and previous research. At an institutional level, questions come from examining audit data and statistics, and making comparisons with other sites. At a national level, a more systematic way has developed of developing topics for research. Research is often determined by policy initiatives, and several general policy initia-

tives are relevant to women's health. For example, the Health of the Nation strategy (Department of Health 1992) set targets for reductions in morbidity and mortality in key areas, the targets in Box 8.1 being particularly relevant to maternity care.

Box 8.1 Relevant Health of the Nation targets (Department of Health 1992)

- To reduce by at least 5% from 1989 the rate of conceptions amongst the under 16s by the year 2000.
- In addition to the overall reduction in prevalence, at least a third of women smokers to stop smoking at the start of their pregnancy by the year 2000.

The Patients Charter (Department of Health 1991) and related initiatives such as the Named Midwife scheme (Department of Health 1993b) aimed to make the NHS more responsive to users' needs and wishes with regard to the delivery, quality and location of services. A systematic evaluation of services and users' experiences is essential to ascertain whether or not these goals are being met. Other policy initiatives are specific to maternity care; for example, *Changing Childbirth* (Department of Health 1993a) outlined 10 indicators of success to be met by the year 2000 and funded projects to develop and evaluate this initiative along with research funded from other sources (McCourt et al 1996, Allen et al 1997).

Policy initiatives are also informed by the Centrally Commissioned Research Programme of the Department of Health (Department of Health 1995a, 1995b), the purpose of which is to provide a knowledge base for health and social policies directed at the health of the population as a whole. The NHS Research and Development (R&D) strategy (Department of Health 1993c, 1995c), in its goal of producing knowledge-based health care, has created a national and regional infrastructure for identifying and prioritizing NHS research requirements. This has resulted in a major research and development programme on NHS and nursing (Department of Health 1993d) priority topics.

The NHS R&D programme defines 'research' as a rigorous and systematic enquiry, conducted on a scale and using methods commensurate with the research question, and designed to lead to generalizable contributions to knowledge. Thus research and development is an overall process of which research and evaluations are a part. Table 8.1 shows the research funded by the Maternal and Child Health programme.

Questions also arise from theoretical considerations, and here, as we have seen, clinicians and social scien-

Table 8.1   Maternity care research funded from the NHS Research and Development programme

Area	Priority topics	Report
Mother and child health	Evaluation of different models of maternity care Short- and long-term outcomes of interventions during labour Evaluation of genetic services Evaluation of services relating to miscarriage Examination of causes, prevention, management and long-term outcome of babies born too early or too small Evaluation of variations in outcome relating to high-risk neonatal care Mental and physical health of mother after birth Impact of maternal and infant nutrition on health	Improving the health of mothers and children: NHS priorities for research and development

Information from Department of Health (1995d).

tists may take quite different approaches to questions relating to health. For example and very simply, the medical approach defines the problem as beginning with a disease or a stage of health care. Psychological approaches are concerned with people's responses to health and illness, while sociologists would look at the

implications of the provision of care both for women and society in general. Table 8.2 highlights the types of question that arise from differing perspectives, using prenatal screening as an example.

Some researchers can also get into a methodological rut, which limits the types of question that they can answer. Well-designed randomized controlled trials answer questions about effectiveness but cannot answer process questions, which are best answered by qualitative research. For example, the Cochrane Database (Update Software 1998) tells us that social support in labour improves maternal and child health outcomes. However, we do not know the mechanism for this, i.e. how and why support during childbirth leads to a better outcome. How do women perceive support from different sources? Only qualitative work may provide these answers, and further trials can answer the question of who is the most effective at providing support during childbirth (Hodnett 1997).

WHAT METHOD IS BEST AT ANSWERING OUR QUESTION?

Different research methods or designs are appropriate for answering different research questions. The research design is largely determined by the research questions and by what is already known about particular aspects of a research topic. As we discuss later in the chapter, more than one research design may be used in any one particular study.

In summary, the types of question we ask demand different methods to answer them. Table 8.3 gives specific examples of how different questions about the induction of labour could most appropriately be answered.

Table 8.2   Different perspectives on prenatal screening

Health professional	Approach
Epidemiologist	What are the uptake, specificity, sensitivity, effectiveness, and efficacy of a particular programme (Wald et al 1998)
Health economist	What is the cost–effectiveness of a prenatal screening programme? What should the outcome measure be? (Mooney & Lange 1993)
Psychologist	What are the effects of antenatal serum screening on pregnant women? (Marteau et al 1992)
Sociologist	How do perceptions of risk differ between the lay public and experts? (Parsons & Atkinson 1992). What is the relationship between prenatal screening and the eugenics movement? (Hubbard 1986)
Midwife	How can midwives support women in making an informed choice about screening? (Smith et al 1995)
Anthropologist	How is the way in which we think about pregnancy being changed by prenatal screening? (Press & Browner 1994)
Ethicist	What are the ethical issues of genetic screening? (Nuffield Council on Bioethics 1993)

Table 8.3 Answering questions

Question	Research method
What is the effect of induction on clinical outcome?	Randomized controlled trial Case control study
What is the effect of induction on psychosocial outcomes?	Randomized controlled trial or survey
What do women feel about induction?	In-depth interviews with women and observation
How are decisions to induce made? Who makes them?	Observation and interviews with clinical staff

How many women are induced in the UK?
  In this hospital?
  Does it vary by class, ethnicity, parity, consultant or hospital?
What are the variations in practice?
	Survey or secondary analysis

What is the history of induction?	Documentary analysis
How did induction become implemented as an innovation?	Interviews with 'experts' and key informants

The research continuum

Within the broader and often-used terms of 'qualitative' and 'quantitative' research, there are categories or groups of research design. One way of describing these is by using a research continuum:

Exploratory→Descriptive→Correlational→
Quasi-experimental→Experimental

However, it must be emphasized that 'progress' along the research continuum may be in either direction.

At one end of the research continuum, if little is known about a particular aspect of a topic, *exploratory* research may be undertaken (Leininger 1985, Rissmiller 1991), the researcher essentially asking individuals about their experiences in a very open-ended, narrative way. For example:

The purpose of this study is to describe the experience of women who have a home birth.

As more information is gathered about a topic, 'progress' is made along the research continuum. Midwives may choose a *correlational* design to investigate relationships between two or more variables (Friedman 1980, Burns & Grove 1993, Smith and Hunt 1997). For example:

Is there a relationship between a women's gratification with her birth experience and her emotional well-being at six weeks after the birth?

At the other end of the research continuum, as more knowledge exists in an area, a *quasi-experimental* or *true experimental* study may be appropriate (Burns & Grove 1993). This allows midwives to test out specific protocols or treatments. For example:

New mothers who receive a debriefing session

following their baby's birth will have significantly higher levels of emotional well-being at six weeks after the birth than those who receive standard postnatal care.

Within each of these broad categories, there are a number of different research approaches or designs. This chapter provides only a brief overview of these approaches.

Exploratory research

Exploratory research largely seeks to observe, describe or explore aspects of a situation. Such studies are conducted in areas where little knowledge exists, largely seeking to describe and explore a person's understanding or experience of given situations (Holloway 1991, Street 1995, Parse 1996). Within the broad category of exploratory research, a number of approaches may be used, for example phenomenological, grounded theory, ethnographic or historical (Glaser & Strauss 1967, Leininger 1985, Crotty 1996). One major focus of qualitative research is to generate hypotheses and develop theories (Hammersley & Atkinson 1995, Smith & Hunt 1997).

Descriptive and correlational research

Descriptive research is used to obtain more information about a particular area or topic. Descriptive–correlational research moves a step further in that it investigates relationships between variables or groups, correlational research seeking to establish a relationship between variables (Friedman 1980, Smith & Hunt 1997).

Within the broad categories of descriptive and correlational research, a number of approaches may be used.

These are described in detail in most good research books (see Further Reading at the end of the chapter). Epidemiologists often use quantitative descriptive designs, which may be either retrospective or prospective. While correlational designs cannot always establish causal relationships, they nevertheless form a critical part of health evaluation (Harper et al 1994). They are rich in realism and can be used for the many problems not appropriate for experimental designs (Polit & Hungler 1991).

Good correlational studies with a careful design and tightly worded hypotheses may be used in prediction (Burns & Grove 1993). For example, in the case of thalidomide, a retrospective approach was used to look at infants born with birth defects who were then identified as having been exposed to thalidomide. However, because no control is possible over the presumed causative factor, the relationship is correlational rather than causal.

It is important to remember that correlation does not prove causation. When a significant correlation exists between two variables, it is not always possible to specify the direction of causation. For example, did the changes in the independent variable cause the changes in the dependent variable, or vice versa.

Experimental designs

Experimental research usually begins with an explanation, predicts what should be found on observation and then tests these predictions. The purpose of most experimental research is to predict a causal relationship between an independent and a dependent variable. That is a change in one 'thing' will be related to a change in another 'thing'.

Within the broad category of experimental research, a number of research designs or approaches are available, for example the randomized clinical trial. Again, these are described in detail in most good books on research (Polit & Hungler 1991, Burns & Grove 1993). The two most common kinds of experimental designs are true experimental and quasi-experimental.

True experimental designs. A true experimental design must have the following features:

- *Random assignment*. Random assignment means each subject in the sample has an equal chance of being in either the treatment or the control group. Methods of random assignment may be simple or complicated. Random selection is different from random assignment; random selection ensures that every subject in the population has an equal chance of being chosen for the study and is used in the survey research.
- *Manipulation*. The researcher must change or manipulate the independent variable. The independent variable may be a treatment, for example a change in routine, such as demand versus 3-hourly feeding for premature infants.
- *Control*. The research design must contain a second group of people who do not receive the treatment or independent variable.

A true experimental design is the most powerful method for testing cause-and-effect relationships. The main advantages of experimental research result from the control, manipulation and random assignment in that it is easier to establish a causal relationship between two variables, thus increasing the trial's internal validity.

The main disadvantage of true experimental designs is that a large number of human characteristics cannot be controlled (Streubert & Carpenter 1995). Ethically, it is often not possible to assign people randomly into two groups. Imagine the possible outcry if women were randomly assigned to give birth at home or hospital regardless of their own wishes. In addition, it is important to control bias by making sure that the analysis includes all the participants who started in the study ('analysis by intention to treat').

Quasi-experimental designs. Quasi-experimental research usually lacks one or more of the characteristics of control, manipulation and random assignment. While it is often not possible randomly to assign individuals into groups, it is still possible in many instances to have a control group. Naturally occurring groups may, however, be non-equivalent (Burns & Grove 1993). In other words (using the home birth example), women who have a home birth may be inherently different from those who give birth in hospital.

There are several advantages of quasi-experimental studies in that they are practical, feasible and more realistic. However, because of a decreased control over competing causes between the independent and dependent variables, there may be alternative explanations for the research results. It is, therefore, more difficult to establish a causal relationship between the independent and dependent variables and to make inferences and predictions from this.

WHAT ARE THE STRENGTHS AND WEAKNESSES OF EACH PARTICULAR DESIGN AND METHOD?

Corner (1991) described a schism in (nursing) research regarding the design of research and the methods used. She felt that research should be more flexible and inventive, moving beyond the quantitative versus qualitative debate. We would like to suggest that the study method is chosen as a result of the research

Table 8.4 Strengths and weaknesses of quantitative and qualitative approaches

Aspect	'Number crunchers': Quantitative	'Navel gazers': Qualitative
Type of research	Randomized controlled trial Case control study Survey Questionnaire	In-depth interview Participant observation Ethnography Conversation analysis
Research questions	How much, how many, how often, what is the effect of…?	What are the experiences, feelings regarding, opinions of…?
Type of question	Precise, requiring a numerical answer	Broad, requiring a verbal answer
Use of hypothesis	Present at the start and tested on data	May emerge as a result of the study
Treatment of data	Isolates and defines variables	Starts with general concepts that may change during research
Sample size	Large	Small
Sampling	Random or representative – to infer from sample to population	Theoretical – to minimize and maximize differences
Issues/items described	Through the eyes of the researcher	Through the eyes of the respondents
Data collection	Extensive Predesigned instrument	Intensive Uses self as instrument
Logic of generalization	Hypothesis-testing against data to see how many cases it explains Statistical generalizability	Examining data to determine an axiom that fits all cases Theoretical generalizability of concepts and categories
Analytical approach	Deductive	Inductive
Strengths	Causal inferences Analysis explicit	Explores lived experience of respondents
Sources of bias	Poor randomization in randomized controlled trial Poor case control Biased sample	Selecting data to fit a preconceived idea Selecting the exotic at the expense of the mundane Sample selection
Weaknesses	Randomized controlled trial – lower external validity, i.e. does it work in the real world	Lower internal validity, difficulty establishing cause and effect Analysis less explicit (before computers)

question. To illustrate this, Table 8.4 has deliberately created a typology of the extreme differences between quantitative and qualitative research. The aim is to demonstrate the strengths and weaknesses of each method rather than to create a hierarchy of evidence as is often presented, with randomized controlled trials given as the 'gold standard'. This is only the case when the question to be answered is one of effectiveness. As we have seen above, there are many other equally valid questions so what we need to reflect on is why the 'effect' questions are so often given priority in research funding.

Similarities between quantitative and qualitative research

All methods of data collection are analysed qualita-

tively insofar as the act of analysis is an interpretation. Qualitative judgements are made each time one moves further away from the point of data collection. For example in a questionnaire, the researcher has to consider whether the question was understood in the way that was intended, whether this class of response is equivalent to that and can be aggregated, and so on. Some procedures, such as factor analysis, depend on an intuitive understanding of the data to identify underlying factors. Some quantitative research is descriptive and does not always test hypotheses, and some qualitative work tests hypotheses.

Multiple methods

From the above discussion, it would appear that using different methods is a good idea, and the term 'triangulation' has been used to describe such a process. The term was originally derived from surveying, where one gets a better idea of where one is with two landmarks rather than one (Denzin 1970). Thus, if different kinds of data produced from different methods come to the same conclusion, our confidence in the results should be increased. We can combine different types of data or different researchers, or test competing theories. Brannen (1995) describes the following ways in which qualitative and quantitative data can be combined:

- **Qualitative work can assist quantitative work by:**
  - the development and piloting of research instruments, questionnaires and scales;
  - the interpretation and clarification of quantitative data;
  - providing exemplars of qualitative data;
  - exploration of subgroups where the quantitative method is inappropriate.
- **Quantitative work can assist qualitative work by:**
  - providing a survey sample that can be used to identify individuals for qualitative study;
  - correcting the 'elite bias' of field methods that overemphasize the articulate and those with high status;
  - providing a background context for qualitative data, often derived from official statistics or the secondary analysis of official data.
- **Qualitative and quantitative approaches are given equal weight:**
  - which may result in two separate but linked studies that are distinct from each other at all stages of the research process; alternatively, they may be integrated into one study, the linkage occurring in the fieldwork, the analysis or the writing up.

Although the idea of using multiple methods seems attractive, there are downfalls (Bryman 1988). Such research is more expensive in researchers' time and the amount of data that is needed, and it may not necessarily provide a better picture. In summary, if you are planning to use multiple methods it is important to remember the following points:

1. Specify the aim of each method, the nature of the resulting data and how the data relate to theory. Most importantly, welcome and explore discrepancies as they may lead to new avenues of enquiry and new theories.

2. Choose one method that describes the context in which the interaction occurs and one that is designed to illuminate the process of the interaction. For example, a study of midwife–woman interaction should also ask itself whether an analysis of the political economy of health care provides an understanding of the constraints and opportunities that determine the parameters of that interaction; i.e. does it differ if you compare the public and private health care systems?

3. Thus, choose one method specifically suited to exploring the structural aspects of the problem and one that can explore the essential elements of meaning to those involved.

Remember that:

- differences between types of data may be important and illuminating; thus, data must never be taken at face value and we need to acknowledge that there is no such thing as 'truth';
- what mixing methods does is to encourage the researcher to view the data critically and test and identify its weaknesses, also highlighting where to test further or carry out more research.
- an agreement of results does not indicate that they are correct – all the results may be wrong.

UNDERTAKING A STUDY: THE ESSENTIAL STEPS

Identifying the problem

Identifying the problem to be studied usually begins with a general topic or a broad question. This is then narrowed down into a carefully worded and concise statement that describes what the researcher intends to study.

Before commencing the research, the following questions should be asked:

- Is the problem an important one?
- Does the problem have significance for midwifery practice?
- Will the knowledge produced benefit patients or the health care system?
- Do the findings have the potential to improve midwifery practice?
- Will the findings contribute to theory?
- Has the problem been studied before? If so, is it worthy of replication?

Literature search

An initial literature search should take place very early in the project. In exploratory research, the review may set the scene for the study without providing great detail (Leininger 1985). However, in descriptive, correlational and experimental research, the literature review helps to narrow down and refine the research problem and provides a justification for the study. Where possible, any study should build upon the findings of other researchers. In some cases, it may be appropriate to replicate a study, for example if there were inconsistent findings or a small sample.

One's own organization may be able to arrange a computer search, or this may be possible through a university library. Defining important concepts and variables in a study is essential, as these are often the key words that will be used in the literature search.

There are several indexes that are valuable for midwives and other health professionals and can be obtained via nursing libraries (Lutley 1994, Smith & Hunt 1997). These include:

- the MIDIRS Data Base
- the Cochrane Library
- the International Nursing Index
- the Cumulative Index to Nursing and Allied Health Literature
- the Nursing Studies Index.

A manual search of the topic area could first be undertaken by looking through the various catalogues. These references can then be used as a basis for a more thorough computer search of the different indexes. If problems arise, staff at the library's information desk are usually very helpful.

When reviewing other research, and when writing the review for a study, the following questions should be asked:

- Is the literature review adequate?
- Are there any major deficits?
- Are primary or secondary sources used?
- Are all the references relevant, or are some merely used for padding?
- Does the literature review only describe research findings or does it critically evaluate?
- Is the review well organized? Are the findings integrated as they relate to each other?
- Does the literature review establish a base or rationale for the research?

Defining variables

Variables are qualities, properties or characteristics of persons, things or situations that are examined in research. In exploratory and often in purely descriptive research, variables emerge from the data collection phase (Patton 1990, Morse 1995). In quantitative research, however, each variable must be defined prior to the study. For example, if one variable is the degree of pain, this must be operationalized to allow it to be measured. The operational definition states how something will be measured, that is, what question-

naire or scale will be used to measure it (Burns & Grove 1993).

Purpose of the study

This is a carefully worded and concise statement describing what the researcher intends to study. The purpose of the study may be written in one of three ways:

- as a *declarative statement* of purpose (often found in exploratory research), which may be followed by specific objectives;
- as a *question* (often found in descriptive/survey research), which may be followed by specific objectives or non-directional hypotheses;
- as *hypotheses* (found in all experimental research), which may be followed by specific directional hypotheses.

Remember that it is the hypothesis which is tested in a study. Therefore, all aspects of the hypothesis must be operationally defined in order that they may be tested (Burns & Grove 1993).

Choosing a research design

An appropriate research design must be selected for the question to be investigated remembering that different designs are appropriate for different research questions (Patton 1990, Rissmiller 1991, Streubert & Carpenter 1995, Parse 1996). Internal and external validity are important concepts relevant to quantitative research designs and sampling methods. The terms are defined rather differently in qualitative research (Pope & Mays 1995).

Internal validity

In correlational and experimental research, internal validity is concerned with the extent to which the independent and dependent variables are truly related. For example, with what degree of assurance can the researcher claim that the independent variable caused or was correlated with the dependent variable? Could other competing causes be responsible for the change in the dependent variable? A higher degree of internal validity is found in true experiments because of the degree of control that can be exercised over extraneous variables or competing causes. Random assignment is the most effective procedure for controlling bias caused by extraneous variables (other variables that are not under investigation but may have a significant effect on the results, for example social status).

External validity

External validity is concerned with the extent to which the research findings can be generalized to other groups of people in the general population. The type of sample selection – where the sample was obtained and how – is a critical feature of the external validity of the study. If a convenience sample was used, it may be difficult to say that the sample was typical of other members of society. Random sampling procedures offer more advantages when generalizing the results of the research (Polit & Hungler 1991, Burns & Grove 1993).

Selecting a sample

It is seldom practical to study an entire population, for example all patients receiving therapy for back pain. Instead, a sample is selected from the total population. Exploratory research usually uses a small convenience sample (Hoffart 1991, Morse 1995). Correlational and experimental studies are more likely to use representative samples (Friedman 1980, Harper et al 1994).

A major question (with reference to the variables of concern in the study) is, how typical or representative is the sample of the total population? In addition, does the sampling framework allow the results to be generalized to other groups?

Choosing the measures

The instrument or tool is a critical feature of the research. In an exploratory study, the researcher may 'act as the instrument' in that only a few very open-ended questions may be asked, for example, 'Tell me about your home birth experience' or 'How did you feel about having your baby at home?' (Appleton 1995, Burnard 1996, Parse 1996).

In correlational or experimental research, however, a highly structured questionnaire or interview schedule may be used. It is imperative that the questionnaire or interview schedule actually measures what the researcher believes it to measure. Estimates of reliability and validity are ways of ensuring that this occurs (Gething 1995). Instruments may be simple or complex, and it may be possible to use existing instruments with good reliability and validity. Questionnaires should be self-coding to make them easier to enter into the computer.

Collecting the data

Data collection procedures should be fully described in the methods section of the report. If data are collected or observations made by more than one person,

steps must be taken to ensure that there is consistency. There are ways of reducing the subjective bias of those collecting data, including measures of interobserver and interrater reliability.

Undertaking the pilot study

A pilot study is almost always necessary during a research project. The pilot may be small but will usually allow any problems to be dealt with before the final study commences.

Data analysis

The type of data analysis undertaken will usually depend on the type of study and may be an analysis of words (qualitative), numbers (quantitative) or both. In qualitative research, a computer software package, for example Ethnograph, may be used, or an analysis of comments undertaken manually. When analysing qualitative data, regardless of the type of analysis, issues of reliability, validity and rigour must be carefully considered (Burnard 1991, Hoffart 1991, Krefting 1991, Beck 1993, Sandelowski 1993, Koch 1994, Appleton 1995, Morse 1995).

Basic quantitative data may be analysed using a hand-held calculator. However, it is more usual to use a computer package, for example Minitab; SPSS-X or SAS.

When using statistical tests, the following questions should be asked (Martin & Pierce 1994, Polgar & Thomas 1995, Smith & Hunt 1997):

- Are appropriate statistical techniques used to analyse the data?
- Is the sample size adequate for the type of data analysis and the number of variables examined?
- Is statistical significance relevant or a chance occurrence?

Writing the final report

If possible, write the final report as each stage of the study proceeds as it is very easy to run out of steam if all the writing is left until the end (Street 1995).

Using the research findings

It is important to share the findings of the study with others. This may be done in a variety of ways (Gething 1995), including:

- hosting informal morning teas for other wards or staff from other organizations;
- in-service education within your organization;

- publishing in appropriate journals;
- sharing the results at conferences and seminars.

ETHICAL CONSIDERATIONS IN THE RESEARCH PROCESS

Research poses ethical dilemmas relating to the interests of individual participants versus the pursuit of knowledge with potential benefit to the population in general. These dilemmas are inherent in *all* aspects of the research process, even at the end, with issues relating to publication and the final storage of data; it is wise to clarify them and resolve potential conflicts prior to starting any study.

There are, however, no simple guidelines. Although the need for ethical consideration is universal, different types of research and each research situation present unique dilemmas that require specific resolution. For a detailed consideration of the issues, readers are advised to consult reputable texts appropriate to the specific research designs (Bowling 1997) and to examine guidelines from professional bodies, for example the British Psychological Society (1991). The following section relates to two of the major ethical principles of research, those of consent and confidentiality.

Practitioner-researchers

Many midwives are now undertaking some forms of research and, in exploring new worlds of midwifery, such 'insider' perspectives can provide valuable insights. However, as Field's (1991) notable quote 'if you want to study water don't ask a goldfish' suggests, these perspectives cannot be exclusive and may prove problematic. The advantages that practitioner-researchers may gain in terms of negotiating access and maintaining an unobtrusive field role have to be considered against the more problematic areas: the danger of imposing a personal 'world view' and the unrecognized hidden assumptions that may bias the data collected.

In ethical terms, there is a need to avoid the potential exploitation of colleagues, clients or students. Practitioner-researchers may also need to resolve conflicting responsibilities that arise from an adherence to a variety of codes of ethical conduct, towards their professional community (colleagues), the research community, the professional bodies (e.g. the UKCC *Code of Professional Conduct*), the research participants and, not least but often forgotten, themselves, as well as from legal restrictions such as observing the Data Protection Act (1989).

All research involves the use of limited resources, particularly time (the participants' and the researcher's)

and funding, so it is important to ensure that these are not used inappropriately. Thus, when undertaking some form of research it may be helpful to consider:

- *Area.* Not all areas are suitable for research. Particular groups, or women attending units with large research communities, need to be protected against being 'over-researched', a situation that can be annoying for the client and can influence the quality of the data collected.
- *Experience:* Matching the researcher to the research is important as research undertaken by people with inappropriate experience can be damaging to women and is unethical. Complex research designs, such as large-scale randomized controlled trials, require more than basic research skills, while working in sensitive areas, for example exploring reactions following a termination for fetal abnormalities, or working with vulnerable groups, such as abused women, requires particular communication skills.

Consent

The idea of gaining 'informed consent' from participants is generally accepted as a principle of research, although it is not universal: midwives may be familiar with laboratory research being conducted on placentae on the basis that, as the tissue is being thrown away, consent is superfluous. Informed consent usually involves the following:

- *Informed:*
  - that all pertinent aspects of what is to occur and what might occur are disclosed to the participant;
  - that the participant should be able to comprehend this information.
- *Consent:*
  - that the participant is competent to make a rational and mature judgement;
  - that the agreement to participate should be voluntary, free from coercion and undue influence.

However, these principles may prove more problematic in practice, as the following discussion shows.

Whose consent?

Although desirable, it may in some situations be considered impossible or inappropriate to gain everyone's consent. For example, in observational research, the consent of authority figures may be gained, but what about the consent of those observed? In institutional and crowd behaviour studies in particular, how do you contact everyone who might be included? It is frequently the less powerful who are ignored: for example, consent for observation in a clinical area may be gained from the doctors, midwives and clients involved but not the cleaners, who are equally essential.

In the maternity services a dilemma may arise if the mother actively wants to participate but her partner disagrees; an example may be the use of the placenta for laboratory research purposes. Whose wishes are paramount? There is also the problem of reactivity. People may feel inhibited and self-conscious as a consequence of being researched so may not behave in the 'normal' manner that the researcher needs to observe.

For what?

Not all research has clearly defined outcomes. Some studies involve a dynamic process and may develop and alter radically, as in, for example, exploratory studies or action research, where the risks and benefits are not necessarily obvious. When the full implications of a study are unknown even by the researcher, at what stage can truly informed consent be sought? In addressing this problem, Munhall (1991) describes a proposal for process consent, which involves a more negotiated, flexible agreement that reflects the reality of the situation and the mutual involvement of the participant and researcher.

Another area to consider involves secondary analysis, in which other researchers may use the data gathered for one study at a later time for a different purpose. Ethically, this may be viewed positively as an appropriate use of a valuable resource, but does anonymity negate the requirement for the participants' consent? In recognition of this reality, funding organizations that store such data (e.g. the Economic and Social Research Council) have developed a consent form for qualitative data that contains different levels of consent. Here, the participant agrees to assist with the primary study, either anonymously or named, and then again for the data to be stored for secondary analysis.

This difficulty relates to the final ownership of data gathered, a point that it may be advantageous to clarify prior to starting the research. This has particular relevance when undertaking government-sponsored research as the results could be modified, delayed or even suppressed if considered unacceptable, the Black Report (Townsend & Davidson 1982) being a notorious example of this.

When?

Identifying the appropriate timing for consent can be difficult. Many midwives will be familiar with the highly undesirable situation of mothers in labour being asked to participate in research. Much potential distress could be avoided by women being informed of possible research participation requests at 'booking' and by a notice board of ongoing research being made available within the hospital or GP practice. Thus, when approached, couples might be more informed and confident in their response. This idea has been promoted within the AIMS/NCT Charter for Ethical Research in Maternity Care (1997).

How?

Consent may be obtained in different ways. Written consent is usually required, especially for intervention studies involving specific clinical procedures. Survey studies may assume consent by the participant completing and returning the questionnaire, and in personal contact situations such as interviews, written consent is increasingly considered necessary.

However, in obtaining any form of informed consent, meeting the language and level of information needs of individual participants is hard to achieve. Can we be sure that translations provided by family and friends ensure an informed consent by the woman? The alternative of providing translated information leaflets does not address the different educational levels of a multicultural clientele – and how much information is it appropriate to give? Some participants may be particularly interested in the research and demand high levels of information, while others readily agree before a full explanation has been provided. In acknowledging a 'right to know', do participants have a 'right not to know'?

By whom?

The dilemma surrounding who is best placed to gain consent from women – the known midwife versus the strange researcher – relates to the timing and place in which the consent is sought. The researcher is better placed to provide information about the study and reassurance that refusal will have no detrimental effect on care. Nevertheless, it is frequently the midwife who is asked to recruit participants, generally for pragmatic reasons but also on the assumption that women prefer not to see many strangers. This itself would provide an interesting area for research.

Confidentiality

The assurance of confidentiality through anonymity is another central principle of ethical research in the belief that:

- participants will respond more openly and honestly if they cannot be identified from the data;
- participants should not be harmed in any way by the research, for example by an individual's views becoming public knowledge.

In much research, identification of the individual is not required. Demographic data about age, sex and so on are sufficient, and confidentiality is achieved through the use of codes and the avoidance of names and addresses. However, in case studies, ethnographies and action research, the situation is more complex. With the current imperative to publish both the evaluations of midwifery service developments and research undertaken by midwives within their own clinical area, these issues are of particular relevance as total anonymity cannot be assured.

Simple strategies such as processing raw data off-site, for example in transcription of tapes, and storing primary data away from the research area, with clearly defined and limited access, may be advisable when undertaking research focusing on professionals in specific units. Nevertheless, this only ensures partial anonymity; studies undertaken in specific areas may be impossible to disguise. For example, publications resulting from the ethnographic study of a high-profile development such as One-to-One midwifery practice require extremely sensitive writing to avoid individuals being compromised.

Discussing these difficulties in her study of ward sisters, Lathlean (1996) notes how her adherence to the principle of anonymity in a nationally recognized innovative development resulted in a very 'bland' presentation and that the 'essence of the experience' had been lost. In research that involves feedback and enables participants to reflect on and react to the findings, Lathlean questions how appropriate it is to guarantee confidentiality, suggesting that it may be more useful to negotiate other arrangements.

A consideration of these ideas is integral to the concepts of greater consumer involvement in research, an approach that has recently been promoted with the development of the Standing Advisory Group on Consumer Involvement in the NHS R&D programme; they are particularly appropriate when considering new worlds of midwifery. Not only are the users and providers of maternity care asked to participate in research, but also their values and views are central to the questions that are posed and explored, and the way in which the results are presented in subsequent publications; they become active participants rather than subjects. This loss of control may appear a risky concept to researchers, but it offers exciting new dimensions for research within the maternity services.

Ethics committees

Very early in the research, the ethical implications of working with human participants must be considered. Most organizations require a proposal to be submitted to them for approval. As well as describing the research, this research proposal shows how human participants will be safeguarded. It may also be necessary to seek approval from more than one ethics committee before the research commences.

All NHS hospitals and some universities now have research ethics committees that, in the interests of safeguarding participants, scrutinize all proposals that come under their jurisdiction (Alberti 1995). Their approval is a requirement of all research undertaken on NHS clients or staff, or in NHS facilities. Ethics committees monitor all areas of research, and their permission may be contingent on certain requirements; for example, participation in clinical research must be noted in the medical records and a letter sent to the participants' GPs. However, Tierney notes that the composition and efficiency of the committees is varied, and much of their work remains framed in a clinical model of research. Also, adherence to their requirements may not be checked, and the committees are often circumvented by small-scale studies conducted under the guise of quality assessment or audit (Tierney 1995). Finally, it is increasingly being considered that poorly designed and poorly disseminated research is unethical; thus, committees may feel that they have a remit to examine the study design as well as the above issues of consent, confidentiality and potential harm.

CONCLUSION

In conclusion, knowledge about research is increasingly becoming part of midwifery practice. Different levels of knowledge are needed depending on where midwives are working. For example, all midwives will need to be critical users of research findings, as women ask them for information about various options for pregnancy and childbirth and as new technologies are introduced. Some midwives are becoming involved in audit and local practice development projects and will need a more in-depth knowledge of the research process. A few may wish to pursue a full-time research career, necessitating a year or two of research training.

For those who are undertaking research, it is important to see the activity of research as a craft, a technical skill, that improves with practice, just as learning to be an experienced midwife takes time. As with learning to do midwifery, research cannot be picked up from a textbook: it is important to learn from and work with experienced researchers.

It is also important to know that research never happens in the way in which it is written up for publication. Research is messy: deadlines overlap, budgets get miscalculated, questionnaires get lost, respondents refuse to cooperate, access to sites is refused and ethics committees refuse to give approval. These 'house-keeping' issues of research are rarely written about, which is why it is so important for novice researchers to pair up with more experienced researchers. Similarly, ethical issues are also rarely acknowledged in published research, often being consigned to working papers and methodology chapters in reports and theses.

Being research minded and basing practice on best evidence requires one consistently to ask why, and to know how to get answers, very often in partnership with women. Many issues that require answers arise from listening to women and observing practice. Sensitization to issues, however, often needs an awareness of the broader literature and the political and social context within which women give birth and within which their health care is provided.

Research has the potential to be a powerful lever for change. It can provide answers that help midwives and women to challenge existing practice. To do this, one needs to understand the strengths and limitations of all the methods to establish what works and what does not, and to find out why and how women receive

---

┌───┐
Pointers for practice

- Ideas for research come from many sources, for example wider society, national policy and research strategies, scientific advances and women's and midwives' experiences of care.
- Different research questions require different methods to answer them, each method having strengths and weaknesses.
- To conduct good research requires high-quality training, varied experience and supportive mentorship, just as being a good midwife does.
- All research should be considered for the ethical impact that it may have on women and their families, students and health professionals, and all research findings need to be disseminated to participants and the wider community.
└───┘

the care they do. However, we also need to recognize that knowledge by itself will not change practice or the organization of care. We also need to be aware of the political dimensions and structural constraints of power relations in organizations when trying to initiate change. Finally, drawing on other disciplines such as anthropology, sociology and social history allows us to place maternity care and childbirth in a wider context and step outside a narrow professional viewpoint.

REFERENCES

AIMS/NCT 1997 Ethical research in maternity care. Association for Improvements in Maternity Care, London

Alberti K G 1995 Local research ethics committees. British Medical Journal 311: 639–41

Alexander J 1996 The Southampton randomised controlled trial of breast shells and Hoffman's exercises for inverted and non-protractile nipples. In: Robinson S, Thomson A (eds) Midwives, research and childbirth, vol. 4. Chapman & Hall, London

Allen I, Bourke Dowling S, Williams S 1997 A leading role for midwives? Evaluation of Midwifery Group Practice Development Projects. Policy Studies Institute, London

Appleton J 1995 Analysing qualitative interview data: addressing issues of validity and reliability. Journal of Advanced Nursing 22(5): 993–7

Baxter C 1996 Working from a multi-racial perspective. In: Kroll D (ed.) Midwifery care for the future, meeting the challenge. Baillière Tindall, London

Beck C 1993 Qualitative research: the evaluation of its credibility, fittingness, and auditability. Western Journal of Nursing Research 15(2): 263

Bowling A 1997 Research methods in health. Open University Press, Buckingham

Brannen J (ed.) 1995 Mixing methods: qualitative and quantitative research. Avebury Press, Aldershot

British Psychological Society 1991 Code of conduct, ethical principles and guidelines. BPS, Leicester

Bryar R 1995 Theory for midwifery practice. Macmillan, London

Bryman A 1988 Quantity and quality in social research. Unwin Hyman, Aldershot

Burnard P 1991 A method of analysing interview transcripts in qualitative research. Nurse Education Today 11: 461–6

Burnard P 1996 Teaching the analysis of textual data: an experiential approach. Nurse Education Today 16: 278–81

Burns N, Grove S K 1993 The practice of nursing research: conduct, critique and utilization. WB Saunders, Philadelphia

Cartwright A 1979 Dignity of labour. Tavistock, London

Chalmers I, Richards M 1977 Intervention and causal inference in obstetric practice. In: Chard T, Richards M (eds) Benefits and hazards of the new obstetrics. Spastics International Medical Publications, London

Chalmers I, Enkin M, Keirse M J N C 1989 Effective care in pregnancy and childbirth. Oxford University Press, Oxford

Corner J 1991 In search of more complete answers to research questions. Quantitative versus qualitative research methods: is there a way forward? Journal of Advanced Nursing 16: 718–27

Crotty M 1996 Phenomenology and nursing research. Churchill Livingstone, Melbourne

Davies J, Evans F 1991 The Newcastle community midwifery care project. In: Robinson S, Thomson A (eds) Midwives, research and childbirth, vol. 2. Chapman & Hall, London

Denzin N K 1970 The Research Act in sociology. Butterworths, London

Department of Health 1991 The patient's charter. HMSO, London

Department of Health 1992 The health of the nation: a strategy for health in England. CM 1986. HMSO, London

Department of Health 1993a Changing childbirth, Part 1. Report of the Expert Maternity Group. HMSO, London

Department of Health 1993b The named nurse, midwife and health visitor. Department of Health, London

Department of Health 1993c Research for health. Department of Health, London

Department of Health 1993d Report of the Taskforce on the Strategy for Research in Nursing, Midwifery and Health Visiting. Department of Health, London

Department of Health 1995a Centrally commissioned research programme. Department of Health, London

Department of Health 1995b Centrally commissioned research programme: commissions in 1995. Department of Health, London

Department of Health 1995c Research and development: towards an evidence based health service. Department of Health, London

Department of Health 1995d Improving the health of mothers and children: NHS priorities for research and development. Department of Health, London

Donnison J 1988 Midwives and medical men: a history of the struggle for control of childbirth, 2nd edn. Historical Publications, New Barnet

Field P A 1991 Doing fieldwork in your own culture. In: Morse J M (ed.) Qualitative nursing research: a contemporary dialogue. Sage, Newbury Park, CA

Flint C, Poulengeris P, Grant A 1989 The 'Know your Midwife' scheme – a randomised controlled trial of continuity of care by a team of midwives. Midwifery 5: 11–16

Friedman G 1980 Primer of epidemiology. McGraw-Hill, USA

Garcia J, Garforth S 1991 Midwifery policies and policymaking. In: Robinson S, Thomson A (eds) Midwives research and childbirth, vol. 2. Chapman & Hall, London

Gething L (ed.) 1995 How to manage research effectively. University of Sydney, Sydney

Glaser B G, Strauss A L 1967 The discovery of grounded theory: strategies for qualitative research. Aldine, Chicago

Graham H, Oakley A 1981 Competing ideologies of reproduction: In Roberts H (ed.) Women, health and reproduction. Routledge, London

Green J M, Coupland V A, Kitzinger J V 1990 Expectations, experiences and psychological outcomes of childbirth: a prospective study of 825 women. Birth 17(1): 15–24

Green V A, Kitzinger J V, Coupland J M 1986 The division of labour: implications for staffing structure for doctors and midwives on the labour ward. Child Care and Development Group, University of Cambridge, Cambridge

Hammersley M, Atkinson P 1995 Ethnography, principles in practice. Routledge, London

Hannam J 1996 Some aspects of the history of the Royal College of Midwives. In: Robinson S, Thomson A M (eds) Midwives, research and childbirth, vol. 4. Chapman & Hall, London

Harper A, Holman C, Dawes V 1994 The health of populations, an introduction. Churchill Livingstone, London

Heagerty B V 1997 Willing handmaidens of science? The struggle over the new midwife in early twentieth-century England. In: Kirkham M J, Perkins E R (eds) Reflections on midwifery. Baillière Tindall, London

Hicks C 1992 Research in midwifery: are midwives their own worst enemies? Midwifery 8: 12–18

Hicks C 1995 Good researcher, poor midwife: an investigation into the impact of central trait assumptions of professional competencies. Midwifery 11: 81–7

Hodnett E D 1997 Support from caregivers during childbirth. In: Neilson J P, Crowther C A, Hodnett E D, Hofmeyr G J, Keirse M J N C (eds) Pregnancy and childbirth module of the Cochrane Database of Systematic Reviews. Cochrane Library, Issue 1. Update Software, Oxford

Hoffart N 1991 A member check procedure to enhance rigor in naturalistic research. Western Journal of Nursing Research 13(4): 522–34

Holloway I M 1991 Qualitative research in nursing: an overview. Journal of Advances in Health and Nursing Care 1(2): 39–58

Hubbard R 1986 Eugenics and prenatal testing. International Journal of Health Services 16: 227–42

Hunt S, Symons A 1995 The social meaning of midwifery. Macmillan, Basingstoke

Kirkham M 1987 Basic supportive care in labour: interaction with and around labouring women. Unpublished PhD thesis, Faculty of Medicine, Manchester University

Krefting L 1991 Rigor in qualitative research: the assessment of trustworthiness. American Journal of Occupational Therapy 45: 214–22

Lathlean J 1996 Ethical issues for nursing research: a methodological focus. Nursing Times Research 1(3): 175–83

Leap N, Hunter B 1993 The midwives tale: an oral history from handywoman to professional midwife. Scarlet Press, London

Leininger M (ed.) 1985 Qualitative research methods in nursing. Grune & Stratton, Orlando

Lewis P 1991 Men in midwifery: their experiences as students and practitioners. In: Robinson S, Thomson A (eds) Midwives, research and childbirth, vol. 2. Chapman & Hall, London

Lutley S 1994 Searching for information. In: Robertson J (ed.) Handbook of clinical nursing research. Churchill Livingstone, London

McCourt C, Page L 1996 Report on the evaluation of One to One Midwifery. Thames Valley University and Hammersmith NHS Trust, London

Macintyre S 1977 The management of childbirth: a review of the sociological research issues. Social Science and Medicine 11: 477–84.

Mander R 1994 Midwifery training and employment decisions of midwives. In: Robinson S, Thomson A M (eds) Midwives, research and childbirth, vol. 3. Chapman & Hall, London

Marland H, Rafferty A M (eds) 1997 Midwives, society and childbirth: debates and controversies in the modern period. Routledge, London

Marteau T M, Cook R, Kidd J 1992 The psychological effects of false-positive results in prenatal screening for fetal abnormality; a prospective study. Prenatal Diagnosis 12(3): 205–14

Martin P, Pierce R 1994 Practical statistics for the health sciences. Thomas Nelson, Sydney

Mooney G, Lange M 1993 Antenatal screening, what constitutes benefit? Social Science and Medicine 37: 7

Morse J 1995 The significance of saturation. Qualitative Health Research 5(2): 147–9

Munhall P L 1991 Institutional review of qualitative research proposals. In: Morse J M (ed.) Qualitative nursing research: a contemporary dialogue, revd edn. Sage, Newbury Park, CA

Neilson J P, Crowther C A, Hodnett E D, Hofmeyr G J,

Keirse M J N C 1997 Pregnancy and childbirth module of the Cochrane Database of Sytematic Reviews. Cochrane Library, Issue 1. Update Software, Oxford

Nuffield Council on Bioethics 1993 Genetic screening: ethical issues. Nuffield Council on Bioethics, London

Oakley A 1980 Women confined: towards a sociology of childbirth. Martin Robertson, Oxford

Oakley A 1984 The captured womb: a history of the medical care of pregnant women. Basil Blackwell, Oxford

Oakley A, Hickey D, Rajan L 1996 Social support in pregnancy: does it have long term effects? Journal of Reproductive and Infant Psychology 14: 7–22.

Parse R R 1996 Building knowledge through: a road much less travelled. Nursing Science Quarterly 9(1): 10–16

Parsons E, Atkinson P 1992 Lay constructions of genetic risk. Sociology of Health and Illness 14: 4

Patton M 1990 Qualitative evaluation and research methods, 2nd edn. Sage, Newbury Park, CA

Polgar S, Thomas S A 1995 Introduction to research in the health sciences, 3rd edn. Churchill Livingstone, London

Polit D, Hungler B 1991 Nursing research: principles and methods, 4 edn. JB Lippincott, Philadelphia

Pollit C, Harrison S, Hunter D, Marnoch G 1990 No hiding place: on the discomforts of researching the contemporary policy process. Journal of Social Policy 19(2): 169–90.

Pope C, Mays N 1995 Reaching the parts other methods cannot reach: an introduction to qualitative methods in health and health services research. British Medical Journal 311: 42–5.

Press N A, Browner C H 1994 Collective silences, collective fictions: how prenatal diagnostic testing became part of routine prenatal care. In: Rothenberg K H, Thomson E J (eds) Women and prenatal testing. Ohio State University Press, Columbus, OH

Rissmiller P 1991 Qualitative or quantitative? Nursing Scan in Research 4(4): 1–4

Robinson S, Owen H 1994 Retention in midwifery: findings from a longitudinal study of midwives careers. In: Robinson S, Thomson A (eds) Midwives' research and childbirth, vol. 3. Chapman & Hall, London

Robinson S, Thomson A 1989, 1991, 1994, 1996 Midwives, research and childbirth, vols 1–4. Chapman & Hall, London

Robinson S, Golden J, Bradley S 1983 A study of the role and responsibilities of the midwife. NERU Report No. 1. Kings College, University of London, London

Sandall J 1996 Continuity of midwifery care in England: a new professional project? Gender, Work and Organization 3(4): 215–26

Sandall J 1997 Midwives' burnout and continuity of care. British Journal of Midwifery 5(2): 106–11

Sandelowski M 1993 Rigor or rigor mortis: the problem of rigor in qualitative research revisited. Advances in Nursing Science 16(2): 1–8

Sleep J 1991 Perineal care: a series of five randomised controlled trials. In Robinson S, Thomson A (eds) Midwives research and childbirth, vol. 2. Chapman & Hall, London

Smith D K, Shaw R W, Slack J, Marteau T M 1995 Training obstetricians and midwives to present screening tests: evaluation of two brief interventions. Prenatal Diagnosis 15: 317–24.

Smith P, Hunt J M (eds) 1997 Research mindedness for practice. Churchill Livingstone, London

Stock J, Wraight A 1993 Developing continuity of care in maternity services: the implications for midwives. Report for Royal College of Midwives. Institute of Manpower Studies, Brighton

Street A 1995 Nursing replay. Churchill Livingstone, Melbourne

Streubert H, Carpenter D 1995 Qualitative research in nursing: advancing the human imperative. JB Lippincott, Philadelphia

Tierney A 1995 The role of research ethics committees. Ethical issues in research. Nurse Researcher 3(1): 43–52.

Townsend P, Davidson N 1982 Inequalities in health: the Black report. Penguin, Harmondsworth

Traynor M, Rafferty A M 1997 The NHS R and D context for nursing research: a working paper. Centre for Policy in Nursing Research, London School of Hygiene and Tropical Medicine, London

United Kingdom Central Council for Nursing, Midwifery and Health Visiting 1992 Code of professional conduct. UKCC, London

Update Software 1998 Cochrane Library. Update Software, Oxford

Wald N J, Kennard A, Hackshaw A, McGuire A 1998 Antenatal screening for Down's syndrome. Health Technology Assessment 2: 1

Wilkins R 1993 Sociological aspects of the mother/community midwife relationship. Unpublished PhD thesis, University of Surrey, Surrey

Williams S A 1997 Women and childbirth in the twentieth century. Sutton Publishing, Stroud

Witz A 1992 Professions and patriarchy. Routledge, London

Wraight A, Ball J, Seccombe I, Stock J 1993 Mapping team midwifery, a report to the Department of Health. IMS Report series 242. Institute Manpower Studies, Brighton

---

FURTHER READING

Bowling A 1997 Research methods in health. Open University Press, Buckingham. *An excellent comprehensive guide to research methods in health, describing the range of methods that can be used to study and evaluate health care.*

Fink A 1995 The survey kit. Sage, London. *Covers planning, how to ask questions, conducting self-administered and postal surveys, designing, conducting telephone interviews and in-*

person, sampling, measuring validity and reliability, analysis and writing the final report.

Herman J L 1988 Program evaluation kit. Sage, London. *A practical guide to planning and conducting programme evaluation. Contains nine volumes that cover planning, design, attitude measurement, tests and scales, qualitative methods and analysis, as well as including a general handbook.*

Transition to parenting

For a while, it seemed that maternity care focused only on physical care and physical outcomes. More recently, there has been an awareness that what has been called 'satisfaction with care' is also important. Yet the concept of satisfaction is not enough. The time around pregnancy, birth and the early weeks of family life is a critical period, when the mother, father and family take the baby into their hearts and lives. It is a time when fundamental psychological and social change is required for the mother and father to take on this new role and responsibility. Midwifery care of the family at this time has profound and longlasting consequences. The chapters in this section examine concepts and research that highlight the critical nature of the transition to parenting and the importance of sensitivity to individual needs.

The first chapter describes the need for a genuine scientific basis to practice, combined with the need for personal sensitivity to the individual needs of the childbearing woman. The next chapter examines in detail the theories and research on adaptation to parenthood and provides practical advice. The chapter on social support examines the need to recognize the social context of birth, the concept of social support and how and why it affects health. Suggestions are made on how to incorporate social support into care. The time of birth marks the beginning of the love affair between the mother, father and their baby. The growth of love and long-term commitment and personal sacrifice by the baby's primary care-giver is crucial to the survival of the infant and the long-term emotional health and pattern for future relationships. Theories of attachment and bonding, both the research and implications for practice are examined in detail. The section ends with a discussion of the dimensions and attributes of caring. A research project to examine the responses of those who may be considered disadvantaged women in two different forms of care is used as a case history. Some clear ideas about what is perceived as 'caring' and 'uncaring' behaviours emerge. Thus, the section ends with the voices of women themselves, emphasizing the need to make all care 'woman focused', responding to their unique needs.

9

Be nice and don't drop the baby

B. Gail Thomas

When I was about to start midwifery training, my husband said, 'Good, now we can find out what all the hot water is for.' Having been reared on black and white movies with birth portrayed as 'women's business' and the man being relegated to stoking the fire and boiling the water, it seemed a mystery to him what all that water would be used for. So, at the end of the first day in the midwifery classroom, I plucked up the courage to ask my tutor. The answer was much simpler than I'd ever imagined – 'Why, it's for the tea!' was my teacher's prompt reply. Now, almost 20 years later, I am beginning to realize that most of birth, and therefore midwifery, is also that simple.

Another memory that highlights relevant issues relates to an experience I had about 5 years ago. I was employed as a midwife teacher in a college that had a contract with the London Ambulance Service to provide updates on childbirth to emergency vehicle crews. These were, in the main, very experienced ambulance personnel with a range of between 3 and 20 years practice behind them. It staggered me to realize that the majority of them would rather be called to a road traffic accident on the M25 than respond to a maternity call. They were very anxious about the uncertainties of birth despite their vast experience of dealing with serious trauma. I found myself teaching them about first aid for obstetric emergencies despite only ever having had to deal with similar situations in the controlled environment of the hospital with all its facilities and experts. It was a humbling experience to listen to them recount stories of the birth of preterm twins in a car in heavy traffic (with a Muslim woman who insisted on blankets being placed over the windows of the car for privacy), coping with a cord prolapse in a tower block where the lifts were out of order and a breech birth with a woman who would not move from the toilet. It made 'calling for medical aid' and preparing a woman for theatre in a hospital emergency seem like a very simple and straightforward (although worrying) option. The 14 different sessions I conducted with these ambulance crew led me to reflect on my practice and conclude that I, like many others midwives, probably had an overinflated opinion of my own self-importance. Birth is, for the majority, a physiological process that will occur regardless of who is present or where the woman is. Birth is normally an intense experience but, basically, really quite simple.

In this chapter, the construct of midwifery will be explored, considering two main perspectives, that of an art and that of a science. A combination of personal reflection and a review of contemporary midwifery literature will be discussed as a means of considering the renewal of midwifery. If we can accept that birth is quite simple, I suggest that there really are only two bottom lines in midwifery practice – be nice, and don't drop the baby.

MIDWIFERY – ART OR SCIENCE?

Birth is a social event. The individual woman becomes a mother and the couple becomes a family; roles and responsibilities inevitably change. The midwife can be pivotal to the success or ease of this change by using a wide variety of skills. These skills fall primarily into two areas: interpersonal skills and practical/clinical skills. This division of abilities highlights the two key aspects of midwifery practice – that of an art and that of a science. The delicate balance between these two areas is an issue of much discussion as many believe that care around childbirth has become dominated by science, to the detriment of both childbearing women and the profession of midwifery.

Science/scientification

The scientific approach does not just relate to childbirth but stems from a much wider set of beliefs surrounding the notion of health and its relationship to medicine. Townsend & Davidson (1988) provide a brief account of the historical development of this relationship. They suggest that, from the times of ancient Greece, there have been two main meanings to the word 'health'. One was derived from the followers of Asclepius, who believed that health was 'freedom from clinically ascertainable disease' and that the main role of the physician was 'to treat disease and to restore health by correcting any imperfections caused by accidents of birth or life' (Dubos, cited in Townsend & Davidson 1988, p. 33). This philosophical approach has escalated throughout the centuries as scientific knowledge has increased and effective treatments have become increasingly available through research

and technology. In contrast, the followers of the goddess Hygeia believed that rational, social organization and rational individual behaviour were all important to the promotion of human health. Happy and harmonious relationships underpin this approach, which accepts that the purpose of medicine is to 'discover and teach the natural laws which will ensure a man a healthy mind in a healthy body' (Dubos, cited in Townsend & Davidson 1988, p. 34).

These two approaches have been popularly described as the 'medical model' and the 'social model' of health (Thorogood 1992). The medical model of health has gained power through the ages as the understanding of the functions and physiology of the human body has increased. It has led to a mechanistic perspective in which the body is conceived as a machine that can be effectively repaired by practitioners with the appropriate knowledge and skills. It relies heavily on scientific knowledge that is generated through experiment and creates the belief that, with enough investigation, the solutions to all health situations can be found.

There can be little doubt that a large component of contemporary midwifery relates to this medical model of health. The improvement of the health of childbearing women and their babies was the impetus behind the Midwives Act of 1902, which made the training of midwives compulsory to stop the perpetuation of the attendance at birth by lay women.

Before the First World War and, in some areas, until the mid-1930's, the majority of working-class women in Britain were attended in childbirth not by a professional but by a local woman. (Leap & Hunter 1993, p. 1)

These women did not receive any formal educational preparation for their work but were apprenticed, often for lengthy periods (Marland 1993), into learning the skills necessary to support women through the birth process. Childbirth was not seen as a medical process requiring the knowledge and skills of the doctor unless a severe emergency occurred. Practice was handed down from generation to generation, with little attempt to study, measure or improve it in any formal way. The Dickensian image of the gin-swilling, unkempt 'Sairey Gamp' type midwife devalued any knowledge base on which practice was established, giving the impression that these women were unscientific and therefore unsafe (despite there now being available evidence of 'unofficial' systems of training from at least the 17th century in London; Evenden 1993). Even though this training existed, it would not have been based on an understanding of human physiology or on the potential value of scientific intervention. The midwives who cared for women giving birth could have been considered as ill prepared or even dangerous by those in the developing scientific community despite the fact that, both historically and internationally, birth was normally successfully accomplished in these conditions.

The move in the USA in the early part of the 20th century to remove midwives from the system of health care was founded on these premises. Dr Henry Garrigues published a book in 1902 (cited in Oakley 1989) that dismissed any sound basis of midwifery practice, suggesting that:

midwives do harm not only through their lack of obstetric knowledge, their neglect of antiseptic precautions, and their tendency to conceal undesirable features, but most of them are inveterate quacks.

It is not surprising that midwifery was all but eradicated in the USA until a resurgence of interest by women in the past few decades led to the creation of the 'nurse-midwife', a being more socially acceptable to the medical community as the practitioner has his or her roots in the scientific base of nursing.

The move to the 'scientification' of birth was based on an assumption that anything that could not be measured could not be scientific and therefore safe. Two philosophical components appear to emerge from this assumption.

First, there is an underpinning belief that reality is a fixed entity that can be reduced to basic components, studied and interpreted objectively and then manipulated in order to improve it. Childbirth, therefore, could be considered to be a process that is fixed; the expectation would be that the length of and progress in the first, second and third stages of labour would be similar in all women and hence predictable. Little attempt would be made to understand the effect of the woman's individual situation and its potential impact on her experience. All first-time mothers would be expected to take roughly the same length of time in labour, need similar support strategies and have a similar outcome. Cassidy (1994), however, suggests that, even though science thinks in simplifications and believes them to be the true reality, these are, in fact, artificial constructs created by man. Straight lines, circles and ellipses for the paths of planets are the result of men drawing a connection between certain points rather than those connections existing in nature. The reductionist or scientist spends time studying the lines, believing them to be the road forward without considering the fact that they are a man-made map. A scientific approach to childbirth would lead to assumptions being made about the expected path to be taken by all women in labour, with landmarks along the way being defined, marked and measured so that the map potentially takes priority over the individual experience.

The second philosophical component relates to the belief that knowledge is only something that can be said. Dalmiya & Alcoff (1993) claim that, traditionally, there has been an acceptance that verbalization is the foundation of insight. Without the ability to articulate what he or she knows, the participant is not knowledgeable. Therefore, midwives practising at a time and in a place where literacy was not accessible to them would be considered to have no knowledge or sound base on which to practise. Dalmiya & Alcoff (1993) challenge this assumption and suggest that some knowledge can only be shown as the words to describe the processes involved are not available, either generally or to those involved. This demonstrable yet not declared knowledge is obviously significantly more difficult to examine and measure and has thus been largely ignored by the scientific community.

Both of these sets of beliefs relate to the lay midwife and the traditional practice of midwifery prior to any attempt at scientification. The lay midwife did not try to measure or quantify her practice but probably provided care on an intuitive basis with its roots in custom and practice. Therefore, the practice was dismissed by scientists who wanted to move to a medical model in order to 'correct imperfections' around birth and improve the health of women and children. Despite the end-point being a worthy one, the means by which it was or is achieved has altered women's experiences of childbirth significantly – and not always for the better.

Medicalization

'Medicalization' is a sociological term first coined by Irving Zola in the 1970s, and it purports that there is an increasing tendency for medicine (and the medical profession) to expand its claims (Hillier 1991). More and more of human life and its social processes have become defined and controlled by medicine. There is an extension of the range of social phenomena mediated by the concepts of health and illness, leading to an expansion of professional power over wider spheres of life (Crawford 1980). Childbirth is an example of this medicalization phenomenon, that has been discussed at length in the literature. Oakley (1980) has shown, in her studies of childbirth, how the medical profession has redefined childbirth as a potentially pathological process, requiring increasing levels of medical intervention and control:

The professional obstetrical view that childbirth is a pathological process and women are passive objects of clinical attention has become an integral part of the way in which the community as a whole sees childbirth. (Oakley 1993; p. 119)

Davis-Floyd (1995) concluded from her interviews with women, obstetricians, nurses and midwives in the USA that the technocratic American society has created a set of obstetric rituals that have completely reframed the birth experience. The symbolic American procedures of seating labouring women in wheel-chairs when they arrive in hospital, putting them to bed on admission to the delivery suite and routinely attaching intravenous infusions all communicate to women the message that they are not just pregnant but sick. This technocratic myth insists that the more nature is controlled, the better it gets and that the ultimate control of nature is not only possible, but also desirable.

There may also be a danger in accepting that 'science' can and does always provide answers to questions in practice. One seemingly appropriate definition of science is 'the exploration of the world around us as a means to increased understanding of it'. If this interpretation is accepted, it follows that the world must be *thoroughly explored* for the subsequent understanding to be scientific. It would seem that, at best, only about 15% of our clinical or management decisions can be considered to be scientific or informed by research evidence (Page 1995) as the remaining 85% of issues have not yet been thoroughly researched or explored. This means that practice is more likely to be 'pseudoscientific' (or appearing to be scientific) as the majority of it is based on tradition and untested theory rather than a thorough exploration. Most midwives are well aware that many interventions have been adopted into common practice with little, if any, scientific exploration prior to their routine use; this applies to, for example, ultrasound examination in pregnancy, continuous electronic fetal heart rate monitoring, artificial rupture of the membranes and the use of the partogram to monitor progress in labour. These interventions have been implemented with the best possible intentions: to improve the outcome for both mother and baby. Those intentions, however, have not always been fulfilled as the 'iatrogenic' effects of the interventions have, at times, caused more harm than good.

The scientific/medical model of childbirth is embodied in the obstetrician, who is defined as the specialist medical practitioner responsible for caring for childbearing women when there is deviance from normality:

Obstetrics is a term used to cover the application of scientific knowledge to assure as far as possible the physical well-being of the mother before and immediately after the birth. (Walker 1976, p. 130)

As childbirth has been increasingly medicalized, obstetricians have increasingly taken control of the care provision for women in pregnancy and labour (but have actually had little interest in the puerperium, leaving the adjustment to parenthood primarily to others, including midwives). Walker (1976) suggests that the roles of the obstetrician and midwife are, in theory, complementary. The former is concerned with 'safe delivery' through the application of scientific knowledge, the emphasis being on the prevention and treatment of the abnormal. The latter is interested in the wider aspects of childbirth as a normal experience, in which the provision of emotional support and preparation for both childbirth and parenthood are integrated into overall care. The midwife, ideally, works with the same clients before, during and after childbirth and develops a close and supportive relationship with those women. When the circumstances surrounding the childbirth experience are no longer considered normal, the obstetrician takes over responsibility and the midwife acts as a nurse under his direction.

Although this appears, on the face of it, quite appropriate, the truth is that, with the increasing tendency towards women giving birth in hospital in Britain since the 1960s, obstetricians have become increasingly involved in normal childbirth. For ease of administration and organization, the majority of women having babies today are 'booked' under the care (and therefore control) of a consultant obstetrician (although midwife-led care initiatives have started to change this). This makes the maintaining of records, the structure of antenatal clinics, covering the delivery suite with a team of doctors and the division of clients on the postnatal wards simpler to coordinate as all the women attending a particular maternity unit are divided into groups based on the number of consultants employed at that unit. The effects reach far beyond administration, however, as these doctors are inevitably schooled in the medical approach to childbirth and therefore affect the type of care offered to women regardless of whether or not their experience is deemed normal.

Although it cannot be assumed that all obstetricians sit firmly in the camp of the medical model of pregnancy (and childbirth), it is easy to see why the majority would. The education of medical students includes a rotation to a maternity unit where they become involved in providing care for labouring women and helping them to give birth. They are expected to 'deliver' approximately 10 women during that period of time and therefore to gain some insight into the experience of normal birth. However, if they then choose to follow a career in obstetrics, they will have little further opportunity to participate in normal birth situations. Midwives 'deliver' over 70% of women in Britain: those whose experience is not complicated. In those cases, the obstetrician is not normally involved in the labour at all. Therefore, by the time the obstetrician reaches the level of consultant, he or she will have spent 6 months as a senior house officer, possibly 2 or 3 years as a registrar and another 2 or 3 years as a senior registrar dealing only with complicated births. The experience as a medical student would seem a distant memory, and the overwhelming sentiment is likely to be that birth is a dangerous experience as there will have been 6 or 7 years of reinforcement that things can, and do, go wrong during labour. There will be little opportunity to contextualize that belief as the experience of participating in normal birth situations will seldom arise. Constant negative feedback will inevitably lead to an image of birth as a 'disaster waiting to happen'.

Just as it cannot be assumed that all obstetricians approach birth from a medical or scientific perspective (although it is understandable why the majority might), it also cannot be assumed that all midwives consider pregnancy and birth to be a normal life event. A midwife's experience will also colour her impression of birth and will influence the type of care that he or she offers women. Experience, however, is only one form of evidence on which practice is or should be based.

The value of science and evidence in midwifery practice

Despite this discussion, highlighting some of the limitations that a scientific or medical approach to childbirth can have on women's experiences of childbirth, there can be no doubt that safe midwifery practice is based on an understanding of physiology. If the midwife is the practitioner who is to define normality and therefore know when it is appropriate to refer to medical colleagues, he or she must understand the underlying processes in order to determine this. I can think of a number of specific examples from my own practice as a midwife that demonstrate the need for in-depth knowledge. I will discuss one personal experience as an example of how practice can be improved when both midwives and women understand the underpinning physiology.

As a student midwife, I received a brief introduction to the concept of breast-feeding in the classroom with a basic description of the physiology of lactation and saw many examples of good and bad practice in the clinical area. At the time I trained (1980), there was little research evidence available, or certainly taught to student midwives, on what led to successful breast-

feeding. Much of what developed as my repertoire of skills came from watching what seemed to work for some mothers and listening to the variety of suggestions that I heard midwives giving. It was not until the publication of *Successful Breastfeeding* in 1988 (Royal College of Midwives 1988) that I was aware of the negative effect that this individual approach to dealing with breast-feeding was having on the overall success of women achieving their chosen method of feeding.

As a new mother in 1982, I breast-fed my own son, but not without problems. As far as I knew, I had positioned him well on my breast when feeding him, but I developed very tender and then bleeding nipples as a result. It probably related much more to my stubborn nature than to truly understanding the physiology of milk transfer that resulted in me breast-feeding for 13 months. Once the evidence was available regarding the importance of the baby forming a teat from breast tissue and not just sucking on the nipple, I realised that my problems had stemmed from poor positioning and that breast-feeding should not be a painful experience. The expectation that breast-feeding should be painful had been reinforced by the practice I had witnessed in my experience both as a student and as a newly qualified midwife. I had heard many midwives suggesting to pregnant women that they should 'toughen up' their nipples in pregnancy by drying them roughly with a towel, by not wearing a bra under rough jumpers, or even by scrubbing them with a scrubbing brush! It was clear that the lack of understanding of the correct positioning at the breast permeated midwifery practice as most midwives whom I knew expected breastfeeding to be painful.

With the publication of *Successful Breastfeeding*, a whole new understanding opened up for me. I do not believe that I was alone.

> I am not imputing negligence or stupidity or malice, or making any other moral judgments. I know that most professionals are hard working, humane and dedicated. I am reporting that there is a degree of professional ignorance which is historically quite understandable, but no longer tolerable. (Minchin 1985)

This Australian author attributed a large part of the responsibility for breast-feeding failure to professional ignorance and, from my personal experience, she was right. Had I understood more accurately the significance of correct fixing at the breast, both my professional practice and my personal experience relating to breast-feeding would have been much more successful. The knowledge of the physiology of lactation and milk transfer has made a positive impact on the way in which I can support women who choose to breast-feed. Science has helped in the provision of effective practice.

Mead (1996) illustrates the lack of a research base for practices such as the routine pattern of antenatal care commonly provided in Britain today. She suggests that midwives and other health care professionals use a variety of sources upon which to base their practice in the absence of research findings; these include tradition, experience, authority, common sense and trial and error. Midwifery as a profession has recognized the value of underpinning practice with research evidence by modifying the Midwives Rules to include a point in Rule 33 (dealing with courses leading to qualification as a midwife) that requires student midwives to 'be able to use relevant literature and research to inform their practice of midwifery' (UKCC 1991). The move towards evidence-based health care (Sackett et al 1996) has been accepted as a positive step by many midwives in an attempt to reduce conflicting advice for women and therefore the confusion that often surrounds decision-making in childbirth. Page (1993) suggests that midwives must become familiar with the scientific evidence available to them and be able to evaluate the costs and benefits of various forms of care if they are to give women the information they need to decide between alternative treatments and approaches. The large increase in both research activity and its reporting (see, for example, Enkin et al 1989, 1996) has led to many aspects of care that have been found to be unhelpful being abandoned despite their having been in common practice. There is clearly a place for scientific understanding in effective care, but it seems that midwifery practice is about more than just the 'appliance of science'.

The current agenda in maternity care has been influenced by the improved understanding of physiology around childbirth and the increase in available research evidence. The emphasis on and availability of research evidence have come about through systematic literature reviews and their publication both as hard text and via computer databases. There is clearly much more scientific knowledge to inform midwifery practice that is easily accessible to the majority of practitioners in the UK today than there has been in the past. However, the contributors to the developing theoretical and conceptual base of midwifery do not appear to be focusing on this scientific side of practice. The literature in which the meaning of midwifery is discussed centres on very different issues: those of the experiences of childbearing women and the role that the midwife plays in them.

Kirkham (1996, p. 166) indicates the need for midwives to have knowledge in order to be able to ensure safety but suggests that this knowledge 'needs to be experienced by the mother as a safety net rather than

the ringmaster's whip. In giving support and exercising skill the midwife's role is an enabling one'. This enabling role appears to be what women are requesting from maternity services. It is clear that they are asking to be able to take control of their childbirth experience, as is demonstrated in the government's *Changing Childbirth* report (Department of Health 1993), and are wanting midwives to have a belief in a woman's ability to give birth without intervention (Hutton 1994). This suggests that a move away from the scientific or medical approach to childbirth is where midwifery should be going if consumer demand is to be met. Does this then mean that the alternative is an 'artistic' approach to the childbearing experience?

The art of midwifery

Unlike the knowledge about the natural sciences, which may be controlled, tested, measured, and replicated, midwifery practice is concerned with humanity or 'unnatural sciences' which cannot be so controlled, because people are unpredictable, individual, have values, attitudes, emotions and feelings which are perceived and expressed in diverse ways and experienced in diverse contexts. (Siddiqui 1994, p. 419)

The need for and ability of midwives to respond to the woman's unique experience of giving birth suggests that there is an artistic element of midwifery practice. Siddiqui (1994) goes on to say that 'to examine midwifery concerns from a cause-and-effect or reductionist outlook, may be to ignore the "art" in favour of the "science" and in doing so, to completely miss fundamental truths about midwifery knowledge'. The essential belief here appears to be not only that there is an artistic component to midwifery practice, but also that it is in fact the element of prime significance.

Bates (1995) suggests that authentic midwifery practice is clearly an art and that it is in the best interests of women that it remains so. Oakley (1989) likens the artistic or caring component of midwifery to love as opposed to technical expertise or science. It seems obvious that these writers are indicating that the interpersonal dimension of midwifery practice is the significant one, the essence of the role that makes midwifery unique. A mother who gave birth in Cambridge in 1987 is quoted to have said, 'I think that in a perfect world every mother should have what I had – a midwife's face that said "look, we have performed a miracle together"' (Oakley 1989, p. 220).

Relationship

It would appear that many of the concepts discussed

in the literature relate to a large theme: that of the relationship between the mother and the midwife. Berg et al (1996, p. 11) suggest that 'it should be the aim of each midwife to provide individualised care and to develop a close and co-operative relationship with each woman'. McCrea & Crute undertook a study of the relationship between the midwife and client based on the belief that 'some "special relationship" is created between the midwife and client. This does not always happen, but when it does, it seems to have a most beneficial healing or therapeutic effect for clients.' (1991, p. 184). Page (1995, p. 229), when discussing the 'new' breed of midwife necessary to improve maternity services, states, 'the new midwife is an experienced clinician who works in and through a relationship with the woman, and who cares effectively, knowing what benefit her actions and advice are likely to have for the woman and her baby, and offering care appropriate to the individuals concerned. This working in and through a relationship is pivotal to the midwife's practice.'

Hutton (1994), having surveyed women's views about the midwives involved in their pregnancy, birth and early parenthood, found that the best memories these women had related to the type of relationship that had developed. The 'best' midwives were those who gave support, encouragement, explanations and progress reports, and who consulted the woman about her wishes. The 'worst' were those who made careless remarks casting doubt on the outcome of the pregnancy, who were insensitive and lacked cooperation and who gave conflicting advice. These comments indicate that midwives have an impact on the woman's experience that can be positive or negative depending on the effort put into developing a therapeutic relationship. Women appear to benefit from having the midwife as a skilled companion (Page 1993) who acts as a guide and counsellor as well as a friend and known point of contact in the health care system.

Personal attributes or qualities are considered by many writers to determine the type of relationship that is likely to develop between mother and midwife. Some of these qualities include honesty (Demilew 1990, Troutt 1994), humility (Isherwood 1992), gentleness (Manning 1994), kindness (Wang 1995), empathy (Schott 1994) and an intuitive nature (Kitzinger 1988). In fact, Davis (1981) claims that the essence of midwifery is 'being humble' and 'paying attention'. Leap & Hunter (1993), in their extensive interviews with handywomen/midwives practising in the early part of this century in Britain, quote some basic attributes that these midwives believed to be important, including common sense, understanding, an ability to get on

with people, kindness, patience, the right attitude (being the mother's friend), cheerfulness, tact and sympathy. The picture of the midwife created through the words of all of these authors is one who is nice to the women she cares for and who is willing to develop a friendly and understanding relationship with them. The ability to form such a relationship may well be influenced by the ability to communicate effectively.

Communication

When I ask you to listen to me and you start giving advice you have not done what I asked…
  When you do something for me that I can and need to do for myself, you contribute to my fears and weakness…
  When I ask you to listen to me and you begin to tell me why I should not feel that way, you are trampling on my feelings…
  So please listen and just hear me. And if you want to talk, wait a minute for your turn, and I will listen to you.

(Anonymous, cited in Kenyon 1991, p. 98)

In Kenyon's research (1991), it was identified that there is a growing awareness of the need for counselling/ communication skills training for midwives. She pointed out that although midwives normally give much advice to the women they care for, fewer than 10% of the midwives' responses demonstrated an acknowledgement of the mother's message. Kenyon's conclusions suggest that a move towards an empathic approach to care in which midwives have the ability and desire to listen would improve the effectiveness of communication in the midwife–woman relationship.

This concept of listening is reinforced by research undertaken by Berg et al (1996). One woman interviewed said, 'This was the first time I felt that someone listened to me and not just to the baby's heartbeat.' The women in this study also felt that encouragement from the midwife to listen to their own innermost feelings was a valuable source of support. Bowland (1995) stresses the need for midwives to listen not only to what the woman says, but also to the sounds of labour, which will increase the midwives' ability to determine normal progress. The notion of effective listening in many contexts appears to be an important component in communication.

Listening is one of many aspects of communication highlighted in the research conducted by Kirkham (1989). Her study of the information that midwives give to women in labour illustrates the fact that women have an intense need for information but that this need is not always met by midwives. Despite the virtually unanimous agreement by the midwives in this study that women want and deserve information, a number of issues constrained their communication.

These included the social class (and therefore perceived ability to understand) of the women, hospital policies and the inexperience of the practitioner. Midwives employed tactics that blocked effective communication, such as routine patter and closed comments that prevented contact with the women's fears or wishes. There were attempts to reassure the women but were rarely based on clear explanations of what was going on in the labour; the midwives appeared to try to minimize the importance of the situation in order to prevent worrying rather than providing the information that would enable women to understand its implications.

Adams (1987) found that women preferred the educating/encouraging midwives' communication style to that of direction. This encouragement can be transmitted verbally or in the form of touch, which Belbin (1996) reports in an account of her labour to have found so very helpful and comforting. Green et al (1990) clearly showed that information helped women to feel in control and consistently led to positive psychological outcomes following birth.

Hughes (1988) claims that midwifery practice is based on the two-way exchange of information. Davis (1994) believes that women need to be well informed about the range, quality and costs of services available to them as part of their decision-making process. She continues to say that a change in the relationship between consumers and professionals must take place, moving from one of control over professional knowledge to one of partnership, in which knowledge and decision-making is shared.

From the authors cited, it can be seen that the ideal communication between midwife and woman is more than just information-giving. It includes listening, empathizing, encouraging, sharing and supporting. Kirkham (1993, p. 15) suggests that:

good communication is two way and likely to be aided by relationships of equality. We must, therefore, aim to give care in such a way that women and midwives work in equal partnership ... [and] we should avoid ways of communicating which reinforce power differences.

Power over and control of the childbearing situation is a further issue that warrants consideration as a key concept in midwifery.

Control

The *Changing Childbirth* Implementation Team was set up as a means of both influencing and monitoring the ways in which the main principles of the Report of the Expert Maternity Group (Department of Health 1993) – choice, continuity and control – were being integrated into maternity services. Cameron (1996) identifies the need for a partnership approach to care in which the decision-making is shared between women and health professionals. This sharing approach to care suggests a redress in the balance of power or control of childbirth. As was suggested earlier in this chapter, the medicalization of childbirth has largely removed women's ability to play an active role in deciding where, when and how to give birth. The Cumberlege report (Department of Health 1993) has set an agenda for empowering women or giving them control over the issues they believe to be important in relation to their childbirth experience.

Empowerment is a transactional concept (Gibson 1991); that is, it involves the powerless taking control as well as the powerful releasing it. In the literature, women are clearly identifying the advantages of feeling in control. Bramadat (1993) found that even 15–20 years after giving birth, women still had vivid memories of the experience. 'Those with high satisfaction scores could be distinguished from those with low scores by their feelings of having accomplished something important, being in control, having an experience that contributed to their self confidence and self esteem' (Bramadat 1993, p. 27). Cooke (1995), in her interviews with women who had experienced continuity of carer during their pregnancy and birth experience, found that making decisions in pregnancy and childbirth enhances a woman's feelings of control and self-esteem. The burgeoning profession of midwifery in Canada (where until recently virtually all births were conducted by doctors in a hospital setting) is based on a client-empowered model in which women are encouraged actively to participate in their care and make informed choices (Farnsworth & Saxell 1993).

A prerequisite of women being able to take control of their experience is for them to have sufficient knowledge and understanding of both the system they are in and the process they are undergoing. It therefore appears to be fundamental for midwives to be able to provide the information that women require in order to make appropriate choices. 'Women who are not informed or who are given inadequate information are unable to be active participants during labour and therefore respond with fear and passivity' (McKay & Yager Smith 1993, p. 140). This belief is supported by Lovell (1996, p. 268), who suggests that 'the prerequisite for being in control is having the power to make decisions; and the prerequisite for decision-making is having full access to information'.

Another relevant issue in the discussion of women's access to information in order to take control relates to the language used by health professionals. The medicalization of birth has led to the creation of a distinct discourse that is often inaccessible to women. There appear to be two main aspects for consideration: a patriarchal approach to women through the language used, and the incomprehensibility of the terminology. Leap (1992) cites a variety of examples of the patter used by midwives around the time of birth that put women in a relatively powerless position. In many cases, the choice of words used places the midwife and/or doctor in the centre of the birth experience ('I delivered Mrs X', 'I think I controlled the pain well'). The woman becomes the passive recipient of midwifery or medical action rather than the person actively birthing a baby.

The medical terminology used in pregnancy and labour may also exclude the woman from being in control of the situation. Bombarded with terms such as 'gestation', 'trimester', 'fundal height', 'biparietal diameter' and 'cephalic presentation', even from the first antenatal appointment women may feel powerless to control an experience that they cannot understand. Hewison (1993), in a discussion of the discourses of childbirth, suggests that the social construction of the whole birth experience is framed by the terminology used in and around it. Scambler (cited in Hewison 1993) states that 'it is quite inappropriate that so many of the pivotal decisions surrounding the bringing of a baby into the world have been redefined as technical and usurped by physicians in their role as experts or agents of formal knowledge.

The move to client-held notes and negotiated parent education classes are two ways in which the negative effects of language are being reduced by midwives. However, these means may not be sufficient to empower women unless there is a fundamental shift in the underlying beliefs held by health professionals of who should be in charge of the birth experience. The empowerment of women requires a release of control by the professional groups who possesses it.

Professional issues

The pros and cons, strengths and weaknesses of midwifery being considered as a profession is a large point of debate and will not be dealt with in detail in this chapter. However, there are a number of issues that arise in the literature about midwifery which could fall into a category entitled professional issues as they are to do with the structure and place of midwifery in society. For convenience, I will use this title but appreciate that it may not be ideal.

Crooke (1991) places a challenge for midwives by suggesting that the public needs to re-establish its confidence in midwives and their practice, not seeing the midwifery model of care as secondary to the obstetric model. The difference between midwifery and the two allied professions of medicine and nursing is sometimes hard to determine. Much medical and nursing knowledge, as well as skills, is used in the practice of midwifery, but there are distinct (if seldom articulated) aspects of midwifery that are unique. Scoggin (1996) interviewed 20 nurse-midwives in the USA in a search for their definition of their occupational identity. It was found that this group used traditional midwifery ideologies of advocacy, normalcy and competency to differentiate themselves from physicians and nurses. There appears to be a general problem, however, with nurses, doctors and some midwives actually understanding these terms and their implications.

Midwives' autonomy is a topical point of debate. The Midwives Code of Practice (UKCC 1994), supported by both the International Confederation of Midwives and the International Federation of Gynaecologists and Obstetricians, clearly defines the role of the midwife as including the ability to:

give the necessary supervision, care and advice to women during pregnancy, labour and the postpartum period, to conduct deliveries on her own responsibility and to care for the newborn and the infant. This care includes preventative measures, procurement of medical assistance and the execution of emergency measures in the absence of medical help.

It would appear that there is considerable responsibility in this role, and a clear sphere of practice is created through this definition, which is determined by the normalcy of the childbearing situation. Once complications arise, the midwife must involve the appropriate medical practitioner. In the absence of problems, she provides the care for woman and child. The concepts of advocacy, normalcy and competency obviously fit into this sphere; on the face of it, the midwives' role is clearly defined.

Where, then, does the confusion come from? The seat of the current dilemma appears to be that the determination of normalcy has been largely taken over by doctors. Downe (1991) claims that often midwives depend on others to make a diagnosis of abnormality and to decide the action to be taken. Kirkham suggests that the midwife is given status only within a very tightly controlled medical system, quoting O'Driscoll et al, who say that 'nowadays, senior registrars are cast firmly in the role of obstetric physicians, rather than surgeons, with most emphasis on the conduct of labour in normal cases' (Kirkham, 1996, p. 187). This being the case, one of the traditional ideologies of midwifery is being challenged by current care delivery patterns, and a midwifery identity crisis appears to be the result.

CONCLUSION

This chapter has freely explored many of the significant issues surrounding midwifery practice in Britain in the 1990s. It has been a broad discussion; the intention has been to contextualize midwifery and start to identify key concepts. The issues have arisen mainly from the literature, but some personal and professional experiences have contributed to the discussion.

The background to the current context of midwifery must begin with historical and political perspectives. This background includes the debate surrounding the art versus science of midwifery and the social model versus medical model constructs in relation to childbirth. The key words that seem to relate to the scientific aspects include 'research', 'evidence-based practice' and 'obstetrics' (and its relation to midwifery); it may be that these ideas can be summed up in the concept of safe practice ('Don't drop the baby'!). This safe practice should be informed by evidence or a 'real scientific' rather than 'pseudoscientific' base.

Although these cannot be dismissed as unimportant issues, the authors currently writing in the midwifery press appear to be focusing much more on the artistic elements of midwifery. I suggest that the word 'relationship' appears to be the pivot in the discussion as the other elements (personal qualities, communication and control) all impact on the woman–midwife relationship. The basic underpinning principle appears to be 'Be nice' to the woman.

Although birth is essentially a simple process, the choices for women that increased technology have provided are not. The renewal of midwifery may come through integrating the scientific and artistic compo-

> **Pointers for practice**
>
> - Midwives need an in-depth knowledge of physiology and the scientific basis of practice.
> - There is a need for scientific understanding in effective care, but midwifery also involves responding to the woman's unique experience of giving birth.
> - The relationship between midwives and women is pivotal to midwifery and should be one of partnership.
> - Communication should include listening, empathizing, encouraging, sharing and supporting.
> - Safe practice should be informed by evidence on a 'real scientific' rather than 'pseudoscientific' base.
> - We should aim for a balance between complicated scientific knowledge and simple acts such as clear explanation.

nents of practice to redefine the advocacy role. This role will not be one in which the power is taken away from women but one in which the midwife protects the woman from the medical system that complicates the birth process. This will entail the interpretation of statistics that are based on populations to provide a meaningful explanation for an individual woman so she can make truly informed choices. It will help women to untangle the complicated web of information with which they are bombarded during pregnancy so that they can decide what is best for them and their families. Midwives must be committed to developing the scientific base of practice and making use of best of available evidence. In doing so, however, they should not overvalue complicated, scientific knowledge to the detriment of simple acts such as clear explanation. The way forward will be in getting the balance right and remembering to 'Be nice and don't drop the baby'.

REFERENCES

Adams M 1987 Deliveries – midwives or mothers? A study of midwifery communication styles. MSc Social Research Methods dissertation, Royal College of Midwifery Library, London

Bates C 1995 Can midwifery be both art and science? British Journal of Midwifery 3(2): 67–8

Belbin A 1996 Power and choice in birthgiving: a case study. British Journal of Midwifery 4(5): 264–7

Berg M, Lundgren I, Hermansson E, Wahlberg V 1996 Women's experience of the encounter with the midwife during childbirth. Midwifery 12(1): 11–15

Bowland K 1995 A description of normal. Journal of Nurse Midwifery 40(6): 466–7

Bramadat I J 1993 Satisfaction with childbirth: theories and methods of measurement. Birth 20(1): 22–9

Cameron J 1996 Parents as partners in care. British Journal of Midwifery 4(4): 218–19

Cassidy C M 1994 Unravelling the ball of string: reality, paradigms, and the study of alternative medicine. ADVANCES: Journal of Mind–Body Health 10(1): 5–31

Chalmers I, Enkin M, Keirse M J N C, (eds) 1989 Effective care in pregnancy and childbirth. Oxford University Press, Oxford

Cooke P 1995 Choice in childbirth. MSc Advanced Health Care Practice dissertation, Oxford Brookes University, Oxford

Crawford R 1980 Healthism and the medicalisation of everyday life. International Journal of Health Services 10(3): 366–88

Crooke L 1991 The rise, fall and rise of midwifery? MA Education dissertation, Royal College of Midwifery Library, London

Dalmiya V, Alcoff L 1993 Are 'old wives tales' justified? In: Alcolff L, Potter D (eds) Feminist epistemologies. Routledge, New York

Davis E 1981 Heart and hands: a midwife's guide to pregnancy and labour. Celestial Arts, Berkeley, CA

Davis K 1994 Responsibilities of choice. Nursing Standard 8(44): 20–1

Davis-Floyd R E 1995 Ritual in the hospital: giving birth the American way. In: Frank Henkart A. (ed.) Trust your body! Bergin & Garvey, Westport, CT

Demilew J 1990 Evolving a midwifery philosophy. Midwifery Matters 45: 11

Department of Health 1993 Changing Childbirth. The report of the Expert Maternity Group. (Camberlege report). HMSO, London

Downe S 1991 Who defines abnormality? Nursing Times 87(18): 22

Enkin M W, Keirse M J N C, Renfrew M J, Neilson S P (eds) 1996 The Cochrane Collaboration pregnancy and childbirth database. Update Software, Oxford

Evenden D 1993 Mothers and their midwives in seventeenth century London. In: Marland H (ed.) The art of midwifery. Routledge, London

Farnsworth D, Saxell L 1993 Midwives and women in partnership – informed choice. Aspiring Midwife (3): 16–17

Gibson C 1991 A concept analysis of empowerment. Journal of Advanced Nursing 16: 354–61

Green J M, Coupland V A, Kitzinger J V 1990 Expectations, experiences and psychological outcomes of childbirth: a prospective study of 825 women. Birth 17: 15–24

Hewison A 1993 The language of labour: an examination of the discourses of childbirth. Midwifery 9(4): 225–34

Hillier S 1991 The limits of medical knowledge. In: Scambler G (ed.) Sociology as applied to medicine. Baillière Tindall, London

Hughes D 1988 Midwifery and models: a high road to nowhere? An evaluation of the place of theory in midwifery practice. MIDIRS Journal (Aug), Pack no. 8

Hutton E 1994 What women want from midwives. British Journal of Midwifery 2(12): 608–11

Isherwood K M 1992 Are British Midwives 'with women'? – the evidence: Midwifery Matters (54): 14–17

Kenyon J 1991 Mothers and empathic responding. MA in Counselling Studies dissertation, Royal College of Midwifery Library, London

Kirkham M 1989 Midwives and information giving in labour. In: Robinson S, Thomson A (eds) Midwives, research and childbirth, vol. 1. Chapman & Hall, London

Kirkham M 1993 Communication in midwifery. In: Alexander J, Levy V, Roche S Midwifery practice: a research based approach. Macmillan, Basingstoke

Kirkham M 1996 Professionalisation past and present: with women or with the powers that be? In: Kroll D (ed.) Midwifery care for the future: meeting the challenge. Baillière Tindall, London

Kitzinger S 1988 Why women need midwives. In: Kitzinger S (ed.) The midwife challenge. Pandora, London

Leap N 1992 The power of words. Nursing Times 88(21): 60–1

Leap N, Hunter B 1993 The midwife's tale. Scarlet Press, London

Lovell A 1996 Power and choice in birthgiving: some thoughts. British Journal of Midwifery 4(5): 268–72

Manning V 1994 The public image of the midwife. MSc Advanced Midwifery Practice dissertation, Royal College of Midwives Library, London

Marland H 1993 The art of midwifery: early modern midwives in Europe. Routledge, London

McCrea H, Crute V 1991 Midwife/client relationship: midwives' perspectives. Midwifery 7(4): 183–92

McKay S, Yager Smith S 1993 'What are they talking about? Is something wrong?' Information sharing during the second stage of labour. Birth 20(3): 140–7

Mead M 1996 Issues in research. In: Kroll D (ed.) Midwifery care for the future: meeting the challenge. Baillière Tindall, London

Minchin M 1985 Breastfeeding matters. Allen & Unwin, Australia

Oakley A 1980 Women confined: towards a sociology of childbirth. Martin Robertson, Oxford

Oakley A 1989 Who cares for women? Midwives Chronicle 102(1218): 214–21

Oakley A 1993 The limits of professional imagination. In: Beatties A, Gott M, Jones L, Sidell M (eds) Health and well-being: a reader. Macmillan, Basingstoke

Page L 1993 Redefining the midwife's role: changes needed in practice. British Journal of Midwifery 1: 21–4

Page L 1995 Renewing midwifery: science and sensitivity in working with women. Lecture to the Australian College of Midwives 9th biennial conference. Sydney, July

Royal College of Midwives (1988) Successful breastfeeding. RCM, London

Sackett D, Rosenberg W M C, Haynes R B, Richardson W S (1996) Evidence based medicine: what it is and what it isn't. British Medical Journal 312: 71–2

Schott J 1994 The importance of encouraging women to think for themselves. British Journal of Midwifery 2: 3–4

Scoggin J 1996 How nurse-midwives define themselves in relation to nursing, medicine and midwifery. Journal of Nurse–Midwifery 41(1): 36–42

Siddiqui J 1994 A philosophical exploration of midwifery knowledge. British Journal of Midwifery 2(9): 419–22

Thorogood N 1992 What is the relevance of sociology for health promotion? In: Bunton R, MacDonald G (eds) Health promotion: disciplines and diversity. Routledge, London

Townsend P, Davidson N 1988 Inequalities in health: the Black report. Penguin Books, London

Troutt B 1994 Choice and control: a midwife's view. Midwives Chronicle 107(1282): 416

United Kingdom Central Council for Nursing, Midwifery and Health Visiting (1991) Midwives rules. UKCC, London

United Kingdom Central Council for Nursing, Midwifery and Health Visiting 1994 A midwife's code of practice. UKCC, London

Walker J F 1976 Midwife or obstetric nurse? Some perceptions of midwives and obstetricians of the role of the midwife. Journal of Advanced Nursing 1: 129–38

Wang M 1995 Communication and negotiation. The consumer's view. Choice for the midwife to meet the challenges of changing childbirth. ENB, London

10

Becoming a parent

Patricia Percival
Christine McCourt

The overall purpose of this chapter is to provide midwives with information that will be useful to new parents during the early months following the birth of their baby. In the second part of the chapter, mini sessions are presented that comprise a parenting series when used with the sessions in Chapter 17. As with the mini sessions in Chapter 17, most of the information in the sessions can be given to parents before and after the birth.

Topics include the everyday and role changes associated with parenthood and how to negotiate these new roles; parenthood romanticized; important issues for men; the mothering role as it is constructed in modern post-industrialized societies, and strategies for surviving this; integrating the birth experience and women's emotional well-being after the birth.

During the antenatal and postnatal periods, the mini sessions can be used to offer information, emotional support and feedback to help men and women to adjust to their new roles as parents (via group or individual teaching). In particular, the sessions provide an opportunity for midwives to dispel some of the myths about parenthood and help parents to have more realistic expectations about their new roles. The sessions also provide men and women with practical information on negotiating new roles and include strategies for surviving the early weeks and months as a new parent.

THE TRANSITION TO PARENTHOOD

For new parents, childbirth is the climax of months or years of anticipation. It is also the beginning of a new life that includes many challenges and adjustments. As we discuss below, becoming a parent has been described both as a major life transition and a major life crisis, a time of crucial psychological adjustment. Becoming a parent requires a couple to make major adjustments as they alter their lifestyle and relationships to accommodate a new family member. New behaviour patterns are necessary as soon as the birth occurs. The weeks and months after the birth have been identified as a time of considerable stress as well as a time of considerable pleasure.

On a scale of major life events and their associated stress, the arrival of a new family member has been rated in the first 20 (Holmes & Rahe 1967). A further survey of 2500 adults found that childbirth was the sixth most stressful life event of the 102 events that were noted (Dohrenwend et al 1978).

Early research

Most of the early sociological research about parenthood used either a crisis or a transition-to-parenthood framework and was based mainly on the experiences of middle-class, first-time parents in the USA and UK. As with any research, the degree of stress or change may well have been underestimated given the problem of respondents making socially desirable responses.

The crisis framework was largely based on Hill's (1949) suggestion that adding a family member constituted a crisis for married couples. Hill defined crisis as:

Any sharp or decisive change for which old patterns are inadequate. A crisis is a situation in which the usual behaviour patterns are found to be unrewarding and new ones are called for immediately.

These early studies found that most couples experienced a degree of crisis that was extensive or severe (LeMasters 1957). These couples appeared to have completely romanticized their view of parenthood. They felt that they had little if any preparation for parental roles, some couples stating that while 'they knew where babies came from', most of them 'didn't know what they were like'. As we will discuss in the mini sessions, many parents in the 1990s feel very much the same: just as unprepared, just as confused and just as 'taken in' by the many romantic myths about being a parent.

Dyer's (1963) findings largely supported those of LeMasters (1957). Women reported feelings of anticlimax or 'being let down' by the mothering experience, of being tied down and having constantly interrupted rest and sleep, as well as decreased house-keeping standards. The men mentioned the necessity of sharing with relatives, the worry of a decreased income and the general adjustments required given the unexpected demands of parenthood. Later research using more representative samples reported a lesser degree of crisis than that found by LeMasters and Dyer

(Hobbs 1968, Russell 1974, Elliott et al 1985). Despite criticisms of the inadequacy of the crisis framework, research from this perspective continued over three decades (Hobbs 1968, Rossi 1968).

The term 'transition to parenthood' was introduced by Rossi (1968) to signify the various changes and adjustments involved in moving from a childless state to parenthood. Using a transition-to-parenthood framework, the sociological literature on first-time parenthood has progressed somewhat from a focus on crisis to a more balanced assessment of the major adjustments required when a dyad is transformed into a triad. Research from a transition framework has included investigations of the family dynamics associated with parenthood, for example changes in marital satisfaction, the household division of labour and social network structures.

Most of these early researchers found that satisfaction with the marriage declines following the birth of the infant (Blum 1981, Feldman & Nash 1984, Belsky et al 1985, Boles 1985, Tomlinson 1987). Again, interviews with parents in the 1990s show that little has changed: couples still report less positive feelings about their relationship following the birth of their first child.

Of importance is the finding that average crisis scores were significantly higher for women than men in most of the early crisis research. Moreover, in some transition-to-parenthood studies, women experienced a greater decline in marital satisfaction following the birth of the infant. This early finding is still present in more recent interviews with parents. We have included this more recent research throughout the chapter, often in the mini sessions.

As well as a decline in marital satisfaction, another consistent finding in both the early and the 1990s research is the more traditional household division of labour that occurs after the birth of the first child. New parents shift away from a view of male and female roles as being equally shared (Ozaki 1986, Tomlinson 1987). The effects of this are also discussed in the mini sessions.

Maternal adjustment

Women have described the early months after the birth as a stressful time of adjustment, when they experience an intense change of self (Mercer 1986, Ruchala & Halstead 1994, Sethi 1995, Barclay et al 1997), a time characterized by considerable physical, emotional and social change (Percival 1990, Gjerdingen & Fontaine 1991). Almost half of the women in Tulman & Fawcett's (1991) study found that the first 6 months after the birth were more difficult than expected. Some women had not fully recovered from the birth by 6 months in that they had not resumed some of their usual prebirth activities, household tasks, physical exercise and usual occupational activities.

There are several reasons why this time is so stressful for women. After the birth, the average new mother must cope with the needs of a new infant as she recovers her own physical and emotional equilibrium. For women, pregnancy, childbirth and parenting are commonly described as events that stimulate identity adaptations, induce the reorganization of interpersonal relations and promote personal maturation (Rubin 1967a, 1967b, 1975). The developmental changes necessary in adapting to first-time or subsequent parenthood require a modification of everyday patterns of functioning. These changes require a great deal of energy and a large investment of time (Mercer 1986, Belsky & Rovine 1990).

The new mother must undertake many new role behaviours as she adjusts to her new role and establishes a relationship with her infant. Such behaviours include learning to care for the infant and the development of a sensitive awareness of the infant's needs and patterns of expressing these needs. There must also be an alteration of lifestyles and relationships to accommodate a new family member (Mercer 1986, Walker et al 1986).

Although some of the changes described in this chapter apply particularly to first-time parents, the parents of subsequent babies also face enormous changes in demands and family relationships as they adjust to the presence of a second, third or subsequent child. Moreover, midwives may expect more experienced parents to need very little support when in fact they also feel uncertain, overwhelmed and exhausted (McCourt & Page 1996).

Rubin (1967a, 1967b) first used the concept of maternal role attainment to describe and explain the psychological processes that occur during pregnancy and after birth as the mother becomes competent and integrates the maternal role into her current role to achieve maternal identity. Mercer (1981, 1986) and Walker et al (1986) also used this term when describing this life change, while Oakley (1980) referred to adjustment to motherhood. This state of maternal role attainment may be achieved as early as 3 months by women in their twenties, and 6–10 months by teenage mothers (Mercer 1981).

Rubin (1967a, 1967b) identified four developmental tasks necessary for maternal adaptation. The first task is seeking and ensuring a safe passage for the mother and her infant during pregnancy and childbirth. The second is the acceptance and support of her baby by significant others. The third is binding in to the infant, and the last giving of herself to her infant.

Mercer (1981) built on Rubin's early work, describing maternal role attainment as a process that had four stages of development: anticipatory, formal, informal and personal. As the mother travels through these stages, she progresses from learning the expectations of the role, to following the directions of others and coping with other role models, to developing her own individual behaviour and finally to gaining confidence and competence in her performance. During the formal stage, the mother relies on others, for example health professionals such as midwives and significant others, to guide her behaviours and expectations.

Theoretical views of adjustment

Researchers have undertaken research on adjustment to motherhood from different theoretical perspectives. Overall, those which emphasize the individual, for example psychoanalytic theory, tend to look at internal attributes as causes of dissatisfaction or lack of adjustment. Conversely, a social perspective focuses on the structure of society and the difficulties associated with the mothering role.

Individual approaches. Psychoanalytic theory is individualistic in that it emphasizes the personality of each woman. It is her conflicts, anxieties and resentments that account for her experience. While this school of thought may acknowledge the mother's social situation, it considers this to be of secondary importance to the mother's internal characteristics in deciding her adaptation. Traditional psychoanalytic theorists tended to see motherhood as being essential for the fulfilment of women; women who experienced dissatisfaction with or problems in adjusting to the maternal role were seen as having problems with their psychosexual development (Deutsch 1944, Benedeck 1959).

Some researchers within the psychoanalytic tradition have emphasized the importance of recognizing pregnancy and new parenthood as major developmental milestones and opportunities for growth (Chodorow 1978, Osofsky & Osofsky 1983). Within this framework, even women who are psychologically well adjusted who want a child may experience considerable psychological upheavals during pregnancy and the adjustment to a new baby. However, women must be able to integrate the maturational changes and adjustments that accompany this period if they are to achieve a new equilibrium. For some women, the adaptation process may result in an opportunity for further growth. For others, the experience may lead to long-term difficulties or poor adjustment.

Social approaches. Inherent in socially based theories of motherhood is the belief that the quality of the mother's experience of motherhood is dependent upon the way in which the role is institutionalized and evaluated. Within a sociological framework, society is seen as shaping and influencing the woman's experience as a mother. In more recent years, there has been an increased emphasis by sociologists on the experience of motherhood (Oakley 1979, 1980). Before this time, most of the research on mothers and children focused almost exclusively on the child, the woman's experience being considered almost coincidentally. During the past two decades, the values of researchers who have omitted the woman's experience of motherhood have been questioned. In addition, although psychoanalysis is certainly individualistic, some later theorists have attempted to respond to these criticisms and integrate their work with more socially orientated approaches.

In their early analysis of parenthood from a conflict framework, LaRossa & LaRossa (1981) concluded that mistaking social problems for individual troubles not only impedes the discovery of solutions, but may also in fact add to the social problem itself. It is, however, easier to treat the individual mother with therapy or medication than it is to address the sociocultural issues surrounding the social role of mother (Oakley 1980) (see also the emotional well-being mini sessions below).

Women, society or both. Within the psychoanalytic traditions, then, it was largely assumed that 'normal' women adapt to and 'cope' with motherhood. Without doubt, the personal attributes that a mother brings to her new role are important in her adaptation. Of enormous importance, however, is the social situation in which she plays out her role. Based on their interviews with women themselves, researchers have concluded that an easy adaptation to first-time motherhood in modern post-industrialized societies is unusual: most women are likely to experience problems (Oakley 1980, Crouch & Manderson 1993).

Factors related to adaptation. Many factors affect the adaptation of women to the maternal role, and research has been undertaken from differing theoretical perspectives. A number of factors are related to the mother's adjustment to the maternal role. These include the following:

- higher levels of social support, which have been shown to be related to easier adjustment to the maternal role: of particular importance is a supportive marital relationship, or support from the husband (Younger 1991, Levitt et al 1993, Reece 1993, Christian et al 1994, Gottlieb & Mendelsom 1995, Halman et al 1995, Hock et al 1995); (see also Chapters 12 and 13);
- the amount of life change, life stress and events: women considered to be most at risk are those with high amounts of life stress and low levels of social support (Mercer 1986, Terry 1991a, 1991b, Grace 1993);
- infant behaviour (Brazleton 1962, Deutsch et al 1988);
- the birth experience (Marut & Mercer 1979, Mercer & Marut 1981, Affonso 1987, Percival 1990, Halman et al 1995);
- maternal health status (Russell 1974, Mercer 1981);
- previous experience with children (Berry 1988, Younger 1991);
- maternal age: older women show a lower level of gratification in the maternal role (Blum 1981, Mercer 1986, Grace 1993, Brown et al 1994);
- maternal age: younger women were found to have fewer psychosocial skills to cope with the maternal role, while older women demonstrated more nurturing behaviours towards their infants (Mercer 1986);
- higher levels of maternal education, which are associated with more difficult adjustment (Russel 1974, Mercer 1981, Younger 1991, Grace 1993);
- the fact that the process of adaptation to the maternal role may be more difficult for career-orientated women (MacDermid et al 1990, Alexander & Higgins 1993, Levy-Shiff 1994);
- personality characteristics such as self-concept, self-esteem, ego strength and individual coping style (Mercer 1986, Percival 1990, Younger 1991, Demyttenaere et al 1995);
- the woman's early relations with her own mother (Benedeck 1959, Deutsch 1944), including separation before the age of 11 years (Frommer & O'Shea 1973);
- the woman's relationship with her mother during pregnancy: the more positive this relationship was, the more the woman reported possessing the characteristics necessary for mothering and the more self-confidence she felt in herself as a mother (Deutsch et al 1988).

Childbirth as social and cultural transition

The above review of research on transition and adjustment to parenthood supports the view that the transition to parenthood is a challenging, often difficult time for the mother and the wider family. The period of transition for the mother has meaning in terms of her entire life experience, family roles and history; for example, as we have discussed, early childhood experiences may have an impact on a woman's adjustment to mothering. In many societies, the birth of a first child marks a point of transition to full adult status and brings with it differing social roles and responsibilities beyond the immediate physical and emotional demands of infant care. The birth of subsequent children prompts further changes to family roles and structures.

Theorists of life changes (Murray-Parkes 1971, Marris 1974) have argued that even positive life changes, such as the birth of a child or a new home, may lead to a sense of loss and grief. In order to cope with change positively and without experiencing undue distress, people need opportunities to make sense of what is happening and to integrate new identities and experiences with previous ones so as to maintain a sense of order in their lives.

Anthropologists have discussed in detail the role of ritual in creating or maintaining such a sense of order within social and cultural groups. Interestingly, the term 'ritual' is often used in a derogatory tone in critical texts in the health services to refer to practices that, in biomedical terms, are felt to be empty and meaningless because they have no direct or apparent curative or caring function.

Recent examples are the routine weighing of women in antenatal clinics, and the preset and habitual manner in which midwife mentors may teach students the right way to lay out a trolley for delivery (McCourt 1999). An anthropological perspective, however, suggests that ritual activity is highly meaningful, but on a primarily symbolic level where meaning is complex and often multivocal. Indeed, functionalist anthropologists in the UK between the 1950s and 70s argued strongly for the functional value of much ritual activity in maintaining social order, or a sense of order within change situations (Gluckman 1962, Douglas et al 1966)

As early as the 1930s, the anthropologist Van Gennep coined the term 'rites of passage' (from the French *rites de passage*; Van Gennep 1960) to describe a clear pattern of ritual activity that is found in a wide range of cultures and social contexts to accompany and manage life changes. The classical rite of passage was particularly associated with puberty and transition to adulthood, which in many societies, particularly where gender roles are strongly separated, has traditionally occurred on an age cohort basis.

Rites of passage surrounding the transition to parenthood are also of major importance in many cultures (see Kitzinger 1989, Vincent-Priya 1992). The classical structure of a rite of passage as outlined by Van Gennep has been remarkably durable and was even strikingly echoed in the accounts of American sociologists in the 1950s of rites of entry to hospitals, prisons and other total institutions (Goffman 1981) as well as in the sociologist Parsons' analysis of the sick role (Parsons 1951). The rite is marked by three phases: separation, liminality and reincorporation. Liminality is derived from the Latin word *limen* (threshold) and conveys well the state of being in transition, betwixt and between two states. Typically, initiates in such rites are separated from ordinary social existence, roles and responsibilities. They may be physically or geographically separated or secluded from everyday social activity, or the separation may be symbolic, as in the removal of hair or everyday clothes. The liminal phase is seen as outside culture and society, and thus fraught with danger.

Rites of passage are paralleled both in traditional cultural rituals surrounding pregnancy, childbirth and the puerperium and in those of hospital childbirth practices. The ways in which the rites of hospital birth approximate rites of passage, particularly the rites of degradation experienced by inmates to long-term hospital care, have been well described elsewhere (Davis-Floyd 1994, Kitzinger 1989). In modern hospital birth, a woman is separated from her ordinary social world, with prepping activities such as the removal of ordinary clothes, admission traces and the withholding of food and drink (actions such as shaving now being largely discontinued in the face of their evidential lack of clinical value), transferred to a labour ward for delivery and thence moved to a postnatal ward, where flowers and visitors are received.

The time period of this transition ritual is short, and increasingly so, the overwhelming interest being in active labour and the delivery of the baby, a transition period that bears a closer relationship to the concerns and interests of maternity professionals than to the significance of the transition in the woman's life. The character of such rituals appears to reflect more closely the needs of the institution and of health professionals for a sense of order and control in a situation characterized by uncertainty, rather than the needs of the woman and her family in this transition. Recent changes in the character and provision of postnatal hospital care bring out this difference particularly clearly, since the significance and meaning of the drama and journey of birth are barely acknowledged in the task-centred and limited character of postnatal hospital care (Simkin 1991, 1992, Ball 1994, McCourt et al 1998).

Sociological research has also indicated that such

attitudes towards the transition of birth are permeating cultural expectations, the implication being that women should make a rapid recovery and return to ordinary life. In a study of the postnatal recovery of women in a US setting, where postnatal home care is not routinely provided as in England, Ruchala & Halstead (1994) found that women were responding to strong expectations that they should be functioning normally within a short period of birth.

The term 'back to normal' seems in itself to deny that a fundamental adjustment in roles and relationships is taking place. An examination of historical and cross-cultural texts, despite the fact that written sources are limited, consistently shows a distinct but different pattern of ritual surrounding birth, with a longer time span of relevance and a much greater focus on the period following birth. The title 'monthly nurse' or 'monthly' was still commonly used in the UK early in this century, referring to the practice of midwives, nurses or handywomen providing care within the home for a month following birth, and cross-culturally prescribed periods or rest and seclusion following birth have ranged from about 10 to 40 days (Towler & Bramall 1986).

Both parents, then, face many challenges during the transition to parenthood as they adjust to their new roles. However, although men and women face the same event, their experiences of the event are unlikely to be comparable. The fathering role varies considerably in different societies. This role has also changed historically and continues to evolve as the roles of men and women change (Edgar 1993, Marks & Lovestone 1995). These changing roles may be a source of stress, confusion and uncertainty for men as they undertake the transition to first-time (and subsequent) parenthood and define their own sense of self as father.

However, women must also face the birth. In addition, in most modern post-industrialized societies, many women also leave the workforce (at the very least for a short time and often for longer) and undertake a new full-time role (Terry 1991a, 1991b). Regardless of recent role shifts (although there are some exceptions), women usually assume the role of primary carer for the new baby. Moreover, most women assume this new role almost immediately after the birth. They no longer have the luxury of being cared for as they recover from the birth, as they would have been earlier in the century; instead, they must become the carers. (See also Chapter 13 for a discussion on the dimensions and attributes of caring.)

The life change that the woman undergoes during the transition to parenthood may be accentuated because it is now usual for her to work until just before the birth of the first child. Fifty years ago, most middle-class women gave up paid work on marriage. In addition (as we discuss in more detail in the mini sessions below), in countries such as the UK, USA, Canada and Australia, a number of broader cultural factors can make life more difficult for both parents, particularly the mother. The way in which the role of mother is constructed in most modern post-industrialized societies makes enormous demands on women and creates difficulties for both parents. Also, the romanticized images that surround the mothering role suggest that it is instinctive and effortless. Moreover, the low status of mothering in society does little for women's self-esteem; many give up 'important' paid work to start their new job and then often feel the need to apologize because they are 'just' a mother (Oakley 1979, 1980).

Midwives supporting parents

Given these many stressors, it is not surprising that the weeks and months after the birth have been identified as a time when the support needs of parents, particularly mothers, are high (Rubin 1967a, Ruchala & Halstead 1994, Sethi 1995, Barclay et al 1997). As we discuss in Chapter 12, this needed support may be available either from informal networks of family or friends, or from formal sources. The formal support available to women and men at this time includes that given by midwives and health visitors (community/ child health/public health nurses). During the antenatal, birth and postnatal period, midwives and health visitors are in an ideal position to provide support to influence all the factors shown by the literature to be important during the transition to parenthood. These include acquiring new skills and incorporating new tasks, acquiring a new self-concept and adapting to changing roles.

There are a number of different ways in which midwives can support or care for women, and these have been discussed throughout the book. In this chapter, we concentrate on the positive ways in which midwives can assist parents to adjust to their new roles. Although adequate research is available that emphasizes the enormous role change occurring at this time, very little of this practical and accurate information actually reaches parents. Instead, they receive a constant barrage of information from the media that emphasizes only the ease, joy and wonder of parenting. In countries such as the UK, USA, Canada and Australia, despite an increase in antenatal education, many parents simply do not recognize how much a baby will change their lives (Ladden & Damato 1992,

Brown et al 1994, Ruchala & Halstead 1994, Sethi 1995, Barclay et al 1997).

Childbirth preparation courses are typically available in most communities, but very few programmes address the mental health and shifting emotional strains of expectant parents. While preparation for the birth itself is essential, Webb (1985) concludes that the courses available do not give attention to the marital relationship and the psychological preparation for parenthood that the significance of this major life event merits. This has changed little in the 1990s. Certainly, the emotional aspects of the birth itself have recently been paid more attention, given the importance of the actual experience of birth to many women. Moreover, as we approach the year 2000, physical outcomes in terms of a live mother and baby are excellent. However, an easy adaptation to first-time motherhood is unusual for most women, and it is more likely to be problematic (Oakley 1980, Crouch & Manderson 1993). In addition (as we discuss later in detail), as many as 1 in 5 women experiences severe and disabling postnatal depression, which in many cases lasts months and even years.

It is now fair to say that, in most developed countries, physical outcomes for mothers and their babies are usually positive; it is unusual for women to die during and after childbirth. However, some women feel so depressed after the birth of their beautiful and healthy baby that they would, at times, like to die (Percival 1998).

The real challenge for midwives is to give the same attention to preparing parents for the overall period of transition as they have given to the labour and birth process. This transition may in reality last months and even years rather than the few weeks 'allocated' by many health professionals. Throughout this chapter, particularly in the mini sessions, we have included ways in which midwives can help parents to experience a more positive period of transition.

THE MINI SESSIONS

The second part of the chapter consists of a number of mini sessions. Most of these have an introductory section, objectives, important teaching points and notes for midwives to refer to when teaching the session. As with the sessions in Chapter 17, the sessions are flexible; most are brief so that more than one session can be used at any given time. At times, the language in the mini sessions is formal and referenced because the overall chapter has tried to fulfil more than one purpose. We have tried to provide midwives with practical information that they can use both in their everyday practice and in running group sessions for parents. The chapter is also intended to be an academic resource that allows midwives to obtain articles for further reading without having to carry out an extensive literature search.

Topics

The mini sessions cover the following topics:

- Parenthood – everyday and role changes
- Negotiating new roles
- Parenthood romanticized
- It's difficult for men too
- The mothering role in modern post-industrialized societies
- Strategies for survival
- Integrating the birth experience
- The 'baby blues' or 'third day blues'
- Postnatal or puerperal psychosis
- Postnatal depression (PND).

Some midwives might argue that it is difficult to get first-time parents to concentrate on anything but the birth. The challenge here is not to abdicate the parenting teaching role but instead to make the group sessions something that parents want to attend. During group sessions, small group sizes, a cosy room, comfortable chairs, refreshments and informal teaching all help. The information in most of the mini sessions in this chapter can be taught before or after the birth to individual parents or to groups of men and women. The mini sessions can also be used as a basis for fathers' or mothers' groups before and after the birth. Some of the changes described in this chapter apply especially to first-time parents. However, overall, the sessions are also appropriate for parents having their second or subsequent child. This latter group is often given less attention both before and after the birth, yet their support needs are very real.

Two sessions are possibly best used for men and women singly: 'Integrating the birth experience' (unless the woman includes her partner) and 'It's difficult for men too'. With respect to the latter session, there is some evidence that men would prefer some fathers-only sessions, or focus groups for men, to look at issues surrounding parenting for men (see Watson 1992, Bader & MacMillan 1994, both cited in Watson et al 1995). It is very important for men (or other partners or friends) to be fully included in all the other group sessions (given that this is considered culturally appropriate). Some fathers have complained how health professionals exclude them (Cowan & Cowan 1992, Belsky & Kelly

1994). Moreover, men need the information in the sessions to help them to understand the difficulties their partners are going through after the birth.

In summary, the information in the mini sessions can be used as a basis for:

- antenatal classes or group sessions in a hospital or community setting;
- antenatal group sessions that are reconvened after the birth to provide postnatal support;
- postnatal group sessions (possibly in parents' homes or a community setting in the early weeks, or in the hospital in countries with longer stays);
- antenatal group sessions followed by individual postnatal reinforcement;
- individual parent teaching after the birth.

Group teaching

Although the information in the mini sessions can be given to parents on a one-to-one basis, health professionals, including midwives, are, because of budgetary constraints, being required to provide increased care with decreased resources. Group teaching by midwives and health visitors is a cost-effective way of increasing family support, with several advantages (Knowles 1990):

- Groups provide an environment of support and empathy.
- Such teaching increases motivation as participants strive to meet shared goals.
- Adults learn better from each other and in a group situation.
- It is an economical way to teach several individuals at one time.

More specifically, researchers have demonstrated the value of groups in increasing support for new parents. Positive outcomes resulting from these groups include (Percival 1990, Henderson & Brouse 1991, NSW Women's Consultative Committee 1994, Watson et al 1995):

- an increase in the confidence of parents in the parenting role;
- a better understanding of the adjustments required during the transition to parenthood;
- a more positive attitude toward infant care;
- an increased use of other resources;
- parents meeting and sharing information and feelings with other couples, and learning from each other's experiences;
- helping parents to develop longer-term informal support networks;

- parents knowing that they are not alone in experiencing difficulties;
- in situations where continuity of carer is not available, antenatal groups provide opportunities for midwives and parents to develop a relationship.

Culturally appropriate support

Women from other cultures need access to education that is culturally appropriate. Ideally, health workers from the women's own or a similar cultural background would deliver this. In addition, after the birth, information and support must also be culturally appropriate. This is particularly important for women from cultures where new mothers receive little assistance from their husbands and are traditionally supported by a network of female relatives and friends. Moreover, it is important that midwives do not view other cultural practices during the transition to parenthood as inappropriate or primitive (NSW Women's Consultative Committee 1994).

MINI SESSION: PARENTHOOD – EVERYDAY AND ROLE CHANGES
Introduction

As we discussed earlier, research suggests that couples do not always have realistic expectations about the impact of parenthood on their lives. Parents may believe that 'good' or 'normal' families experience only the joys of having children. They may, therefore, feel they have to pretend that they are coping with all the tasks of parenthood. This may well apply after the birth of the first and subsequent children. It is essential that parents know that enormous life changes occur for most couples. If midwives tell parents that life is usually very different after the birth, they are less likely to feel that they are failing as a mother, father or lover when things are no longer the same as they were. Parents who are aware that many couples experience role changes during the early years of parenting are more likely to cope positively with these changes. For example, those parents who feel less happy with their partner will also realize that they are not unusual or alone.

Objectives

- Men and women will have an increased understanding of the everyday practical changes that occur after the birth.

- Women and men will have an increased understanding of the role adjustments that often occur after the birth.

Important teaching points

- *Antenatal*. Describe the everyday life changes and role adjustments that occur for most couples after the birth.
- *Postnatal*. Ask group members about the changes that have occurred in their lives since their baby's birth and encourage them to share these with the group.

Midwives' teaching notes

Parenthood: the everyday changes

However much a new baby is loved and wanted, and regardless of the joy experienced by new parents, the impact on their everyday lives is great. As most parents know 'pre-parenthood' and 'post-parenthood' are very different. Most men and women find that the following changes occur after the birth of their baby:

- There is usually a major disruption in their lives, with very little routine, particularly in the early weeks.
- Parents have insufficient time and a lack of personal space.
- With their new, constantly changing responsibilities, parents have less time for each other, to talk, to go out, to make love or just to enjoy being together.
- Many couples find that the new baby takes all of the spontaneity out of their social life. Things have to be planned, baby-sitters have to be found, and at the end of the day there has to be the energy to go out.

It's so different now. Pre-parenthood staying at home (after work) may have meant relaxing with a good book and enjoying being alone or together.

Post-parenthood is very different. The many and varied needs of a new baby result in parents having less (or no) time for themselves or each other. It may be difficult for a woman alone in the house to have a shower, wash her hair or even eat a meal in peace. Sleep becomes an almost forgotten luxury, one that is replaced by feeding, bathing, changing and consoling a new infant, not to mention the many and varied tasks required to keep a household running smoothly.

The changes are even more obvious when attempting to leave the house. Pre-parenthood, going out for a cup of tea involved saying goodbye to the dog (or cat) and locking the front door, possibly with a jacket flung casually over one arm in case of cooler weather. Post-parenthood going out of the house is quite a different matter. The casually flung jacket is replaced by arms full of carry bags, nappies, flannels, changes of clothing (several), bibs, wet wipes, spare sheets and blankets. It is difficult to imagine that such a small person could possibly require such a large amount of baggage. But he or she does. And what is more, it can be guaranteed that the arrival of the long-awaited and planned-for cup of tea will coincide with the baby waking up.

On occasions, a baby-sitter may be an alternative to always leaving the house with such full arms. Some parents may be fortunate enough to have grandparents or aunts and uncles who are prepared to baby-sit. Others may have to rely on a paid baby-sitter. For many parents, the cost of hiring someone reliable may mean that outings as a couple are rare.

Women's own words

…It's a whole different life now…

I need to have a long shower or just go to the toilet in peace.

Well none of your time is your own … you've got this tiny little thing that runs your whole life 24 hours a day. It just doesn't stop.

…I was just having breakfast at one o'clock in the afternoon.

(Percival 1990, Sethi 1995, Barclay et al 1997)

Different friends and seeing more of family

Becoming a parent is also associated with changes in the couple's social network structure. Overall, there is decreased interaction with mutual husband-and-wife friends and increased contact with couples who have children under the age of 2. There is also increased contact with the couple's own parents and decreased contact with friends in the same age range as the new parents. These changes suggest that parents are mobilizing supports that can help them with parenting (Belsky & Rovine 1990, Reece 1993).

Parenthood: relationship changes

Research has shown that many couples experience similar changes during the early years of parenting. These include changes in satisfaction with their own relationship, the division of labour and the couple's social networks. Many new parents may feel that they are unusual or abnormal when these changes occur.

Feeling less satisfied. Most 1990s research largely agrees with earlier work with respect to the couple's satisfaction with the quality of their relationship or marital adjustment. Interviews with parents have found that most couples feel less satisfied with their relationship in the early years after the birth (Belsky & Rovine 1990, Tomlinson & Irwin 1993; Belsky & Kelly 1994, Levy-Shiff 1994, Hock et al 1995). Couples mentioned such things as less sexual intimacy, fewer expressions of affection and greater conflict in their relationship, as well as increased economic stresses.

Belsky & Kelly (1994) interviewed couples over a 4-year period and assessed such aspects as feelings of love towards the spouse, feelings of ambivalence, and levels of conflict and communication in the relationship. They found that:

- 13% became 'severe decliners', that is, they suffered dramatic and negative alterations in their relationship;
- 38% became 'moderate decliners';
- 30% experienced no change;
- 19% were 'improvers'; this group experienced increased feelings of love towards their spouse, less ambivalence and conflict, and better communication in the relationship.

Women's own words. Women described the situation in the following terms (Percival 1990):

I think having the baby has brought my husband and me closer.
 I feel having a baby can bring you closer to your husband and yet at the same time it can pull you apart.
 My neighbours looked after the baby for an afternoon and we went out for lunch. It was bliss. My husband and I really value our time alone now and we appreciate each other's company more.

Who does what. Overall, women can expect to have to do 'much more with much less' when they have a baby: both partner and family support decline during the first year after the birth. As we discuss below, this drop in support comes at a critical time for women. New mothers with appropriate amounts of situation-specific support may be less depressed, anxious, angry and/or fatigued than other mothers (Gottlieb & Mendelsom 1995).

Couples in LaRossa & LaRossa's (1981) study had set up child care arrangements that created a scarcity of valued free time, and more often than not it was the wife who 'came out on the short end of the stick' (investigator's quote). This appeared to occur whether or not the wife was employed. Moreover, at that time, while women viewed these imbalances as illegitimate, they did not push for equality of responsibility for children.

In the 1990s, following the first birth, many new par-ents shift away from a more contemporary view of male and female roles as shared to a more traditional one (Gjerdingen & Chaloner 1994, Levy-Shiff 1994). Some have even argued that the father's contribution is minimal (Fishbein 1990, Blair & Lichter 1991). Moreover, when women also work outside the home, they still contribute more to household chores, and this increases during the first year after the birth (Gjerdingen & Chaloner 1994).

Couples in conflict. This greater gender differentiation is a source of difficulty and conflict for couples, with negative consequences for both the quality and the stability of the marriage. Entwistle & Doering (1981) argued that a couple's egalitarian ideals are severely tested with the birth of the first child. LaRossa & LaRossa's (1981) interview transcripts led them to comment upon the amount of conflict behaviour in marriage and the conflicting views of men and women in their study. Conflict between parenting and other family roles is related to a more difficult adjustment for both men and women (LaRossa & LaRossa 1981, Hinkley 1986). Interviews with parents in the 1980s found that this traditional division of labour was related to women feeling less positive about the maternal role (Blum 1981, Duncan 1984, Hinkley 1986, Ozaki 1986, Tomlinson 1987).

More recent interviews with women revealed that their satisfaction with their partner's contribution to housework declined during this first year (Reece 1993, Gjerdingen & Chaloner 1994). Women's feelings about their partner 'doing his share' are very important; satisfaction with their partner's contribution to housework can be related to their own mental health (Gjerdingen & Chaloner 1994). As well, depressed mothers in Hock et al's (1995) study had partners with more traditional views of role segregation. However, the findings of early interviews with couples suggested that it was the couple's comfort with their role that was more important than the equality of the division of labour (Belsky et al 1985, Boles 1985).

We used to be equal. In early research, couples with an egalitarian or equal relationship before the birth of their first child experienced more problems adjusting to parenthood than did couples with more gender-role segregated relationships (Oakley 1980, Entwistle & Doering 1981, Feldman & Nash 1984). Given recent role shifts for women, more couples may view their relationship as being egalitarian or equal and more couples may therefore be affected when things become more traditional after the first birth (MacDermid et al 1990). Moreover, in the 1990s, couples may delay marriage and parenthood (Glezer 1993). Their interdependence with each other may be even more disrupted when a third person enters the relationship, leading to greater stress in the marriage (Alexander & Higgins 1993).

It may be not only the amount of the workload that women respond to, but also the absence of equity and feelings of shared closeness that the couple had before the birth. In addition, women may see men's involvement with the child as a loving, caring act towards themselves (Levy-Shiff 1994). Certainly, if women feel cared for and happy with their partner's expressions of caring, they may also be more satisfied with their contribution to housework (Gjerdingen & Chaloner 1994).

To conclude

Although the baby's arrival is usually a joyous event, many couples feel less satisfied with their own relationship during the early years of parenting. The birth of a first baby results in a shift towards a more traditional household division of labour in which women have responsibility for most of the childcare and household tasks. This can result in new mothers feeling less happy with their new role and may also be one of the reasons why both parents feel less happy with their relationship after the birth of their first child.

Where to from here?

Some ways in which midwives can help parents to reconcile their different wants and needs during the transition to parenthood are discussed below in the mini session 'Negotiating new roles'.

MINI SESSION: NEGOTIATING NEW ROLES

Introduction

As we discussed in the last session, the more traditional household division of labour after the birth may be one reason why couples feel less happy with their relationship after the birth of their first child. The ongoing quality of the couple's relationship is important as conflict between parents may cause some men to withdraw and decrease their involvement (Gottman 1994) at a time when the woman's need for practical and emotional support is very high.

The couple's feelings about their relationship or marital adjustment may also interact with depression in the mother; that is, women who are less happy about their partnership are more likely to experience postnatal depression (PND) (Christian et al 1994). In addition, some women with PND have partners who report being less satisfied with their marriage (Hock et al 1995). In turn (as we discuss later), PND has an adverse effect not only on the woman, but also on her child and partner.

Belsky & Kelly (1994) have concluded that 'The chief hallmark of couples who transform the His and Hers transition into the Our transition is the ability to reconcile the conflicting priorities of their individual transitions.' During the following session, midwives can help in the resocialization of men towards an expanded parenting role (Fishbein 1990) and help them to recognize their partner's increased need for practical and emotional support. If this increases men's participation, it may in turn decrease the likelihood of PND and also prevent the deterioration in the marital relationship (Belsky & Kelly 1994).

This expanded role is one in which couples work out what is fair as far as caring for the baby, cooking meals, doing housework and earning a living are concerned, so that neither partner works more hours than the other. It is important that midwives point out to parents that caring for the baby is a full-time job (Sethi 1995). It is, therefore, unrealistic to expect women also to manage the household (Terry et al 1991). As well as making life easier for his partner, the father's involvement may increase his awareness of the difficulties of the role and increase his empathy towards the mother (Levy-Shiff 1994). Women also need help to see their partner's equal involvement as a positive thing and not a threat to their own role. They may also need to recognize their partner's need for recognition for his commitment.

Objective

- The new parents will recognize the importance of supporting each other as they learn their new roles.

Important teaching points

- Discuss the things that new parents can do to help each other and maintain a positive relationship in the early weeks and months of being a parent.
- If possible, copy the pamphlet (see below) and go through this.
- Ask couples what else they could do to help each other.

Midwives' teaching notes

Men and women becoming parents

Over the years, interviews with parents have found

several important differences between the experiences of men and women following the birth of the first infant.

Stress and anxiety. Stress and anxiety patterns have been described:

- From the earliest interviews, women have experienced a degree of anxiety and stress or crisis that is greater than that experienced by their partners (Hobbs 1968, Russell 1974, Elliott et al 1985, Terry 1991a, 1991b).
- While men's stress levels off after 1 month, women's continues to rise throughout the first year (Belsky & Kelly 1994).
- Women who are dissatisfied with the level of spouse support experience higher stress in the parenting role (Leventhal-Beifer et al 1992).

Relationship. The following have been found with respect to relationships:

- Women experience a greater decline in their satisfaction with their relationship following the birth of the infant (Levy-Shiff 1994).
- The decline in satisfaction is less for women when fathers are more involved in childcare (Levy-Shiff 1994) or if women feel more satisfied with their partners' contributions to household activities (Terry et al 1991).
- Women also experience less decline in their satisfaction with their relationship when they perceive that their needs for emotional support, affection, interest and shared time have been met (Levitt et al 1993).
- Men's satisfaction with marital quality is also higher when they are more involved in childcare (Nugent 1991).

Other differences. Other differences that can be seen are listed below:

- Women have also been shown to experience more parenting joys than men, as well as more restrictions (Elliot et al 1985, Hinkley 1986, Ruchala & Halstead 1994, Sethi 1995).
- The imbalance of free time (time available for activities other than child or household care) may also favour men (LaRossa & LaRossa 1981).
- Women experience lower levels of emotional well-being (Terry 1991a).

Needing different things. Belsky & Kelly (1994), from their interviews with parents over a 4-year period, found that men and women wanted and needed quite different things during the transition to parenthood:

- Women fundamentally wanted a partner rather than a helper – someone to take an active role in childcare and housework, someone who would also offer emotional support by listening to doubts, anxieties and frustration.
- However, while they recognized the workload had increased dramatically, men also wanted some affection and attention for themselves, a reasonable social life and some freedom for hobbies, sports and friends.

If couples are able to compromise, a more positive outcome is possible. Some possible strategies to help them do this are included in the following pamphlet.

Pamphlet: your midwife's advice for new parents – working together

Negotiating roles

Remember, as a couple, you are more likely to survive becoming a parent and keep a happy relationship if:

- men can recognize that, during the early weeks and months, women's needs for physical and emotional support far outweigh their own needs;
- women are able to meet partners halfway by recognizing their need for attention and giving them some of the gratitude they would like for their commitment (Belsky & Kelly 1994).

Doing the work

- From the very beginning, recognize that this baby is a 'joint venture'.
- For most couples, one person working 8 hours outside the home and the other working 24 hours at home is probably the fastest possible route to an unhappy relationship (not to mention a possible separation or divorce).
- Remember that learning to care for a baby is a full-time job. If the woman is the one at home doing this, it is very important to remember that, in the early weeks, she is also recovering from the birth.
- Work out what is fair as far as care of the baby, cooking meals, doing housework and earning a living is concerned. As far as possible, make sure that neither partner works more hours than the other.
- Both of you need to be involved in all aspects of caring for your baby. This way, both of you gain confidence and overcome any fear of handling your precious new baby. And it also means that both of you get a break.
- Remember that doing something is the best way of learning, and doing something often enough leads to competence and feeling good.

- Take it in turns. If the baby is crying and little has helped, one of you take time off and one of you stay with the baby. For example, if the partner takes the baby out for a pram or car ride, this gives a woman time alone.

Your relationship

- Grit your teeth and accept that this is a time when most parents have very little time for each other.
- The loving relationship you had before the birth is still there. You are both just too tired to express it at the moment.
- Be honest about how you are feeling with your partner.
- Tell each other how you feel. Talk to each other even if this is in shorthand.
- Try to make a few rules. For example, if one of you is angry, overwhelmed or exhausted, ask the other to try to be calm for this short time. The order will always be reversed later. Two upset people may result in a quarrel that uses more energy and rarely solves anything.
- Don't demand perfection of each other. You are both only human.
- Above all, be kind to each other (however hard this might be when you are both exhausted from lack of sleep). It really is important.

The 'Supermum' myth

- Remember that, however joyful having a new baby is, it is also a time of enormous change for both of you.
- Keep reminding yourself of the 'Supermum' myth – that it is just that, a myth.
- Women, *don't ever* think that you are 'not coping': the many tasks that go with being a parent in the early weeks are too much for one person. And men, *don't ever* think of your partner as 'not coping'.
- Concentrate on maintaining the *status quo* and avoid any unnecessary changes. Don't add other strains such as moving house or renovating.
- And remember, life will never be the same as it was before the birth, but eventually, with this gorgeous new person in your lives, it may be better.

To conclude

Encouraging both parents to negotiate and compromise is possibly one of the most helpful things that midwives can encourage them to do at this time.

Where to from here?

Some ways in which midwives can help parents to understand why they have unrealistic expectations of parenthood are discussed below in the mini session 'Parenthood romanticized'. (Alternatively, this latter session can be used as the first parenting session to set the scene.)

MINI SESSION: PARENTHOOD ROMANTICIZED

Introduction

In countries such as the UK, USA and Australia, parent roles (particularly the role of mother), although not necessarily held in high esteem, are nevertheless surrounded by romanticized, idealized images. As early as 1971, Janeway argued that motherhood is so entangled in mythical thinking that it is difficult to distinguish the myth from reality. Because of the mystique that surrounds motherhood in modern post-industrialized societies, women may have a highly romanticized picture that contrasts sharply with the actual experience of motherhood (Rossi 1968, Oakley 1979).

The romanticized image of parenting sets standards that are impossible for parents to achieve. Inherent in society's romanticized image of motherhood is the 'Supermum' myth. In discussing this 'Supermum' myth, Sears (1985) comments that never before have mothers been required or expected to do so much, for so many, with so little support. Grossman et al (1980) argue that this 'myth of parenthood' tyrannizes most new parents in their efforts to at least approximate to the idealized image. According to this idealized image, a wanted pregnancy is always undertaken joyfully, the couple are united more strongly during pregnancy, and the birth is uncomplicated. The myth continues after the birth, only minor adjustments being required before parents feel comfortable and natural in their unambiguous roles (Grossman et al 1980). Because of the mystique surrounding motherhood, individual women may find it necessary to maintain a pretence of coping with the often overwhelming tasks of the mothering role as it is constructed in modern post-industrialized society (Oakley 1979).

Grossman et al (1980) found that while women in their research, when interviewed 2 months after the birth, vividly described the difficulties they had experienced since the infants' birth, they nevertheless carefully stated they felt 'out of the woods now'. However, the research team felt that most parents were presenting an image consistent with the cultural stereotype or idealized image of parenthood: that well-functioning families experience only the joys of having a newborn and are easily able to incorporate the arrival of a new baby. In reality, the emotional disequilibrium occasioned by the birth was still very much in evidence. Most of the couples were still experiencing various degrees of difficulty. However, the couple's fears of being a dysfunctional family, or the woman's fear that she was having an unnatural psychopathological reaction, precluded their admitting to these difficulties. More recently, women who expressed guilt because they did not feel elated at the birth of their perfect baby were relieved to find that they were not 'odd' (Painter 1995). Moreover, as we discuss below in the mini sessions on emotional well-being, many women in the 1990s still feel the need to 'put on a front'.

Midwives exploding the myths

Perhaps the most important part of exploding the myths of parenthood is constantly reinforcing the non-existence of the three mythological beings 'Perfect Mother', 'Perfect Father' and 'Perfect Baby'. Because the media will continue to present a romanticized image of parenting, parents need to be able to acknowledge these images, talk about them and, more importantly, laugh at them. Before and after the birth, midwives can encourage parents to do this. Parents need midwives to tell them that they do not need to live up to the impossible standards set by the romanticized image of parenting and indeed that most parents physically and emotionally cannot live up to these standards.

Objective

- The new parents will be aware of the myths that may result in a romanticized view of the parenting role and that these can affect couples.

Important teaching points

- Clarify through discussion the fact that society promotes a highly romanticized picture of parenthood that is quite different from the actual experience.
- In a humorous way, discuss the three 'perfect beings': Perfect Mother, Perfect Father and Perfect Baby.
- Encourage group members to discuss how they feel that this romanticized image of parenting may affect new parents.

Midwives' teaching notes

Parenting: the myths

These three mythological beings – Perfect Mother,

Perfect Father and Perfect Baby – are a large part of the romanticized image of parenthood promoted by society. In reality, of course, these three 'perfect beings' do not exist.

Perfect Mother. Perfect Mother (alias 'Supermum') is that imaginary glamorous creature who resembles the tissue or toilet soap advertisements. Perfect Mother had a perfect birth and bonded with her Perfect Baby immediately, with no real need for change in her life. Her breasts never leaked, she could sit down immediately because she did not have an episiotomy, and she certainly did not have breast engorgement. As for haemorrhoids and varicose veins – well what do you think? This perfect being also immediately (before leaving the birth suite) went back to her prebirth weight; her figure was once again perfect and her stomach never, ever stuck out.

Perfect Mother's hair and make-up are always perfect, her clothes stunning and her house immaculate. She never feels exhausted or fed-up, or wishes that she had not had the baby, and she definitely, never, ever, ever stays in her dressing gown until lunchtime (or teatime). Her hair is always clean, her clothes are always tidy, her house is immaculate, and she provides gourmet meals for her husband every night. Of course, as well as all this, she works full-time outside the home.

Perfect Father. Perfect Father (or should we call him 'Superdad'?) also immediately adjusted to the birth of his children and became a perfect father. He gazes adoringly at Perfect Baby and Perfect Mother all of the time when he is not working at his perfect, stress-free job. He is of course such a help to 'Supermum' (not that she needs his help). And he never, ever loses his temper or shouts at his children. Oh, and of course he always looks perfect in his immaculately clean and ironed clothes (courtesy of Perfect Mother).

Perfect Child Within the idealistic, romanticized myth of parenthood, Perfect Baby gains exactly the right amount of weight every week, never vomits, never ever has colic, rarely cries, slept through the night from 1 week onwards and smiles at everyone all the time. In turn, Perfect Child is always endearing, sweet, cooperative, quiet and lovable. Sweet, endearing Perfect Baby and Perfect Child do not require their parents to make any changes in their well-ordered existence, and they never, ever disrupt their lives.

Parenting: the realities

Of course, Perfect Mother, Perfect Father and Perfect Baby are only a figment of society's imagination – mythical beings. So will the non-perfect parents please stand up and bring their non-perfect baby with them?

Non-perfect parents. The reality of the matter is that parents are real people, with real stresses. To begin with, despite everyone's best efforts, women may not always have the perfect birth that they had expected. They may end up with a painful episiotomy or tear, cracked and sore nipples, engorgement and leaking breasts. Stretch marks and a protruding abdomen are sometimes inevitable.

As for bonding immediately with their baby, Oakley (1979) found that as many as 70% of mothers were not interested in their babies when they first held them. A similar number sometimes felt angry with their babies for not doing what the textbooks said they ought to in the early weeks. It is not abnormal for women to feel trapped and to have second (third, or even more) thoughts about having had their baby. In the early weeks, despite all the hard work and very little rest, there is actually very little to show at the end of the day. This may be made worse by the fact that, at the end of the day, babies are often irritable and crying.

It is quite normal for non-perfect parents to feel stressed and frustrated by the demands of parenthood. In addition to being parents, they may both have full-time jobs and even study commitments. Indeed, as previously stated, Sears (1985) commented that never before have parents been required or expected to 'do so much, for so many, with so little support'.

Non-perfect baby. The further reality is that babies and children are usually a source of great disruption to their parents. Babies do cry, do not sleep through the night, need to be fed frequently, do vomit and sometimes have colic. And they always know when their parents are about to sit down for a hot meal or a cuddle. Small children are often inquisitive, noisy or disobedient and may also at times be demanding and disruptive.

Back to the myths

Regardless, however, of these realities about children, and the changes that are experienced by most couples, society continues to promote a highly romanticized picture of parenthood that is quite different from reality. This romanticized picture is quite different from the actual experience of being a mother (Rossi 1968, Oakley 1979).

So how is it done? This highly romanticized picture is promoted in various ways. For example, women's magazines and advertisements always present a very romantic picture of motherhood. Stories of the actresses and singers who fit this romantic picture are regular features. These stars tell us how easy, wonderful and natural being a mother is for them. However, they often forget to mention how helpful it is to have three nannies, at least one housekeeper, a cook, several gardeners, a good plastic surgeon and, of course, a personal trainer.

Just imagine. On a lighter note, imagine reading the following quotes in *Women's Weekly* or *Women's Day* magazine (and further imagine that they were made by Melanie Griffiths, Jerry Hall, Elle McPherson or even Jane Seymour):

My hemorrhoids were terrible ... I was walking hunched over ... I could not believe it ... I was walking to the nursery ... with my legs apart and all hunched over...

The episiotomy, basically was my worst problem. I just felt like I couldn't walk around and do things ... It was really hard.

(interview quotes, Ruchala & Halstead 1994)

It would actually be difficult to imagine famous actresses telling readers about their haemorrhoids – but it would be so kind to women if they did.

A specific example. The following were included as part of a feature in a recent Australian women's magazine that talked about the birth of the star's newest (and fourth) new baby.

The first picture shows a woman (the star) and three other children having dinner at a round table (complete with starched white tablecloth, arranged flowers and wine glasses). In the foreground of the picture, a baby is sleeping in a bassinette. The second picture shows a portrait perfect mother with a sleeping new baby in her arms and a small child sitting quietly on her lap. Both children are wearing frilly white dresses.

First, a serious discussion of these images. The routine and ordered existence of new motherhood is suggested by the seemingly content, sleeping new baby and the well-behaved older children. This suggests that new babies sleep at family mealtimes while older children sit obediently in chairs and listen to adult conversation. Natural motherhood is implied by the mother's appearance. Her shawl and long flowing hair suggest an earthiness and lack of sophistication, a naturalness and motherliness. Moreover, the baby is next to the mother, showing her as the natural carer.

The purity and glamour of motherhood are emphasized by the abundance of white and light surrounding the mother and baby in both pictures. The white tablecloth, bassinette cover and flowers have connotations of purity, while the light and the beautiful white clothes of the baby and child present a glamorous and romantic image of 'mother and child'.

The 'right' place and responsibility of the new mother is portrayed by the position of the baby and by the lighting in the picture. The baby is placed next to the mother, and the lighting in the foreground emphasizes the mother and baby; indeed, mother and baby are almost linked by the light. Although the mother's attention is ostensibly on the others at the table, this link reminds us that the baby is still her responsibility. The illustration presents mothering as the right and natural function of a woman: the father of the child can be away, but the new mother's 'right' place is with her baby.

Both pictures are typical of the way the media portray motherhood. Such texts may seem harmless and even pleasant, but by presenting a picture that emphasizes the ease, routine, order, purity and glamour of being a new mother, they invoke myths of motherhood that are idealized and romanticized, hiding from readers the reality of being a new mother.

And now, a fairy story about these texts.   Starring Perfect Mother and Perfect Children (Perfect Father being away). The mythological beings Perfect Mother and Perfect Baby (who later becomes Perfect Child) are the stars of our story and a part of the romanticized and idealized image of motherhood presented by both illustrations.

Perfect Mother (alias 'Supermum') is that glamorous creature who, after feeding, burping, bathing, changing and settling the baby (and attending to the needs of the three older children) had time to arrange flowers, had time to cook a gourmet meal, had time to wash (and iron and starch) a beautiful white tablecloth, had time to eat a relaxed meal, and had time to enjoy a glass of wine. And, judging by her long, shiny locks, Perfect Mother also had time to wash her hair. The ease of mothering for 'Supermum' is shown in the first picture by the presence of the starched white tablecloth, the arranged flowers, the wine glasses and the mother's relaxed attitude as she talks to her family.

Moreover, within the idealized, romanticized myth of motherhood presented in the pictures, Perfect Baby obligingly sleeps while Perfect Mother enjoys her relaxed meal. In turn, each Perfect Child sits obediently in a chair and listens patiently to adult conversation. As shown in the texts, Endearing Perfect Baby and Sweet Perfect Child are cooperative, quiet and lovable little people who fit into their mother's routine and ordered existence.

Alas, the fairy story just ended.
To end the fairy story, we simply replace the mythical characters in the picture with a non-perfect new mother and her non-perfect baby and children. A different picture emerges, a picture that is quite incompatible with the previous idealized and romanticized myth of motherhood. The relaxed evening meal certainly disintegrates following this, as does the portrait perfect representation of Perfect Mother, Perfect Baby and Perfect Child.

Our real non-perfect new mother is now poised gingerly on an air ring that has been placed on her chair. She is desperately ignoring the demands of her non-perfect children as she tries to eat while consoling her non-perfect crying baby. In both pictures, her demeanour is one of fatigue as she wonders which pain is worse: that from her sore nipples, her engorged and leaking breasts, or her haemorrhoids. Her open-fronted dress is covered with breast milk (courtesy of her leaking breasts), vomit (courtesy of our non-perfect baby) and chocolate (courtesy of a non-perfect older child). Non-perfect baby and the non-perfect older children in the first picture are all shouting loudly, refusing to eat, spilling food and drinks, and generally vying with the baby for their mother's attention.

In the second illustration, the chocolate (used by non-perfect new mother as a bribe to keep her older child quiet) is now smeared all over our non-perfect child's face, her white dress and the baby's white dress (from non-perfect older child pinching him when her mother wasn't looking). Our non-perfect baby is crying loudly. This could be because he is hungry and wants feeding, because he has been fed and has wind, because he is irritable at the end of a long day or just because, after all, that is what most small babies do at mealtimes and when their parents dress them up.

The condition of the baby's white dress has also deteriorated somewhat. As well as being stained with his sister's chocolate handprint, the front of the dress was also adversely affected when he vomited after his dear sister tried to feed him the pearls from around the toy dog's neck as a special treat (which quite possibly also contributed to his crying). Or could it have been caused when she pinched him – who knows?

Back to the reality

One thing, however, is certain. The text now more closely mirrors the reality of motherhood, a reality in which children are usually a source of great disruption to their parents. However much a new baby is loved and wanted, and regardless of the joy experienced by a new mother, the impact on her everyday life is, as we discussed earlier, great. As most mothers come to know, there is usually very little routine in their lives, particularly in the early days. The many and varied needs of a new baby result in a new mother having less (or no) time for herself. In the early weeks, fatigue and exhaustion are usual as sleep becomes an almost forgotten luxury.

The idealized and romanticized myths of motherhood promoted by such texts hide from ordinary women the reality of being a mother. However, neither text is able to sustain these myths in the presence of non-perfect new mother, non-perfect baby and non-perfect older child. Motherhood begins to look like what it really is – hard work.

In our society, the idealized and romanticized myths of motherhood presented in such texts are particularly powerful as, before their own child is born, men and women are largely unaware of the reality of parenting. Within the nuclear family, girls and women have limited sources of knowledge when learning about being a new mother. Indeed, some may have no reality other than the 'reality' presented by the media. They may be aware of what it is like to look after babies or small children for a few hours; they are, however, usually not aware of the reality of having another human being depend on them for their every need for 24 hours of every day (Oakley 1980).

Women readers with limited experience of children are unlikely to see that the reality of motherhood is being hidden, let alone how this is being done. Therefore, such images as these are, like cigarettes, harmful to women and children.

I'm failing. Romanticized images of parenting can make life much more difficult for parents, particularly women, in a number of ways (Rossi 1968, Bernard 1975, Oakley 1979, 1980, Grossman et al 1980, Painter 1995):

- Parents may succumb to the popular belief that the parenting role is instinctive and may see preparation as unnecessary.
- Women can feel cheated if motherhood does not live up to their expectations.
- Because women may feel that they should be able to live up to these standards, they may feel guilty, unhappy and depressed when they find that this is difficult or impossible. They may also feel that they have failed as a mother.
- Men may feel that their partner is 'failing' as a mother if she is not able to manage the multitude of roles expected of her.
- Women may also find it necessary to pretend that they are 'coping' with all the tasks of motherhood.
- New parents may believe that 'good' families experience only the joys of having a newborn. Women are more likely to express negative feelings once they know that other women also experience these feelings.

To conclude

Although the romanticized images of parenting may appear harmless, they are actually very insidious in the way in which they 'set up' new parents; thus, they need to be recognized and exposed.

MINI SESSION: IT'S DIFFICULT FOR MEN TOO

Introduction

The role of father has changed historically and also varies considerably between different societies (Marks & Lovestone 1995). Some social theorists have argued that, in the 1990s, in countries such as Australia, the UK and the USA, the meaning of parenthood is being transformed in concert with the reconstruction of marital relationships. Men and women today want not only more equal and satisfying partnerships in marriage, but also shared parenting (Edgar 1993). Such changes can only be positive given the conflict that occurs in many relationships when parents assume more traditional roles after the birth of their first child.

Other social theorists have, however, challenged the 'ideology of the new domesticated male' and have argued that, although the general feeling in the 1990s is that before the first birth most couples share household chores equally, this may not always be so. Interviews with couples suggest that, in many households (with or without children), women generally contribute more or even assume most of the responsibility for household chores (Shelton 1990, Blair & Lichter 1991).

What is positive is that research from the Australian Institute of Family Studies 'has flagged a decreasing gap between men expressing the "correct" values about equality in marriage and their actual behaviour' (Edgar 1993). On a less positive note, 15–20% of couples are separated or divorced by the time the infant is 4 years old. Men and women have given several reasons for this high separation rate. These include marital conflict and difficulty adjusting to the profound relationship changes, the father's lack of involvement in chores and jealousy of the mother's preoccupation with the baby. Men complain that women exclude them, and women feel overwhelmed and taken for granted (Cowan & Cowan 1992, Belsky & Kelly 1994).

In addition, some men say that health professionals exclude them. For example: 'Feels like we've been forgotten at times … they don't usually worry about us …' (Barclay et al 1996). They have also complained of not being warned about the possible emotional changes that they might experience during their partner's pregnancy and birth (Henderson & Brouse 1991, Hyssala et al 1993). For men, a large part of the benefit of antenatal classes was meeting and sharing information and feelings with other couples (Henderson & Brouse 1991). Several researchers have suggested that, given their changing roles, men may benefit from men-only groups before or after the birth, or both. Men have found such groups helpful and have requested fathers-only sessions with experienced fathers as speakers, or focus groups for men to look at men's issues (Watson 1992, Bader & MacMillan 1994, cited in Watson et al 1995).

Objectives

- Before the birth, men will have the opportunity to discuss their concerns about the pregnancy, birth and their role as a father.
- After the birth, men will have the opportunity to share with other men what becoming a father is like.

Important teaching points

- *Antenatal.* Briefly discuss the research findings on becoming a father.
- Encourage men to talk about how they feel about becoming a father.
- *Postnatal.* Ask men about the changes that have occurred in their lives since their baby's birth and encourage them to share these with the group.
- If possible (and appropriate), include experienced fathers who are prepared to talk about the highs and lows of being a parent.

Midwives' teaching notes

Men becoming fathers

In countries such as the UK, USA and Australia, societal expectations of men are changing. This can lead to stress and confusion for men, particularly during the transition to parenting. For example, their partner may want (and need) an equal relationship, but their own parents (and possibly some male friends) may discourage their involvement in household chores and childcare. It is important not to underemphasize the effects of men's own parents in influencing how they become fathers (Cowan & Cowan 1992). For example, fathers may be pressured by their own parents into not participating in parenting classes: 'my husband's father asked him why he was going to antenatal classes when he already knew where the maternity ward was at the hospital' (NSW Women's Consultative Committee 1994).

I really want to be involved. An increased involvement of men in childcare could lead to better parenting and improved relationships, and a healthier family environment (Watson et al 1995). A father's involvement in the care of his baby may increase his awareness of the difficulties that his partner experiences and increase his empathy towards his partner (Levy-Shiff 1994). Certainly, men are equally competent at infant care, but they are poorly socialized for the role (Fishbein 1990).

As we have previously discussed, but need to emphasize further, men's involvement after the birth is important both for women and for men themselves. Men's own satisfaction with marital quality across the transition to parenthood was higher when the father was involved in childcare (Nugent 1991). However, (based on their interviews with men and women), researchers have identified a number of obstacles to men's full participation in childcare (Lamb et al 1986, Cowan & Cowan 1992, Russell 1994):

- limited role models of men as primary carers of new babies;
- insufficient role models of men as nurturers;
- some men not feeling as competent as their partners at looking after the baby (even small amounts of criticism can lead to them giving up caregiving);
- their own parents, who may offer mixed or negative feedback when men have high levels of involvement;
- some women's strong feelings about losing their role as primary caregivers, or their feeling threatened if men become too skilled at looking after the baby. Women may erect barriers to prevent this happening.

Who teaches men? There is evidence that men rely on women (who are themselves learning a new role) for help with infant problems and parenting information or for support (Humenick & Bugen 1987, Stevens 1988). However, some researchers have found that many parents are so distressed that they are unable to support each other (Henderson & Brouse 1991). This situation bears a marked resemblance to a recent episode of 'Superman' when the hero flew to break Lois's fall from a multistorey building. Superman said to Lois, *'I've got you'*. And Lois replied, *'Yes, but who's got you?'*

Important issues and conflicts. Some issues that have been identified by men as being important during the transition to parenthood include:

- resolving conflict

- spending time with the children
- sharing household tasks
- their perception of their relationship.

In addition, a number of areas have emerged as sources of conflict for some men as they adjust to their new role (Cowan & Cowan 1992, Bader & MacMillan 1994, Belsky & Kelly 1994):

- the division of household labour – who does what;
- difficulties in the couple's relationship, with less time together and decreased communication and affection;
- a lack of free time;
- social isolation;
- financial pressure;
- balancing family life and career.

Some researchers have found that a substantial number of fathers report experiencing some negative physical or emotional symptoms such as depression following the baby's birth (Raskin et al 1990, Ballard et al 1994, Watson et al 1995). However, as we have previously discussed, after the birth men report less stress or crisis than their partners (Terry 1991a), and their stress levels off after 1 month (Belsky & Kelly 1994).

Father's adjustment.   Jordan (1990) suggested that fathers go though three developmental processes or stages as they adjust to their new role:

1. grappling with the reality of the pregnancy and child;
2. struggling for recognition as a parent;
3. persevering in the role of involved parenthood.

To conclude

Midwives have an important role to play in helping men to adjust to their role. One way of doing this is to organize men's groups (for men who would like these), where men can share their experiences.

MINI SESSION: THE MOTHERING ROLE IN MODERN POST-INDUSTRIALIZED SOCIETIES

Introduction

Midwives and health visitors are in an ideal position to help women to adjust in a positive way to being a new mother. During the antenatal period, midwives can make the future of mothering experience easier and more joyful for women by helping both parents to recognize and deal with the way in which the mother-

ing role is structured in our culture. When used during the antenatal months, the information in this session will also help both parents to have a better idea of what really happens after the birth for most families. If the antenatal session is continued (or even used for the first time) during the postnatal period, this will give women the opportunity to share with other women what being a new mother is really like. This sharing will help women to realize that they are not alone in any difficulties they are experiencing. It may also help them establish a network of friends who are in a similar situation.

Some may argue that actually exposing the unfairness of the way in which motherhood is structured in countries such as the UK, USA, Canada and Australia can make women angry at a time when they are very vulnerable. However, anger reflected outwards is more positive than guilt displaced inwards, certainly for the women.

Objective

- The new parents will be aware of the different factors that can make the mothering role more difficult for women in modern post-industrialized societies.

Important teaching points

- *Antenatal.* Discuss the many challenges and changes faced by women when they become mothers.
- *Postnatal.* Encourage group members to share the highs and lows of their new life.

Midwives' teaching notes

Becoming a mother is, in any society, the most powerful physical, emotional and social challenge that most women will ever experience. Carrying new life within one's own body is extraordinary and unique (Broom 1994).

Gains and losses

Women both gain and lose when they become mothers. In recent interviews, women spoke of the things that they had gained and the things that they had lost when they had a baby. Gains included their amazement at the wonder of being a mother, their happiness with their role and the depth of love that they felt for their baby. Losses included a loss of time, a loss of energy (feeling fatigued, exhausted and drained), a loss of company (being alone), a loss of their personal freedom (feeling trapped and confined) and, for some women, even a loss of their sense of self (Percival 1990, Gjerdingen & Fontaine 1991, Gjerdingen et al 1993, Pugh & Milligan 1993, Ruchala & Halstead 1994, Sethi 1995, Barclay et al 1997):

I don't know how to put it into words what motherhood is like. It is the most true love I have experienced in my life. It is happiness, it is frustration too and it is devotion and sacrifice.
   I mean motherhood is an amazing thing…
   As much as I love her and she's wonderful and good and everything, it's a big change. It really is.
   The severe anxiety lump in my stomach that I had earlier on when I was first at home has subsided. I think that is because my confidence has grown and I am very happy in the mother role.
   The most important adjustment is not being able to do things on the spur of the moment…
   It's very demanding … sometimes I crave for that time of freedom and peace and quiet.

For women, the early weeks and months are a time requiring many adjustments that cause stress and increase vulnerability (Caplan 1957, Rubin 1975).

Physical stresses

Getting over the birth. The typical events of a first or subsequent pregnancy and birth can make the early weeks after the birth a time of decreased physical strength for many women (Gjerdingen & Fontaine 1991, Gjerdingen et al 1993, Pugh & Milligan 1993). Pregnancy is physically demanding for women, bringing about radical alterations in body shape and sensation. Women pregnant for the first time may have worked full time outside the home until just before the birth. Those having a second or subsequent child may have combined working full time outside the home with meeting the needs of toddlers or older children. Both groups would have had few opportunities for rest during pregnancy. Even without complications, birthing is hard work. Moreover, the physical changes immediately after birth are as radical (and more rapid) than those during pregnancy (Broom 1994). Life is even more difficult for women who may have had interventions such as an episiotomy or an instrumental or caesarean birth.

Women may experience a number of physical stressors in the early weeks after the birth of the infant. These include perineal healing, uterine drainage, mild contractions, the onset or inhibition of lactation, endocrine fluctuations, the re-establishment of normal bowel and bladder functions, and assorted neuromuscular discomforts (Gjerdingen & Fontaine 1991, Gjerdingen et al 1993).

Has my figure gone forever? The mother's appearance in the early weeks is also drastically transformed from its prebirth state (Perfect Mother, of course, being the exception to this rule). This may cause women great emotional discomfort in a society that emphasizes the appearance of the female body. The continuation of physiological discomforts may well lead to stress concerning body image. Stretch marks, a protruding abdomen, leaking nipples (and sometimes haemorrhoids) may conflict with the return to normal that many women expect as soon as the birth is over.

This is so hard. While recovering physically and emotionally from the first or subsequent birth, however, women must also care for their new baby. Caring for a new baby is very demanding: infants make heavy and continuous claims on time, attention and energy, and it is particularly difficult when most of the caring is done by one person (Broom 1994). At this time, all women face enormous challenges to their physical and emotional well-being. First-time new mothers are also 'learning on the job'. Mothers of a second, or subsequent, child are caring for a new and individual baby (who may have a very different personality and temperament from previous children) while also meeting the needs of toddlers or older children. The women in Percival's (1990) study spoke of the difficulties of caring for their baby when they really needed someone to care for them:

I didn't realize that the care would be 24 hours around the clock on constant demand. It's very frustrating having to put the baby first when you are really not feeling 100 percent well yourself.
   You wonder how you are going to cope. It is so terrible not having any sleep. I feel like a zombie but you get used to it and I try to sleep during the day.

I'm so exhausted. The early weeks after the birth are characterized by considerable physical, emotional and social change (Gjerdingen & Fontaine 1991). Interviews with women in the 1990s also show that these weeks are a time of intense fatigue and exhaustion for most women (Gjerdingen & Chaloner 1994, Ruchala & Halstead 1994, Sethi 1995, Barclay et al 1997). Fatigue is often caused by physical and emotional demands (Pugh & Milligan 1993). It is, therefore, hardly surprising that women experience exhaustion in the early weeks after the birth, given the many demands upon their time and energy. To quote: 'It's like you're drained' (Barclay et al 1997).

Becoming a juggler. During the early weeks after the birth, women become jugglers as they try to do everything that they are expected to do. The following comments reflect the many competing demands made on the new mother's time as she adjusts to her new role (Percival 1990):

Looking after the baby is okay if I leave other things but on occasions the things I have to leave really get me down.

I am not overwhelmed by the work. I rest while he is sleeping. Naturally I get a bit peeved but it is nothing I can't cope with.

I am always busy with the baby non-stop. Sometimes I get really frustrated that I can't get my housework done.

Sociocultural stresses

As we have previously discussed, as well as being a time of great joy, the early weeks of mothering may also be a time of great stress for the new mother. Apart from the physical demands of childbirth, a number of broader sociocultural factors may contribute to the difficulty that women have in adjusting to motherhood. These include the myths surrounding motherhood, the lack of a realistic preparation for the role, the abruptness of the transition, the low status of mothering and the way in which the social role of mother is constructed in modern post-industrialized societies.

Oh no, not those myths again. As we have discussed, women may have a highly romanticized view of parenthood, leading to unrealistic expectations of the role of mothering: 'they all said to me "oh it's so easy" ... and then all of a sudden I realised it wasn't quite that easy' (Barclay et al 1997). As we discuss below, this romanticized image of parenting has the potential to affect women's self esteem and emotional well-being. The results of her interviews with new mothers led Oakley (1980) to conclude that women are less likely to be depressed following the birth of their infant if they are able to enjoy motherhood for what it is rather than trying to live up to an idealized image.

Help, I'm not prepared. Women may commence motherhood with limited preparation and no real role models to follow. Moreover, women are expected to cope well with new parenthood while men are expected to be unprepared (Terry 1991a, 1991b). Barnett (1991) argued that, in our culture (especially if one is the mother), parenting expertise is supposed to 'arrive' with the baby (see also Chapter 17). As we have previously discussed, women in the 1990s may lack a knowledge of and preparation for the changes involved in being a parent (Percival 1990, Barclay et al 1997):

I went to all the classes but I don't really know what to do. I am in the dark. When she cries at night I try all different things. At the moment my night times are pretty harrowing.

There's nothing about after [the birth]. Its like you know, you should know what to do ... but it was one huge black hole.

She takes up all of my time. None of the antenatal classes mentioned the amount of time the baby would take up, and they never discussed difficult babies.

And I'm certainly not ready. Many women, then, begin the mothering role with unrealistic expectations and inadequate preparation. The problem may be compounded by the abruptness of the transition to the maternal role. Rossi (1968) described how the birth of a child is not followed by any gradual taking on of responsibility, as in the case of a professional work role. While a period of courtship usually precedes marriage, parenthood arrives abruptly. When a woman brings a new baby home, it is as if she is shifted from the position of graduate student to a professor without any apprenticeship experience of slowly increasing responsibility. The new mother's 24-hour duties commence immediately when she must assume responsibility for an infant who is, usually, totally dependent on her care.

Motherhood devalued. In Western societies, mothering is a job that demands a unique combination of management responsibilities, manual labour and skilled work. However, it has also been argued that motherhood has low status in our society, parenting functions being held in lower esteem than other work roles (LeMasters 1974, Bernard 1975). Because the myths (about motherhood in particular) present parenting as effortless, it may well be that society does not give credit to parents or value parenting functions. Traditional family organizations obligate most new mothers to set aside their role of 'importance' (paid employment) for the tasks of mothering, which are not valued (Oakley 1979, 1980). In addition, motherhood limits the woman's earning capacity and increases her dependency (Broom 1994).

Does it have to be so difficult? As is any other role, the mothering role is a product of each culture and refers to the acts a mother is expected to perform in relation to her child (Koniak-Griffin 1993).

A number of social theorists have argued that modern post-industrialized societies (such as the UK, USA and Australia) do not compare well with other cultures in the way in which motherhood is structured. In his comparison of British and Bushman societies, Blurton-Jones (1974b) argues that countries such as the UK make life more difficult for, and place barriers in the way of, new mothers. These barriers include the spacing of children, the isolation from other adults and the lack of ongoing support from older women. In addition, in her discussion of motherhood throughout the ages in different cultures, Bernard (1975) concluded:

It is as though we had selected the worst features of all of the ways motherhood is structured around the world and combined them to produce our current design. We make it all but impossible for so many well-meaning and conscientious women to perform the maternal role in an optimum manner.

For the most part, then, women in many modern post-industrialized societies who become mothers are isolated within the nuclear family, with total responsibility for the continuous care of their children, often with little or no adult contact from one day to the next. However captivating and rewarding babies and children are, nothing can substitute for adult interaction. This social isolation represents another significant cost of motherhood (Broom 1994).

Also, women and men often lack the support of an extended family to give practical help and provide role models. Grandparents may live in another county or state, or may themselves have full-time jobs. This lack of support can place enormous strain on women (and men) as they try their best to be committed parents as well as to juggle their many other commitments.

I'm so alone. Bernard (1974, 1975) has argued that both mother and infant are harmed by isolating them within the nuclear family and assigning the mother total responsibility for the continuous care of the infant. For example, 'It's very isolating these first few weeks', 'I feel confined' (Sethi 1995, Barclay et al 1997). The social isolation associated with motherhood may also cut women off from the intellectual stimulation that they might have had while they were working (Kitzinger 1978). If the new mother has left the paid workforce (temporarily or permanently), she suffers not only a loss of income, but also a loss of the daily social contact that most workplaces provide. These changes alone usually bring with them a loss of identity (NSW Women's Consultative Committee 1994).

What about me? Women are faced with mutually incompatible requirements: for tender loving care around the clock, and of exclusive responsibility for children. This situation may lead to anxiety, guilt and fatigue on the part of the mother (Bernard 1974, 1975). Oakley (1979) argues that a lack of harmony exists between the needs of women and the requirements of motherhood as a social role. One-third of the women in her (1979) research expressed dissatisfaction with the social role of mother, including such factors as isolation and the work of childrearing. This finding is supported by more recent interviews with women (NSW Women's Consultative Committee 1994, Ruchala & Halstead 1994, Sethi 1995, Barclay et al 1997).

Motherhood thus constructed is difficult to reconcile with many other social responsibilities, including those of wife, let alone paid worker. The identity of 'mother' displaces many or even all the woman's previous social positions (Broom 1994). Given recent role shifts for women (MacDermid et al 1990), this all-encompassing 'mother identity' may result in women feeling that they have gained a great deal – but at what cost?

Many women struggle to reconcile the multiple roles of career woman, mother and wife. Women's experience is one of negotiating multiple roles or walking a tightrope (Moen 1992, Barclay et al 1997). Women who have spent considerable time building a career may be subjected to even greater stress (Alexander & Higgins 1993), as may those who place a high priority on paid employment (Levy-Shiff 1994). Women may experience high levels of guilt and tension surrounding the need to return to work (Terry 1991b, Russell 1994). For example, a woman in Sethi's (1995) study commented:

It isn't as if we can't manage with one income but the thing is, I don't want to lose my work experience (tears in her eyes) ... My husband says 'I don't think you should go back to work' ... I believe I am sacrificing my needs ... I hope I don't have to sacrifice my being just to be a mother.

Finally, Nicholson (1983) reports that one of the greatest of the many wrongs inflicted on mothers has been to give them the worst part of the deal and then make them feel guilty about it.

To conclude

Following the birth, a woman in Western society must cope with the 24-hour needs of a new infant as she recovers her own physical and emotional equilibrium. Apart from the physical demands imposed by childbirth, a number of broader sociocultural factors may make it harder for women to adjust to motherhood. Motherhood is highly romanticized, and women may be unprepared for the reality of day-to-day mothering, as well as for the abruptness of the transition to the mothering role. Women are further disadvantaged by the low status of their mothering role. Finally, the way in which this role is structured compares unfavourably with the situation in other cultures in its expectations of women. This results in social isolation and may lead to anxiety, guilt and fatigue on the part of the mother.

Where to from here?

Some ways in which women can make life easier in the early weeks are discussed in the mini session 'Strategies for survival' below. This session links with and follows the previous session.

MINI SESSION: STRATEGIES FOR SURVIVAL

Introduction

In countries such as the UK, USA and Australia, the person at home full time with the baby in the early weeks is still more likely to be the woman. However, in the interest of being fair to those men who are at home full time, it must be noted that the following strategies work equally well for both men and women. As well as providing practical information, the session also reinforces for parents midwives', views that it is not only acceptable to ask for help, but also a positive thing to do.

Objective

- The parent at home will be aware of and able to use strategies to make life easier in the early weeks and months of being a parent.

Important teaching points

- Discuss the things that the person at home with the baby can do to make life a little easier in the early weeks and months of motherhood.
- If possible, copy the pamphlet and go through this.
- Ask couples what else they could do to make life easier.

Midwives' teaching notes

Pamphlet: Your midwife's advice for surviving the early weeks

Remember that survival is the name of the game during the first few weeks until things settle down.

Accept help

- Accept all offers of help. If friends and relatives wish to do the cleaning, cook meals or baby-sit, accept gratefully. Remember that giving makes others feel good, so you are doing them a favour too. You can always give back to them later.
- If the budget allows, employ a cleaning and ironing person and use a nappy wash service.

Short cuts

- Become expert at doing a quick, superficial clean and tidy around the house. Learn to 'love the weeds', or in this case the dust and unwashed dishes.
- Women, buy a couple of kaftans (front opening if breastfeeding) to put on in the morning, and wear one instead of a dressing gown. Men, pull on a loose pair of non-iron trousers and a T-shirt.

Be kind to yourself

- You *must* have some time on your own without the baby each week, even if it is just 2 hours in bed, a trip to the hairdressers or time to read a book.

- Be selfish. Recognize that this is a tough time of enormous change and look after yourself. If your baby is asleep, unplug the phone, put a sign on the door and go to bed.
- Make sleep a *number one priority*. It is quite unlikely that your baby will remember whether the dishes were done or the house dusted.
- Share the experience of parenthood by teaming up with another parent whom you can ring if things are getting you down.

Look after yourself

- Eat nutritious food. To increase physical and emotional well-being, have easy meals and snacks that include fruit, vegetables and protein.
- Take a good multivitamin tablet to ensure lots of vitamin B and minerals.

Change your thinking

- Don't feel guilty about the things that don't get done. Keep reminding yourself that, if they are being perfectly honest, most parents cannot get through everything that has to be done (except 'Supermum' of course).
- Don't feel guilty if you feel depressed, fed up or trapped, hate being a parent, and yearn for those free, independent days before your baby was born. At one time or another, most women (and men) feel like this.
- When people give unwanted advice (as they will), nod and smile.
- Don't waste energy arguing with others about the way in which you are going to do things; just accept the advice and do things your own way.

To conclude

Making life easier is the most important thing for parents to do in the early weeks. Midwives are the best people to tell them that it is OK to do this.

MINI SESSION: INTEGRATING THE BIRTH EXPERIENCE

Introduction

Affonso (1987) emphasized the importance of the woman engaging in the important psychological task of integrating the events surrounding pregnancy, labour and birth into a functional whole. She argued that women must resolve conflicts or unfulfilled expectations surrounding the labour or birth. The meaning that a woman attributes to childbirth may be an important clue to the presence of ambivalent feelings (Affonso & Domino 1984, Affonso & Arizmendi 1986). In emphasizing the importance of the clarification of the labour and birth, Affonso (1987) argued that these ambivalent feelings can be a precursor to the conflicts that compromise maternal adaptation.

The ideal situation for most women is one in which they are guaranteed continuity of carer throughout the pregnancy, birth and postnatal time as well as the continuous presence of a known midwife throughout labour (see McCourt & Page 1996). In such situations, even when the woman has interventions, she is more likely to feel in control as she has emotional support from a familiar midwife. She will then also almost certainly have someone she knows who can review the birth with her. Sadly, for many women, this ideal situation will simply not be available. Moreover, research by Percival (1990, 1998) suggests that, for many women (certainly in Australia), their ideal image of an intervention-free birth will not be realized. These studies found a high incidence of forceps and caesarean births, particularly among first-time mothers.

It is important, therefore, that women are given the opportunity to resolve conflicts or unfulfilled expectations about the labour and birth. Midwives are in an ideal position to assist women in integrating their birth experience. This can be done on a one-to-one basis, ideally with the midwife who was with the mother during the birth (see Clement 1995). Alternatively, the midwife may use the following mini session as the basis for a group to debrief women. Both approaches have their advantages. Some women may feel more comfortable talking to one midwife, particularly if they know her well, whereas others may benefit from listening to the shared experiences of other women.

Objectives

The new mother will:

- have the opportunity to discuss how she feels about her birth;
- begin to have more positive feelings about her birth experience;
- begin to appreciate that the birth experience is not an indicator of self-worth or success as a mother.

Important teaching points

- Discuss the importance of the woman talking about and working through the events surrounding the labour and the birth until she feels comfortable.

- Encourage women to share their feelings about their birth experience.
- Clarify that a poor birth experience is not an indicator of self-worth, and emphasize that the birth is not related to success as a mother.

Midwives' teaching notes

As we approach the year 2000, it is perhaps difficult to envisage that, at the beginning of the century, there was a real chance that either the mother or the baby would not survive the birth. In recent years, as physical safety is almost always assured, the emotional aspects of childbirth have increased in importance for women. For many women, the birth is no longer only a means to an end, that is, a live, well infant: the actual experience of the birth itself is also important.

Researchers have emphasized the importance of women working through and resolving the events surrounding the pregnancy, labour and birth until they feel comfortable with them. It has been argued that women's emotional well-being and adjustment to their new role may be affected by conflicts or unfulfilled expectations surrounding the labour or delivery. Some women may experience negative feelings if they have a complicated birth. However, it is not necessarily the type of birth that results in positive or negative feelings. Instead, it is the woman's feelings about the birth that seem to be important. For example, one woman may view a caesarean birth (particularly an elective one) as a positive experience. Another who had a vaginal birth but who needed pain relief may well view the birth negatively. Other women feel negative about having a caesarean birth. Any complicated birth in which the mother also feels she has no say may well predispose her to feelings of inadequacy and lack of control after the birth (Brown et al 1994).

Women who feel lower levels of gratification or who view their birth experience negatively may also:

- feel that they have 'failed' because they were unable to have a 'natural' birth;
- see their performance in labour as being indicative of their adequacy as a mother, leaving them at risk of compromised maternal adjustment;
- possess lower levels of confidence in, and satisfaction with, motherhood and infant care during the postnatal period;
- have lower levels of self-esteem and emotional well-being;
- view their baby in a less positive way;
- experience delayed attachment to the baby.

In addition, some women who have undergone cae-sarean births may:

- view the labour process as being ineffective or the experience as being incomplete;
- have less positive perceptions of the birth experience;
- experience a feeling of numbness and disappointment at the loss of the happy, natural birth they had anticipated;
- see their inability to give birth vaginally as being a sign of weakness: women in Marut & Mercer's (1979) research viewed 'pushing the infant out' as the hallmark of strength;
- feel that they have 'lost face' before husbands, relatives and friends; for example, women in research carried out by Cranley et al (1983) felt that they had let their husbands down by being unable to give birth vaginally;
- have a less positive perception of their infants (Mercer & Marut 1981).
- possess decreased self-esteem;
- have a higher level of postnatal depression. For example, women in Hamilton's (1986) research who experienced a significantly higher level of PND also had a higher caesarean section birth rate.

(Marut & Mercer 1979, Mercer & Marut 1981, Cranley et al 1983, Affonso & Domino 1984, Affonso & Arizmendi 1986, Hamilton 1986, Affonso 1987, Percival 1990)

To conclude

Factors such as high levels of intervention during labour, and assisted and caesarean births, have been associated with decreased self-esteem and PND, as have dissatisfaction with labour and birth, having no say in decisions and the presence of unwanted people at the birth. It may well be that it is not the type of birth, but the woman's feelings about the birth that may be the critical factor. Encouraging women to review the birth can, therefore, be very positive

WOMEN'S EMOTIONAL WELL-BEING AFTER THE BIRTH

In the UK, the Department of Health has identified mental health as one of five key priority areas in improving the health of the nation (Department of Health 1992). As we have previously discussed, becoming a parent is a time of great psychological and physical upheaval. The changes that women experience at this time have the potential to be detrimental to their emotional well-being (Terry 1991a, 1991b). Indeed, women are more likely to develop disturbances in their emotional well-being during the first year after the birth than at any other time.

Postnatal mood disorders have been recognized since the time of Hippocrates. However, until the 1960s, all postnatal mood disorders were classified as a single phenomenon. The medical profession's interest was largely in psychosis (this previously being viewed as the most severe manifestation of postnatal mood disorder). It is now widely accepted that three distinct and different types of mood disorder can affect women during the 12 months after the birth of their baby (Barnett 1991, NSW Women's Consultative Committee 1994, Pope 1994):

- The 'baby blues' or 'third day blues' affects as many as 80% of women during first 2 weeks of their baby's life.
- Puerperal psychosis is the least common of the postnatal mood disorders, affecting 1 or 2 in every 1000 women.
- PND affects as many as 1 in 5 women after their baby's birth. It is a severe and disabling depressive illness that may last months or years.

We have prepared mini sessions for all of these postnatal mood disorders. It is important that prospective parents are given some information on all three. In particular (as postnatal mood disorder was previously classified as a single condition), it is important that men and women understand there are *three* distinct types of mood disorder, which have different symptoms and need different management. They may have heard 'horror stories' about postnatal psychosis that may make them reluctant to admit to feelings of depression after the birth. We have placed more emphasis on PND as it is often more difficult to recognize than puerperal psychosis and its effects are more far reaching and devastating than those of the 'baby blues'.

MINI SESSION: THE 'BABY BLUES' OR 'THIRD DAY BLUES'
Objective

- The new parents will understand the emotional changes that most women experience during the first 2 weeks after the birth.

Important teaching points

- Explain that, after the baby's birth, most women

experience emotional changes such as the 'baby blues' or 'third day blues'.

Midwives' teaching notes

Most women suffer acute emotional lability and some degree of anxiety or depression after childbirth. The 'blues' is the most common and least serious of the postnatal mood disorders. It has been called the 'third day blues' because it usually occurs within a few days of childbirth.

Summary

- Up to 80% of women experience 'normal' baby blues during the first 2 weeks of their baby's life.
- Women may have emotional concerns ranging from feeling down, tense and irritable to being depressed. They may experience mood swings from elation to increased sensitivity and frequent episodes of crying.
- The mood disturbance does not usually last very long and goes away without treatment. Beck et al (1992) found that the severity of blues scores began to increase on day 2, peaked on the fifth day and then decreased.
- Women need special understanding and support from midwives; in particular they need to be listened to, have their feelings acknowledged and be given clear information and practical assistance.
- One theory attributes the cause to the rapid changes in hormone levels that occur in the transition from pregnancy to non-pregnancy.
- Early studies found most women experienced some depression developing within a short time of being in sole charge of the infant for the first time (Oakley 1979, Entwistle and Doering 1981).
- Some researchers have argued the depressive interludes experienced by 70–80% of mothers following the birth could in part be attributed to the grief that accompanies role change: the woman may experience a grieving for her old childless self.
- A significant relationship has been found between depression scores 1 week after the birth and depression levels at 6 weeks postpartum.

(Kitzinger 1975, Oakley 1980, Beck et al 1992, Pope 1994, Ruchala & Halstead 1994)

MINI SESSION: POSTNATAL OR PUERPERAL PSYCHOSIS

Objective

- The new parents will understand that postnatal *psychosis* occurs in only 1 or 2 in every 1000 births.

Important teaching points

- Explain that postnatal or puerperal psychosis is a rare condition.
- Emphasize that postnatal or puerperal psychosis is quite distinct and different from postnatal depression.

Midwives' teaching notes

Unlike the 'baby blues' or postnatal depression, postnatal psychosis is a rare condition: (NSW Women's Consultative Committee 1994, Pope 1994, Marks & Lovestone 1995)

- It is the least common of the postnatal mood disorders, occurring in only 1 or 2 of every 1000 births.
- It is the most serious postnatal problem in terms of the treatment required.
- The onset is rapid, symptoms appearing 2–4 weeks after the birth.
- The condition often occurs in women who have a personal or family history of psychiatric illness and is usually considered to be a form of manic-depressive illness that is precipitated by childbirth.
- The condition is relatively easy to recognize.
- The woman may experience disorganized thoughts or confusion, indecision, periods of elation, hallucinations and being out of touch with reality.
- Prompt psychiatric treatment is required; this usually includes hospitalization and medication.

MINI SESSION: POSTNATAL DEPRESSION

Introduction

Effects of postnatal depression

PND can have far reaching effects on women, their partners and their children (Pope 1994).

Effects on women. The following quote is an excerpt from a diary kept by a journalist (Cornes 1999) during the time she experienced PND:

In a former life I swam with turtles and rafted grade four rapids bellowing like Red Sonja. I interviewed celebrities and made folk grin at my witty ripostes. Today there is vomit on my dress and mashed pumpkin in my hair. In a former life, the irony of it would have made me laugh but I have postnatal depression and instead I cry with self pity.

The bottom line for 1 out of 5 women is that they feel terrible at a time when their family, friends and society expect them to be happy – and not only happy, but also able to take care of themselves, an infant and possibly a partner. As Broom (1994) describes:

Our cultural prescription stipulates that women are 'made' to have babies, that 'normal' women want babies, and that mothering is a happy experience. If a woman disrupts this prescription by being depressed, she challenges our fundamental understanding of femininity and maternity.

The woman's own husband, family and friends may not only be unable to understand her feelings, but may also feel that she has no 'right' to be depressed.

Effects on infants. Oakley (1980) argued that PND is a significant contributory factor to the behaviour patterns displayed in insensitive and unresponsive mothering. The results of a recent meta-analysis of 19 studies (Beck 1995a) showed PND had a moderate-to-large effect on mother–infant interaction during the first year after the birth.

Effects on men. Interviews with men have shown that they may experience a loss of intimacy in their relationship when their partner has PND. They feel depressed, often in response to the relationship change, and are stressed with economic and career responsibilities and opportunities. They may also fear for the future and wonder whether their partner will ever get better (Williams 1994).

Rates of postnatal depression

The incidence of postpartum depression varies somewhat in different studies. During the 1990s, some research has suggested a rate of between 10 and 15% (Carothers & Murray 1990, Campbell & Cohn 1991, Beck et al 1992, Thorpe et al 1992, Painter 1995).

Other research using the Edinburgh Postnatal Depression Scale (EPDS) has suggested the rate may be higher: up to 20% (Brown et al 1994, Maloney 1995). In their research, Brown et al (1994) used an EPDS score of 12 and acknowledged that they may have missed some women who were depressed.

Kowalski (1994) reported an astoundingly high PND rate of almost 58% as measured by the EPDS (using a score of over 12). McIntosh (1993) found that 63% of women reported having experienced depression (defined as 'depressed mood lasting for at least 2 weeks during the first 9 months after the birth of their baby). Of respondents to the NSW Women's Consultative Committee survey (1994), 38% of women said that they had experienced postnatal depression.

In summary (based on research using the EPDS in countries such as the UK, USA and Australia), it is appropriate for midwives to tell parents that as many as 1 in 5 women (and possibly more) will experience a severe and disabling depressive illness after their baby's birth that may last months or even years.

Diagnosis of postnatal depression

One of the greatest barriers to helping women with PND is that it is often not diagnosed. The diagnosis of PND can be difficult for a number of reasons. Midwives and health visitors may not recognize PND. Moreover, as we discuss in the mini session, women themselves may not recognize PND or may feel that they need to keep silent or 'put on a front'.

Not recognized. PND is often not recognized or diagnosed by health professionals (Cox et al 1987). Holden (1994) found that when the EPDS was used to screen women, in 60% of instances health visitors were not aware that women in their care were depressed. Additionally, in Painter's (1995) study, none of the women identified with depression (using the EPDS) had been referred by or previously referred themselves to any agency. The health visitors involved felt that some women would have remained undetected had the EPDS not been used.

The development of the EPDS allows a more accurate diagnosis of PND to be made. This 10-items scale is easy to complete, taking about 5 minutes. Each question has four possible answers that relate to how the woman has been feeling in the past 7 days (see Cox et al 1987 for a copy of the scale). Scores of zero to 30 are possible on the EPDS. A score above 12 usually identifies women who are depressed or on the borderline of depression. Women whose scores are above 9 are probably depressed. It must be noted that a score of 12 is conservative. This score is usually used when there is no follow-up interview that can confirm the woman's feelings, for example in research settings. Using scores above 9 or 10 has been recommended in clinical settings, a follow-up interview usually taking place to confirm the depression (Cox et al 1987).

The EPDS has been validated with a number of different populations, including North American (Roy et al 1993) and Australian (Boyce et al 1993). It is also acceptable to English-speaking women from culturally and ethnically diverse populations (Brown et al 1994, Percival 1998) and has been successfully used following its translation into different languages (Dragonas et al 1992).

How can midwives and health visitors help?

Both midwives and health visitors have an enormous role to play in the prevention of PND. As previously discussed, midwives are the health professionals who have the most to do with women before the birth and for the first month after the birth. They are key people in identifying and helping to prevent depression in new mothers. However, as some women may not present with PND until after their discharge from midwifery care, strong links with health visitors are essential. The following strategies are based on the literature presented in the different mini sessions. In addition, most of the suggestions we have made throughout the chapter on the ways in which midwives can help parents to adjust to their new role can only be helpful in preventing PND.

Provide continuity of care. The ideal situation for most women is one in which they have continuity of carer throughout the pregnancy, birth and postnatal period as well the continuous presence of a known midwife throughout labour (as is found, for example, in the 'One-to-one' practice described in Chapter 6). If this is not possible it should at least be ensured that the woman has met the midwife who will be present at the birth (possibly at antenatal classes). Giving birth 'in the company of strangers' is possibly something that only occurs in modern post-industrialized societies.

Inform men and women. Tell all women and their families about PND; the topic may not be adequately covered in antenatal classes in order to avoid frightening couples (Mills & Kornblith 1992). In addition, provide parents with information (verbal and written) on the changes that arrive with the baby, and include strategies for dealing with these changes (such as those incorporated in this chapter) as well as details of appropriate community resources. Include men (or other partners and friends) in all aspects of teaching (rather than just the birth), whether this be on role changes or nappy changes.

Reassess antenatal classes. Have consistent group leaders, as participants are more likely to seek help from someone they know. In addition, make sure that both male and female health professionals are available to facilitate groups. Reconvene the antenatal classes after the babies have been born, trying to ensure that the people who lead the antenatal groups also have continuing contact with parents after the birth of the baby (for example, as a combined midwifery and health visitor effort). Have smaller groups or classes and look carefully at the venue – is a hospital really the best place to learn about being the parent of a healthy child?

Assess risk factors. Make an early assessment of risk factors in the pregnancy and postnatal period, for example depression during pregnancy or insufficient support (see causes of PND below).

Optimize the birth experience. Do everything humanly possible to make the birth as positive as it can possibly be. For example, ensure a continuous presence during labour (preferably a known midwife),

discourage people from 'popping in and out', explain what is going on, and encourage the woman to be involved in all decisions: she is, after all, the one having the baby.

Listen to women. Incorporate structured 'listening visits' into clinical practice for all women. These may serve an important debriefing role, for example in listening to women talk about their labour and birth. For women with PND, the opportunity to talk about their feelings to a sympathetic listener is very important. Structured 'listening interventions' by health visitors have been found to be positive for women with PND (see Clement 1995 for a review).

Be a myth-exploder. At every opportunity, discourage the myth that motherhood means only happiness, and give women permission to speak about their negative feelings.

Give consistent advice. Giving conflicting advice to women, particularly when it is offered as being 'right' or 'wrong', is one of the most destructive things that midwives can do to women (apart from dropping the baby or telling women to 'pull themselves together' when they are exhausted and crying during the first week after the birth).

Offer extra support. Provide the parents with additional support if the infant is premature or sick, or if the mother has had a multiple birth. Similarly, if the mother suffered complications during the pregnancy or birth, or after the birth, additional support will be needed.

Acknowledge the problem. A prompt and adequate diagnosis is essential. (This is more likely to be made by the health visitor, although midwives may diagnose PND before women are discharged from midwifery care.)

Have sufficient knowledge. Midwives and health visitors need to have sufficient knowledge about PND to make an accurate diagnosis. The EDPS is a useful screening tool for identifying PND. A brief screening tool such as the EPDS may also 'give women permission' to talk about their own feelings. It has been recommended that health visitors screen women at 6 weeks after the birth (Holden 1994, Painter 1995).

Be kind to women and their partners. Perhaps more than anything, all parents need people to be kind to them. Aspects of caring or support have been emphasized throughout the book; these aspects are important for all women and are particularly important in preventing PND. From her interviews with women with PND, Beck (1995b) identified a number of acts that women felt were caring (see Further reading below). Women are, in the early weeks after the birth, often performing a balancing act. All midwifery acts that are kind and caring can help to prevent the scales from being tipped towards PND; the opposite, of course, is also true.

Run PND postnatal support groups. Some women (although not all) may benefit from support groups. These may be useful as one way of providing increased social support and contact (Morse 1993).

Extra help. Encourage parents to obtain as much domestic and childcare support as possible. Investigate all voluntary and subsidized sources of help, and make parents aware of these.

Midwifery research and postnatal depression

Midwives and health visitors also have an important role in future research, particularly in designing and using strategies that may reduce levels of PND. However, Broom (1994) argues that research on PND 'should not become part of the problem it is supposed to be studying'. When doing research, the way in which questions are phrased is very important. For example, Broom (1994) suggests that researchers ask the questions:

- How can mothers (all mothers) be helped to enjoy their mothering and be successful at it?' *rather than* 'How are women with PND different from those who do not have it?'
- 'What kinds of society, community and social arrangements protect and support mothers and babies? *rather than* 'What kind of women are at risk of PND?'

Objective

- The prospective parents will understand what postnatal depression is, how it presents and where to seek help.

Important teaching points

- Tell women and their partners that, in the 12 months after the birth, as many as 1 in 5 women will experience PND.
- Emphasize that PND is not the woman's 'fault' and that it is not a sign of 'failing' or 'not coping' with the mothering role. Guilt is unnecessary.
- Explain how PND presents, and emphasize that it is imperative that help is sought if PND is suspected.
- Inform parents of the community resources in their area that can help with PND.
- If possible, show a video that shares the experience of families in which the woman has experienced PND.

Midwives' teaching notes

Definition of postnatal depression

PND refers to an episode of clinical depression that occurs during the first 12 months after the birth of a baby. Its onset may be sudden, but is more often insidious and the mood changes last for more than 2 weeks. These mood changes can affect women's physical, psychological and social functioning, and noticeably interfere with the usual patterns of their lives (Barnett 1991, NSW Women's Consultative Committee 1994, Pope 1994). As well as being disabling, PND may also last a considerable time, with 30–50% of women remaining depressed after 12 months (Cox et al 1987).

'Symptoms' of postnatal depression

Clinical perspective. Symptoms of postnatal depression can include (Barnett 1991, Pope 1994, NSW Women's Consultative Committee 1994, Williams 1994):

- despondency, sadness, crying and loss of control when usually competent;
- poor self-image, low self-worth and a feeling of failure as a mother;
- exhaustion, being overwhelmed by the responsibility of motherhood and wanting to flee;
- being overwhelmed by life events, with past problems being reawakened;
- being unable to think clearly or find the right words;
- difficulty sleeping even when the baby is settled;
- being agitated, fast-talking, anxious and irritable, as well as rushing from one activity to another or being apathetic;
- the inability to undertake household tasks;
- a poor appetite or overeating;
- being afraid of being alone or having a fear of social contact;
- exaggerated fears about the health of the self, baby or partner, with a reluctance to leave the baby;
- feelings of loss and unanticipated loss;
- suicidal thoughts, plans or actions.

For the most part, the symptoms of PND are the same as those of any clinical depression. However, because they present following the baby's birth, these symptoms may be seen or acted upon differently by mothers and health professionals. For example (Pope 1994):

- Sleep and appetite disturbances, lethargy and fatigue may be seen as 'normal' for new mothers.
- Decreased sexual desire might seem acceptable following childbirth.

- A lack of confidence and feelings of poor self-worth could be attributed to the isolation that often comes with being a mother.
- Increased uncertainty, anxiety and crying may be dismissed as 'neurotic'.

Women's own experiences. Williams (1992) reports that the language women use to describe depression is critical and does not conform to psychiatric terminology. Women's own descriptions are perhaps the best way of describing PND to parents. Women in Maloney's (1995) research made such comments as:

I was just confused because I didn't know why I was feeling this way.
  I'm an extremely organised person and had a very high position in my job and I always coped. This was different ... I was disorganised in my mind ... my mind gets very fogged up.
    ...lack of sleep. I thought I needed to go somewhere to get away from them ... I thought that I was going into a big black hole...
    ...Oh we went through a terrible time ... it was basically like a big black hole...
  I just felt like there was no future and there was nothing to look forward to. I couldn't do anything. I just wanted to sleep all day.

The women in Beck's (1992) research spoke of having 'minds filled with cobwebs and concentration levels decreased'.

The following quotes are taken from a group programme in which women were asked 'What has your depression meant for you? (Williams 1994):

- Feelings of failure, I must cope, at all costs
- Anxiety, is this me not managing, being frightened of me
- Overwhelming feelings of loss
- Hard to eat, problems of feeding
- Confusion about who I am
- I was disappointed I was not trained to be a mother
- Emptiness, nowhere to go after baby
- Lonely, physically difficult to get out of house
- Why didn't I get help earlier?
- Guilt about husband helping, jealous of husband's work
- Nightmares and daymares.

Diagnosis of postnatal depression

As discussed above, diagnosing PND can be difficult. Women may not recognize PND, or they may feel that they need to keep silent or 'put on a front'.

Not recognizing PND. PND may not be recognized by the mother herself (Mills & Kornblith 1992, Buist 1993). Pope (1994) has argued that the biggest obstacles to women receiving appropriate treatment for PND are not recognizing what is happening and not knowing what to do about it. Moreover, Williams (1994) found that men also had a limited or poor understanding of PND and believed that it was only related to hormonal changes. Some women in Maloney's (1995) research said:

If I had known the symptoms to look for in postnatal depression, I wouldn't have gone through the hell I went through, maybe my marriage would have survived....
  I didn't know about PND at all. I thought it was a load of rubbish really.

Keeping silent. Sometimes, however, women may find it difficult to confide their negative feelings or talk about depression (Beck 1995c). More than two-thirds of the women in Painter's (1995) research (who were later diagnosed as having PND) had not mentioned their feelings during the health visitor's two home visits. Of the respondents to the NSW Women's Consultative Committee (1994) survey who said that they had experienced PND, over half did not seek any help for their problems.

Some women remain silent or 'put on a front' because they are ashamed and concerned that others will judge them: 'On the worst of days ... I dared not show my desire to escape from my beautiful new child, my caring husband of 16 years. I had it all, yet I felt I had nothing. Still now it is almost too shameful to articulate' (Cornes 1999).

This silence is part of the larger 'conspiracy of silence' surrounding motherhood that we discussed earlier in the chapter. Some women with PND actually isolate themselves in an attempt to maintain their silence. Other mothers remain silent because they feel that people are only interested in the baby (Beck 1992, Maloney 1995).

Putting on a front. Women may also be aware that something is wrong in their lives but may feel that they have to 'put on a front' to maintain the appearance of 'coping' or being a 'good mother' (Maloney 1995):

I took it as a reflection upon myself that they were obviously thinking I could not cope...'
  You compare yourself to a lot of other girls and you think she's such a good mum and I'm not a good mum.

Moreover, women with PND (Williams 1994):

- rarely present with a request for self-help;
- often seek help for physical rather than emotional symptoms;
- may appear to be managing well;
- may be well dressed, well made-up, smiling a great deal, very talkative and rigidly in control;
- often present with an over concern about the baby.

These responses suggest that women have believed and are bound up in the myths about motherhood and what motherhood is supposed to be. Women may also 'put on a front' because of their partners' attitude. For example, Williams (1999) found that men felt strongly that other women managed; that it was only their own partner who was failing as a mother. The enormous sadness of PND is that many women do not even feel angry when they have PND; instead, they feel guilty because they are 'failing', and blame themselves.

Causes of postnatal depression

The causes of PND are not clearly defined despite a great deal of research having being undertaken. The causes may be social, physiological, psychological or all three. A 'medical model' of PND regards it as a disease with possible physical and perhaps psychological causes (although these have not yet, despite ongoing research, been fully determined). Within this model, a woman with PND would be 'treated' so that she 'copes' with the 'mothering role' (as constructed in our culture) without it being considered that the role itself needs to be changed.

As we discussed in the section on maternal adjustment above, those who support a social explanation of 'poor' maternal adjustment (or PND) believe that viewing PND as a disease transfers responsibility away from society and the community and onto the individual woman. Welburn (1980) aptly sums up these different approaches:

After we have given birth it is as if we wake up to discover that a mountain of sand has been deposited in front of the doors of our home. Some women get to work energetically to dig routes out. They have friends who come along and help. They work round the sand and over the sand; they find marvellously inventive ways to cope with the situation. Some women find one difficult route out and stick to that. Some try to dig a way through and get buried, others just look at it, feel defeated, retreat within their four walls and give up.

Psychologists concern themselves with the reasons why some of us can be energetic and find routes out and others get buried. The latter are often called 'inadequate personalities' and ways to help them are suggested. This ignores the essential question of why the sand needs to be there in the first place.

So much sand. As previously discussed, learning to care for the baby is a full-time job for most women. Yet women in countries such as the UK, USA, Canada and Australia (while recovering physically and emotionally from the birth and learning a new role) are expected to take care of themselves, an infant, a partner, a house and possibly an older child. Women with PND have spoken of juggling their many roles and keeping up with the expectations of others (Maloney 1995):

He loves the house to be all organised and to come home to a cooked meal and things like that.

My husband didn't understand me, he expected me to do all the things in the house as I did before.

… friends who don't have children would come to visit. They'd expect you to run around after them.

It has been argued that the symptoms of PND experienced by women may be pleas for help in their efforts to cope with emotional distress during pregnancy and after the birth (Affonso 1992). Certainly, the physical and psychological stress that new mothers experience can lead to a downward spiral of increasing helplessness and hopelessness (Morse 1993). Moreover, a person facing so much change and so many challenges is within her rights to feel depressed. Broom (1992) argued there is nothing irrational about depression after having a baby and that 'perhaps we should be more surprised that any women escape PND rather than being puzzled that many or most women have some transient distress'.

As we described earlier, women undertake a process of adjustment during the transition to motherhood. One wonders whether some women really 'adjust to', 'adapt to' or 'attain' the maternal role as it is constructed in our culture. Certainly, women adjust to their (usually much loved) baby. Instead, perhaps, some women finally 'get used to' the mothering role itself. Others simply 'get depressed'.

Not enough people digging. Recent research suggests that, overall, new mothers with appropriate amounts of situation-specific support are less depressed, anxious, angry and/or fatigued than other mothers (Gottlieb & Mendelsom 1995). Social support is associated with higher levels of emotional well-being in women (and, as we discussed earlier, also with easier maternal adjustment). Support from the husband or a supportive marital relationship is particularly valuable (Nicolson 1990, Percival 1990, Thorpe et al 1992, Kowalski 1994, Beck 1995c, Demyttenaere et al 1995). (See also Chapters 12 and 13.)

Higher levels of marital satisfaction after the birth are associated with higher levels of emotional well-being in women (Duncan 1984, Christian et al 1994), as are high levels of marital satisfaction before the birth (Grossman et al 1980). These higher levels of satisfaction with the relationship for both partners are important as they possibly mean that women have more support and less stress after the birth. Depressed mothers have partners who report poorer marital adjustment and a more traditional view of gender roles (Hock et al 1995). Many participants in the NSW Women's Consultative Committee (1994) consultations said that a supportive partner made the difference between coping and descending into despair and helplessness.

The following comments also reflect the importance of practical and emotional support from partners, family and friends (Percival 1990, Maloney 1995):

My husband has been on holidays for a week and that has been a good help.

There were times when I rang him at work and just said 'I cannot do this any more' and he'd come straight home.

I have my mum staying with me at the moment and I found her a wonderful help. She takes over the daily household chores and I deal with the baby.

[I have appreciated the availability] of monetary support from my father when I have been really desperate.

However, midwives may need to encourage or 'give permission' to women to ask for support. Some women have viewed having to ask for help as an admission of inadequacy or dependence: 'I always try to handle things on my own. I don't want to bother anybody, I feel like I'm whining again.' Others have expressed a reluctance to ask for support and preferred others to offer without being asked (Harrison et al 1995).

So many losses. As we discussed earlier in the chapter, women who have recently had their first baby speak of the things that they have lost: the loss of time, personal freedom, company, employment and even of their sense of self (Ruchala & Halstead 1994, Sethi 1995, Barclay et al 1997). Women with depression in Nicolson's (1990) study spoke about the loss of former identity, the loss of sexuality, intellectual ability and occupation, and the change from a 'liberated' woman to a 'traditional' woman. Women with PND in Maloney's (1995) research mentioned the isolation of mothering, their exhaustion, their lack of sleep and a loss of self-image.

Loss was also a dominant theme in Driscoll's (1990) interviews of women with depression: loss of relationships and lifestyle, loss of energy and self-esteem. Early research also suggests that women's self-esteem drops when they leave paid employment and take up full-time child care (Rossi 1968, Bernard 1974, 1975).

Kitzinger (1975) referred to the fourth trimester as a transitional period of some 3 months after the birth when many women are vulnerable and may experience confusion and despair. As discussed above, a woman may during this time experience a grieving for her old childless self and may also fear that she will never be normal again (Kitzinger 1975, Beck 1992). More recently, the results of Driscoll's (1990) work also suggest that the depression experienced by women following the birth could in part be attributed to the grief that accompanies role change. It takes considerable time for women (and men) to realize that while the old sense of what was normal will not return, a different kind of normality will occur.

The birth experience. A good labour and birth or positive feelings about the experience are associated with higher levels of emotional well-being in women (Russell 1974, Grossman et al 1980, Percival 1990). Factors such as high levels of intervention during labour, assisted delivery and caesarean birth have been associated with PND, as have dissatisfaction with labour and birth, having no say in decisions and the presence of unwanted people at the birth (Brown et al 1994). It may well be that it is not the type of birth but how the woman feels about this and how much of a say she has that are the critical factors (see the above session on integrating the birth experience).

Too many myths. As we have previously discussed, Oakley (1979, 1980) concluded that women are also less likely to be depressed following the birth of their infant if they feel in control and able to enjoy motherhood for what it is without seeking an idealized image.

Other factors. Research has identified several other factors that have been associated with PND and higher levels of anxiety and stress after the birth. These include:

- women's age over 34 years (Brown et al 1994);
- previous depression or depression in pregnancy (Gotlib et al 1991, O'Hara et al 1991, Thorpe et al 1992);
- depression levels 1 week after the birth, are related to depression levels at 6 weeks after the birth (Beck et al 1992);
- lower life adaptation scores and higher socio-economic status (Grossman et al 1980);
- individual coping style (at 6 months only) (Demyttenaere et al 1995);
- stressful life events during pregnancy or the postnatal period, including moving house, the death of a close relative or friend, financial problems, caring for three or more other children (NSW Women's Consultative Committee 1994);
- conversely, the use of feminine adjectives to describe oneself or a more traditional role orientation were associated with *lower* levels of PND (Grossman et al 1980, Duncan 1984).

Prevention and treatment

Even if PND is not an illness in the medical sense, it has been argued that many women are happy when their 'condition' is 'diagnosed' as their feelings are validated (NSW Women's Consultative Committee 1994). The currently recommended treatment for PND is counselling or psychotherapy for the woman, and possibly for her partner. Antidepressant medication may also be prescribed (Pope 1994). The midwifery and health visitor role in preventing PND is presented in the introduction section of this mini session.

Community resources

In most communities, there are a number of resources available to help new parents. In addition, there are usually resources and support groups that specifically help with PND. It is very important for midwives to give parents the details of such resources in their community. In addition, parents need to be empowered actually to feel to be able to ask for help; making support available is of little value if individuals believe that they have failed in their role if they seek this support. Isolated within the nuclear family, individuals often do not realize that other families also experience negative feelings and have difficulty with their roles.

Pointers for practice

- Midwives have most to do with women and their partners before and after the birth. Accept the challenge of emphasizing the overall transition to parenthood and help men and women to adjust to their new roles.
- The way in which the social role of mother is constructed in modern post-industrialized societies is unfair, particularly for women. Tell women this so that they do not feel they are the ones who are 'failing'.
- Look at ways to work within this mothering role in order to make life easier for individual women. Also, be aware that this role can be changed by the culture that created it (and that you are part of that culture).
- Expose the myths that surround motherhood and make fun of them.
- Accept that, as well as being a time of great joy, the early weeks of mothering are also a time of great stress. Give women 'permission' to feel miserable without them also having to feel guilty. And never, ever, ever tell them that they should be thankful to have a healthy normal baby – they already know this.
- Where possible, include men or other partners and friends when teaching. Not doing this reinforces the fact that caring for the baby is the women's job.
- Incorporate structured 'listening visits' into clinical practice for all women in order to give them an opportunity to talk about their feelings with a sympathetic listener.
- Work smarter not harder; groups are a really cost-effective way of teaching parents and they help parents to get to know each other.

CONCLUSION

In conclusion, midwives have a major role in empowering parents during the transition to parenthood by making them aware that they are normal people who are going through a time of great change in their lives. Moreover, they need to know that most parents experience the same changes and challenges.

Women and men also need to know that it is a positive thing to break the 'conspiracy of silence' that surrounds parenthood. Breaking this 'conspiracy of

---

Activities

1. Identify community resources in your area that assist parents in adjusting to their new roles. These may include 'drop-in' centres, childcare facilities, outreach or day programmes, residential facilities and after-hours emergency telephone lines.
2. Obtain information on support programmes and groups for women (and their families) who experience PND.
3. Make a list of these community resources for your area, including telephone numbers and addresses. Give this list to parents before they are discharged from midwifery care.
4. Obtain leaflets on PND if they are available. These may include a contact telephone number in your area that women can call if they prefer to speak to someone anonymously.
5. Identify appropriate videos that emphasize the emotional aspects of adjusting to parenthood.
6. Get together with the health visitor in your area and investigate how you can work together to provide antenatal and postnatal group sessions to help parents. How can you optimize your individual skills to make the best use of the times when you are both available during the overall period of the transition to parenthood?
7. Review the 'preparation for parenthood' component of your antenatal classes. Can you use or adapt some of the sessions in this chapter?
8. Encourage parents to continue meeting after the birth in their own homes to share their experiences and support each other. Attend the first meeting.
9. Work towards making continuity of carer (throughout the antenatal, birth and postnatal periods) available for all families so that they can develop an ongoing relationship with the midwife. Can you run a trial scheme in your area?
10. If you are a student midwife, negotiate with your lecturers to do some of the above as an assignment.

silence' means that parents can talk about the difficulties they are experiencing; they can talk about their need for extra support; and they do not have to pretend that they are managing alone for fear that others will believe they are a 'bad' or 'abnormal' family. Moreover, parents need to be able to ask for help without the spectre of the three 'Perfect Beings' hanging over them. Midwives can tell parents that being able to ask for support from either family, friends or professionals is a positive move, one meaning that they are good parents who want to be even better. Most importantly, as they forge ahead to become the real non-perfect parents of their real non-perfect baby, men and women need to be encouraged to recognize that they are only human and can only do their best.

REFERENCES

Affonso D 1987 Assessment of maternal postpartum adaptation. Public Health Nursing 4(1): 9–20

Affonso D 1992 Postpartum depression: a nursing perspective on women's health and behaviors. IMAGE: Journal of Nursing Scholarship 24: 215–21

Affonso D, Arizmendi T 1986 Disturbances in postpartum adaptation and depressive symptomatology. Journal of Psychosomatic Obstetrics and Gynecology 5: 15–32

Affonso D, Domino G 1984 Postpartum depression: a review. Birth 11(4): 231–5

Alexander M, Higgins T 1993 Emotional trade-offs of becoming a parent: how social roles influence self-discrepancy effects. Journal of Personality and Social Psychology 65(6): 1259–69

Bader E, MacMillan M 1994 Fathers – partners in parenting: different ways to be strong and supportive fathers. Final report. North York Inter-Agency & Community Council, North York, Ontario

Ball J 1994 Reactions to motherhood: the role of postnatal care. Cambridge University Press, Cambridge

Ballard C G, Davis R, Cullen P C, Mohan R N, Dean C 1994 Prevalence of postnatal psychiatric morbidity in mothers and fathers. British Journal of Psychiatry 164: 782–8

Barclay L, Donovan J, Genovese A 1996 Men's experiences during their partner's first pregnancy: a grounded theory analysis. Australian Journal of Advanced Nursing 13(3): 12–24

Barclay L, Everitt L, Rogan F, Schmied V, Wyllie A 1997 Becoming a mother – an analysis of women's experience of early motherhood. Journal of Advanced Nursing 25: 719–28

Barnett B 1991 Coping with postnatal depression. Lothian, Port Melbourne

Beck C T 1992 The lived experience of postpartum depression: a phenomenological study. Nursing Research 41(3): 166–70

Beck C T 1995a The effects of postpartum depression on maternal–infant interaction: a meta-analysis. Nursing Research 44(5): 298–304

Beck C T 1995b Perceptions of nurses' caring by mothers experiencing postpartum depression. Journal of Obstetric, Gynecologic, and Neonatal Nursing Clinical Studies 24(9): 819–25

Beck C T 1995c Screening methods for postpartum depression. Journal of Obstetric, Gynecologic, and Neonatal Nursing Principles and Practice 24(4): 308–12

Beck C T, Reynolds M A, Rutowski P 1992 Maternity blues and postpartum depression. Journal of Obstetric, Gynecologic, and Neonatal Nursing Clinical Studies 21(4): 287–93

Belsky J, Kelly J 1994 The transition to parenthood: how a first child changes a marriage. Delacorte Press, New York

Belsky J, Rovine M 1990 Patterns of marital change across the transition to parenthood: pregnancy to three years postpartum. Journal of Marriage and the Family 52: 5–19

Belsky J, Lang M E, Rovine M 1985 Stability and change in marriage across the transition to parenthood – a second study. Journal of Marriage and the Family 47(4): 855–65

Benedeck T 1959 Parenthood as a developmental phase. Journal of the American Psychoanalytic Association 7: 389–417

Bernard J 1974 The future of motherhood. Dial Press, New York

Bernard J 1975 Women, wives, mothers: values and options. Aldine Press, Chicago

Berry S J 1988 The role of maternal expectations and infant characteristics in the transition to parenthood. Dissertation Abstracts International 48(12-B, Part 1): 3669

Blair S L, Lichter D T 1991 Measuring the division of household labor. Journal of Family Issues 12(1): 91–113

Blum M E 1981 The relationship of marital satisfaction, sex role attitudes, and psychological intervention in prepared delivery classes to the transition to parenthood: a short term longitudinal study of middle-income couples. Dissertation Abstracts International 42(5-B): 2094–5

Blurton-Jones N G 1974 Ethology and early socialization. In: Richards N (ed.) The integration of a child into a social world. Cambridge University Press, London

Boles A J 1985 Predictors and correlates of marital satisfaction during the transition to parenthood. Dissertation Abstracts International 46(2-B): 634

Boyce P, Stubbs R, Todd A 1993 The Edinburgh postnatal depression scale: validation in an Australian sample. Australian and New Zealand Journal of Psychiatry 27: 472–6

Brazelton T B 1962 Crying in infancy. Pediatrics 29: 579–88

Broom D 1994 Mothers and babies in a social context. In: Carter J (ed.) Postnatal depression: towards a research agenda for human services and health. Proceedings from the Postnatal Depression Workshop 1992. Commonwealth Department of Human Services and Health Research Advisory Committee, Issues for Research 2: 17–19

Brown S, Lumley J, Small R, Astbury J 1994 Missing voices: the experience of motherhood. Oxford University Press, Oxford

Buist A 1993 The management of postnatal depression. Australian Family Physician 22(11): 2025–9

Campbell S, Cohn J 1991 Prevalence and correlates of

postpartum depression in first time mothers. Journal of Abnormal Psychology 100: 594–9

Caplan G 1957 Psychological aspects of maternity care. American Journal of Public Health 47(1): 25

Carothers A D, Murray L 1990 Estimating psychiatric morbidity by logistic regression: application to postnatal depression in a community sample. Psychological Medicine 20: 695–702

Chodorow N 1978 The reproduction of mothering: psychoanalysis and the sociology of gender. University of California Press, London

Christian J L, O'Leary K D, Vivian D 1994 Depressive symptomatology in maritally discordant women and men: the role of individual and relationship variables. Journal of Family Psychology 8: 32–42

Clement S 1995 'Listening visits' in pregnancy: a strategy for preventing postnatal depression? Midwifery 11(2): 75–80

Cornes J 1999 Oh baby. West Australian (Big Weekend), 9 January, p. 1.

Cowan C, Cowan P 1992 When partners become parents: the big life change for couples. Basic Books, New York

Cox J, Holden J, Sagovsky R 1987 Detection of postnatal depression: development of the 10 item Edinburgh postnatal depression scale. British Journal of Psychiatry 150: 782–6

Cranley M S, Hedahl K J, Pegg S H 1983 Women's perceptions of vaginal and cesarean deliveries. Nursing Research 32(1): 10–15

Crouch M, Manderson L 1993 New motherhood. Cultural and personal transitions. Gordon & Breach, Camberwell, Australia

Davis-Floyd R 1994 The ritual of hospital birth in America. In: Spradley J P, McCurdey D W (eds) Conformity and conflict. Readings in cultural anthropology. 8th edn. HarperCollins, New York

Demyttenaere K, Lenaerts H, Nijs P, Van Assche F A 1995 Individual coping style and psychological attitudes during pregnancy predict depression levels during pregnancy and during postpartum. Acta Psychiatrica Scandinavica 91: 95–102

Department of Health 1992 The health of the nation: a strategy for health in England. HMSO, London

Deutsch F M, Ruble D N, Fleming A, Brooks-Gunn J 1988 Information-seeking and maternal self-definition during the transition to motherhood. Journal of Personality and Social Psychology 55(3): 420–31

Deutsch H 1944 The psychology of women, vol. 1. Grune & Stratton, New York

Dohrenwend B, Krasnoff L, Askenasy A, Dohrenwend B 1978 Exemplification of a method for scaling life events. Journal of Health and Social Behavior 19: 205–29

Douglas M 1966 Purity and danger: an analysis of concepts of pollution and taboo. Routledge & Kegan Paul, London

Dragonas T, Thorpe K, Golding J 1992 Transition to fatherhood: a cross-cultural comparison. Journal of Psychosomatic Obstetrics and Gynaecology 13: 1–19

Driscoll J W 1990 Maternal parenthood and the grief process. Journal of Perinatal and Neonatal Nursing 4: 1–10

Duncan S W 1984 The transition to parenthood: coping and adaptation of couples to pregnancy and the birth of their first child. Dissertation Abstracts International 45(5-B): 1600

Dyer E D 1963 Parenthood as crisis: a restudy. Marriage and Family Living 25: 196–201

Edgar D 1993 Parents at the core of family life. Family Matters 36: 2–3

Elliott S A, Watson J P, Brough D I 1985 Transition to parenthood by British couples. Journal of Reproductive and Infant Psychology 3(1): 28–39

Entwistle D R, Doering S G 1981 The first birth. A family turning point. John Hopkins University Press, Baltimore

Feldman S S, Nash S C 1984 The transition from expectancy to parenthood: Impact of the firstborn child on men and women. Sex Roles 11(1–2): 61–78

Fishbein E G 1990 Involvement with a newborn by attitude toward women's roles. Health Care for Women International 11: 109–115

Frommer E A, O'Shea G 1973 The importance of childhood experience in relation to problems of marriage and family building. British Journal of Psychiatry 123: 157

Garfinkel H 1956 Conditions of successful degradation ceremonies. American Journal of Sociology, LXI

Gennep A Van 1960 The rites of passage. Routledge & Kegan Paul, London

Gjerdingen D K, Chaloner K 1994 Mothers' experience with household roles and social support during the first postpartum year. Women and Health 21(4): 57–75

Gjerdingen D K, Fontaine P 1991 Family-centered postpartum care. Family Medicine 23: 189–93

Gjerdingen D K, Froberg D G, Chaloner K M, McGovern P M 1993 Changes in women's physical health during the first postpartum year. Archives of Family Medicine 2: 277–83

Glezer H 1993 Pathways to family formation. Family Matters 34: 16–20

Gluckman M (ed.) 1962 Essays on the ritual of social relations. Manchester University Press Manchester

Goffman E 1968 Asylums. Essays on the social situation of mental patients and other inmates. Penguin, Harmondsworth

Gotlib I, Whiffen V, Wallace P, Mount J 1991 A prospective investigation of postpartum depression: factors involved in onset and recovery. Journal of Abnormal Psychology 100: 122–32

Gottlieb L N, Mendelsom M J 1995 Mothers' moods and social support when a second child is born. Maternal–Child Nursing Journal 23(1): 3–14

Gottman J M 1994 Why marriages succeed or fail. Simon & Schuster, New York

Grace J T 1993 Mothers' self-reports of parenthood across the first 6 months postpartum. Research in Nursing and Health 16(6): 431–9

Grossman F K, Eichler L S, Winickoff S A 1980 Pregnancy, birth, and parenthood. Jossey-Bass, San Francisco

Halman L J, Oakley D, Lederman R 1995 Adaptation to pregnancy and motherhood among subfecund and fecund primiparous women. Maternal–Child Nursing Journal 23(3): 90–100

Hamilton J H 1986 Postpartum depression, social support, and life events. Dissertation Abstracts International 47(3-B): 1273

Harrison M J, Neufeld A, Kushner K 1995 Women in transition: access and barriers to social support. Journal of Advanced Nursing 21(5): 858–64

Henderson A D, Brouse A J 1991 The experiences of new fathers during the first 3 weeks of life. Journal of Advanced Nursing 16(3): 293–8

Hill R 1949 Families under stress. Harper, New York

Hinkley K R 1986 An interdisciplinary approach to the

transition to parenthood. Dissertation Abstracts International 47(6-A): 2332

Hobbs D F 1968 Transition to parenthood: a replication and an extension. Journal of Marriage and the Family 30(3): 413–17

Hock E, Schirtzinger M B, Lutz W J, Widaman K 1995 Maternal depressive symptomatology over the transition to parenthood: assessing the influence of marital satisfaction and marital sex role traditionalism. Journal of Family Psychology 9(1): 79–88

Holden J M 1994 Using the Edinburgh Postnatal Depression Scale in clinical practice. In: Cox J L, Holden J M (eds) Perinatal psychiatry: use and misuse of the Edinburgh Postnatal Depression Scale. Gaskell, London

Holmes T, Rahe R H 1967 The social readjustment rating scale. Journal of Psychosomatic Research 11: 213–18

Humenick S S, Bugen L A 1987 Parenting roles: expectation versus reality. Maternal–Child Nursing 12: 36–9

Hyssala L, Rautava P, Sillanpaa M 1993 Opinions and expectations of fathers of young families of family counselling. Scandinavian Journal of Caring Sciences 7: 237–42

Janeway E 1971 Man's world: woman's place, a study in social mythology. William Morrow, New York

Jordan B 1993 Birth in four cultures. A crosscultural investigation of childbirth in Yucatan, Holland, Sweden and the United States, 4th edn., revised and expanded by R. Davis-Floyd (ed.) Waveland Press, Illinois

Jordan P L 1990 Laboring for relevance: expectant and new fatherhood. Nursing Research 39(1): 11–16

Kitzinger S 1975 The fourth trimester? Midwife Health Visitor and Community Nurse 2: 118–21

Kitzinger S 1978 The experience of childbirth, 4th edn. Penguin Books, Harmondsworth

Kitzinger S 1989 Childbirth and society. In: Chalmers I E, Enkin M, Keirse M J N C (eds) Effective care in pregnancy and childbirth. Oxford University Press, Oxford

Knowles M 1990 The adult learner: a neglected species, 4th edn. Gulf Publishing, Houston

Koniak-Griffin D 1993 Maternal role attainment. IMAGE: Journal of Nursing Scholarship 25(3): 257–62

Kowalski J 1994 Local support structures. In Carter J (ed.) Postnatal depression; towards a research agenda for human services and health. Proceedings from the Postnatal Depression Workshop 1992. Commonwealth Department of Human Services and Health Research Advisory Committee, Issues for Research 2: 70–1

Ladden M, Damato E 1992 Parenting and supportive programs. NAACOG's Clinical Issues 3(1): 174–87

Lamb M E, Pleck J, Levine J 1986 Effects of paternal involvement on fathers and mothers. In: Lewis C, O'Brien M (eds) Reassessing fatherhood. Sage, Beverly Hills

LaRossa R, LaRossa M M 1981 Transition to parenthood: how infants change families. Sage, Beverley Hills

LeMasters E 1957 Parenthood as crisis. Marriage and Family Living 19: 352–5

LeMasters E 1974 Parents in modern America. Dorsey Press, Chicago

Leventhal-Belfer L, Cowan P A, Cowan C P 1992 Satisfaction with child care arrangements: effects on adaptation to parenthood. American Journal of Orthopsychiatry 62(2): 165–77

Levitt M J, Coffman S, Guacci-Franco N, Loveless S 1993 Social support and relationship change after childbirth: an expectancy model. Health Care for Women International 14(6): 503–12

Levy-Shiff R 1994 Individual and contextual correlates of marital change across the transition to parenthood. Developmental Psychology 30(4): 591–601

McCourt C, Page L 1996 Report on the evaluation of one-to-one midwifery. Hammersmith Hospitals NHS Trust, London

McCourt C, Page L, Hewison J, Vail A 1998 Evaluation of One-to-One midwifery: women's responses to care. Birth 25(2): 73–80

McCourt C 1999 Interim report: evaluation of the implementation of evidence-based learning in the curriculum. Unpublished thesis. Thames Valley University, London

MacDermid S, Huston T, McHale S 1990 Changes in marriage associated with the transition to parenthood: individual differences as a function of sex role attitudes and changes in the division of household labor. Journal of Marriage and the Family 52: 475–86

McIntosh J 1993 Postpartum depression: women's help-seeking behaviour and perceptions of cause. Journal of Advanced Nursing 18(2): 178–84

Maloney M M 1995 Postnatal depression: a study of mothers in the metropolitan area of Perth, Western Australia. Curtin University Press, Perth

Marks M, Lovestone S 1995 The role of the father in parental postnatal mental health. British Journal of Medical Psychology 68: 157–68

Marris P 1974 Loss and change. Routledge & Kegan Paul, London

Marut J S, Mercer R T 1979 A comparison of primipara's perceptions of vaginal and cesarean births. Nursing Research 28(5): 260–6

Mercer R T 1981 Factors impacting on the maternal role: the first year of motherhood. In Lederman R P (ed.) Perinatal parental behavior: nursing research and implications for newborn health. Alan R Liss, New York

Mercer R T 1986 Predictors of maternal role attainment at one year postbirth. Western Journal of Nursing Research 8(1): 9–32

Mercer R T, Marut J S 1981 Comparative viewpoints: cesarean versus vaginal birth. In Affonso D (ed.) Impact of cesarean. F A Davis, Philadelphia

Mills J B, Kornblith P R 1992 Fragile beginnings: identification and treatment of postpartum disorders. Health and Social Work 17(3): 192–8

Moen P 1992 Women's two roles: a contemporary dilemma. Auburn House, New York

Morse C A 1993 Psychological influence in postnatal depression. Australian Journal of Advanced Nursing 10(4): 26–31

Murray-Parkes C 1971 Psycho-social transitions. A field for study. Social Science and Medicine 5: 101–15

Nicholson J 1983 The heartache of motherhood. Penguin Books Australia, Ringwood, Victoria

Nicolson P 1990 Understanding postnatal depression: a mother-centred approach. Journal of Advanced Nursing 15: 689–95

NSW Women's Consultative Committee 1994 'If motherhood is bliss, why do I feel so awful?' Community consultations on post natal stress and depression in NSW. NSW Ministry for the Status and Advancement of Women, Woolloomooloo

Nugent J K 1991 Cultural and psychological influences on the father's role in infant development. Journal of Marriage and the Family 53: 475–85

Oakley A 1979 From here to maternity: becoming a mother. Penguin Books, Harmondsworth

Oakley A 1980 Women confined: towards a sociology of childbirth. Martin Robertson, Oxford

O'Hara M, Schlechte J, Lewis D, Varner M 1991 Controlled prospective study of postpartum mood disorders: psychological, environmental, and hormonal variables. Journal of Abnormal Psychology 100: 63–73

Osofsky H J, Osofsky J D 1983 Adaptation to pregnancy and new parenthood. In Dennerstein L, Burrows G D (eds) Handbook of psychosomatic obstetrics and gynecology. Elsevier Biomedical Press, Amsterdam

Ozaki M M 1986 Marital role performance during the transition to parenthood. Dissertation Abstracts International 47(2-B): 801

Painter A 1995 Health visitor identification of postnatal depression. Health Visitor 68(4): 138–40

Parsons T 1951 The social system. Free Press, New York

Percival P 1990 The relationship between perceived nursing care and maternal adjustment for primiparae during the transition to motherhood. Unpublished Doctoral dissertation, Curtin University of Technology, Western Australia

Percival P 1998 Research in progress. Edith Cowan University, Western Australia

Pope S 1994 Postnatal depression. Centre for Women's Health, Perth, Western Australia

Pugh L, Milligan R 1993 A framework for the study of childbearing fatigue. Advances in Nursing Science 15: 60–70

Raskin J D, Richman J A, Gaines C 1990 Patterns of depressive symptoms in expectant and new parents. American Journal of Psychiatry 147: 658–60

Reece S M 1993 Social support and the early maternal experience of primiparas over 35. Maternal–Child Nursing Journal 21(3): 91–8

Rossi A S 1968 Transition to parenthood. Journal of Marriage and the Family 30(1): 26–9

Roy A, Garg P, Cole K et al 1993 Use of the Edinburgh postnatal depression scale in a North American population. Progress in Neuropsychopharmacology and Biological Psychiatry 17: 501–4

Rubin R 1967a Attainment of the maternal role. Part 1: Processes. Nursing Research 16(3): 237–45

Rubin R 1967b Attainment of the maternal role. Part 2: Models and referents. Nursing Research 16(3): 342–6

Rubin R 1975 Maternal tasks in pregnancy. Maternal–Child Nursing Journal 4(3): 143–53

Ruchala P L, Halstead L 1994 The postpartum experience of low-risk women: a time of adjustment and change. Maternal–Child Nursing Journal 22(3): 83–9

Russell C S 1974 Transition to parenthood: problems and gratifications. Journal of Marriage and the Family 36(2): 294–301

Russell G 1994 Sharing the pleasures and pains of family life. Family Matters 37: 13–19

Sears W 1985 The fussy baby. La Leche League International, Franklin Park, ILL

Sethi S 1995 The dialectic in becoming a mother: experiencing a postpartum phenomenon. Scandinavian Journal of Caring Science 9: 235–44

Shelton B A 1990 The distribution of household tasks: does wife's employment status make a difference? Journal of Family Issues 11(2): 115–35

Simkin P 1991 Just another day in a woman's life: women's long term perceptions of their first birth experience. Birth 18(1): 203–10

Simkin P 1992 Just another day in a woman's life?: nature and consistency of women's long term memories of their first birth experiences. Birth 19(2): 64–81

Stevens J H Jr 1988 Shared knowledge about infants among fathers and mothers. Journal of Genetic Psychology 149: 515–25

Terry D 1991a Predictors of subjective stress in a sample of new parents. Australian Journal of Psychology 43(1): 29–36

Terry D 1991b Stress, coping and adaptation to new parenthood. Journal of Social and Personal Relationships 8: 527–47

Terry D J, McHugh T A, Noller P 1991 Role dissatisfaction and the decline in marital quality across the transition to parenthood. Australian Journal of Psychology 43(3): 129–32

Thorpe K J, Dragonas T, Golding J 1992 The effects of psychosocial factors on the mother's emotional well-being during early parenthood: a cross-cultural study of Britain and Greece. Journal of Reproductive and Infant Psychology 10: 205–17

Tomlinson P S 1987 Spousal differences in marital satisfaction during transition to parenthood. Nursing Research 36(4): 239–43

Tomlinson P S, Irwin B 1993 Qualitative study of women's report of family adaptation pattern four years following transition to parenthood. Issues in Mental Health Nursing 14(2): 119–38

Towler J, Bramall J 1986 Midwives in history and society. Croom Helm, Beckenham

Tulman L, Fawcett J 1991 Recovery from childbirth: looking back 6 months after delivery. Health Care for Women International 12: 341–50

Vincent-Priya J 1992 Birth traditions and modern pregnancy care. Element Books, Dorset

Walker L O, Crain H, Thompson E 1986 Maternal role attainment and identity in the postpartum period: stability and change. Nursing Research 35(2): 68–71

Watson W J, Watson L, Wetzel W, Bader E, Talbot Y 1995 Transition to parenthood: what about fathers? Canadian Family Physician 41: 807–12

Webb N B 1985 Transition to parenthood: a time-limited mutual aid group to facilitate a major role change. Special Issue: Time as a factor in groupwork: time-limited group experiences. Social Work with Groups 8(2): 29–41

Welburn V 1980 Postnatal depression. Manchester University Press, Great Britain

Williams S S 1994 A social work view. In: Carter J (ed.) Postnatal depression: towards a research agenda for human services and health. Proceedings from the Postnatal Depression Workshop 1992. Commonwealth Department of Human Services and Health Research Advisory Committee. Issues for Research 2: 27–30

Younger J B 1991 A model of parenting stress. Research in Nursing and Health 14(3): 197–204

FURTHER READING

Beck C T 1995 Perceptions of nurses' caring by mothers experiencing postpartum depression. Journal of Obstetric, Gynecologic, and Neonatal Nursing Clinical Studies 24(9): 819–25
Lists specific action that women with PND see as caring.

Clement S 1995 'Listening visits' in pregnancy: a strategy for preventing postnatal depression? Midwifery 11(2): 75–80

11

The growth of human love and commitment

Barbara C. Mills

Section on 'Implications for the midwife'
Lesley Ann Page

In Western society today, as social and emotional ills are of ever-burgeoning concern, it behoves each of us as professionals to examine the role we might play in the promotion of the long-term emotional and social health of individuals and of society. This chapter is predicated upon the tenet that the early years of life are of critical import in determining the long-term mental health of the individual. The midwife is a facilitator not only of the physical birth, but indeed also of the birth of the self, the family and the potential for human love. The midwife, therefore, is in a unique position to play a critical role in the areas of both mental health promotion and the screening of parents and infants at risk of long-term social and emotional problems.

This chapter acknowledges the role of the midwife in facilitating the optimal circumstances for the birth of life and of human love. We address the influence of the early parent–child relationship upon the long-term emotional and relational health of the growing and developing infant. The human infant's attachment to the mother (or other primary care-giver) is seen as a prerequisite for survival and a test-bed for all the other attachments that he or she will make in the future.

In this chapter, Bowlby's attachment paradigm will be used to explore the concepts of the attachment system and of the development of early internal representational models of self and of self in relation to others that form the template for the long-term mental health of the individual. Research will be explored that will shed light upon the connection between the sensitivity of early parenting and the subsequent developmental trajectory of the child. The midwife's role in facilitating the early parent–child attachment will be examined, as will her role in screening and intervening when the relationship puts the child at potential risk.

BIRTH AND THE FOUNDATION OF HUMAN LOVE

Birth marks the beginning of a great love affair between the parents and their new infant (Klaus et al 1975). It is a love affair orchestrated by nature to ensure that the newborn human infant receives what it needs: the longest period of nurturing required by any species on the face of the earth. Fortunately, there are very few new parents who are not ready and committed to love their tiny newborn infant. Indeed, both parent and infant are primed at birth to fall in love. Most full-term healthy newborns are programmed with amazing capacities to capture the love, attention and commitment of their parents. Despite a harrowing journey, healthy neonates are able to turn to the familiar voice of the mother. They gaze at their father's face with great intent, grip the finger placed in their tiny palm and, if given the opportunity, will slowly but surely crawl up the length of the mother's abdomen to latch on to her nipple (Klaus et al 1995). The cry of the newborn is one that is difficult for the adult to ignore. The pitch, tone and intensity stir within us an urge to respond and to soothe.

There are few parents who are not ready to love this small, dependent miracle that has emerged from the mother's body. The 9 months of pregnancy and the mother's changing body and psyche have normally built within her a set of hopes and expectations for this child and their future relationship together. By the time labour begins, the mother is usually anxious to deliver and to begin to love and bond with her new infant. The early postpartum period is frequently characterized by the magic of this early intimate and intense relationship.

A variety of researchers have demonstrated the import that the first hours and days of life hold for the bonding between parent and infant. The work of Klaus et al (1995) has poignantly demonstrated the significance of such factors as the support and empowerment of parents during labour and delivery, and the provision of an atmopshere following birth that facilitates the natural process by which parents fall in love with, and become committed to, their infants. Pearce (1993, p. 119) asserts that when bonding is facilitated and successful:

behavioural changes in the bonded mother include a new sense of personal power, physical strength, and an intuitive knowledge of her infant's need. She acts out of the vast intelligence through which our species has survived for untold aeons. This is the intelligence of the heart, a nonverbal knowing. She has in bonding to her infant, bonded to her own heart and come into her own power, unlocking the insights on which our species has depended for millennia.

What we do know, however, is that the ability to sustain the commitment to an infant, and to sustain the sacrifice and skill that are necessary to raise the child to be a healthy, loving, sociable individual, takes more than the initial love, magic and physiological changes of the perinatal period. Like any human relationship, the relationship between parent and infant is influenced by a myriad of factors. Such factors include the parents' own experience of being parented, their lifelong history of relationships, their own ability to love and support each other, perinatal factors, environmental stress. The quality of the emotional support received by the parents, as well as infant factors such as health and temperament. In fact, a variety of recent research studies have concluded that it is those relationship factors occurring long before the birth of the infant which have the most profound effect upon the long-term quality of the parent–infant relationship (Lyons-Ruth et al 1990, Zeanah 1993). Similarly, this same research also demonstrates that the quality of the early parent–child relationship is the most consistent factor that influences the long-term mental, emotional and social health of the individual.

In this era, wherein our Western society is becoming increasingly alarmed over the rise in child abuse and neglect, as well as the social and emotional problems of both adults and children, it behoves professionals to examine the part that those of us involved in the early parent–child relationship can play in the early prevention, detection and intervention of mental health problems. This chapter is written on the premise that the quality of the early parent–child relationship is a key determinant of the long-term mental health of the individual. Within this chapter, we will examine the various factors that influence the ability of a parent to bond with, nurture and remain sensitive to her infant. We will examine relevant theory and research, primarily influenced by attachment theory (Bowlby 1988), that traces the impact of the early parent–child relationship upon the long-term mental health of the infant, the child and later the adult. Finally, we will combine this information in an exploration of the role that the midwife might play in recognizing parents and infants who are at risk of developing problems in parenting. The final intent will then be to suggest interventions that might be implemented in order to interrupt the transmission of destructive attachment patterns and parenting practices from one generation to the next.

Principle to the focus of this chapter is the repeated finding that the factors most strongly influencing the quality of the mother–child relationship are already in place long before pregnancy or labour begin. The focus on attachment theory and research is intended to confirm the import of the first years of life in determining the nature of the child's relational and developmental trajectory. Attachment research is additionally presented to demonstrate the link between the mother's history of relationships and her ability to provide the quality of parenting needed by her infant. The ultimate goal is to provide a theory base from which the midwife can chart an approach for assessing and intervening for the purpose of the primary prevention of problems in the early parent–child attachment.

ATTACHMENT THEORY AND RESEARCH

Attachment theory, as we currently know it, arises from the work of John Bowlby and Mary Ainsworth. Bowlby was a child psychotherapist who found current mental health theories of his day to be entirely inadequate for understanding and treating the problems in his own practice. Turning to the fields of ethology, cybernetics and psychoanalysis, as well as to his own detailed research, he formulated the basic outline and principles of attachment theory. His seminal works, the three volumes of *Attachment and Loss* (Bowlby 1969, 1973, 1980), form the basis for understanding the impact of an infant's early experience upon the development of self and relationship patterns. Ainsworth furthered the usefulness of attachment theory by:

- translating its basic tenets into empirical findings;
- developing infant observational instruments;
- expanding the theoretical concepts of attachment theory.

This section will introduce the reader to the basic tenets of attachment theory.

Attachment theory essentially states that the quality of the early relationship between parent and child is an essential determinant of the long-term social and emotional health of the individual. Bowlby (1988) explains that the power of the attachment system arises from the absolute and long-term dependency of the human infant upon the care-giving figure. Because of this dependency, the attachment relationship is key to the survival of the infant. Since maintaining contact with the parent is a survival need, the infant will over time adapt his or her behaviour and ways of being in the world to ensure that parental rejection or abandonment does not occur. For this reason, attachment relational patterns learned during this early preverbal stage of life are powerful and influential in determining future behaviour. Subsequently, the behavioural patterns that evolve from the early parent–child relationship reflect the infant's developing internal representational model of self and of self in relation to others. Bowlby proposes that these early internal models have a profound influence on the long-term interactional, exploratory and social behaviour of the individual over time.

Ainsworth's research (1967, 1973) extended our understanding of the interface between attachment and the quality of the mother–infant relationship. She followed mothers and infants in both the USA and Uganda, using detailed systematic observations over the first 18 months of life. Her findings provide a more detailed understanding of the relationship between early maternal care and sensitivity and the ongoing relational pattern of her infant. From these early data, Ainsworth developed an observational/assessment instrument (the Strange Situation procedure) that has allowed researchers both to operationalize the concept of internal representational models and to track the stability of individual attachment patterns over time.

The Strange Situation procedure is a standardized observational instrument that assesses the attachment patterns of infants between 12 and 18 months of age. The procedure documents an infant's interactional patterns with a care-giver during a series of observations in which the parent and infant are in a play situation, followed by a separation and then a reunion with the care-giving figure. Depending upon the infant's response and interactional patterns with the parent, the infant is classified into a category of secure attachment or one of three different categories of insecure attachment. The assessment can be utilized with either parent or a consistent care-giving figure. Attachment patterns may be different depending upon the relational history that the infant has with the individual parent or care-giver.

Internal representational models and attachment security

Attachment theory (Bowlby 1988) and research tell us that the early mother–child relationship provides a prototype upon which all future intimate relationships are modelled. Furthermore, the way in which the mother or primary care-giver interacts with the child provides continuous feedback to the child of his or her lovability, worth and competence. Through repetitive, emotionally laden interaction with the care-giving figure, the infant slowly but surely forms an internal image or internal representational model of self, of others and of self in relation to others. This concept of internal representational models is one of the most useful concepts within attachment theory, allowing researchers to operationalize attachment concepts.

Ainsworth et al's (1978) research demonstrated that infants form consistent internal representational models of attachment by the age of 18 months. An internal representational model is defined as a series of feelings, beliefs, expectations and behavioural strategies used by the child when under stress or in relation to others.

Working models can serve a useful purpose for the child, making unnecessary the construction of a new set of expectations for each new situation. The child can use existing models to appraise and guide behaviour in new situations. For example, a child who has a working model of his mother as available when needed may spend less time monitoring her movements than a baby unsure of his mother's availability. Although Bowlby views working models as open to new input, he believes that because they tend to operate outside consciousness, they become increasingly resistant to change over time. Thus, when working models are no longer appropriate or necessary in a relationship, they may remain influential, guiding an individual's behaviour in repetitive and even pathological ways.

For Bowlby, there is an inextricable interwining of the working model of self and the working model of relationship to the primary attachment figure. Individuals are seen as developing either secure or insecure attachments depending upon the sensitivity of their early care-giving experience. If the child experiences a positive early parenting relationship in which needs are met with sensitivity and consistency, a secure attachment relationship is formed, and positive internal representational models ensue. These representational models are of attachment figures as positive, available, safe, responsive and helpful. Similarly, the internal representational model of self is one of self as worthy, loveable and capable. In contrast, if early care is inconsistent, insensitive, hurtful or frustrating, an insecure attachment to the care-giver will develop. The resultant internal model will be of the self as unlovable, incapable and unworthy. The representational model of others in relationships will be of others as dangerous, hurtful, unpredictable or unreliable.

Thus, Bowlby's attachment theory suggests that the types of parent–infant relationship that are most likely to yield secure attachments and therefore emotionally healthy individuals are the ones in which the parent is sensitively receptive to the child's signals and contingently responsive to them. For secure attachment to be sustained, parental sensitivity changes as the child's needs for both security and for exploration change with development. Subsequent research by Ainsworth et al (1978) further delineated parental sensitivity as parenting that is readily available to the child and freely giving of comfort and close bodily contact when requested, particularly when the child is frightened, ill or distressed.

In one of his later writings, Bowlby (1991) spoke eloquently about the developmental trajectories that the child's early attachment patterns set in motion. He summarized a variety of longitudinal research demonstrating that insecure attachments in infancy were found to predict disturbed developmental patterns, and thwarted potential in later life. These long-term studies, fuelled by Ainsworth's Strange Situation procedure, have generally confirmed the link between the quality of early parenting and the child's ongoing mental health and relationship patterns (George et al 1985, Troy & Sroufe 1987, Colin 1996). The next section will review selected studies demonstrating the relational and developmental impact over time of early attachment security.

Sequelae of infant attachment patterns in later childhood

If, as Bowlby suggests, the early parent–infant attachment relationship serves as an internal, perhaps tacit, model for future relationships, one would expect the pattern to repeat itself in childhood relationships as well as within later parenting relationships. This hypothesis has indeed been tested in a number of studies, using the Strange Situation as the base. This section will highlight studies that track relationship patterns from infancy into early and middle childhood, in the 'typical' as well as the maltreated population.

Early studies sought to determine the stability of the Strange Situation classification at 12 and 18 months of age. More stability was found in securely attached children and within stable families with minimal stress. In stable, middle-class homes, most studies found a very high stability of attachment patterns over time. Connell (1976) found that 81% of the infants in the sample received the same attachment security classification using the Strange Situation Instrument at 12 and 18 months of age. Similarly, Waters (1978) assessed 50 middle-class babies and found a 96% consistency in classification between 12 and 18 months old. Main & Weston (1981) also found an 87% consistency when following 15 babies over time.

Of more relevance, however, are the studies that follow children over time in order to understand the developmental consequences following early insensitive parenting and insecure attachment in infancy. One of the most impressive and informative of these is the Minnesota longitudinal study that followed 267 high-risk families from the prenatal period through early adolescence. At the current time, the most recent findings track children with both secure and insecure attachments into early adolescence. Much of this section will discuss some of the most remarkable findings from this seminal work.

As part of the Minnesota sample, Troy & Sroufe (1987) examined the association between 38 preschool children's attachment histories and their interaction with their peers in a preschool setting. All the children (20 males and 18 females) had been previously assessed using the Strange Situation procedure at 12 months of age and were routinely in contact with each other in a preschool setting. After at least 6 weeks of preschool attendance, the children were observed playing in a specifically designated playroom for seven different sessions of 15 minutes each, spread over many weeks. The data were analysed comparing the play behaviour of different combinations of children with varying classifications of attachment security.

An analysis of the children's play by three different judges showed a significant difference in the quality of play and quantity of aggression between dyads containing insecurely attached children and those containing securely attached youngsters. The analysis revealed that the presence of a child with an insecure attachment history was significantly associated with victimization such as aggressive, hurtful or coersive play. Five out of seven pairs in which at least one child had an insecure attachment history showed victimization, whereas none of the seven pairs without a history of insecure attachment showed victimization ($P<0.01$).

In contrast, the presence in the dyad of a child with a secure attachment history was definitively associated with a non-victimizing play relationship. None of eight such pairs showed victimization, whereas victimization was found in five out of the six pairs containing exclusively insecurely attached children ($P<0.005$).

Troy & Sroufe's (1987) research sheds light on a number of important findings in the clinical abuse and attachment literature. It is a well-known fact in abuse and neglect research that maltreated children are more likely than well-treated children to be the victims of further abuse or serious aggression. They are also more likely in adult life to aggress against others within intimate relationships. This research, however, is the first to document the connection between the quality of the early attachment relationship (rather than the specific abusive act) and the child's predisposition towards continuing both the victim and the victimizer roles within relationships. This finding alone has major implications for early preventive intervention. It

is relevant not only for the prevention of abuse in further generations, but also in relation to the consistent finding in the clinical literature that disturbed peer relationships in childhood are one of the most powerful predictors of pathology in adulthood.

In addition, if these data are assessed strictly in relation to the concepts of internal working models (Bowlby 1988), it strongly suggests that the child re-enacts not only the model of self, but also the part of the parent in the relationship model. Although the above study included some abused and neglected children, subjects were selected on the basis of the Strange Situation rather than on a history of maltreatment. The following study specifically traces the relationship patterns of children coming from maltreating homes.

Egeland & Erickson (1993) identified 80 preschool children from their longitudinal study of 267 high-risk children, whose care-taking experience fits into four different patterns of child maltreatment. The four maltreatment groups were divided into groups characterized by parenting behaviour histories of:

- physical abuse;
- hostility/verbal abuse;
- psychological unavailability;
- physical neglect.

A control group of children and mothers who provided adequate care were selected from the remaining high-risk sample. The two groups were assessed in order to compare the children's developmental pathways and behavioural patterns during the first 5 years of life.

In general, the insecurely attached children from maltreated groups were characterized by patterns of:

- diminishing IQ scores over time;
- increasingly hostile and negative affect and interactional patterns;
- lack of self-esteem, concentration, creativity and ego control in comparison to their non-maltreated securely attached peers.

The authors found some significant differences between the patterns of response, depending upon the type of maltreatment to which the children were subjected. Nonetheless, the most striking generalizable consequence of maltreatment was the ongoing declining level of functioning displayed by all the groups of abused and neglected children over time.

Egeland et al (1990) documented another stage in the Minnesota longitudinal study. Their analysis of data sought to determine which symptoms and behaviours seen in high-risk preschool children were predictive of later demeanour in the early school years. They followed 96 of the preschool children already followed from birth and continued to assess them yearly through until the third grade. They found a high degree of continuity between the children's preschool behaviour and that seen in the first 3 years of school. Insecurely attached children who had demonstrated relationship problems in preschool were likely to also have relationship problems in primary school, and children who were socially and academically competent in preschool were also found to be competent in their school years. In fact, 80% of the children identified as insecurely attached and aggressive in preschool were also identified as aggressive towards their peers in 2 out of their 3 years of elementary school. Similarly, 71% of the youngsters labelled as withdrawn in preschool were also judged to be withdrawn in primary school. Furthermore, the children who were classified as aggressive or withdrawn at 4 years of age scored significantly below the academic achievement levels of the competent children.

Although the continuity of behaviour in this study (Egeland et al 1990) is striking, the exceptions are of equal interest. There were a number of intervening factors that correlated with a decrease in behavioural problems. Improvement in behaviour, and movement from an insecure attachment category to a secure one, corresponded with:

- a lessening of maternal depression;
- a reduction in the number of stressful family life events;
- an increase in the quality of stimulation in the child's home environment.

The severity of maternal depression appeared directly to affect the quality of the relationship between the mother and her child while indirectly impacting on the quality and organization of the home environment.

In the most recent publication from the Minnesota study, Sroufe (1991) summarized the alternate developmental and relational pathways taken by the insecurely attached children. Data were derived from:

1. parent–child observation sessions;
2. preschool observations;
3. the first 3 years in grade school;
4. a summer camp experience in their tenth and eleventh years of age.

Sroufe concluded that the relational and developmental patterns that each group followed reflected their internal representations of self and of self in relation to others.

His summarized findings of the longitudinal study

to date concluded that children who displayed secure attachment during the 18 month Strange Situation assessment tended to continue to exhibit higher functioning and healthier relationship patterns during the subsequent 10 years of study. As preschoolers, they were characterized by greater confidence, resourcefulness, self-direction, enthusiasm, positive affect and problem-solving ability than their insecurely attached peers. They were also likely to be more curious, resourceful and forceful in pursuing tasks and goals.

In the preschool and school years, the secure children were less likely to sit beside the teacher, more likely to initiate positive contact with their peers and more likely to greet their teachers and peers. When confronted with rejection from peers, they were more likely to reframe it into a positive message and to continue to seek contact with other children.

As 10- and 11-year-olds, these securely attached children were more likely than their insecure peers to be confident and flexible, and were better able to manage their impulses, feelings and desires. As in the earlier years, these preteens were more likely to display positive affect in all relations with others. In addition, they came across as more socially competent and better able to establish and maintain deeper relationships. Their interaction with peers was generally characterized by reciprocity and fairness.

The contrasting description of the insecurely attached children maintained a consistent profile throughout the 11 years of the study. Insecurely attached children were characterized as being more aggressive, avoidant and sensitive to rebuff at all stages of development. As early as the preschool years, they showed decreased confidence and less curiosity, and were either unable or unwilling to engage in challenging tasks. Although they were more likely to cling to teachers, they were also less likely to ask a counsellor or teacher for assistance when experiencing difficulty.

In the preadolescent years, the insecure children's peer relationships were more often marked by hostility and a lack of commitment. They tended to choose friends who were also insecurely attached and within those friendships, often played either the victim or victimizer role. The interactions tended to be characterized by hostility, teasing, rejection and exploitative behaviour.

The play of insecurely attached children was also distinctive at each age. As early as the preschool years, their play lacked the fantasy and complexity of securely attached children. When make-believe themes did occur in later years, conflict or problems more often tended to move towards unsuccessful or negative resolution. Although the profile of the insecurely attached child is certainly discouraging, Sroufe (1991, p. 303) concludes this article by saying that:

This strong data on the continuity of adaptation over time should not lead to pessimism concerning change. The organizational perspective (on the self) is also useful for conceptualising intervention and change. The inner organisation of self is a derivative of organised vital relationships and, as such most likely will undergo change in the context of other significant relationships.

With the reality of the long-term impact of inadequate parenting becoming clear, the logical next step is to ask whether individuals' early parenting then goes on to influence how they parent their own children. With the goal of exploring this question, Main and colleagues developed the Adult Attachment Interview (AAI; Main & Goldwyn 1985). This instrument, in conjunction with the Strange Situation procedure, has allowed researchers to examine the relationship between adults' resolution of attachment experiences and their own ability to parent their child with the sensitivity and consistency necessary to foster secure attachment and consequently a healthier developmental trajectory.

The AAI reflects Sroufe's belief that adult attachment represents more than the individual's early experiences. It allows for the influence of a variety of vital relationships in the individual's life in addition to the early care-giving relationship. The AAI has been used in a variety of studies to assess parents' working models in clinical and non-clinical populations of infants, young children and school-age children.

The AAI has been useful in exploring the transmission of parenting styles and attachment patterns from one generation to the next. Of key import is how particularly aberrant parenting, such as abuse and neglect, is transmitted across generations. The next section will examine research relevant to these questions.

Transgenerational cycle of parenting styles

In today's Western society of working couples and isolated nuclear families, many new parents approach the complex task of parenting their newborn as novices. One might suppose that they must learn their new parenting skills 'on the job' as they inevitably become immersed in the all-consuming task. On the contrary, the reality is far from this intuitive conclusion. A variety of research concludes that parenting style, methods and the degree of responsiveness are powerfully preconditioned by factors present long before the infant's birth. A number of family research teams have concluded that the father and mother's psychological adaptation and quality of marriage before the birth of the first child predicts the quality of parenting during the early years (Belsky et al 1985, Lewis et al 1988). Another body of attachment research concludes that the parents' role in the parent–child interaction reflects relationship patterns that have evolved from, and been influenced by, a wide variety of experiences, thoughts and insights learned within intimate relationships over time (Colin 1996, Kaufman & Ziegler 1987).

A multitude of studies have also reported the transmission of parenting attitudes, models and behaviours across generations. The earliest of this research evolved from the child maltreatment literature. Authors have long reported the statistical tendency for individuals who were abused as children to have a higher likelihood of abusing their own children (Herrenkohl et al 1983, Kaufman & Ziegler 1987, Belsky & Pensky 1988, Ney 1988). The intergenerational repetition of parenting behaviours is, however, not exclusive to those who maltreat their children. Caspi & Elder (1988) have concluded that parental personality is directly related to parenting style and child behaviour. They found that unstable, irritable, conflicted parents who experienced marital discord produce irritable, explosive children. If, however, parents were able to transcend their own marital problems enough to provide positive parenting, the children showed little negative behaviour.

In the theory of adult attachment, it is posited that parenting behaviour and sensitivity most often dates back to the parents' own experience of being parented. This early experience leads to internal representational models that influence the degree and manner of responsiveness they will be able to show their children (Main et al 1985, Bowlby 1988). Parents who were raised with sensitivity as infants are expected to be more open and responsive to their infant's needs than abused, rejected or insensitively reared parents (Colin 1996). Recent reviews also conclude, however, that these early models may also be altered during or after childhood through prolonged experience with another attachment figure or a supportive partner, or within a therapeutic relationship (Egeland et al 1988, Werner 1989, Colin 1996).

This section will explore a number of useful studies that add to our understanding of both the transgenerational cycle of parenting and those factors that interrupt the transmission of negative or insecure internal representational models across generations. The AAI (Main & Goldwyn 1984) is used in most of these studies and will now be reviewed.

The adult attachment paradigm presents a unique

way of looking at the intergenerational transmission of parenting. Rather than supposing that a parent's own childhood experiences translate literally into a child-rearing style, this theory is based upon the belief that it is the *currently held* internal representation, and therefore the current interpretation of the past, that affects the quality and transmission of parenting. The previously held simplistic assumption that insensitively raised, abused or neglected parents automatically repeat the experience with their own children is, within this paradigm, replaced by a more dynamic interpretation in which change through insight, external variables and significant other relationships can facilitate a conscious reworking and alteration of early experience.

The AAI subsequently assesses the adult's 'state of mind' with respect to attachment relationships, rather than purely past experience. Although this instrument requires extensive training for the actual classification of the subjects, the concepts and methodology of the interview are useful for any health professional who wishes to assess a woman's attachment patterns and history. For this reason, it will be described in some detail and referred to later under suggestions for assessment and intervention.

In the AAI, subjects are asked a series of questions and probes designed to elicit as full a story as possible about the individual's childhood attachment experiences. The manner in which these experiences are conveyed, rather than the nature of the experiences themselves, yields an overall classification of the adult's *current* state of mind with respect to attachment. During the interview, the individuals are asked to describe childhood experiences with their own parents and how they feel the experiences affected their adult personality and their current behaviour with their children. On the basis of the experiences described, and the ways in which the subject discusses them and derives meaning from them, the adult is classified into one of three groups – secure/autonomous, insecure/dismissing and insecure/preoccupied – that most accurately characterizes his or her state of mind regarding attachment relationships (Main & Golwyn 1984).

A significant association has been demonstrated between the mother's classifications in the AAI and the observed behaviours of her infant in Ainsworth et al's (1978) Strange Situation. Main et al (1985) have demonstrated that the mothers of securely attached children, in describing their childhood experiences, share the common characteristic of having achieved some integration between current feeling and past experiences relevant to attachment, unlike the parents of insecurely attached children. Securely attached mothers are objective and show balance in their evaluation of childhood experiences in much the same way that securely attached children steer a middle course between attachment behaviours and autonomous exploration in the Strange Situation. The mother's autonomy from her experience is thought to leave her free to respond sensitively to her child's needs instead of being entangled in her own. Dismissing (insecure) adults on the other hand share in common a history of some rejection and an organization of thought that permits attachment to be relatively deactivated or avoided through self-deception (leading to high idealization and poor recall), grandiosity (leading to a derogatory attitude) or denial (leading to a view of the self as unaffected by malignant experiences). They are cut off from attachments in much the same way as insecurely attached infants ignore care-giver cues.

Van Ijzendoorn (1992) performed an extensive review of the literature related to the intergenerational transmission of parenting in non-clinical populations. Reviewing four studies using the AAI, she concluded a strong concordance between the parent's view of his or her attachment biography and his or her attachment relationship to the infant. An example is found in Main et al's (1985) study of 40 mothers and their 6-year-old children. These children had been assessed as infants using the SSI at 12 and 18 months of age. In this 6-year follow-up, the parents completed the AAI. The correspondence between the mother's state of mind with respect to attachment and her infant's attachment classification from the Strange Situation procedure 5 years earlier was 75%.

Similarly, in their European study, Grossman & Fremer-Bombik (1988) found an 88% correlation between the parent's AAI classification and her behaviour toward the infant as well as the infant's patterns of attachment to her using the Strange Situation procedure. The authors concluded that it was not just the mother's experience as a child that was important, but also the parent's conscious awareness and insight into her experience of being parented. Mothers who had received inadequate parenting but as an adult had a clear image of how they were treated by their parent, and were able to discuss its impact, were able to relate to their infants in a sensitive way that promoted attachment security. They concluded that (Grossman & Fremer-Bombik 1988, p. 255):

a mother who remembers well how she felt when something bad happened to her and how her parents responded to comfort her, will listen empathically to her infant's distress signals. A mother who cannot remember much of her childhood distress, or remembers only in a distorted form, seems less able to listen openly and feel sympathetic with her infant. She may push aside memories of her own distress by ignoring her infant's distress.

In researching 'problematic populations', Ainsworth & Eichberg (1991) found an 80% correspondence in classification between mother and infant classification when studying infants and their mothers who had experienced loss and were in the process of mourning.

A number of studies are of particular value in understanding some of the factors involved in the transmission of aberrant parenting behaviours. De Lozier (1982) assessed adult attachment using the Wallace–DeLozier attachment questionnaire in addition to a separation anxiety test. Her population consisted of 18 mothers who were known to have abused their children, and 18 matched controls. In comparing the participants' childhood experiences, she found significant differences between the samples. Abusive mothers were found to have experienced a greater incidence of threat of separation or withdrawal of care-giving during childhood than were the controls. Such threats included ones of abandonment, harsh punishment and being sent away. There was also the perception by the maltreating mothers that they, as children, were expected to care for their care-givers. In adulthood, these women saw significant others as being essentially unavailable. The quality of support around the birth of the maltreated child was also a distinguishing factor. The abusing mothers reported feeling fearful, alone, unsafe and dissatisfied with the availability and support of significant others.

The Minnesota longitudinal study (Egeland et al 1988), with its rich data, also provides a particularly useful insight into the transmission of maltreatment as well as the factors related to its repetition or interruption. Of the 267 high-risk families involved in this research, 47 of the mothers were classified as having been abused as children. During the first 5 years of the study, 18 (38%) of these mothers were found to maltreat their own children. Twelve (25%) were reported as giving clearly adequate care to their children. The remaining 17 could not be definitively classified into either category. The research team analysed factors differentiating the two 'classifiable' groups. The results of the analysis showed that mothers who broke the abusive cycle were significantly more likely to have:

- received emotional support from a non-abusive parent or other close adult during childhood;
- participated in individual or group therapy for at least 1 year;
- had a stable emotionally supportive relationship with a partner.

Finally, Ney (1988) followed 154 families, 32 of which were known to have abused their children, in order to identify those factors which could distinguish abusive from non-abusive parents. He found that women who were battered by their partners were more likely to abuse their children. He also found a significant correlation between mothers who were physically or sexually abused as children and those who verbally abused their children.

In summary, recent research tells us that parenting, like any important relationship, is influenced by a myriad of factors, many of which are present long before conception. The mother's relationship history is of particular importance in influencing the sensitivity and ease with which she nurtures her infant. This relationship history includes her own experience of being parented, her relationship with other important adults in her life and her adult relationship history. Of special relevance is her ongoing relationship with her partner. The adult attachment paradigm stresses that we must assess the level of insight that the parent has into his or her own experience of being parented if we are going to anticipate the quality of parenting he or she will provide to the infant. Given the place of insight in this equation, it is not surprising therefore that a parent's participation in therapy is influential in determining his or her ability to interrupt the cycle of insensitive or hurtful parenting.

The place of infant factors in attachment security

Winnicott (1987) has poignantly remarked that 'there is no such thing as a baby in the absence of a sustaining caregiving relationship'. Similarly, we would be remiss in examining the development of attachment and the birth of love without examining the role that the infant temperament plays in this process.

The newborn infant is a product of his or her genes as well as 9 months in the intrauterine environment. Some babies are easy to love and a parent's dream. They are strong, healthy, cuddly, clear in their demands and easy to comfort and settle. It is easy to react to these infants with sensitivity and consequently to feel competent as a parent. But not all babies (or their parents) are so fortunate. Many otherwise healthy, full-term babies may be difficult to nurture and parent, either because of their level of adaptability or cuddliness, or because of an unusual level of hypersensitivity to stimuli. These infants require a greater level of parental skill, creativity and commitment in order for them to settle and feel consistently nurtured and contained. Because of their unique nature or physiology, the hypersensitive may send confusing signals of rejection to their parents. Without assistance, parents may grow to feel inadequate and discouraged in the task of parenting these infants. A number of theorists have examined the impact of and continuity in infant temperament and its relationship to the child's developmental trajectory. The work most useful to those working in the perinatal period is that of Dr Barry Brazelton (1979, 1981, 1984).

Brazelton (1984) developed the Neonatal Behavioural Assessment Scale (NBAS) to help both parents and professionals better understand and identify the individual variations in the newborn's behavioural responses to the environment. The stimuli used to assess the baby are the same that parents use in interacting with their infant. During the assessment, the baby is evaluated while being held, talked to, touched, rocked and cuddled. The newborn's responsiveness to stimuli, as well as irritability and 'soothability', is assessed. A profile of the infant as well as how to support, soothe and contain him or her arises from the information.

Many researchers had hoped to find early indices of an infant's ongoing temperament in the responses to items on the NBAS. Cumulative data now show only a weak relationship between NBAS scores and later behaviour (Brazelton & Cramer 1990). Subsequently, this assessment tool has been most appropriately utilized as an assessment of the newborn's early capability for interaction with the care-giver. Assessment information can be used to help parents to understand the unique and sometimes idiosyncratic needs and responses of their infant. Not only is it important for parents to learn about how to meet the unique needs of their baby, but this kind of objective assessment also allows them to understand infant behaviour without subjective misinterpretation. For example, it is very easy for parents to interpret the behaviour of a stiff, non-cuddly baby who is easily upset and hard to settle as being rejecting of them as parents. If the parents are not helped to meet the unique needs of this temperamentally difficult baby, the infant may experience parental confusion as non-support and insensitivity. Insecure attachments may result.

During the 1980s, developmental psychologists researched and questioned the relationship between infant temperament and later attachment behaviour (Kagan 1982, Belsky & Rovine 1987). They hypothesized that attachment security was influenced by the infant's innate temperamental characteristics rather than the care-giver's level of sensitivity or responsiveness. A variety of research has, however, demonstrated that attachment security shows much greater stability than does infant temperamental classification (Colin

1996). Indeed, in her research, Colin found that even characteristics such as cuddliness and adaptability were more dependent upon, and varied according to, which parent or care-giver held the baby than the baby's innate characteristics.

In 1987, Goldsmith & Alansky published a meta-analysis from a variety of studies that compared the impact of infant temperament and maternal sensitivity on determining infant attachment patterns. They concluded that it was the mother's sensitive responsiveness rather than infant measures that predicted attachment security. Van Ijzendoorn (1992) came to similar conclusions in his more recent meta-analysis of 34 clinical studies. He concluded that when maternal problems (such as a history of abuse, mental illness or poor social support) were present in a study group, there was an increase in insecure attachment in the infant. In contrast, there were few demonstrated effects of a child-related factor (e.g. prematurity, developmental disability or illness) on the attachment distribution. He summarized that (Van Ijzendoorn 1992, p. 90):

Our data suggest that if mothers suffer from mental illness or engage in disturbed caregiving behaviour (e.g., maltreatment) their children cannot compensate for the resulting lack of maternal responsiveness and are vulnerable to insecure forms of attachment. However when children are impaired (physically or mentally in various degrees) their mothers are generally capable of compensating for this potential handicap in the dyadic relationship.

There are, however, exceptions to this conclusion, when other variables are factored in. For example, Crockenberg (1981) used the NBAS to study 46 mother–infant pairs. The infants were assessed for irritability on the fifth and tenth days of life. A 4-hour home visit was made when the babies were 3 months old, wherein the mother was assessed for maternal responsiveness. During the same visit, mothers were interviewed in relation to their sources of support and the levels of stress in their life. The babies were later assessed for attachment security at 12 months of life. High infant irritability, as measured by the NBAS, was only associated with an increased incidence of insecure attachment when the mother also experienced poor social support and high stress. The authors concluded that when the infants were relatively undemanding and easy to comfort, the mother could provide responsive care even in the absence of good social support. If the baby was difficult, emotional and material support from others could make a critical difference in the mother's ability to provide responsive care.

In another review, Vaughn et al (1992) concluded that attachment and temperament could be more usefully conceptualized as overlapping domains because child behaviour and affect regulation occur and are measured in a social context. In her review, Colin (1996, p. 114) concludes that the emerging consensus is as follows:

Infants differ from each other at birth and in the early weeks because of genetic and prenatal factors. Differences such as irritability, sociability, fearfulness, proneness-to-distress, and being 'easy' or 'difficult' may certainly affect the tone of parent–infant interactions. Such differences are subject to change with maturation and social experience and are unlikely in themselves to determine the security of the infant's emerging attachment. However, in interaction with other factors, such as the parent's responsiveness and the social support available to the parent, congenital differences in temperament may influence attachment.

In summary, we might conclude that the assessment of a newborn's adaptability, soothability and response to stimuli is an important part of the postpartum assessment. It allows the midwife to individualize the teaching of infant care to the unique needs of both the mother and the newborn. If, during this assessment, we find a difficult baby in addition to vulnerabilities in the mother's history or current environmental support, additional support and intervention are advised.

THERAPEUTIC INTERVENTION RESEARCH

A variety of therapeutic intervention programmes have been inspired by the link between insecure parent–infant attachment and an increased risk of malfunctioning in the emotional–social domain. The majority of these programmes have been aimed at either enhancing parental sensitivity to infant cues or processing maternal representational models. Studies relevant to the midwife will be reviewed below.

The first category of study reviewed here will be of those attempting to influence parental sensitivity to infant cues. These are based on previously described hypotheses that parental responsiveness and sensitivity are key factors in the development of secure attachment in the infant (Ainsworth et al 1978). Two categories of research have addressed this issue: the first being more behavioural, and the second aimed at the mother's internal representational models of attachment.

Anisfeld et al (1990) designed a simple yet intriguing behavioural approach. They hypothesized that a mother's sensitivity to her infant would be enhanced quite easily by increased physical contact with her infant. They assumed that greater sensitivity would lead to secure attachment. They divided 49 mothers of low socio-economic status between an experimental and a control group. Upon discharge from hospital, mothers in the experimental group were given soft infant carriers and encouraged to use them daily with their infants. Those in the control group were given plastic infant seats. At 3.5 months, the mothers and infants were visited in their home, and the mothers were rated on their sensitivity of response to their infants. Additionally, the Strange Situation procedure was used at 13 months to assess the quality of infant–mother attachment. Although mothers who had used the infant carriers were found to score higher in maternal sensitivity, the results did not reach statistical significance. The difference in infant attachment was, however, phenomenal. In the experimental group (using the soft infant carriers), 83% of the infants appeared to be securely attached, whereas only 38% of the control group were secure. The authors concluded that the infant's experience of being carried close to the mother seemed to have affected the infant's attachment security to a degree far beyond that attributable to increased maternal sensitivity.

A preventive intervention study was designed by Lyons-Ruth et al (1990) to determine whether a year of a trustworthy, accepting, professional relationship during the infant's first year of life could counteract the impact of poverty, maternal depression and an inadequate care-giving history. The intervention group of 10 high-risk families received weekly home visits designed to support the mother and provide modelling and reinforcement of developmentally appropriate exchanges between mother and infant. A secondary goal was to decrease social isolation. At 18 months of age, scores of maternal sensitivity, covert hostility and flatness of affect in the mothers, and from the Strange Situation procedure in the infants, were compared with those of a matched control group. Although the study found no significant effects of treatment on maternal sensitivity, there was a marked difference in attachment security of the infants. Eighty per cent of the infants in the non-treated group were rated as insecurely attached compared with only 43% in the treatment group.

Van Ijzendoorn et al (1995) reviewed a number of studies from the Netherlands. One by Van den Boom (cited in Van Ijzendoorn et al 1995) is of particular interest to this review. One hundred highly irritable infants from lower-class families were selected for the evaluation of a short-term intervention for enhancing maternal sensitivity to difficult infants. Interveners visited the control mothers three times at home between the infant's sixth and ninth month of life. The intervener assisted the mothers in adjusting to the infants' unique cues, particularly negative signals such as crying. The mothers were rated on maternal sensitivity pre- and post-test using a number of instruments. The quality of the infant–mother attachment was also evaluated at 12 months of age using the Strange Situation procedure. Mothers who received coaching were found to be significantly more responsive to their infants on the post-test than were the control mothers. In addition, 68% of the experimental group infants were found to be securely attached at 12 months compared with only 28% of the control group.

Van Ijzendoorn et al (1995) also conducted a meta-analysis of 12 different intervention studies designed to influence both maternal sensitivity and the security of infant attachment. The analysis involved a total of 900 mother–infant dyads using a variety of modes of intervention. Overall, the authors concluded that the families profited by the intervention, the greatest impact being in the form of increased maternal sensitivity to the infants' needs and cues. A highly significant combined effect size for maternal sensitivity ($d = 0.58$) was reported. The combined effect size for infant attachment was, however, less encouraging and was considered to be weak ($d = 0.17$). The authors suggest that the discrepancy in the combined effect size may be explained by the immediacy of impact. They hypothesize that the interventions for enhancing maternal sensitivity are inevitably more successful as the goal is more proximal and more easily achieved. The impact on infant security is, however, more complex and may require more time to measure change.

IMPLICATIONS FOR ASSESSMENT AND INTERVENTION DURING THE PERINATAL PERIOD

So far in this chapter, we have reviewed attachment-related theory and research with the purpose of establishing a conceptual and research base from which to examine the midwife's role in the screening of, promotion of and intervention in the early parent–infant relationship. The research to date has made a credible link between:

- the mother's attachment security and that of her infant;
- the quality of the early parent–infant relationship and the later security of the infant's attachment to the mother;
- insecure attachment in the infant and suboptimal developmental and relational patterns in the child.

The literature has additionally provided us with a number of focal points for assessment and potential intervention. This section will begin by providing a synopsis of those factors shown to be influential on the quality and sensitivity with which a mother relates to her infant. Particular emphasis will be placed upon information that can be reasonably assessed in the course of the midwife's interaction with the mother. Focal points of assessment will be organized according to the most appropriate time in the perinatal period for optimal screening and intervention. Figure 11.1 summarizes the proposed pathway of factors influencing attachment and the parent–infant relationship.

Focus of assessment in the early prenatal period

The assessment of the mother's 'state of mind' in relation to attachment should begin early in pregnancy. The importance of this early screening to the long-term mental health of the child can be likened to the importance of early screening for such physiological stressors as maternal substance abuse in terms of the long-term physical health of the child. In the early screening, we are assessing for insecurely attached mothers who will be unable to meet their infants' needs with sensitivity and consistency as a result of their own negative experience of being parented. In addition, we are screening for such environmental factors as high levels of stress, social isolation and a lack of support systems that would further compromise the mother's ability to tend to her infant's needs. Table 11.1 summarizes the historical and environmental factors that have the potential to counteract the influence of early abuse or insensitive parenting on the mother's ability to respond with sensitivity to her infant. Table 11.2 outlines the historical and environmental factors that may negatively influence the quality of the early parent–child relationship.

Early prenatal screening interview

The literature tells us that the mother's own early caregiving experience has a profound impact upon her ability to parent her child. Her early experience of being parented provides the foundation of her long-term relationship patterns. As Sroufe (1996) remarks, these patterns are not laid in stone. There are a variety of relational, cognitive and/or therapeutic experiences that can serve to modify a parent's attitudes, insight and internal representational models with respect to attachment experiences. Because the process of influencing a parent's internal representational models, and therefore her insight into her relational history and patterns, is complex, assessment and intervention should ideally begin early in pregnancy.

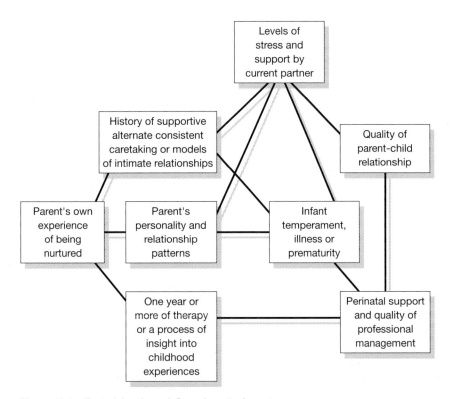

Figure 11.1   Factorial pathway influencing attachment

Although the AAI (Main & Goldwyn 1984) is a tool that requires extensive training and would therefore be unrealistic for the practising midwife to use, its approach provides a format and philosophy that can be used by any professional in screening for unresolved attachment problems. The interviewing process is intended to 'surprise the unconscious' into providing a snapshot of adults who are either *preoccupied* with their experience of insensitive parenting or have in contrast *blocked* the experience from conscious processing. Either situation leaves the parent unable to respond to infant demands based upon her infant's needs without her own attachment needs interfering.

This section will briefly describe an interview strategy that will guide the midwife in her interview and assessment of the mother's relational history and her current insight into its impact upon her. The interview should occur once the midwife has developed a trusting relationship with the mother. The interview should be unhurried and be conducted with sensitivity and in an atmosphere of support. The goal of the assessment is to screen for those mothers who should be referred to therapy or for extra nurturance, modelling and support during pregnancy and the early postpartum period.

The interview strategy will be discussed in overview at this time, the more specific details of a suggested interview schedule being outlined in Box 11.1. The midwife can begin by saying something like, 'When they become pregnant, women often think about their own experience of being parented. I would like to spend the next little while asking you about some of your own childhood experiences and about your dreams for your own child.' Beginning the interview by asking about demographic data such as where she lived, the number of children in the family, the frequency of moves and contact with extended family will allow the woman to begin slowly and provides a context to the topic.

The second part of the interview is very important as it provides the mother's conscious, often defended or edited, view of her family. The questions are general ones, and the woman's initial answers often reflect the 'acceptable family line' if the parenting has been hurtful or insensitive. These initial responses will later be compared and contrasted with her answers to the more specific questions of the third part of the interview, which provide a 'truer' picture of the parenting she actually received. The consistency or inconsistency

Table 11.1 Checklist of mother's childhood 'historical' risk factors

Risk factor	Degree of risk	Presence of risk (+ or −)
Relationship history		
Physical, sexual or emotional abuse by the care-giver	High	
Physical or emotional neglect	High	
Death of parent or abandonment by parent or primary care-giver	High	
Loss of parent through abandonment or apprehension	High	
Frequent changes of primary care-givers (relatives, nannies, foster parent)	Moderate	
Prevalent parental inconsistency or unavailability	Moderate	
Parental mental illness that prevented parent from nurturing	High	
Parental alcoholism or drug abuse that interfered with availability or consistency of care	High	
Current memory distortions of childhood attachment		
Inability to remember significant periods of childhood	Moderate	
General or global memory of parenting contradicts specific memories	High	
Obsessed with childhood memories	Moderate	
No insight into impact of negative parenting on self. Unable to imagine parenting role with child or unable to imagine parenting differently. No goals for child's well-being.	High	

Table 11.2 Checklist of current risk factors

Risk factor	Importance of risk	Presence of risk (+ or −)
Current relationship factors		
Abusive partner	High	
Highly conflictual or unsupportive relationship with partner	Moderate	
Single parent with minimal support from family or friends	Moderate	
Other risk factors		
Social isolation of mother or family	Moderate	
Significant environmental or economic stressors	Moderate	
Substance abuse by mother or partner	High	
Psychiatric diagnosis in mother or partner that interferes with relationships	High	

between the answers in the two sections will provide us with information on whether:

- her 'current state of mind' in relation to attachment includes insight and a conscious processing of childhood experiences;
- her internal representational models have been altered and transformed over time.

If the woman's childhood experiences are ones of abuse, neglect or parental insensitivity and unavailability, and she has no insight into their impact upon her, she is at risk of repeating the same mistakes with her own child. If the mother is so preoccupied with her own treatment as a child that it is difficult to talk about her infant or gain insight into how she wants to parent

differently, her infant will also be at risk. A preoccupied parent is so wrapped up in her own needs that she is indeed likely to resent her infant for demanding her attention.

As briefly described in Box 11.1, the third part of the interview asks specific questions that elicit facts rather than the broad feelings or opinions. The midwife's task in analysing the responses is twofold. She must first determine whether the mother's own experience as a child reflects hurtful, neglectful or insensitive parenting. Second, if it does, she must then ask three questions in assessing the mother's responses to questions:

1. Is there a discrepancy between the woman's overall view of the quality of her childhood experiences and the detailed answers to the more specific questions?

2. Does the mother have a conscious insight into the impact that her childhood experiences had upon her?

3. Does she know how she wants to parent differently with her own child?

Box 11.1 provides suggested questions and a proposed order for the interview. The first part of the interview schedule assesses the mother's current internal representational models, as discussed above. The second part assesses current stressors or relationship patterns in the mother's life. The checklists allow the midwife succinctly to identify the number and severity of risk factors that are present in the mother's life.

If the midwife begins working with the mother early

Box 11.1 Suggested questions for the early prenatal interview

Part I: Mother's experience of being parented as a child

A: Demographic data

1. Could you tell me a little about your family when you were small? Maybe you could begin by telling me where you were born, where you lived and what family members lived in the house while you were growing up.
2. How many brother and sisters did you have? Where were you in the birth order? Do you live close to your siblings now?
3. Did your parents stay together through your childhood? If not, what was your pattern of visiting?
4. Did you see your grandparents much when you were small?

B: Broad questions about early parenting

1. How would you describe your relationship with your parents as a young child? Start with as far back as you can remember. (Encourage the parent to go back in memory to at least age 5 and younger if possible. Take as much time as you need to help her to explore this question as fully as possible.)
2. Could you think for a minute and choose four or five adjectives that would be most descriptive of your relationship with your mother during childhood?
3. Choose four or five adjectives that would best describe your relationship with your father as a child.
4. Which parent did you feel closest to and why?

C: Questions specific to parenting practices

1. Separately select each of the adjectives that the mother has used to describe her relationship with her own mother and explore these in more detail. (For example, 'You said that your relationship with your mother could be described as …; could you give me an example how it was…?')
2. For each of the adjectives used to describe the mother's relationship with her father, ask the same questions as in 1.
3. Could you describe whom you would go to for comfort in your family when you were upset? How did they comfort you? Was there anyone else who supported you?
4. Could you describe how you were disciplined as a child? Who was the disciplinarian? For what were you punished?
5. What happened when you were mad or acted out in your family?
6. Did you experience any death or separation from significant family members as a child?
7. Was there any other important nurturing or care-giving figure in your life (nannies, neighbours, grandparents, siblings who assumed major care-giving roles)?
8. How has your relationship with your parents and siblings changed as you have become an adult?

D. Insight- or transformation-orientated questions

1. In what ways would you like to be like your parent as you parent your child?
2. In what ways would you like to parent your child differently from how you were parented?
3. Is there anyone in your life other than your parents who has influenced your dreams about how you want to parent your child?
4. Is there anything that you have learned from your experiences as a child?

Part II: Current stressors

A: Mother's current support and relational situation

1. Who else lives with you?
2. Is there anyone who is a special support to you during your pregnancy?
3. Who do you plan to have help you during the labour, delivery and postpartum period?
4. Is there anyone particular in your life at the moment that you turn to for help, support or guidance?
5. Could you describe your relationship with the baby's father?
6. How will your partner be involved in the baby's care?

Table 11.3 Attachment-related strengths checklist

Maternal history and current positive factors	Level of importance	Presence of strength(+ or −)
Mother shows insight into affect of negative parenting on self. She is clear how she wishes to parent differently	High	
History of care-giving figure other than parents who provided a consistent sensitive and supportive relationship	High	
Has had long-term consistent relationship with partner	Moderate	
Has engaged in a year or more of therapy that has explored attachment issues and or abuse issues	Moderate	
Has supportive 'others' in life to nurture and help with baby	Moderate	

in pregnancy, the quality of this professional relationship has the potential to provide, at least in part, an alternative model of nurturing that the mother may be able to internalize in order to influence the sensitivity of care that she shows her infant. The year that a midwife spends with a set of parents, including both the prenatal and the postpartum period, may well be enough to alter the internal working models of a mother or couple to the degree that the transgenerational cycle of insecure attachment or dysfunction can be interrupted. If, however, the mother has a difficult attachment history and many risk factors, without evidence of resolution or insight, it would be optimal to refer the mother to counselling. If the referral is specific in identifying the attachment risks, an appropriate mode of therapy can be selected. Alternatively, one can enlist the support of professional home health visitors who can visit the mother weekly throughout her pregnancy, providing support as well as assistance in examining the mother's own history and its implications for her experience of motherhood.

Finally, the time of labour and delivery, as well as the immediate postpartum period, is an essential time in which the midwife can make a profound difference. Sensitive support and care of the mother and father during the perinatal period lead to a greater sensitivity in the mother's willingness and ability to care for her infant. Allowing for peaceful, undisturbed time for the parent and infant to get to know each other during the immediate postpartum period provides for an optimal start in the parent–infant bonding process.

Assessing an infant's cuddliness, soothability and temperament takes an additional sensitivity and knowledge on the part of the midwife but really no additional time. An experienced midwife can easily identify those infants who will be more difficult to parent, to nurse or to soothe. By being aware of how much a temperamentally difficult infant can influence the quality of parental comfort and commitment, the midwife can learn to allot a higher priority to a difficult mother – infant pair. Much of the task of promoting the parent–infant attachment is a matter of insight and dedication on the part of the professional. The results of such efforts may be life altering.

Finally, the midwife is not expected to be all things to all parents and their infants. However, a keen awareness of the importance of the early parent–infant relationship for the long-term health of the individual and of society will enable her to, within all aspects of her interaction with the family, maintain an alert eye to assessment for those clients who will need extraordinary scrutiny and intervention. An awareness of her unique opportunity to influence the long-term physical and emotional health of the individual and society will give her the commitment to the awesome responsibility she holds in her unique role in the life of a family.

IMPLICATIONS FOR THE MIDWIFE

The relationship between midwives, women and families

Midwives work with women at a critical point in the development of this greatest and most fundamental love affair of human life and society, the initiation and growth of the love between the mother, the father and their child. Parents will bring to pregnancy and the birth of their child the history of their own relationships, life circumstances and mind set. This history will be the most powerful determinant of the relationship trajectory between parents and child. Nevertheless, the actual pregnancy and birth of the baby is the birth of the family. The woman's care and her experience of it will be an important characteristic in influencing her relationship with her baby. It is important for midwives to be aware of both the opportunity to support the growth of love and the possibility of disturbing it. This growth of love, in the right circumstances, will be the foundation for the enduring commitment that helps the parents to make the necessary sacrifices and adjustments to provide physical, emotional and spiritual care, guidance and support until the child reaches independence. Most important of all, this commitment will be tied with bonds of love and affection that become the root of the child's sense of self and a pattern on which all his or her future relationships may be shaped.

The literature reviewed in this chapter makes clear the importance of secure attachments to the future survival and well-being of children and their development to become competent and happy adults. There are a number of important implications for midwives. Specific suggestions to help to provide support for the process of attachment have been given throughout the chapter. It is recognized that many of the patterns for parenting were laid down long before the mother became pregnant and before the midwife met the parents. Nevertheless, because of the dynamic nature of the development of maternal or paternal sensitivity, there are still opportunities for the midwife to influence the development of family relationships in a number of ways. These include nurturing and supporting the mother through the pregnancy and birth, screening for families who have the potential for greater problems than others, assessing the behaviour of the newborn and teaching the parents on the basis of this assessment, and extra support for and referral of high-risk families.

Developing sensitive systems

However, these suggestions, described in detail earlier in the chapter and summarized above, require appropriate organizations and cultures of care for their implementation. Unfortunately, many systems of care work against such individual sensitivity. Most babies in the industrialized world are born in hospital. As Klaus & Kennell (1976, p, 2) note:

crucial life events surrounding the development of both attachment and detachment have been removed from the home and brought into the hospital over the past 60 years. The hospital now determines the procedures involved in birth and death. The experiences surrounding these two events in the life of an individual have been stripped of the long established traditions and support systems built up over centuries to help families through these highly meaningful transitions.

It is all too easy, in busy hospital systems, to forget the significance of birth as a transition. It is all too easy to lose sight of the individuals who are in our care. Especially where care is fragmented between many different care-givers, and there is no one professional who gets to know the woman and her family as individuals, care is likely to become routine and the individual needs of women and their families be unknown or ignored.

Despite the heightened awareness of the importance of the development of attachment between mother, father and baby, problems that are likely to disturb or distort the development of attachment persist in many hospitals. Labour and delivery rooms are often like intensive care units, engendering a high level of anxiety. There is often a tendency to leave women alone in labour (Garcia et al 1998) and then, after the birth, rush to transfer the mother and baby to a postnatal ward, giving the new mother and father no chance to enjoy and get to know their baby in those first precious and irreplaceable moments. In Britain particularly, there is an acknowledged and widespread problem in postnatal wards, where many mothers and babies spend the first 2 days of family life. New mothers are reporting what amounts to a sense of neglect (McCourt and Page 1996, Garcia et al 1998) at a vulnerable time when they deserve to be, and would benefit from, being cherished.

Over recent decades, we have seen the beginning of two important changes that are directly or indirectly related to an awareness of the need to support the process of bonding or attachment. These deserve further consideration because they may be the most important basis on which midwives will be able to alter the structure and approach of their practice, particularly within the hospital setting.

Interventions to support bonding

The first of these changes is the increased awareness, which first became apparent in the 1960s, that hospital routines may be interfering with and have a negative effect on the development of family bonds and affection. It was common during that time for the mother and baby to be separated, often for many days after birth (Klaus & Kennell 1976). Barrera & Rosenbaum (1992), in their overview of randomized controlled trials, describe the enormous popularity in the late 1960s of the concepts of 'bonding' and 'attachment'. Although these words are often used interchangeably, they are usually used to refer to slightly different concepts (Klaus & Kennel 1976, p. 221):

Bonding usually refers to the affectional tie or bond of mother to infant believed to occur immediately after birth, perhaps to a sensitive or critical period.

As such, 'bonding is conceived as a rapid, mainly unidirectional, process and is thought to be facilitated by skin to skin contact'. The authors define attachment, on the other hand, as referring to:

the infant's development of an affectional bond, affective tie, or psychological bond to the primary caregiver, usually the mother during the last half of the last year of life. Infant attachment is thought to have a biological function to ensure infant survival, security and protection; it is considered a hypothetical construct of affection manifested by attachment behaviours which develop over time through a process of parent–child interaction.

The overview of randomized controlled trials of interventions aiming to support parents and promote attachment describes the evaluation of a number of approaches. The work of Klaus & Kennell stimulated much of the early work on bonding. This explored the broad question, 'Does early contact of mother with newborn infant enhance bonding, and lead to measurable changes in maternal attitude and behaviours?' (Barrera & Rosenbaum 1992, p. 222). The research studies reviewed in this chapter cover a number of categories of intervention including:

- increased mother–newborn contact in the immediate postnatal period;
- extended early mother–infant contact;
- increased father–infant contact;
- educational and supportive interventions prior to hospital discharge;
- supportive interventions during the transition from hospital to home;
- centre-based and home-based parental support.

Many of these evaluations assumed a linear cause-and-effect process and did not take into account the dynamic nature of the process, which is multifactorial.

Many were restricted to the hospital, although some extended to the community.

While recognizing the limitations of some of the research reviewed, in terms of methods, limited interventions and different outcome measures, the authors provide some important conclusions. In brief, they observe first that there is an increasing recognition of the multiple factors that contribute to the development, continuity, nature and strength of attachment between parent and child. This is certainly clearly reflected in the review of studies reported earlier in this chapter and is an important consideration for midwives in their practice. In their approach to supporting parents, it is important to remember this complexity.

Of great importance is the issue of 'consistency among studies regarding the positive effect of supportive intervention on socio economically disadvantaged families or less experienced parents' (Barrera & Rosenbaum 1992, p. 240). Where there is a question of the equitable use of resources, midwives would do well to offer extra support to parents in these groups.

Finally, the authors comment (Barrera & Rosenbaum 1992, p. 241) that:

despite the multitude of studies on maternal 'bonding' and 'attachment', and intervention studies to promote development and to support families, there is a paucity of intervention literature describing the actual promotion of attachment between mother/father and child.

Given the potential importance of the 'marital' relationship to the child (Clulow 1989), this is an important area for further consideration and research.

Such research is often perceived as indicating that bonding is an instantaneous event and that if the chance of bonding at birth is lost, it will not be regained. There has been concern expressed about the guilt feelings aroused in mothers if they do not 'bond' instantly with their baby (Littlewood & McHugh 1997). Inevitably perhaps, because of the hospital context in which the implications of the research have been implemented, 'bonding' and the provision of 'bonding time' have become another procedure for the mother to follow and the midwife to observe. Such an approach denies its complexity, the number of factors that affect it and the lengthy nature of the development of attachment between parents and child. Of course, as Niven recommends (in Littlewood & McHugh 1997), the woman's contact with her baby should be determined by her needs. A mother exhausted by a long and difficult labour may well not want to look at, let alone hold, her baby for a while. But while we ensure that procedures for 'bonding' are not imposed on the mother and baby against the mother's needs, we must ensure that the experience of receiving the baby directly into their arms and against their heart is not denied to those many women who want it.

In critiquing the research and considering its consequences, it will be important that midwives do not dismiss the theories and findings of years of painstaking and sound research.

Developing supportive, woman-centred care

The second change we have witnessed over the past 20 years is a more general change to systems of care that will provide more individually sensitive and supportive care. These alternative systems have included the provision of a known and named midwife to care for individual women and their families throughout the system of care (continuity of carer), and birthing centres. Although the goals of such schemes have not always been explicitly or solely concentrated on support for the development of attachment between parents and baby, they have included a number of factors that will be important in this aim. For example, some schemes include an element of extra social support by midwives, visits to the woman and family in their home, a community presence and a known and trusted midwife for care during labour and birth (McCourt & Page 1996).

Some of the evaluations have included indicators of positive responses of the mother to her experience of care, as well as to pregnancy and birth, and to her baby. These indicators are in part related to the nature of the attachment, at an early stage, between the mother and her baby. For example, one study undertaken in London evaluated an innovation in which the key component was the provision of a One-to-One named midwife who cared for individual women through the whole of pregnancy, labour and birth and the early weeks of the life of the baby (see Chapter 6). This evaluation of women's responses to the new form of care took the form of a controlled study including women ($N = 728$) who received the new service (the study group) and women in the control group, who received conventional care ($N = 675$).

The new service was set up in a neighbourhood that was the most deprived area served by the local maternity service. More women in the study group were in low social and occupational classes and were living in rented rather than privately owned accommodation. They were less likely to have the support of a partner and less likely to be white and English speaking. A clinical audit revealed no significant clinical differences between the groups in terms of parity or risk status. The study used a wide range of methods, including quantitative and qualitative, to ensure participation by a wide cross-section of women.

Questionnaires included validated psychosocial scales to assess any possible impact on women's psychological well-being and feelings of confidence and preparedness for giving birth and caring for the baby. Study group women were more likely to feel 'very well prepared for the birth' (18%) than control group women (12%). Feelings of preparedness for the birth were matched by feelings of confidence and preparedness for motherhood. Study group women were more likely to be very confident (51%) than control group women (39%) even though they were less likely to have a planned pregnancy (7% versus 3% initially being 'not very happy' or 'very unhappy') or the support of a partner (McCourt et al 1998).

Moreover, such systems of care allow more sensitive and personal assessments than would be possible in one-off visits in a hospital setting. Earlier, it was proposed that the assessment of the mother's 'state of mind' in relation to attachment should begin early in pregnancy. It was also suggested that if the midwife begins working with the mother early in pregnancy, the quality of this professional relationship has the potential of providing, at least in part, an alternative model of nurturing that the mother may be able to internalize to influence the sensitivity of care that she shows her infant.

It is difficult to imagine how these proposals may be be implemented if care is fragmented. Getting to know the woman over time, making visits in her own home and developing a relationship of trust are a prerequisite to this approach.

However, although such alternative systems of care may be necessary for screening for and assessing factors that are likely to support the growth of attachment between parents and baby, they may not be sufficient in themselves. Midwives practising in such new systems may well have come from settings that do not recognize the importance of issues such as attachment. They may need further education to develop a theoretical basis and the degree of personal sensitivity and wisdom to undertake the assessment, interpret the findings and provide support.

Many midwives who continue to practise in more conventional settings in which fragmented care is the norm will find that the extent of their ability to assess and support the development of attachment is limited. Nevertheless, they will find opportunities to make some assessments and supportive interventions. Importantly, an awareness of the importance and power of a secure attachment, and the negative effect of an insecure attachment, is necessary to midwives whatever their style of practice. Such an awareness should, given the possibility of supporting or distorting the development of attachment, remind them to act with respect in all of their contacts with mothers, fathers and babies.

CONCLUSION

This chapter provides an extensive review of the literature that acts as a theoretical basis for understanding the growth of love and the development of attachment between parents and their baby. The nature of understanding over years of painstaking research has evolved to show that the development of attachment is complex and interactional.

Cycles of abuse and neglect have been acknowledged over recent years. However, the recently discovered indication that the lack of a secure attachment in itself may be associated with more negative relationship patterns over many years, and also with victimization and aggression in dyads and in groups may have important and profound consequences not only for individuals, but also for society at large.

Although the early experiences of the parents in their primary relationships are the most powerful predictor of the quality of their maternal/paternal sensitivity and relationship with their own children, it is now known that other factors may ameliorate earlier negative influences. This is an important piece of

---

Pointers for practice

- Screening to identify families who may need extra support or referral includes the assessment of a number of factors, including the history of the parents' own experience, ameliorating factors in a high-risk history, present life circumstances, the behaviour of the newborn and the quality of perinatal care.
- In her provision of sensitive care and working with the mother from early in pregnancy, the midwife may, through the quality of this relationship, provide a model of care that the mother may internalize to influence the sensitivity of care she shows her infant.
- It is important to remember that the nature and behaviour of the baby will be a factor in the development of attachment. The use of a newborn behavioural assessment scale and its interpretation to the parents may help to prevent the parents feeling rejected by their baby.
- It is important to bear in mind the effect of postnatal depression on the mother's ability to respond to the needs of her child and, indirectly, on the organization and quality of the home.

information for midwives, who may otherwise believe that there is little they can do to support the development of attachment.

A number of specific approaches to the assessment of families and to support for the process of attachment have been proposed for midwives to integrate into their practice. Many may be reluctant to become involved in such approaches, being fearful of interfering in the private domain of family relationships and of labelling parents from an early stage, yet the importance of laying down a secure attachment should make such an approach as important as is the assessment of parents with high-risk pregnancies, for example. It should be remembered that this is a unique opportunity, and may be the only opportunity, to identify parents who may need extra support.

Many midwives practise in institutions that are dominated by machines, strict medical protocols, routines and a lack of time to do those things which matter. It may be difficult in such situations to remember that the way in which we treat women and their partners, and their babies when they are born, may have profound and longlasting consequences. However, the power of the attachment between the parents and their baby, and of the need for enduring commitment for survival and well-being, as well as the ability of the midwife to support, disturb or distort its development, is fundamental to the birth of the family.

The midwife may, through the sensitivity of her care, particularly influence the mother, and perhaps also the father, aiding the development of the parental sensitivity that is fundamental to the future of the baby.

REFERENCES

Ainsfield E, Casper V, Nozyce M, Cunningham N 1990 Does infant carrying promote attachment: an experimental study of the effects of increased physical contact on the development of attachment. Child Development 61: 1617–27

Ainsworth M D 1967 Infancy in Uganda. Johns Hopkins Press, Baltimore

Ainsworth M D 1973 The development of infant–mother attachment. In: Caldwell B M, Ricciuti N (eds) Review of child development research, vol. 3, University of Chicago Press, Chicago

Ainsworth M D, Eichberg C 1991 Effects on infant–mother attachment of mother's unresolved loss of an attachment figure. In: Parkes C M, Stevenson-Hinde J, Marris P (eds) Attachment across the life cycle. Routledge, London

Ainsworth M D, Blehar M C, Water E, Wall S 1978 Patterns of attachment: a psychological study of the strange situation. Lawrence Erlbaum, Hillsdale, NJ

Barrera M E, Rosenbaum P L 1992 Supporting parents and promoting attachment. In: Sinclair J C, Bracken M B (eds) Effective care of the newborn infant. Oxford University Press, Oxford

Belsky J, Pensky E 1988 Developmental history personality and family relationships: toward an emergent family system. In: Hinde R A, Stevenson-Hinde J (eds) Relationships within families: mutual influences. Oxford University Press, New York

Belsky J, Rovine M J 1988 Nonmaternal care in the first year of life and security of infant–parent attachment. Child Development 59: 157–67

Belsky J, Lang M, Rovinge M 1985 Stability and change in marriage across the transition to parenthood: a second study. Journal of Marriage and the Family 47: 855–65

Bowlby J 1969 Attachment and loss, vol. 1. Basic Books, New York

Bowlby J 1973 Attachment and loss, vol. II. Basic Books, New York

Bowlby J 1980 Attachment and loss, vol. III. Basic Books, New York

Bowlby J 1988 A secure base. Basic Books, New York

Bowlby J 1991 Ethological light on the psychoanalytical problems. In Bateson P (ed.) Development and integration of behaviour. Cambridge University Press, Cambridge

Brazelton T B 1979 Behavioural competence of the newborn infant. Seminars in Perinatology 3: 35–44

Brazelton T B 1981 On becoming a family. Delacorte, New York

Brazelton T B 1984 Neonatal behavioural assessment scale. JB Lippincott, Philadelphia

Brazelton T B, Cramer B C 1990 The earliest relationship: parents, infants and the drama of early attachment. Addison-Wesley, Reading, MA

Clulow C F 1989 To have and to hold: marriage, the first baby and preparing couples for parenthood. Aberdeen University Press, Aberdeen

Colin V L 1996 Human attachment. Temple University Press, Philadelphia

Connel D B 1976 Individual difference in attachment: an investigation into stability, implications and relationships to structure in early language development. Unpublished doctoral dissertation, Syracuse University, Syracuse

Crockenberg S B 1981 Infant irritability, mother responsiveness, and social support influences on the security of infant–mother attachment. Child Development 57: 857–69

DeLozier P 1982 Attachment theory and child abuse. In: Parkes C M, Stevenson-Hinde J (eds) The place of attachment in human relationships. Basic Books, New York

Egeland B, Jacobvitz D K, Sroufe L A 1988 Breaking the cycle of abuse. Child Development 59: 1071–88

Egeland B, Kalkoske M, Gottesman N, Erickon M F (1990) Patterns of aggression beyond the preschool years. Journal of Child Psychology, Psychiatry and Related Disciplines 31: 891–908

Garcia J, Redshaw M, Fitzsimons B, Keene J 1998 First class delivery: a national survey of women's views of maternity care. Audit Commission and the National Perinatal Epidemiology Unit, London

George C, Kaplan N, Main M 1985 The adult attachment interview. Unpulished manuscript. Department of Psychology, University of California at Berkely

Goldsmith H H, Alansky J A 1987 Maternal and infant temperamental predictors of attachment: a meta-analytic review. Journal of Consulting and Clinical Psychology: 805–16

James B 1989 Treating traumatized children: new insights and creative interventions. Lexington Books, Lexington, MA

Kagan J 1982 Psychological research on the human infant: an evaluative summary. WT Grant Foundation, New York

Kaufman J, Ziegler E 1987 Do abused children become abusive parents? American Journal of Orthopsychiatry 57 (2): 186–191

Klaus M H, Kennell J H 1976 Maternal–infant bonding. CV Mosby, St Louis

Klaus M H, Kennell J H 1982 Parent infant bonding. CV Mosby, St Louis

Klaus M H, Kennell J H, Klaus P H 1995 Bonding: building the foundations of secure attachment and dependence. Addison-Wesley, New York

Littlewood J, McHugh N 1997 Maternal distress and postnatal depression: the myth of Madonna. Macmillan, Basingstoke

Lyons-Ruth K, Connell D B, Gruenbaum H U, Botein S 1990 Infants at social risk: maternal depression and family support services as mediators of infant development and security of attachment. Child Development 37: 671–4

McCourt C, Page L A 1996 Report on the evaluation of One-to-One midwifery practice. TVU, London

McCourt C, Page L A, Hewison J, Vail A 1998 Evaluation of One-to-One midwifery: women's responses. Birth 25(2): 73–80

Pearce J C 1993 Evolution's end. Harper, San Francisco

Sroufe L A 1991 An organizational perspectie on the self. In: Cicchetti D, Beeghly M (eds.) The self in transition. University of Chicago Press, Chicago

Sroufe L A 1996 Emotional development: the organization of emotional life in the early years. Cambridge University Press, Cambridge

Troy M, Sroufe L A 1987 Victimisation among preschoolers: role of attachment relationship history. Journal of American Academy of Child and Adolescent Psychiatry. 26: 166–172

Van Ijzendoorn M H 1992 Intergenerational transmission of parenting: a review of studies of nonclinical populations. Developmental Review 12: 76–92

Van Ijzendoorn M H, Femmie J, Duyvesteyn G C 1995 Breaking the intergenerational cycle of insecure attachment: a review of attachment based interventions on maternal sensitivity and infant security. Child Development 63: 463–73

Vaughn B E, Stevenson-Hinde J, Waters E et al 1992 Attachment security and temperament in infancy and early childhood. Developmental Psychology 28: 463–73

Waters E 1978 The reliability and stability of individual differences in infant-mother attachment. Child Development. 49: 483–494

Werner E 1989 High risk children in young adulthood: a longitudinal study from birth to 32 years of life. In Hinde R, Stevenson-Hinde J (eds.) Relationships within families: mutual influences. Clarendon Press, New York

Zeanah C H 1993 Handbook of infant mental health. Guildford Press, London

FURTHER READING

Beeghley M, Cicchetti D 1994 Child maltreatment, attachment and the self system: emergence of an internal state lexicon in toddlers at high social risk. Development and Psychopathology 6: 6–30

Belsky J, Newzworski T 1988 Clinical implications of attachment. Lawrence Erlbaum, Hillsdale, NJ

Berger A M, Knutston J F, Mehm J G, Perkins K A 1988 The self-report of punitive childhood experiences of young adults and adolescents. Child Abuse and Neglect 12: 251–62

Bloom K C 1996 The development of attachment behaviours in pregnant adolescents. Nursing Research 44: 284–9

Brazelton T B, Yogman M W 1986 Affective development in infancy. Ablex, New Jersey

Caspi A, Elder G H 1988 Emergent family patterns: the intergenerational consturction of problem behaviour and relationships. In Hinde R & Stevenson-Hinde J (eds.) Relationships within families: mutual influences. Clarendon Press, Oxford

Cicchetti D, Barnett D 1991 Attachment organization in maltreated preschoolers. Development and Psychopathology 3: 397–441

Cicchetti D, Beeghly M 1991 The self in transition: infancy to childhood. University of Chicago Press, Chicago

Cicchetti D, Carlson V 1989 Child maltreatment. Cambridge University Press, New York

Cicchetti D, Greenberg M T 1991 The legacy of John Bowlby. Development and Psychopathology 3: 347–50

Crittenden P M, Ainsworth M D S 1989 Child maltreatment and attachment theory. In: Cicchetti D, Carlson V (eds) Child maltreatment: theory and research in the causes and consequences of child abuse and neglect. Cambridge University Press, New York

Crittenden P M, DiLella D L 1988 Compulsive compliance: the development of inhibitory coping strategy in infancy. Journal of Abnormal Child Psychology 16: 585–99

Donavan D M, McIntyre J M 1990 Healing the hurt child. New York: Norton

Egeland B, Erickson M F 1993 Attachment theory and findings: implications for prevention and intervention. In: Kramer S, Parens H (eds) Prevention in mental health: now, tomorrow and ever? Jaon Aronson, Northvale, NJ

Erickson M F, Egeland B, Pianta R 1989 The effects of maltreatment on the development of young children. In: Cicchetti D, Carlson V (eds) Child maltreatment. Cambridge University Press, New York

Erickson M F, Sroufe L A, Egeland B R 1992 The relationship between quality of attachment and behaviour problems in preschool in a high-risk sample. In Bretherton I & Waters E (eds.) Growing points of attachment theory and research. Monographs of the

Society of Research in Child Development, 50 (1–2, serial no. 209): 147–166

Fraiberg S, Adelson E, Shapiro V 1975 Ghosts in the nursery: a psychoanalytic approach to the problem of impaired infant–mother relationships. Journal of the American Academy of Child Psychiatry 14: 387–423

Gil G, Fisher K W 1996 Development and vulnerability in close relationships. Lawrence Erlbaum, Makaway, NJ

Greenberg M T, Cicchetti D, Cummings E M 1990 Attachment in the preschool years. University of Chicago Press, Chicago

Grossman K, Fremer-Bombik E 1988 Maternal attachment representation as related to patterns of mother-infant attachment and maternal care during the first years of life. In Hinde R & Stevenson-Hindle J (eds.) Relationship within families: mutual influences. Clarendon Press, New York

Guidano V F 1987 Complexity of the self. Guildford Press, London

Herrenkhol E C, Herrenkhol R C 1983 Perspectives on the intergenerational transmission of abuse. In Finkelhor D (ed) The dark side of familes. Sage, New York

Holmes J 1993 John Bowlby and attachment. Routledge, London

Jacobson S W, Frye K F 1991 Effect of maternal social support on attachment. Child Development 62: 572–82

Lamb M E, Thompson R A, Gardner W, Carnov E L 1985 Infant–mother attachment. Lawrence Erlbaum, NJ

Leifer M, Wax L, Morrison M 1989 The use of multitreatment modalities in early intervention: a quantitative case study. Infant Mental Health Journal 10: 100–16

Lewis J M, Owen M T, Cox M J 1988 The transition to parenthood: III. Incorporation of the child into the family. Family Process, 27: 411–421

Lieberman A F, Weston R R, Pawl J H 1991 Preventive intervention and outcome in anxiously attached dyads. Child Development 62: 199–209

Lynch M, Cicchetti D 1991 Patterns of relatedness in maltreated and nonmaltreated children: connections among multiple representational models. Development and Psychopathology 3: 207–26

McCrone E R, Egeland B, Kalkoske M, Carlson E A 1994 Relations between early maltreatment and mental representation of relationships assessed with projective storytelling in middle childhood. Development and Psychopathology 6: 99–120

Mahler M, Pine F, Bergman A 1975 The psychological birth of the human infant. Basic Books, New York

Main M, Goldwyn R 1984 Predicting rejection of her infant from mother's representation of her own experience: implications for the abused-abusing cycle. Child Abuse and Neglect, 8: 203–217

Main M, Goldwyn R 1985 Adult attachment classification rating system. Unpublished manuscript, University of California, Berkely

Main M, Weston D 1981 The quality of the toddler's relationship to mother and father: related to conflict behaviour and readiness to establish relationships. Child Development, 52: 932–940

Main M, Kaplan N, Cassidy J 1985 Security in infancy, childhood and adulthood: a move to the levels of representation. In: Bretherton I & Waters E (eds) Growing points in attachment theory and research. Monographs of the Society for Research in Child Development, 50: 66–104

Ney B G 1988 Transgenerational abuse. Child Psychiatry and Human Development, 18 (3): 151–168

Parkes C M, Stevenson-Hinde J 1982 The place of attachment in human behaviour. Tavistock Publications, London

Parkes C M, Stevenson-Hinde J, Marris P 1988 Attachment across the life span. Routledge, London

Stern M H, Goldberg S, Kroonenberg P M, Oded J F 1992 The relative effects of maternal and child problems on the quality of attachment: a meta-analysis of attachment in clinical samples. Child Development 63: 840–58

West M L, Sheldon-Keller A 1994 Patterns of relating: an adult attachment perspective. Guildford Press, New York

Winnicott D W 1987 The child, the family and the outside world. Addison-Wesley, Reading, MA

Zeanah C H, Zeanah P D 1989 Intergenerational transmission of maltreatment: insights from attachment theory and research. Psychiatry 52: 177–98

12

Social support in childbirth

Christine McCourt
Patricia Percival

Birth in its social context

In chapter 10, we learnt about the importance of viewing pregnancy and birth as part of the life course of a woman and her family. From the woman's point of view, birth is not so much a medical event as a major transition in her life, a transition that implies major changes in personal and social identity and roles (Kitzinger 1989). The meaning of pregnancy and birth is broad and complex, taking its form within a web of cultural and social influences, and within a life history.

We have noted how ritual processes, in all cultures and in a range of situations, are involved in the management of transition. Although much medical treatment has a ritual basis or a ritual aspect (Jordan 1993, Davis-Floyd 1994), this is generally out of the context of the lives of patients and their families or communities (McCourt-Perring 1993, Good 1994). Rituals of hospital birth in particular do not necessarily provide social or emotional support to the woman and her family but may respond to the particular needs of the institution or those working within it (Kirkham 1989, Hunt & Symonds 1995).

Since birth takes place in a social context and, as anthropologists have emphasized, is a social as well as physiological act, social support has been an important aspect of pregnancy and birth care historically and in most, if not all, cultures (Towler & Bramall 1986, Kitzinger 1989, Jordan 1993). Medicine in European and North American societies, which social scientists refer to as biomedicine, is unusual in the degree to which such aspects of care have been overlooked in its development (Young 1981). For example, Kitzinger points out that, although in most societies, women kin and neighbours have important roles in supporting women giving birth, with the development of obstetrics, lay women were gradually excluded from birthing environments. She notes that, as recently as 1975, popular obstetric texts advised against the presence of birth companions, suggesting that 'old wives tales' and stories would frighten women giving birth (Bourne 1975, quoted in Kitzinger 1989). This approach is linked to the mind/body dichotomy in biomedical thinking (Helman 1994) and practice, in which, instead of being seen as part of life, childbirth in the modern obstetric unit is set apart from the context of the woman's life. When such a view of birth prevails, an understanding of social or cultural issues, if sought at all, is often geared to understanding the way in which beliefs, attitudes and behaviour may impede the practice of medical care (Young 1981, 1982).

However, an increasing amount of social science and midwifery research has explored the issue of social support for childbearing women and the role that the maternity services might play in offering or facilitating rather than undermining such supports to women. Reviewing key areas of this research, this chapter explores the concept of social support, what it means, why it appears to influence health and how it might be incorporated more fully within maternity care.

What is social support?

The term 'social support' sounds vague and catch-all, something that we assume to be, by definition, a good thing, without really understanding what it is or whether it has any measurable value. Its meaning is taken for granted in such a way that it is rarely discussed, yet concepts of support are likely to be culturally and socially variable. This produces problems in researching social support since the underlying assumptions or theoretical frameworks of the work are not always spelt out (House 1981, Tilden 1985). Wheatley, discussing psychosocial support in pregnancy and birth, refers to the broad but simple definition used by the psychologists Schumaker & Brownell (1984, p. 13):

an exchange of resources between at least two individuals perceived by the provider or recipient to be intended to enhance the well-being of the recipient.

Similarly, Madge & Marmot (1987, quoted in Oakley 1992, p. 26) note that:

there seems to be little controversy … that something about social relationships can be good for health, although quite what is important remains unclear.

Critical reviews of social support research have identified several conceptual and methodological flaws that are inherent in many social support studies. These include the overall atheoretical stance; a lack of definitional consensus; the consideration of social support as a single rather than a multifaceted measure; measures with limited reliability and validity; an emphasis on the quantity rather than the quality of support; and a tendency to ignore the negative side of social interactions (Cohen & McKay 1983; Rook 1984; Schumaker & Brownell 1984; Kessler et al 1985, Thoits 1985, Heller et al 1986).

The problem with many definitions is that they appear tautological, implying simply that social support is a relationship that is perceived as supportive. It is helpful, therefore, to break such general definitions down into different attributes and operationalize them. The simplest distinction that is commonly drawn is by describing social support as either emotional or practical in nature. Because of the importance of the emotional elements of support, it tends to be described quite interchangeably as either social or psychosocial support. Research on what people understand as social support has consistently identified a set of key components of the concept (House 1981):

- *Emotional support.* This is probably the aspect most commonly associated with the concept of social support. The term implies a warm or caring relationship, but emotional support may be as simple as presence or companionship and a willingness to listen. Some commentators also emphasize the role of conveying esteem in emotional support.
- *Informational support.* Being given good information and advice is widely perceived as supportive. It underlies the ability to make positive choices, as well as increasing confidence and a sense of security. It may also help by increasing the personal sense of control.
- *Practical or tangible support.* The type of practical support may vary widely, and its importance should not be underestimated. It may include financial support for a pregnant woman or physical comfort measures during labour and birth, for example.

The features of social support also overlap considerably with those identified for caring, and these terms are often used interchangeably. Like words such as 'community' or 'support', 'care' is a term commonly used by those providing services, one that has overwhelmingly positive associations. It is a very broad concept that, despite being central to the philosophy and practice of nursing and midwifery, is often left undefined (Leininger 1988). The sociologist Bulmer (1987), discussing the problems of what we mean by such terms, described care as having two key forms:

1. *caring for*, which may include physical tending or providing material and psychological resources, depending on the person's need;
2. *caring about*, which may not mean providing direct

care but involves concern that is supportive, on an individual or a more general level.

The first is a form of labour and is generally more onerous and involved. The second may also have valuable support functions, but it is important to conceptually distinguish different forms of support that may be more or less relevant for different people and situations. Additionally, it is important to distinguish quality of support from the number or simple existence of social relationships (Hall et al 1987).

What does social support do?

Social support is widely assumed to be beneficial by its very nature, but evidence from psychological, sociological and health research indicates that it is possible to measure and identify particular benefits of such support. As we shall see later in this chapter, much of the midwifery and maternity research evidence focuses on possible benefits for the physical health of mothers and babies. This represents, perhaps, a desire to investigate what will be regarded as 'hard' evidence of benefit (Oakley 1992). There is also research evidence of psychological health benefits, although these are not in any case entirely distinct outcomes: psychological benefits may enhance physical health and vice versa. This will be discussed below in looking at concepts of health. Equally, the importance of the more intangible, difficult to measure, aspects of well-being should not be underestimated. If providing supportive care enhances a woman's happiness or satisfaction with the experience of pregnancy, without incurring risks or other losses for her, perhaps this should be viewed as sufficient in its own right (Elbourne et al 1989).

Oakley (1992) reviews a range of studies providing evidence that social support influences physical and psychological health. Among the best known is a large-scale, community-based study of patterns of mortality in the USA (Cohen & Syme 1987). This study showed that long-term survival correlated with social support independently of other potentially related factors such as initial physical health, social status or habits such as smoking. Generally, social involvement predicted better survival, but the types of involvement that mattered differed for men and women. Similar patterns of correlation have been found for psychological health (Cobb 1976, Ganster & Victor 1988).

The mechanisms by which social support 'works', for example to have a positive impact on health, are not clearly understood, but there is a great deal of evidence that social support works on a number of levels because health is multifaceted and influenced by a wide range of physiological, environmental and social factors. The approach of biomedicine has been rooted in an epistemology that tends to view such issues as separate. Research into social support and health adds weight to the alternative view that such factors are closely interrelated – what some commentators have described as an ecological view of health (Arney 1982, Scheper-Hughes & Lock 1987, see also the philosophy adopted and set out in the 1997 UK government White Paper on the health service, NHSME 1997).

How does social support work?

Although, as noted above, the precise mechanisms by which social support may influence health are unclear, psychologists have outlined several theories of the functions of social support. These include the key hypotheses that:

- social support acts as a buffer against stress (Cobb 1976);
- it assists the development of coping strategies that support health (Wheatley 1998).

Such theories are relatively individualistic, focusing on ways in which individual choices or behaviour may influence health. They also rely on the concept of stress as a key factor in health and illness (Young 1980, Pollock 1988). Oakley (1992) adds to the stress theory two hypotheses that are more sociological in orientation:

- that social support makes the experience of stress less likely;
- that it facilitates recovery from illness.

Social support, therefore, is widely viewed as protective against the negative effects of psychosocial risk factors on health. These risk factors include demographic characteristics (such as being poor or old), psychological factors (such as a previous history of depression) and adverse health habits (such as smoking) (Culpepper & Jack 1993; see also Chapter 7). Stress is part of everyday life and is increased during periods of considerable change, for example pregnancy, changing home or job, or bereavement (Murray-Parkes 1971, Marris 1974). Such psychological risk factors appear to play a role in reducing the person's ability to cope with stress, or encourage responses to stress that may not benefit health. The 'buffering' hypothesis suggests that psychosocial supports can help to counteract such negative effects (Wheatley 1998).

Aaronson, discussing the stress-buffering hypothesis, highlights Broadhead's argument that social support is both an outcome of healthy social competence and a contributory cause of good health (Broadhead et al 1983, Aaronson 1989). In this view, the effects of social support (or a lack of it) are likely to be iterative and self-confirming: those with good health or social resources are more likely to obtain social support, encouraging a cycle of positive health benefit. This hypothesis is supported by the longer-term research conducted on social support in pregnancy, suggesting that receiving supportive services may enhance a woman's ability to obtain and draw on other potential sources of support (Olds et al 1986, Oakley et al 1996).

It has also been argued that social support has direct health-enhancing effects: take, for example, Henderson's (1977) view that support is a basic human need that must be satisfied for an individual to enjoy a sense of well-being. Biomedical research on stress suggests that the mechanism by which social support may mediate the effects of stress, or directly influence health, may be endocrinological (hormonal), biochemical or via the immune system. For example, Teixeira, Fisk & Glover's (1999) study of umbilical blood flow indicates lower levels of blood flow in mothers who are stressed or anxious, pointing to links between stress, anxiety and relevant physiological processes. Psychological researchers have also argued that the majority of beneficial effects of support are cognitively mediated, in that perceptions of support may influence a person's interpretation of stressors, knowledge of coping strategies and self-concept (Cohen & McKay 1983, Procidano & Heller 1983).

Perceived and received support

In attempting to define social support so that it can be measured or studied, it is helpful to distinguish between perceived and received support, since support that is given but not perceived as such may be ineffective (Cohen & Wills 1985, Kessler & Mcleod 1985), and it is the perceived adequacy of support that has been found, in some studies, to relate positively to mental or physical health (Barrera 1986, Hirsch & Rapkin 1986). Perceived support – that which the person recognizes as support – may differ from what might be counted by another person as support given. In a study of what influences women's health behaviour during pregnancy, Aaronson (1989) found that both perceived and received support had independent positive effects on women's ability to modify behaviours such as drinking alcohol or smoking. This research supported the argument that social support may act as a buffer against stress but also suggested that social support may 'work' by enhancing an adherence to 'healthy' behaviour (Cobb 1976). Perceptions of support may also be enhanced by clarifying what

support is expected or available, since a difference between expectation and experience is likely to be unhelpful (Levitt et al 1993).

Wheatley (1998) points out that the type of support that is helpful, and whether quantity or quality of support is more important, is likely to vary. The support needs of first- and second-time parents, for example, are likely to be different (Jordan 1989, Gottlieb & Mendelson 1995). The psychological concept of person–environment fit is related to the potential for difference between perceived and received support (Cohen & McKay 1983). Whereas a good fit between the support offered and what is perceived as supportive enhances its effectiveness, a poor fit may be ineffective or have negative results, for example by undermining a person's sense of confidence or personal control. Increasing research emphasis is now being placed on understanding the influence of 'negative support' (Henderson 1980, Strauss 1980, Wellman 1981, Fiore et al 1983, Rook 1984, Shinn et al 1984, Antonucci 1985, Paykel 1985, Barrera 1986, Lehman et al 1986, Tilden & Galyen 1987). Support may be viewed negatively, for example if it is perceived to be overprotective or lacking in understanding. Additionally, expectations of support that are not met may have negative consequences (Gore 1978). Social ties or relationships – either personal or professional – cannot simply be assumed to be beneficial. Similarly, Oakley (1992) highlights the possibility of health professionals offering support or care that is not helpful. This issue will be discussed when considering the roles of maternity services – and their limitations – in offering social support.

HEALTH AS A SOCIAL CONCEPT
What is health?

In this volume, we refer to a broad definition of health that fits closely with the philosophy and approaches of midwifery and with the weight of sociological and clinical evidence. The World Health Organization (1946) has promoted such a view, defining health as:

a state of complete physical, mental and social well-being, and not merely the absence of disease or infirmity.

While this definition outlines an ideal, perhaps reflecting the optimism and reforming focus of the post-war years in Europe, it acknowledges the broad range of possible influences on health and advocates a positive rather than reactive approach. More recently (World Health Organization 1986), the organization has increased its focus on community action rather than just education or preventive health care for the promotion of health (Crafter 1997).

Anthropological concepts

Jordan, in her cross-cultural study of midwifery, argued for a *biosocial* framework, an integrated approach recognizing that the spheres of physiology, psychology, culture and social science 'constantly challenge all our efforts to separate them' (Jordan 1993, p. 3).

The assumption that mind and body are separate, so can be treated and studied separately – described as *dualism* – has played an important role in the origins of biomedicine in Euro-American society. This approach to knowledge formed part of enlightenment thinking in the Europe of the 18th century and was set out most clearly in the work of the French philosopher, Descartes (1912). What has become known as Cartesian theory set out a mechanical view of the body, with a metaphor of the body as a machine in which mind or spirit and body were consequently viewed as separate (Helman 1994). Scheper-Hughes & Lock (1987) describe the need to use such terms as 'biosocial' or 'psychosocial' as reflections of the fragmentation caused by Cartesian epistemology. Such integrated approaches, viewing physiological processes as not readily separable from a host of other influences on health, reject Cartesian philosophy and is more closely in line with post-modern thinking in the natural sciences (Capra 1983).

Anthropologists studying health care systems have drawn a theoretical distinction between the concepts of illness, sickness and disease (Young 1982, Stacey 1988). In this model, the concepts of illness, disease and sickness are understood as normatively defined, despite their biological base, so are culturally variable.

- *Illness* is understood in terms of the experience of the person who is ill. It is primarily a personal and psychological state. People may experience illness without any external or symptomatic evidence of disease.
- *Disease* is a pathological condition defined in terms of indicators agreed between biomedical practitioners. Disease may exist without a state of illness, where no symptoms are experienced by the person with the disease or where the symptoms are culturally defined as normal.
- *Sickness*, a concept working on a social or societal level, often focusing on the functional consequences of illness or disease. Put simply, a person is defined as sick when illness or disease prevents the performance of normal social roles.

This theoretical approach is useful for health professionals in terms of understanding that illness is multi-faceted and that its definition, prevention and treatment are far from simple. It also provides a cultural framework for understanding why pregnancy and birth can be viewed differently – as a normal state or as pathological, a state of sickness – according to the varying perspectives of those involved.

Influences on health

It is a common but misconceived assumption that the study of health is primarily about the study of medicine or the health services. Social historians and epidemiologists (McKeown 1979, Stacey 1988) have established that the factors influencing health are varied and complex, medicine playing a relatively peripheral role in public health.

The issues are complex, and the particular roles of different factors influencing health are difficult to pick out, so that questions and arguments remain about the ways in which the many factors are at play in influencing the health of an individual or a population. These arguments are set out clearly in epidemiological work on inequalities in health (Whitehead 1987, Townsend et al 1988, Wilcox et al 1995).

The health of individuals, when they are viewed as part of a population or a social group, form clear patterns that correlate with socio-economic and cultural patterns such as those of social class. The concept of class, like that of health or community, is difficult to pin down and define clearly. Most people have a feel for what it means and can identify some criteria for defining class, but it shares properties of symbolic systems in being multivocal, having a range of meanings at different levels, which are implicit rather than explicit and assumed to be shared. This stems from the fact that class is not an entity in itself – a thing that can cause something, such as good or bad health – but a form of categorization (Oakley 1992) that refers to the processes of people's lives as much as the structures. It is important, therefore, to try to understand which aspects of the life experiences and conditions of people in different 'classes' may make a difference to health. In the UK, the Registrar General's definition, based on occupational criteria, is used in the collation of health and other government statistics. The Jarman index (Jarman 1991) is an alternative measurement system, focusing on area-based indicators of socio-economic deprivation. These statistics have consistently revealed that, in the UK, people in social class V, or with higher deprivation scores, have far higher mortality and morbidity than those in higher social classes. The epidemiology of health is discussed more fully in Chapter 16.

THE ROLE OF HEALTH SERVICES

Maintaining health and preventing illness?

We have noted above the historical and epidemiological argument that health services play a relatively peripheral role in reproducing health, however important particular medical interventions may be to individuals with health problems. In discussing the importance of choice, continuity and control in the maternity services, Sandall (1995) reminds readers that assumptions are made in health policy documents about social support (Department of Health 1993) that may ignore the importance of social structure and inequality in maternal and child health (National Children's Home and Maternity Alliance 1995, Wilcox et al 1995, Roberts 1997). Sandall notes that successive government reports have assumed that medical intervention will compensate for the health effects of adverse social circumstances. The Winterton Report's (House of Commons 1992) advocacy of wider social policy changes alongside maternity services reform was not reflected in the brief of the Expert Maternity Group, which was confined to maternity services (Department of Health 1993).

The area in which services seek to influence public health is primarily in the prevention of illness and the maintenance of health, through health education, promotion and screening or immunization programmes. Preventive health care has been described as working on three levels (Robertson 1988, Turton & Orr 1993):

1. *primary*: before a disease process starts, for example immunization or advice on nutrition or accident prevention;
2. *secondary*: to alleviate or arrest disease, such as screening, early diagnosis and treatment, and dental checks;
3. *tertiary*: to limit or alleviate the effects of disease or illness, for example rehabilitation.

Since midwives focus on both the care of normal pregnancy and birth and the prevention or detection of possible health problems, their work spans all three.

Health promotion is described by Crafter as a broader concept than health education, which primarily seeks to change individual behaviour (Crafter 1997, Jones & Sidell 1997). A focus on health education alone relates closely to the behavioural/cultural theory of social patterns of health, a perspective that assumes that health is mainly influenced by individual lifestyles and behaviour, without acknowledging the impact of social and political conditions on the choices that people make. Health promotion, recognizing the complexity of influences on health, also includes community action, aiming towards structural changes. This approach is supported by evidence from recent research on the problems and limitations of health education (Graham 1984, Farrant & Russell 1986).

Treatment – caring or curing?

Once a person becomes ill, or identifies themselves as ill, the role of the health services is to provide treatment aimed at the diagnosis, cure or alleviation of the illness symptoms. Treatment can be conceptually divided into *curing* and *caring*, a distinction that follows closely the traditional gender divisions in society and the different roles of medical and nursing staff. The distinction is, of course, often blurred in practice, particularly where people suffer from long-term illness or disability. Curing is conventionally viewed as active, while caring is viewed as supportive (Leininger 1988).

In UK maternity services, the distinction has been marked out particularly clearly as the boundary between the primary roles of midwifery and obstetrics. While the encroachment of obstetric practices into care for 'normal' pregnancy and birth has weakened the boundary set up by the 1902 Midwives Act, recent policy shifts back in the direction of community-based services could be said to have shifted the caring/curing division towards one between hospital and community-based care (Robinson 1989, McCourt 1998).

The enduring importance of *care* in the provision of health services reflects the nature of health needs, including the need for social support. As Oakley (1993), has highlighted the use of placebo effects (from the Latin for 'I please') in medical research highlights the importance of providing care and support in the maintenance or restoration of health. The ways in which the placebo has been understood in biomedicine reflect an artificial dichotomy between pleasing the patient and benefiting the patient. Oakley reviews a range of studies to illustrate this point in which placebos have shown health benefits, in a number of cases benefits as effective as those gained from recognized biomedical treatments (Oakley 1992). Evidence that levels of social support influence health illuminate the enduring importance of *care* as an aspect of all healing.

THE ROLE OF SOCIAL SUPPORT IN MATERNAL AND CHILD HEALTH

Although it is clear that material conditions have an

important influence on health, the multidimensional nature of concepts such as social class shows that factors such as occupation, for example, influence experiences as diverse as social isolation (Brown & Harris 1978) and responses to stress (Paine 1982) as well as people's material conditions. Social networks form an important component of people's social position (Bott 1971), which may make a profound difference to how they cope with their living conditions.

What service users perceive as support

Research findings on how 'ordinary people' view social support correspond well with social and psychological theories. Gottlieb, for example (1978, quoted in Oakley 1992), found that what people valued most were:

- emotionally sustaining behaviours, for example listening, showing concern and conveying intimacy;
- problem-solving behaviours such as material and financial help.

Studies of women's experiences and perceptions of pregnancy and birth are highly consistent in indicating what they see as supportive maternity care. This includes good communication: not only being given information, but also being listened to and being able to discuss concerns, options and so on, being treated as individuals, having a sense of choice and control over what happens to them (Green et al 1988, Reid & Garcia 1989, Hirst et al 1998). Being focused on the role of services, such studies tend to overlook the important role of informal sources of support, personal networks or non-health services, but the general principles could be applied to lay (informal) or professional (formal) support.

In a comparative study of women's responses to maternity care (McCourt et al 1998), the authors found that a number of features of care were related to women's feelings of being supported by the maternity services. These included good mutual communication and exchange of information, knowing carers and feeling known by them. Such relationships appeared to enhance the women's sense of trust, confidence and control in both themselves and service providers, and the perception of professionals as sensitive and caring. Importantly, this pattern of responses was found across a range of social and ethnic groups (Harper-Bulman & McCourt 1997).

Studies of women in different social class and ethnic groups (MORI 1993, Handler et al 1996, Laslett et al

1997, Hirst et al 1998) suggest that such core principles are relevant to a wide range of women rather than being confined to an articulate minority. Women's specific concerns about support do vary, however, as do their specific experiences of health care, many women in minority groups, for example, experiencing greater communication problems with service providers (see above) and evidence showing that women in lower social-class groups receive poorer information from service providers (Cartwright 1979, Reid & Garcia 1989, Walker et al 1995).

In a US study of women's views about nursing support during labour, the most helpful behaviours identified included: feeling cared about as an individual and treated with respect, praise, staff appearing calm and confident, and assistance with breathing and relaxing. The study used an instrument listing 25 potentially supportive behaviours, which a group of four nurse-midwives were asked to categorize as emotional, informational or tangible support. The women regarded all the categories as important, but behaviours categorized as emotional support were perceived as the most helpful by the women (Bryanton et al 1994). The authors note that these findings were highly consistent with those of previous studies of women's views of support, even when different methods, samples and terminology were used.

Who can provide it?

It is easy for health or other service providers to assume that they are the main sources of support for those who use the service. The majority of women will look for and gain most of their support from 'informal' sources: family, friends and neighbours. The importance of ordinary social networks is such that women who are socially isolated – those with a limited number of contacts, or who have a lack of close and supportive relationships with their social contacts – are more likely to suffer depression (Brown & Harris 1978). This means that much social support does not and need not come from professionals or formal service providers. This argument is backed up by those trials of support in labour that have used lay rather than professional companions and by studies of additional pregnancy support provided by non-professionals. This does not detract, however, from the importance of service providers offering supportive care, either to complement women's ordinary social networks, to substitute for them in specific ways where they are lacking or to work in such a way as to enhance or back up the informal sources of support on which women rely.

Formal and informal care

Care or support provided by professionals and 'lay' people is often referred to in the policy literature as formal and informal care respectively (Willmot 1986). These two forms of care have been much discussed in terms of community care policy for people who need long-term support, such as older people. Social scientists have explored the implications of community care policy by studying the role of kin, friends and neighbours as carers. In many cases, informal carers will be women, but men may also play an important role in providing care for their partners. Abrams, in his seminal study of neighbourhood care (Bulmer 1986), argued that kin, friendships and neighbourhood relationships are of overwhelming importance in social support, so that public services should seek to facilitate such support networks where possible and avoid undermining or bypassing them.

Social network analysis

Social network analysis was first developed by social anthropologists as a route into understanding and describing social relationship patterns, both in small-scale and urbanized societies (Barnes 1954, Bott 1971). It is also widely used by sociologists and by social policy analysts, who see it as a way of avoiding an over-reliance on the concept of community, with all its problems of definition. A social network is simply a representation of the relationships or ties that any person has. It may be recorded and presented in the form of a topographical map or diagram, which may look like a spider's web, with 'ego', the individual concerned, at the centre and different individuals as points in the web.

Network analysis has been useful for tackling the methodological problems of asking people to rate their levels of social support, those with good health being more likely to rate their social support more positively. It requires researchers and respondents to be more specific about the relationships involved. Social networks can be classified or measured in various ways including according to their:

- *extent*: the number of ties or relationships and how far ranging they are;
- *density or interconnectedness*: the degree to which people in the network are linked to each other;
- *quality*: the nature and significance of relationships and whether they are close or distant;
- *type*: for example, whether they are formal or personal;

- *frequency*: how often contacts are made;
- *duration or durability*: how stable the relationships are;
- *direction or symmetry*: for example, whether the relationships are mutual or involve dependency in one direction.

For particular individuals, it may be possible to draw one network, including all types of tie, or several different networks, for example distinguishing primary or personal ties (kin, friends, some neighbours, etc.) from secondary ties (such as helping relationships with professionals or volunteers and mutual support networks).

Community theorists have noted that densely connected, durable and frequent networks are often characteristic of a traditional notion of community – as one within a discrete area and with close knit ties. Social changes such as occupational and geographical mobility mean that most people now have more extensive and loose-knit networks, with far less overlapping of ties. In an early qualitative study of 41 middle- and upper-class mothers, Abernethy (1973) examined the effects of a tight or loose social network in predicting a woman's attitude to her children and her response to the demands of the maternal role. She concluded that women in loose networks appeared to suffer from insufficient feedback and were therefore likely to be exposed to a confusing array of variance in childrearing theory. She argued that this profusion of opinion led to inconsistent maternal behaviour as well as diminishing confidence in any particular technique of childcare. Women embedded in a tight network were more likely to have confidence in their maternal competence, while those in loose networks were more likely to be frustrated by motherhood and to feel unsure of how to relate to their children.

Although such loose networks are often associated with the 'loss' of traditional communities, with all their connotations of social support (Young & Willmott 1957), sociologists have argued that they have many positive attributes and do not necessarily imply a lack of social support (Bulmer 1987). Very close-knit communities have often been associated with adverse social circumstances and conditions, and may be a response to such situations 'which diminished with rising levels of affluence, mobility and choice' (Abrams, discussed in Bulmer 1987, p. 33). Such changes may nevertheless mean that many women are now more dependent on the health services for practical and informational support than they might have been in the past.

Types of relationship in social networks are also commonly divided into those with kin (nuclear and more distant family), friends, neighbours, volunteer helpers and paid service providers. In very close-knit networks, such categories often overlap considerably. Generally, however, the nature of such relationships and the types of support they conventionally involve differ. This is important to note since the types of social support that will be offered to or seen as acceptable by an individual will differ accordingly, and they cannot generally be substituted. For example, neighbour relationships are generally called on for emergency help, short-term and reciprocal support, and general 'looking out for' or concern rather than support involving close, time-consuming contact. In contrast, kin tend to be relied on most readily for long-term support and more intimate forms of care. Where kin are not available to provide such care, professional support is most likely to be considered appropriate. Friendships are more likely to be called on for informational support and occasional or sporadic practical and personal support.

It should also be noted, as suggested above, that social ties or networks are not necessarily or always helpful or supportive. Maintaining social networks may entail personal costs such as burdens of time and resources, either practical or emotional (Tilden & Stewart 1985), that are not necessarily fully reciprocated. It is likely, in such situations, that a woman will not perceive her personal ties as supportive (Paykel 1985). Some networks or relationships may also have direct negative effects – such as in sustaining self-harming behaviours – (Strauss 1980), and the simple presence of a marital tie, which may not necessarily imply a close, confiding relationship (Brown & Harris 1978, Brown & Bifulco 1985), cannot be assumed to be supportive. It is important, therefore, to consider the quality as well as the number of social relationships when assessing social support.

Although, in many cases, midwives will not be closely concerned with the personal support networks of women in their care, it is important to remain aware of the fact that social support is, for most women, something that will come primarily, and in the longer term, from personal rather than professional sources. The support that a midwife can and should offer does not encompass the entire support network of the woman in her care. Where a woman appears to lack social support, it will be useful to bear in mind the types of relationship that are relied upon for different forms of support. Midwives can also link women to sources of support that effectively bridge professional and personal relationships, for example voluntary schemes such as Homestart or Pals in Pregnancy (a *Changing Childbirth*-related project being developed and evaluated in Coventry, UK; see Useful addresses below) or by facilitating women's mutual support groups.

In a survey of Finnish mothers, Tarkka & Paunonen (1996) found that women had a wide range of people in their social support networks, but spouses and partners, followed by parents and then friends, were the most important source of support in pregnancy. In contrast, midwives were rated as being the most important source of support during the birth. These authors divided the types of support (following Kahn 1979) into:

- *affect*: appreciation, respect or love, and creating a sense of security;
- *affirmation*: reinforcement, feedback and advice;
- *aid*: such as objects or money, or spending time to help someone.

They found that women received most support from midwives in labour in the domain of affect, and least in affirmation, younger and first-time mothers receiving more support overall. The mothers identified reception and treatment by the staff, encouragement, a sense of security, the alleviation of pain, the individuality of treatment, and continuity (the number of different midwives taking over care and overall care from a named midwife) as being important to their experience of birth. Emotional support (affect) was associated with a positive birth experience (Tarkka & Paunonen 1996).

WHAT CAN MATERNITY SERVICES DO TO OFFER SUPPORT?

Although maternity services cannot have a major impact on the factors that make some women more vulnerable than others to ill-health, midwives can make a difference – positively or negatively – as a result of their key role in supporting women in pregnancy, birth and the perinatal period. This section sets out some of the ways in which services can enhance social support and examines the evidence from research on social support and midwifery or maternity care.

Two key principles can be applied to midwifery care in this respect:

1. Avoiding harm:
   - the importance of avoiding practices that undermine support or self-esteem;
   - the need for communication and dialogue, especially when interventions are needed;
   - appreciating the impact of knowledge, choice and control on women's self-esteem and confidence, and the degree to which a

perception of a lack of control can undermine women's experience of pregnancy and birth (Green et al 1988).

2. Helping:
   - finding out what forms of support are appropriate and helpful for different women;
   - considering the meaning and impact of social support in maternity care and for individual women.

Ball, in her study of postnatal care (1994), argues that midwifery research and practice should focus on the areas of need for support that maternity services are in a position to influence, both positively and negatively. During pregnancy and the perinatal period, women have close contact with midwives and are likely to look to them, in addition to family and friends, for support. However, a number of care practices that undermine or simply make support more difficult have become routine in the past few decades. Although research has identified the lack of evidence basis for some routine practices, the impact of organizational 'cultures' tends to work against the discontinuation of established practices. One example of such developments is the routine use of continuous electronic fetal monitoring. Recent overviews of trial evidence suggest that this form of monitoring is not justified for routine use on grounds of safety (MIDIRS 1997, Thacker & Stroup 1998). More qualitative studies of its use have identified that the use of electronic monitors may decrease the personal attention and thereby support given to women (Grant 1989, Lewison 1993, Page 1993). For example, in a recent observation study (T. Stevens, unpublished report, 1998) data gathered on the delivery suite ward round, in an obstetrically orientated maternity unit with a high use of electronic monitors, revealed a strong tendency of health professionals to give attention to the monitor before giving attention to the mother herself.

In the antenatal period, one of the key areas of support identified by women (Green et al 1988, MORI 1993, Brown & Lumley 1994, McCourt & Page 1996, Proctor 1998, Hirst et al 1998) is good communication. This involves both providing clear, relevant and (as far as possible) unbiased information and most crucially, listening to the woman. Listening is a fundamental skill since it is a foundation for good communication and will give the best idea of what a woman wants and needs to know. The giving of advice is secondary to the giving of good basic information and should follow on from this if the woman seeks it.

Such communication is also a component of emotional and practical support. A midwife is unlikely to be the woman's main source of emotional support in pregnancy but may have a valuable role by showing interest, being responsive to worries or concerns and being available to discuss them. Such a role emerged as an important aspect of why women in continuity of carer schemes value such continuity so highly and why it appears to be associated with greater maternal confidence (McCourt et al 1998).

The importance of practical support should also not be underestimated. Again, midwives may have a limited role to play in providing such support, but good information or practical help with getting information, advice or referrals (e.g. for housing or financial problems) may make a difference. During the perinatal period, midwives are in a particularly good position to provide greatly needed practical support. Since, as we have noted in the previous chapters, birth is a time of tremendous social, physical and psychological upheaval, there is a great deal that can be done. Key areas of support are in physical recovery from birth, caring for the newborn and establishing breast-feeding. Research evidence on support in this period will be discussed in the section to follow.

The research evidence

Research on the effects of social support in pregnancy and birth fall into three main stages, social support during

- pregnancy
- birth
- the postnatal period.

Additionally, researchers have investigated the possible impact of different forms of support offered by 'lay' and professional helpers.

There is also a range of research approaches used in such studies. Much of the basic evidence on social support comes from epidemiological work, which mainly relies on studying patterns of health in a whole population or community. This can be very powerful in establishing the correlation between different variables, for example class and health. Such observational studies are more limited in establishing precise cause-and-effect relationships, for example the direction of cause in a correlation or whether a third unknown factor explains a relationship between two variables. For these reasons, randomized controlled trials are widely accepted as having the best chance of establishing cause-and-effect relationships. Health databases, systematic reviews and meta-analyses of studies therefore tend to focus entirely on such trials. Trials should never be viewed uncritically, however, since they are difficult to perform well, particularly when the intervention or relationship is complex and difficult to define and control in a precise manner. Social support is one such area, so that some trials of interventions – health education, for example, or additional home visits – may be weak or difficult to interpret. Trials are also often characterized by a lack of attention to process, which, in the case of social support, is central to the nature of the intervention. This focus in databases and overviews of research also tends to overlook the important contributions of qualitative research to understanding how women experience and respond to care.

The trials and observational or comparative studies described here all have an important component of social support but are difficult to compare since they cover a wide range of interventions that could be classified as social support, as well as seeking still to investigate the concept itself and establish what is effective social support in the context of maternity care. Additionally, not all studies have clearly established whether the support provided was perceived as such by women using the services, a factor that we have noted is likely profoundly to influence the effectiveness of any support offered.

Social support during pregnancy

Some researchers have argued that there is no evidence of antenatal maternity care having any measurable benefit (Hall et al 1980). Similarly, a number of commentators (e.g. Oakley 1992, Hirst et al 1998) have pointed out that the pattern of antenatal care delivery grew out of assumed benefits, rather than any knowledge base, during the 1920s and has remained largely unchanged (albeit with different technology) since then. While it is important not to assume that a service has a benefit simply because it is provided on this basis, the key outcomes measured in research have been primarily clinical, orientated towards risk assessment and safety at birth, and leading to gaps in the research evidence. Several commentators have also pointed out that risk assessment in maternity care has relied overwhelmingly on biomedical indicators, which are largely untested and give little or no weight to psychosocial risk factors (Oakley 1992, Lane 1995; see also Chapter 4). In antenatal care generally, it seems that the lack of clarity regarding the purpose of care is reflected in a lack of agreement about what constitutes a risk and how 'risk' should be managed.

Sikorski et al's (1996) study of a reduced schedule of antenatal care showed that although clinical safety was not compromised, satisfaction with care was decreased, suggesting that many women were seeking more from maternity care than birth safety alone. Hirst et al (1998) argue that reassurance is a major attribute that women seek from maternity care, a need that is not always met since health checks can cause anxiety as well as reassurance and the content of care, for example communication or support versus routine checks, has not been given sufficient consideration. Similarly, Oakley argues that receiving health care can have a negative impact and notes that criticisms of the services began to emerge as maternity care became increasingly depersonalized and fragmented (Oakley 1992).

In an overview of trials of social support during pregnancy, Elbourne et al (1989) found that the provision of additional support by the maternity services generally reduced anxiety and psychological and physical morbidity as well as, in most cases, increasing satisfaction with care. The 14 trials included all had social and psychological support as the main focus or as one objective. They involved a range of forms of support, from the provision of information to more comprehensive support packages including home visits. The interventions were also applied to a range of women, including minority ethnic women, socially disadvantaged women and women with high obstetric risk status. The overview concluded that social support may have a range of positive effects, which cluster around feelings (e.g. confidence, nervousness, fear or positive feelings regarding birth), communication, satisfaction with care and sense of control. The interventions had no significant impact on labour interventions or outcomes, but the support measures involved were not extended to labour and birth.

The authors concluded that, given the positive impact of social support on women's feelings about pregnancy and birth, and the lack of negative effects found in these trials, such support should be seen as integral to good maternity care. However, they noted that increasing fragmentation of care had made this more difficult, and linked such developments to the artificial separation by the obstetric services of the interests of the mother and the fetus/child. Obstetric developments in preceding years had tended to focus on child rather than maternal health, ignoring the close relationship between the two and encouraging a tendency to tell women what to do, an approach that ignores the complexities of circumstances and decisions influencing health (see also Chapter 4). They suggest, drawing on this research, that having one's perspective ignored can itself be detrimental to health.

Following a set of 'hunches' developed in earlier

qualitative work on women's experiences of maternity care (Oakley 1979, 1980, 1984), Oakley and colleagues set up a large-scale randomized controlled trial designed to test whether social support in pregnancy could have an impact on health. Low birth weight was selected as the main outcome measure since it is a strong indicator of maternal and child health that is amenable to relatively reliable measurement (Oakley 1992) and that was expected to be sensitive to any positive effects of social support in pregnancy, since it tends to be associated with social disadvantage, poor maternal health and health-related behaviours such as smoking (National Children's Home 1995, Wilcox et al 1995). The trial, therefore, was a good example of the range of relevant research approaches, using a randomized controlled trial to test hypotheses developed over time through more qualitative forms of enquiry.

Women who had one or more previous low birth weight babies (defined as weighing less than 2500 g) were invited to participate and were subsequently randomized into an intervention group, receiving additional support from midwives (in the form of at least three home visits/research interviews and two brief visits or telephone contacts, plus access to the research midwife at all times via the telephone) and a control group receiving conventional care (Oakley 1992). Although the intervention did not significantly increase birth weight, it was associated with a number of positive outcomes, including fewer very-low birth weight babies. Women in the intervention group had fewer antenatal hospital admissions, a lower use of epidural pain relief and more spontaneous labours and spontaneous vaginal births, and babies needing special care required less invasive resuscitation methods and less intensive care. The women reported better physical health for themselves and their babies, and less use of health services, 6 weeks after the birth. They were positive about the intervention, emphasizing the importance of the midwife listening to them (Oakley et al 1990).

A follow-up study conducted 7 years after birth found that important differences between the groups had been maintained. In particular, intervention group mothers reported fewer health problems in their children and fewer concerns about their social well-being. They showed greater personal well-being and also appeared more able to seek and obtain social support from others, particularly their partners (Oakley et al 1996). Such long-term follow-up studies are rare, mainly because of funding constraints, but may be of great value in considering influences on health. The researchers concluded that social support during pregnancy can have a number of benefits, without carrying some of the risks associated with pharmacological or biomedical treatment. They note, however, that social support is unlikely 'to override the cumulative effects and problems of social disadvantage' (Oakley et al 1990, p. 161). The nature and degree of these effects are well illustrated by the histories of women involved in the study, explored in the qualitative research interviews (Oakley 1992).

A systematic review of trials of social support in high-risk pregnancies (Hodnett & Roberts 1997) indicates that the clinical benefits found in such trials have been marginal and that interventions have not achieved significant increases in birth weight. The reviewers point out that such interventions may not be adequate to counter the well-researched effects of poverty and social disadvantage on health. In a commentary on one major trial (Villar et al 1992), which did not find a statistically significant increase in birth weight with additional support, Hodnett suggests that an exclusive or undue focus on birth weight could be missing the point (Hodnett 1993) and that the outcomes measured in such trials may not be the only ones that matter. The author notes that, although receiving prenatal care is generally associated with a better health outcome, little is known about what components of care are useful or effective.

This argument is also supported by the findings of Sikorski et al's (1996) trial of a reduced schedule of antenatal visiting in the UK which indicated that, although clinically safe, the reduced schedule decreased women's sense of confidence and satisfaction. Since these trials were not designed to examine other possible effects of professional support, they do not provide clear evidence on what its effects may be. In a re-analysis of women's questionnaires and case records, to investigate the reasons for maternal dissatisfaction, the authors found that women who were satisfied with the reduced schedule were less likely to be depressed and more likely to have had a care-giver who listened and encouraged them to ask questions. The authors concluded that care should safeguard social support for depressed women and that improving the psychosocial quality of care might improve the acceptability of reduced schedules. They recommended an individualized approach to visiting schedules, related to the needs and wishes of mothers (Clement et al 1997).

A more recent trial of prenatal social support by social scientists aimed to identify more clearly women whose risk was likely to be related to a lack of social support. The study randomized African-American women who lacked the support normally provided by mothers or partners into an intervention group offered additional support, designed to substitute for this, and a control group receiving the usual care. The authors note that, contrary to previous studies, this intervention was effective in reducing the rate of low birth weight in a group with a higher than usual prevalence of this (Norbeck & et al 1996). These more promising findings may have been linked to a more precise targeting of an appropriate study group, i.e. women who lacked support, and possibly to the nature of the support offered.

Although it is possible to conclude from the overview of trials (Hodnett & Roberts 1997) that social support in pregnancy does not have a significant impact on infant health (see, for example, Langer's commentary on this overview in the World Health Organization reproductive health library; World Health Organization 1997), there remains a great deal of work to be done. Trials that have shown benefits have been those looking at related outcomes such as psychological health or satisfaction of the mother, or less easily measurable aspects of infant health, in addition to birth weight. In addition, social support is difficult to specify precisely in the manner that an effective trial requires, for example as in a pharmacological intervention. Studies have included a range of types and levels of support, offered by different people, some focusing only on particular aspects of support, such as information, others being broader. Bearing in mind the distinction drawn between perceived and received support, trials have not always sought the perceptions of the mothers involved about whether the care or intervention offered has been perceived as supportive. This is particularly the case where trials involve educational interventions, which may be perceived as supportive by professionals but not by service users.

Educational interventions vary widely in approach, and it has been suggested (Arney 1982) that they are often about educating women to accept services rather than 'empowering' or supporting them. The heavy reliance on educational programmes of some trials that showed little effect of social support (Villar et al 1992) indicates the importance of clarifying what is meant by social support. A further methodological problem noted is in defining the concept of risk (Gabe 1995). Despite the basic importance of risk assessment as a rationale for antenatal care provision, and the reliance of many social support studies on the concept of risk, little attention has been given to how risk is defined or measured and what constitutes risk (Hirst et al 1998). Maternity services show a tendency to classify risk in terms of medical and obstetric history, whereas much social support research relies on sociological and epidemiological definitions of risk.

Continuity of carer throughout the maternity period

Since the publication of *Changing Childbirth* in the UK, a number of schemes have been piloted to establish and evaluate ways of implementing the core principles of *choice*, *continuity* and *control* for women using maternity services. These principles have been viewed by midwives and others concerned with maternity care as crucial elements of woman-centred care since they have been identified as important in a range of studies on women's experiences of maternity care. The concept of continuity is interesting because, although it is distinct from that of social support, existing research suggests that the two overlap in practice in important ways. A review of the history of midwifery in Euro-American societies during the 20th century suggests that the shift towards hospital- and obstetrically based maternity care has been linked to both fragmentation of care and a reduction in the social support offered to women (Towler & Bramall 1986). This has also been accompanied by an increasing encouragement of reliance on 'expert' advice and help rather than that provided by personal relationships.

As noted by Sandall (1995), the thrust of policy throughout the 20th century in the UK has been towards tackling problems by the use of technology rather than by reducing social inequality or offering greater social support to mothers. Histories of midwifery (Leap 1993, Allison 1996) demonstrate that the role of midwives has changed considerably, and that although nostalgia for the working conditions of traditional community midwives and their precursors – lay midwives or handywomen – is unwarranted, their role encompassed a considerable degree of community knowledge and social support to women. Studies of schemes aiming to reintroduce elements of that traditional role suggest that enabling midwives to provide continuity of carer is not just about continuity *per se* but about restoring to midwives, measures of personal control and satisfaction, which go hand in hand with a more supportive and enabling relationship with the women in their care (Sandall 1997).

Studies of caseload midwifery (which include both team and individual caseloads) provide evidence that is consistent with that found in studies of social support (Flint 1987, 1993, Rowley et al 1995, McCourt & Page 1996, Turnbull et al 1996, Benjamin 1997, Jowett & al 1997). On the whole, trials and comparative observational studies have shown similar findings:

- Women offered continuity of carer are more satisfied with their care.
- They have a reduced likelihood of receiving epidural anaesthesia or episiotomy.
- They show some evidence of increased confidence and preparedness for the birth and care of the baby.

Continuity of carer schemes can, however, be distinguished in terms of whether they provide continuity of antenatal and postnatal care only (which is arguably little different from the community midwifery practised in many areas of the UK) or whether they provide continuity throughout care, including birth. The evaluation of One-to-One midwifery looked at a caseload practice scheme in which midwives carried a personal rather than team caseload, working in partnerships and with back-up support to provide cover when needed (McCourt 1998). Very high rates of continuity of carer were achieved, even though, in this obstetrically orientated setting, women usually saw a high number of carers (McCourt & Page 1996). The study explored women's responses to care using quantitative and qualitative data, and compared the experiences of women receiving caseload and conventional ('shared' or hospital-based) care.

An analysis of statistical data showed that women preferred continuity of care with known carers, mainly midwives, and community-based visits. The qualitative data revealed far more about the meaning of continuity of carer to the women themselves and about the degrees of unhappiness they experienced, which was not necessarily expressed as dissatisfaction. Unsurprisingly, these women tended to think less in terms of terminology such as 'continuity of care', or carer, or 'social support' but described the ways in which knowing their main carer(s), seeing them at each visit (usually the named midwife but sometimes the partner or GP, or the consultant in high-risk cases) and experiencing consistency in this way made them feel known, understood and supported. It appeared to generate greater confidence in themselves, as new mothers, and in their carers. Mothers also described the importance of a known midwife being with them throughout labour and birth in terms of feeling understood and respected, being relaxed and confident, and feeling comforted (McCourt et al 1998). Confidence applied to feelings about the midwives as good and competent carers, as well as to themselves as being able to cope with the challenge of birth, and was linked to a sense of control over their experiences. Women who lacked such continuity of support were more likely to describe feelings of anxiety, fear and confusion in their accounts of pregnancy and birth.

This scheme differed from the main trials on continuity of carer in its emphasis on personal caseloads for midwives – creating an enhanced degree of autonomy and 'ownership' for midwives – and in catering for women of all obstetrically defined risks, serving a relatively socially disadvantaged population. Many of the women receiving caseload midwife care were not regarded, biomedically, as high risk but suffered a range of other problems such as poor housing, substance misuse, poverty, lack of partner support and migration as refugees. An analysis of the interviews with ethnic minority and younger mothers in the study suggested that, contrary to popular stereotypes (Green et al 1990, Bowler 1993), these women were more dissatisfied with conventional maternity services, particularly with regard to the lack of support or personal and sensitive care, and they valued the support of a known midwife particularly highly.

It could be argued that these mothers' accounts are primarily about feeling supported by their midwife carers, a support that should be achievable by ensuring continuity of care – a consistent approach rather than known carers – or simply by good midwives (Garcia 1995, Allen et al 1997, Lee 1997, Green et al 1998). However, the lack of such accounts, except in a very few cases, in women receiving shared or conventional consultant-led maternity care suggests that the supportive or caring qualities of midwives cannot be readily separated from the organization of their work. The manner in which services are organized and provided may have an important impact on their quality via the impact they make on workers (Gyllenhammar 1977, Sandall 1997). The organization of services around midwife caseloads facilitates more woman-centred care than is feasible with an organization of care around clinics and wards, or even teams (Wraight et al 1993), and the continuity of relationship that results may enhance the midwife's job satisfaction and capacity to provide supportive care.

Support in labour

A series of randomized controlled trials and observational studies has been conducted in a range of contexts to test the hypothesis that support in labour has benefits for women. One of the key features of these studies is that they look at the impact of *continuous* support, by either trained or untrained people. These studies are reviewed and summarised by Hodnett (1997a) in the Cochrane Library, providing strong evidence for the importance of the continuous presence of a supporter during labour. Although the precise details of support, as well as the contexts of each study, differ, the interventions shared key features of social support that are summed up by Hodnett & Osborn (1989) as follows:

- emotional support, for example reassurance, comfort and a continuous physical presence;
- informational support, such as the giving of explanations and advice;
- tangible support, for example massage and ice chips,
- advocacy: conveying and negotiating women's wishes with professionals.

The first such trials were conducted in South America by Sosa and colleagues (Sosa et al 1980, Klaus et al 1986). They drew on the indigenous tradition (found in a range of cultures; see Kitzinger 1989, Jordan 1993) of support and companionship by experienced local women, referred to in these studies (drawing on the Greek term for a female labour supporter) as doulas. Cross-culturally, the practice of labouring without such companionship has been particular to biomedical practice. A controlled trial was conducted in a busy Guatemalan hospital, allocating eligible women (healthy women admitted without a companion in early but established labour) randomly to an intervention or a control group. Those in the intervention group were supported by a doula, while control group women received standard care. The study found significant reductions in the intervention group in the duration of labour, oxytocic augmentation, the rate of caesarean section, admission to the neonatal unit and perinatal complications. Additionally, regression analysis suggested that the effects were greater in women living alone. The study indicated that very large, clinically as well as statistically significant differences could be achieved with 'poor women who routinely undergo labour alone on a crowded ward' (Klaus et al 1986, p. 586).

To test its applicability to the North American context, with high prevailing intervention rates and a greater access to pain relief, the study was replicated in a busy, obstetrically orientated unit in the USA (Kennell et al 1991). This unit catered for a large proportion of women who were socially disadvantaged and non-English speaking. The labour supporters were bilingual local lay women with personal experience of a normal birth, given 3 weeks of preparation. Similar results were obtained. Women admitted in labour without a companion fared better with the support of a doula. This study included both an observed group without a support and a control group, assessed by a review of the hospital notes after birth. Interestingly, similar differences but of a smaller magnitude were found

between the control group with a review of notes only and the group unobtrusively observed by a researcher. This unexpected finding suggested that even a continuous presence without active engagement or support could have a protective effect.

The authors noted that mechanisms for such effects are not known but pointed to research on the effects of adrenaline, levels of which are related to stress, on uterine contractions and blood flow (Teixeira & Glover 1999). They hypothesized that social support may 'work' by reducing such stress responses. The impact of the physical presence of an observer also suggested that the presence of a companion might have modified the actions or responses or professional carers.

In a similar study, in a South African hospital (Wolman et al 1993), women without access to private medicine and without a birth companion were randomized to a support or control group. Women with the support of a volunteer labour companion showed lower rates of postnatal depression and higher rates of self-esteem at 6 weeks postnatally than did those in the control group. This study differs, therefore, in that psychological benefits were included as a key outcome. The authors concluded that companionship modifies factors in a clinical labour environment that contribute to the development of postnatal depression and recommended that more attention be paid to the psychosocial environment of birth.

These studies were conducted in settings very different from those experienced by many women giving birth in hospitals in the UK and other European countries, particularly since the practice of allowing women to have chosen companions in labour has been reinstituted in most units. Hodnett & Osborn's (1989) trial of continuous professional support in labour was conducted in a Canadian teaching hospital serving a mainly white, middle-class group of women, who were routinely allowed the companionship of their husband or partner. This hospital had a high level of routine intervention in labour, typical of North American and many UK teaching hospitals at the time, and good staff-to-patient ratios. The study examined the impact of continuous support by a familiar, trained care-giver, using a self-employed 'coach' who was either a lay or a student midwife. Although the results of this study were less dramatic than those of previous trials, significant reductions were found in the use of pain relief medication and the incidence of episiotomy. The authors note that factors such as the duration of labour were difficult to assess in a context with a routine acceleration of labour: only eight women (out of the 103 women included in the trial) laboured with no intervention. The study showed some improved outcome in women who should have had low levels of problems generally, the main predictor variables being the provision of support and high expectations of personal control. The authors suggested that providing continuous support may not require additional staffing so much as a rethinking of priorities on labour and delivery suites.

In her overview, Hodnett (1997a) identified 11 trials, including the trials outlined above. The interventions were provided by both professionals and lay people, in a wide range of cultural and medical settings, some of which excluded other companions or support persons, such as partners or kinswomen. The overview indicated that continuous support in labour (by lay or professional companions) led to reduction in:

- the duration of labour;
- the likelihood of medication being needed for pain relief;
- the incidence of operative vaginal delivery;
- the number of 5-minute Apgar scores below 7.

Additionally, in those settings where companions were not normally admitted, the interventions reduced the probability of a caesarean section birth. Individual trials also found evidence of greater satisfaction with birth; for example, women were less likely to find labour worse than expected and felt greater personal control during the birth. Certain trials also found a longer duration of breast-feeding and lower rates of perineal trauma, postnatal depression and difficulty in mothering.

The reviewer recommended that, given the evidence of benefits and lack of known risks associated with intrapartum support, all women should receive such support, not only from those close to them, but also from specially trained care-givers (nurses, midwives or lay women). This support should include a continuous presence, the provision of hands-on comfort and encouragement. Hodnett argues that, to facilitate such provision of support, the priorities and routines of labour wards will need reconsideration, so that staff are able to spend less time on ineffective activities and more on support, and can be deployed to match needs more closely. Additionally, staff will need continuing education (Hodnett 1997a).

A more recent trial of one-to-one labour support (Gagnon 1997) found a significant reduction in the incidence of oxytocin stimulation but no other clinical differences in a Canadian hospital setting where other birth companions are usually present. The authors noted features of the context that could have reduced the impact of support in relation to some outcomes. For example, many women were already receiving epidural anaesthesia by the time of randomization, and its use was strongly encouraged in this unit. The limitations of such findings should alert us to the need to take both the context and the type of intervention into account when studying the effects of social support. In this case, the women selected were not those likely to be in the highest need of social support from professionals, but the setting also placed limitations on the capacity of supportive care to influence interventions in birth. In a commentary on the findings of this study, Hodnett questioned the effectiveness of the support given, viewing the role of the nurses as constrained by hospital policies. She reminds the reader that 'a randomised trial tells you what happened not why it happened' (1997b, p. 78). Referring to a work sampling study conducted in a Canadian hospital (McNiven et al 1992), Hodnett noted how little time was spent in direct supportive activities and argued that nurses need education to provide support, since direct caring work is devalued (see also Gagnon & Waghorn 1997).

Although these trials did not usually or necessarily include support persons already known to the woman, trials and observational studies of continuity of carers during pregnancy and birth have found some similar benefits. Hodnett's (1988a) review of the continuity of care-givers during pregnancy and birth identified the following benefits

- increased maternal satisfaction;
- less use of anaesthesia for pain;
- a reduced probability of episiotomy, but an increased probability of tears;
- a lower rate of neonatal resuscitation.

Although the relationships are unclear, and it is very difficult to tease out the importance of different components of care, it appears probable that continuity of care-giver, which has normally been introduced with the overall aim of enhancing woman-centred care, increases both perceived and received social support for women.

Most of these studies have been focused on 'uncomplicated' labour. A small trial of (34) women in preterm labour showed similar findings, extending the possible advantages of social support to preterm labour and birth (Cogan & Spinatto 1988). Similarly, in a study of women's experiences of induced labour, Cartwright (1979) found that women in many cases lacked adequate information or personal support. These findings were echoed in the evaluation of One-to-One midwifery, where women who did not have a named midwife described considerable anxiety and distress related to a lack of good explanation, social support or medical checks in early induced labour. In contrast, women with a known midwife found the experience less distressing. Women admitted for induction of labour in this Trust were routinely separated from their partners or companions for early labour because of the restrictions of the shared wards to which they were admitted (McCourt et al 1998). No trials have been conducted on the effects of social support for women in induced or otherwise complicated labour, but qualitative evidence suggests that any effects of support are likely to be increased.

Cartwright's and other studies (e.g. Reid & Garcia 1989) have also indicated that the quality of communication with professionals varies widely, women in lower social classes and minority ethnic groups generally receiving less adequate information from and dialogue with health professionals (Phoenix 1990, MORI 1993). Such findings suggest that women in greater need of support receive less from the maternity services.

Postnatal support

We have noted in Chapter 10 the importance of pregnancy and birth as a time of adjustment and change, a major life event, which precipitates a need for, and has traditionally generated a high level of, social support. Despite the high levels of clinical support provided in many countries, biomedical systems of care have shown a tendency to focus on labour and birth as a transition while overlooking the broader and longer-term transition of which they form a key part. This approach to birth, and a tendency to view the needs or interests of mother and infant as separate, has been reflected in an increasing investment in the technologies of pregnancy and birth, and a reduction in hospital provision for the postnatal care of mothers and babies. Ironically, while the use of many diagnostic and monitoring technologies has become routine – applied to women regarded as being of low clinical risk – postnatal maternity services are being withdrawn from such 'low-risk' mothers. Cross-culturally, rules and customs concerning the care and support of postnatal mothers have been central concerns around birth. Even in the UK, where length of the postnatal hospital stay has declined dramatically in the recent past (Department of Health 1997), a 'lying-in' period was culturally the norm in the recent past.

In a study of the support needs of 347 mothers, from 36 weeks of pregnancy to 6 weeks postnatally, Ball (1994) noted the historical role of midwives as female companions to mothers and the importance of pregnancy and birth as a life event, the impact of which will vary according to the woman's social supports and life circumstances. Ball emphasized that maternity services have the capacity to undermine as well as to enhance support. For example, the experience of hospitalization may, in itself, be stressful to women 'as it causes them to relinquish control of their patterns of daily living' (1994, p. 2), so that it is important for service providers to avoid creating additional stress.

Ball noted that traditions regarding the postnatal period are culturally variable but are generally marked by some form of seclusion. In many cultures, this may be for a month or as long as 40 days, during which the mother and child receive protective care or observe protective ritual practices (Kitzinger 1989, Vincent-Priya 1992, Jordan 1993). A 'lying-in' period of 10 days was written into the 1902 Midwives Act in the UK and carried over into the tradition of midwife visits for 10 days following birth. A range of studies have shown that some form of unhappiness or depression following birth is common, precise rates varying according to the definition of depression (Romito 1989, Cox & Holden 1994). Whether unhappiness after birth is perceived as 'normal' or as 'pathological', it is inherently undesirable for women to suffer such symptoms in response to what they hope will be a happy and fulfilling experience. See also Chapter 10.

Ball's (1994) study looked at the impact of hospital practices on mothers' experiences, noting that they often worked against the provision of social support, for example practices and routines that led to the unnecessary separation of the mother and baby soon after birth. Ironically, now that maternal–infant bonding has been recognized as an issue by health professionals, these practices have often been replaced by a practice of 'rooming-in' coupled with a loss of practical support. Ball noted the following as common aspects of maternity care that are not supportive to women:

- fragmentation of care;
- task- rather than person-based work and routines;
- a didactic style when giving help or advice;
- care focused mainly on the physical examination of the mother and feeding of the baby;
- observed inadequacies in the support for feeding.

She also noted a mismatch between midwives' summing-up of women's emotional states and their more specific comments, for example on the numbers of women who had been crying or showing sleep or appetite disturbances, suggesting that they either see this as 'normal' or give low priority to emotional states.

Factor analysis in Ball's study showed that emotional well-being and satisfaction with motherhood were associated with:

- antecedent factors
- other stress factors
- self-confidence on the return home.

Women's experiences of other stress factors were strongly influenced by postnatal care practices, the key factors being feelings at the time of birth, self-image in feeding the baby in hospital and conflicting advice or lack of rest in hospital.

With the reduction in the length of postnatal hospital stay in recent years, there is some evidence that the expectation of a period of rest and recovery following birth has also declined. In a US study, Ruchala & Halstead (1994) found that a predominantly middle-class group of white women, with partners (i.e. not at a high risk of lack of social support), were suffering considerable symptoms of fatigue, unhappiness and incongruence of their experience with their expectations. The mothers described physical, psychological and social difficulties in recovery and adjustment after birth, these being stronger in first-time mothers. Although women were able to call on their mothers and partners for primary sources of support, this was generally for limited periods, and the women were affected by feelings that they should be able to cope normally within a short period after birth. Postnatal home visits by health professionals are not normally provided in the USA, in contrast to the UK, where women expect home visits by midwives, and to the Netherlands, where maternity aides are also available to provide practical support. The authors suggest that more postnatal care is needed but point out that much of what the women needed did not require professional support *per se* although it might not be available from family, friends or community.

In a qualitative study of young, working-class mothers, experiences of postnatal care and support for feeding (Hodinott & Pill 1999) described the cycle of loss of confidence that often takes place in new mothers. Lack of practical and moral support, or support given in an undermining manner, led to feelings of not coping and a loss of confidence, precipitating a change in feeding method. Hodinott drew on the anthropological concept of embodied, as opposed to theoretical, knowledge to describe the ways in which social change had made women more vulnerable to inadequacies or inconsistencies in the provision of professional advice or support. Young women with a direct personal experience of contact with newborn babies held more embodied knowledge so were less vulnerable to loss of confidence. Similarly, women valued an 'apprenticeship' style of personal support and being given adequate information, rather than receiving direct advice, to help them make their own decisions.

A recent national survey by the Audit Commission (1997, Garcia et al 1998) confirmed the lack of postnatal support felt by some women. Within a context of generally quite high levels of expressed satisfaction with maternity services, women were least likely to be satisfied with postnatal care. Among the problems noted were a lack of rest, inconsistent advice, fragmentation of care and busy, rushed staff.

In the evaluation of One-to-One midwifery (McCourt & Page 1996), women described considerable gaps in support during their postnatal hospital stay, which involved some hospital midwives being unavailable in both a literal sense – being too busy – and in a metaphorical sense – being off-hand or uninterested or unsympathetic – as well as a tendency when giving help or advice to undermine rather than enhance women's self-confidence. Commenting on postnatal care, only about half of the women reported that they had received all the help they needed or attention from the staff when they needed it, and fewer than this (39% of the One-to-One and 33% of the control group) felt that they had received enough rest. Views of postnatal care at home were more positive, although some control group women complained of receiving conflicting advice from different midwives, and a number of women would have preferred visits over a longer period than the 10-day UK norm for postnatal care. Interestingly, women who received One-to-One (caseload midwifery) care were more likely to say that they would have liked visits over a longer period, even though they were more positive about the home support they received and the caseload midwives were able to visit selectively for up to 28 days after the birth. This view may have been linked to higher expectations of care in women who received a more flexible service. This group of women was also less likely than those in the control group to live with a partner or to have paid support at home. Just over half of the women in each group received support at home from their mother, and 16–25% received support from sisters, friends and/or mothers-in-law.

Practices regarding the type and level of postnatal support (if any) given by professionals or others at home vary widely between different countries. As we have seen in Chapter 10, in traditional cultural settings, a high level of support, encompassing periods of seclusion, rest and protective ritual practices, is the norm even though this is not always experienced by women who are poor or socially isolated. In European societies with socialized systems of medical care, home-based support from professionals is common, although the sort of practical support available in contexts where home birth remains common, such as the maternity aide system in the Netherlands, is not widely available. In the UK, women have a legal right to assessment for 'home help', for example (Department of Health 1990, Palmer 1996), but this is rarely obtained in practice and may be charged on a means-tested basis. In non-socialized systems of care, such as the system in the USA, postnatal home care is not part of normal service provision and is thus more likely to be seen as an additional intervention.

This is reflected in an overview of trials of home-based postnatal support for disadvantaged women. Most trials were conducted in the USA and were geared towards the prevention of child abuse and child health or service utilization problems, only rarely focusing on the psychosocial or physical health effects for the mother (Hodnett & Roberts 1997). The reviewers concluded that there is some evidence of a beneficial effect – for example, a better take-up of immunizations and a reduced number of hospitalizations – and no evidence of harmful effects from such support. They suggest that schemes using the skills of experienced mothers living in those communities may well provide less expensive and more culturally sensitive support than hospital-based programmes led by a team of health care professionals (Schafer et al 1998). Examples in the UK, generally developed in the voluntary sector, include Homestart and Newpin (see Useful addresses below), schemes that match isolated and vulnerable parents with volunteer supporters, generally local women with childcare experience.

Studies of women's experiences of postnatal care have highlighted the degree of support that many women need in breast-feeding and the perceived inadequacies and inconsistencies in the support provided by maternity services, in hospital or at home (Rajan & Oakley 1990, Stamp & Crowther 1994). A small-scale pilot study of the impact of placing health care assistants in the community to provide additional support to new breast-feeding mothers is currently being planned in the UK. Similarly, a study of women's functional status after birth found that a significant number of women did not feel that they had returned to normal functioning, in a range of ways including self- and infant care, 6 months after giving birth (Tulman et al 1990).

Given the awareness of high levels of some degree of distress or depression following childbirth (Romito 1989), postnatal care is also perceived as having an important potential role in the prevention of postnatal depression. Although much of this care may be provided or coordinated by other professionals, for exam-

ple health visitors (Cox & Holden 1994), the work of Ball and others has shown that the manner in which postnatal care is provided, and whether it is supportive, may influence women's experiences of depression. An overview of trials of care-giver support for postpartum depression (Ray & Hodnett 1997) suggests that additional support may be beneficial in reducing depression. Since little experimental research has been carried out in this area, the overview included only two trials, involving a small number of women, indicating caution in practice and the need for more research. Both trials involved counselling in a primary care setting. The reviewers note the lack of evidence for high rates of postnatal depression in non-Western cultures, suggesting that, in societies with lower rates of social isolation among new mothers, mothers may be protected from such depression (Romito 1989). However, this view may be based simply on lack of research or a lack of sensitivity to cross-cultural variations in the expression of distress, which biomedicine classifies as depression.

Although the aetiology and nature of postnatal depression is subject to debate, it is currently viewed by psychiatrists (Cox & Holden 1994) as involving a range of physiological, psychological and sociocultural factors, which include previous life experiences and forms of support as well as matters such as hormonal changes. Taking this view, although it may not be possible for maternity services to prevent all postnatal depression, or even to make a major impact on all women's experiences, supportive services may be able to reduce the impact of precipitating factors that, as Ball says, load the dice for a woman. At a more basic level, they have an obligation to avoid practices that are harmful rather than beneficial to women's psychological health.

CONCLUSION

The range of studies supporting the hypothesis of a link between support and responses to stress suggest that it is important to understand the ways in which women themselves perceive the provision of support. Research on women's views and experiences of maternity care consistently show that women respond positively to care that they perceive as supportive – knowing their carers and being known by them – to continuity of care and carer, and to good communication, showing greater confidence in their carers and in their own ability to cope with birth and parenting when offered social support, at all stages of care.

Not all research has shown similar effects of social support, some trials suggesting limited clinical impact

---

Pointers for Practice

- Birth is a major transition in a woman's life and is a social as well as a physiological act. Social support aids a healthy transition to motherhood.
- Much social support will come from personal sources; however, social support should be integral to maternity services and particularly to midwifery services.
- There is a correlation between social support and physical health.
- Women respond positively to care that they perceive to be supportive, knowing their carers and being known by them, to continuity of care and carer, and to good communication.
- Women who have received positive social support at all stages of their care show greater confidence in their carers and in their ability to cope with birth and parenting.
- The supportive or caring qualities of midwives cannot be readily separated from the organization of their work.

(Hodnett 1998b). The results of studies that focus on those most lacking in social support suggest that the benefits are greater and wider in such cases. This suggests that there is a need for maternity services to reconsider and redefine concepts of risk to include more psychosocial indicators of need. However, it is worth noting Elbourne et al's (1989) argument that support should be seen as integral to good care rather than the subject of special schemes with added support, even though the latter may be beneficial for certain women.

It is also important to take care in research to clarify and define the type and quality of support offered since needs and perceptions of support differ. Such variations, or lack of conceptual clarity, as well as variations in the context and recipients of support may explain the range of findings in the research. It is equally important to remember that maternity services cannot do it all and may also have the capacity to undermine as well as to enhance support to women.

REFERENCES

Aaronson L S 1989 Perceived and received support: effects on health behavior during pregnancy. Nursing Research 38(1): 4–9

Abernethy V D 1973 Social network and reponse to the maternal role. International Journal of Sociology and the Family 3: 86–92

Allen I, Bourke Dowling S, Williams S 1997 A leading role for midwives? Evaluation of midwifery group practice development projects. Policy Studies Institute, London

Allison J 1996 Delivered at home. Chapman & Hall, London

Antonucci T C 1985 Social support: theoretical advances, recent findings and pressing issues. In: Sarason I S, Sarason B R (eds) Social support: theory. Martinus Nijhoff, Dordrecht

Arney W 1982 Power and the profession of obstetrics. University of Chicago Press, Chicago

Audit Commission 1997 First class delivery: improving maternity services in England and Wales. Audit Commission, London

Ball J 1994 Reactions to motherhood: the role of postnatal care. Cambridge University Press, Cambridge

Barnes J A 1954 Class and committees in a Norwegian Island Parish. Human Relations 7(1): 39–58

Barrera M 1986 Distinctions between social support concepts, measures, and models. American Journal of Community Psychology 14(4): 413–45

Benjamin Y 1997 An evaluation of an alternative organisation of midwifery care: partnership caseload holding within a midwifery group practice. Interim report. Unpublished document, Leicester Royal Infirmary

Bott E 1971 Family and social network: roles, norms and external relationships in ordinary urban families. Tavistock, London

Bowler I 1993 'They're not the same as us': midwives

stereotypes of South Asian descent maternity patients. Sociology of Health and Illness 15(2): 157–78

Broadhead W T, Kaplan B H, James S A, Wagner E H, Schonbach V J 1983 The epidemiological evidence for a relationship between social support and health. American Journal of Epidemiology 117(5): 521–37

Brown G W, Bifulco A 1985 Social support, life events and depression. In: Sarason I G, Sarason B R (eds) Social support: theory. Martinus Nijhoff, Dordrecht 370

Brown G W, Harris T 1978 Social origins of depression: a study of psychiatric disorder in women. Tavistock, London

Brown S, Lumley J 1994 Satisfaction with care in labor and birth: a survey of 790 Australian women. Birth 21(1): 4–13

Bryanton J, Fraser-Davey H, Sullivan P 1994 Women's perceptions of nursing support during labor. Journal of Gynaecological and Neonatal Nursing 23(8): 638–44

Bulmer M 1986 Neighbours: the work of Philip Abrams. Cambridge University Press, Cambridge

Bulmer M 1987 The social basis of community care. Allen & Unwin, London

Capra F 1983 The turning point. Science, society and the rising culture. Flamingo, London

Cartwright A 1979 The dignity of labour? A study of childbearing and induction. Tavistock, London

Clement S (ed.) 1998 Psychological perspectives on pregnancy and childbirth. Churchill Livingstone, Edinburgh

Cobb S 1976 Social support as a moderator of life stress. Psychosomatic Medicine 38(5): 300–14

Cogan R, Spinnato J A 1988 Social support during premature labor: effects on labor and the newborn. Journal of Psychosomatic Obstetrics and Gynaecology 8: 209–16

Cohen S, McKay G 1983 Social support, stress and the buffering hypothesis: a theoretical analysis. In: Baum A,

Singer J E, Taylor S (eds) Handbook of psychology and health, vol. 4. Lawrence Erlbaum, Hillsdale, NJ

Cohen S, Syme S L 1987 Social support and health. Academic Press, New York

Cohen S, Wills T A 1985 Stress, social support, and the buffering hypothesis. Psychological Bulletin 98: 310–57

Cox J, Holden J (eds) 1994 Perinatal psychiatry. Use and misuse of the Edinburgh postnatal depression scale. Gaskell/Royal College of Psychiatrists, London

Crafter H 1997 Health promotion in midwifery: principles and practice. Edward Arnold, London

Culpepper L, Jack B 1993 Psychosocial issues in pregnancy. Primary Care 20(3): 599–619

Davis-Floyd R 1994 The ritual of hospital birth in America. In: Spradley J P, McCurdey D W (eds) Conformity and conflict. Readings in cultural anthropology. Harper-Collins, New York

Department of Health 1990 The NHS and Community Care Act. HMSO, London

Department of Health 1993 Changing childbirth. Report of the Expert Maternity Group (Cumberlege report). HMSO, London

Department of Health 1997 NHS maternity statistics, England: 1989–90 to 1994–95. Department of Health, London

Descartes R 1912 A discourse on method. Meditations and principles (trans. J Veitch). Everyman's Library, London

Elbourne D, Oakley A, Chalmers I 1989 Social and psychological support during pregnancy. In: Chalmers I, Enkin M, Keirse M J N C (eds) Effective care in pregnancy and childbirth. Oxford University Press, Oxford

Farrant W, Russell J 1986 The politics of health information. Institute of Education, London

Fiore J, Becker J, Coppel DB 1983 Social network interactions: a buffer or a stress. American Journal of Community Psychology 11: 423–40

Flint C 1987 The know your midwife report. 49 Peckermans Wood, London

Flint C, Poulengesis P 1993 Midwifery teams and caseloads. Butterworth-Heinemann, London

Gabe J 1995 (ed.) Medicine, health and risk. Sociological approaches. Blackwell, Oxford

Gagnon A 1997 A randomized trial of one-to-one nurse support of women in labour. Birth 24(2): 71–7

Gagnon A, Waghorn K 1997 Supportive care by maternity nurses: a work sampling study in an intrapartum unit. Birth 23(1): 1–6

Ganster D C, Victor B 1988 The impact of social support on mental and physical health. British Journal of Medical Psychology 61: 17–36

Garcia J 1995 Continuity of carer in context: what matters to women? In: Page L (ed.) Effective group practice in midwifery. Blackwell Science, Oxford

Garcia J, Redshaw M, Fitzsimons B, Keene J 1998 First class delivery: a national survey of women's views of maternity care. Commission/National Perinatal Epidemiology Unit, Abingdon

Good B 1994 Medicine, rationality and experience. An anthropological perspective. Cambridge University Press, Cambridge

Gore S 1978 The effect of social support in moderating the health consequences of unemployment. Journal of Health and Social Behaviour 19: 157–65

Gottlieb L, Mendelson M 1995 Mothers' moods and social support when a second child is born. Maternal Child Nursing Journal 23(1): 3–14

Graham H 1984 Women, health and the family. Harvester Wheatsheaf, Brighton

Graham H, Oakley A 1981 Competing ideologies of reproduction: medical and maternal perspectives on pregnancy. In Roberts H (ed.) Women, health and reproduction. Routledge & Kegan Paul, London

Grant A 1989 Monitoring the fetus during labour. In: Chalmers I, Enkin M, Kierse M J N C (eds) Effective care in pregnancy and childbirth. Oxford University Press, Oxford

Green J, Coupland V, Kitzinger J 1988 Great expectations. A prospective study of women's expectations and experiences of childbirth. Childcare and Development Group, Cambridge University

Green J, Curtis P, Price H, Renfrew M 1998 Continuing to care: the organisation of midwifery services in the UK. Hochland & Hochland, Hale

Green J, Kitzinger J, Coupland V 1990 Stereotypes of childbearing women: a look at some evidence. Midwifery 6: 125–32

Gyllenhammar P 1977 People at work. Addison Wesley, Reading, MA

Hall L A, Schaefer E S, Greenberg R B 1987 Quality and quantity of social support as correlates of psychosomatic symptoms in mothers with young children. Research in Nursing and Health 10(4): 287–98

Hall M, Chang P, McGillivray I 1980 Is routine antenatal care worthwhile? Lancet ii: 78–80

Handler H, Raube K, Kelley M, Giachetto A 1996 Women's satisfaction with prenatal care settings: a focus group study. Birth 23(1): 31–7.

Harper-Bulman K, McCourt C 1997 Report on Somali women's experiences of maternity care. Centre for Midwifery Practice, Thames Valley University, London

Heller K, Swindle R W, Dusenbury L 1986 Component social support processes: comments and integration. Journal of Consulting and Clinical Psychology 54(4): 466–70

Helman C 1994 Culture, health and illness. Butterworth-Heinemann, Oxford

Henderson S 1977 The social network, support and neurosis. British Journal of Psychiatry 131: 185–91

Henderson S 1980 A development in social psychiatry: the systematic study of social bonds. Journal of Nervous and Mental Disease 168: 63–9

Hirsch B J, Rapkin B D 1986 Social networks and adult identities: profiles and correlates of support and rejection. American Journal of Community Psychology 14(4): 395–412

Hirst J, Hewison J, Dowswell T, Bashington H, Warrilow J 1998 Antenatal care: what do women want? In: Clement S (ed) Psychological perspectives on pregnancy and childbirth. Churchill Livingstone, Edinburgh

Hodnett E D 1993 Social support during high-risk pregnancy: does it help? commentary on: Villar J, Farnot U, Barros F, Victora C, Langer A, Belizan J. A randomized trial of psychosocial support during high-risk pregnancies. New England Journal of Medicine 1992; 327: 1266–1271. Birth 20(4): 218–19

Hodnett E D 1997a Support from caregivers during childbirth. In: Neilson J P, Crowther C A, Hodnett E D, Hofmeyr G J, Keirse M J N C (eds.) Pregnancy and Childbirth Module of the Cochrane Database of Systematic Reviews, Issue 3. Cochrane Collaboration. Update Software, Oxford

Hodnett E D 1997b Are nurses effective providers of labor support? Should they be? Can they be? Commentary on Gagnon in same volume. Birth 24(2): 78–80

Hodnett E D 1998a Continuity of caregivers during pregnancy and birth (Cochrane Review). In: Neilson J P, Crowther C A, Hodnett E D, Hofmeyr G J, Keirse M J N C (eds) Cochrane Library, Issue 3. Update Software, Oxford

Hodnett E 1998b Support from caregivers during at-risk pregnancy. Cochrane Review. In the Cochrane Library, Issue 2, updated quarterly. Update Software, Oxford

Hodnett E D, Osborn R W 1989 Effects of continuous intrapartum professional support on childbirth outcomes. Research in Nursing and Health 12: 289–97

Hodnett E D, Roberts I 1997 Home-based social support for socially disadvantaged mothers. In: Neilson J P, Crowther C A, Hodnett E D, Hofmeyr G J, Keirse M J N C (eds) Pregnancy and childbirth module of the Cochrane Database of Systematic Reviews, Issue 3. Cochrane Collaboration. Update Software, Oxford

House J S 1981 Work, stress and social support. Addison-Wesley, Reading, MA

House of Commons 1992 Maternity services: government response to the second report from the Health Committee, Session 1991–92 (Winterton Report). HMSO, London

Hunt S, Symonds S 1995 The social meanings of midwifery. Macmillan, London

Jarman B 1981 A survey of primary care. Paper 16. Royal College of General Practitioners, London

Jones L, Sidell M 1997 The challenge of promoting health. Exploration and action. Macmillan/Open University, Basingstoke

Jordan P 1989 Support behaviors identified as helpful and desired by second-time parents over the perinatal period. Maternal Child Nursing Journal 18(2): 133–45

Jordan B 1993 Birth in four cultures. A crosscultural investigation of childbirth in Yucatan, Holland, Sweden and the United States, 4th edn. Waveland Press, Prospect Heights, IL

Jowett C and colleagues. Caseload midwifery. Audit of caseload care, November 1996–June 1997. Unpublished document. Royal Shrewsbury Hospitals NHS Trust

Kahn L 1979 Ageing and social support. In: Riley M (ed.) Ageing from birth to death: interdisciplinary perspectives. Westview Press, Boulder, CO

Kennell J, Klaus M, McGrath S, Robertson S, Hinckley C 1991 Continuous emotional support during labor in a US Hospital: a randomised controlled trial. Journal of the American Medical Association 265(17): 2197–201

Kessler R C, McLeod J D 1985 Social support and mental health in community samples. In: Cohen S, Syme SL (eds) Social support and health. Academic Press, New York

Kessler R C, McLeod J B, Wethington E 1985 The costs of caring: a perspective on the relationship between sex and psychological distress. In: Sarason I G, Sarason B R (eds) Social support: theory. Martinus Nijhoff, Dordrecht

Kirkham M 1989 Midwives and information-giving in labour. In: Robinson S, Thomson A (eds) Midwives, research and childbirth. Chapman & Hall, London

Kitzinger S 1989 Childbirth and society. In: Chalmers I, Enkin M, Keirse M J N C (eds) Effective care in pregnancy and childbirth. Oxford University Press, Oxford

Klaus M H, Kennell J H, Robertson S S, Sosa R 1986 Effects of social support during parturition on maternal and infant morbidity. British Medical Journal 293: 585–7

Lane K 1995 The medical model of the body as a site of risk. In Gabe J (ed.) Medicine, health and risk. Sociological approaches. Blackwell, Oxford

Laslett A, Brown S, Lumley J 1997 Women's views of different models of antenatal care in Victoria, Australia. Birth 24(2): 81–9

Leap N 1993 The midwife's tale: an oral history from handy women to professional midwife. Scarlett Press, London

Lee G 1997 The concept of 'continuity' – what does it mean? In: Kirkham M, Perkins E (eds) Reflections on midwifery. Baillière Tindall, London

Lehman D R, Ellard J H, Wortman C B 1986 Social support for the bereaved: recipients' and providers' perspectives on what is helpful. Journal of Consulting and Clinical Psychology 54(4): 438–46

Leininger M 1988 Caring, an essential human need. Proceedings of the three national caring conferences. Wayne State University Press, Detroit

Levitt M, Coffman S, Guacci-Franco N, Loveless S 1993 Social support and relationship change after childbirth: an expectancy model. Health Care Women International 14(6): 503–12

Lewison H 1993 The consumer's reaction to the technology of the labour ward. In: Spencer J, Ward R (eds) Intrapartum fetal surveillance. Royal College of Obstetricians and Gynaecologists, London

McCourt C 1998 Concepts of community in changing healthcare: a study of change in midwifery practice. In: Edgar I R, Russell A (eds) The anthropology of welfare. Routledge, London

McCourt C, Page L 1996 Report on the evaluation of One-to-One midwifery. Centre for Midwifery Practice, TVU, London

McCourt-Perring C 1993 The experience of psychiatric hospital closure: an anthropological study. Avebury, Aldershot

McCourt C, Page L, Hewison J, Vail A 1998 Evaluation of One-to-One midwifery: women's response to care. Birth 25(2): 73–80

McKeown T 1979 The role of medicine: dream, mirage or nemesis? Blackwell, Oxford

McNiven P, Hodnett E, O'Brien-Pallas L L 1992 Supporting women in labour. A work sampling study of the activities of labour and delivery nurses. Birth 19(1): 3

Marris P 1974 Loss and change. Routledge & Kegan Paul, London

MIDIRS and NHS Centre for Reviews and Dissemination 1997 Informed choice leaflet on continuous electronic foetal monitoring. MIDIRS, Bristol

MORI 1993 A survey of women's views of the maternity services. Maternity services research study. Department of Health, London

Murray-Parkes C 1971 Psycho-social transitions. A field for study. Social Science and Medicine 5: 101–15

National Children's Home and Maternity Alliance 1995 Poor expectations. Poverty and undernourishment in pregnancy. NCH/Maternity Alliance, London

NHSME 1997 A new NHS: modern and dependable Cm 3807. Stationery Office, London

Norbeck J S, De Joseph J F, Smith R T 1996 A randomized trial of an empirically-derived social support intervention to prevent low birthweight among African American women. Social Science and Medicine 43: 947–54

Oakley A 1979 Becoming a mother. Martin Robertson, Oxford

Oakley A 1980 Women confined: towards a sociology of childbirth. Martin Robertson, Oxford

Oakley A 1984 The captured womb: a history of the medical care of pregnant women. Basil Blackwell, Oxford

Oakley A 1992 Social support and motherhood. The natural

history of a research project. Blackwell, Oxford

Oakley A 1993 Essays on women, medicine and health. Edinburgh University Press, Edinburgh

Oakley A, Rajan L, Grant A 1990 Social support and pregnancy outcome: report of a randomised controlled trial. British Journal of Obstetrics and Gynaecology 97: 155–62

Oakley A, Hickey D, Rajan L et al 1996 Social support in pregnancy: does it have long term effects? Journal of Reproductive and Infant Psychology 14: 7–22

Olds D, Henderson C, Chamberlin R, Tatelbaum R 1986 Preventing child abuse and neglect: a randomized trial of nurse home visitation. Paediatrics 78: 65–78

Page L 1993 How and who should be monitored: the midwife's view. In: Spencer J, Ward R (eds) Intrapartum fetal surveillance. Royal College of Obstetricians and Gynaecologists, London

Paine W (ed.) 1982 Job stress and burnout. Sage, Beverley Hills

Palmer C 1996 Maternity rights. Legal Action Group/Maternity Alliance, London

Paykel E S 1985 Life events, social support and clinical psychiatric disorder. In: Sarason I B, Sarason B R (eds) Social support: theory. Martinus Nijhoff, Dordrecht

Phoenix A 1990 Black women and the maternity services. In: Garcia J, Kilpatrick R, Richards (eds) The politics of maternity care. Clarendon Press, Oxford

Pollock K 1988 On the nature of social stress: production of a modern mythology. Social Science and Medicine 26: 3

Procidano M E, Heller K 1983 Measures of perceived social support from friends and from family: three validation studies. American Journal of Community Psychology 11(1): 1–24

Proctor S 1998 What determines quality in maternity care? Comparing the perceptions of childbearing women and midwives. Birth 25(2): 85–93

Rajan L, Oakley A 1990 Infant feeding practice in mothers at risk of low birth weight delivery: Midwifery 6(1): 18–27

Ray K, Hodnett E D 1997 Caregiver support for postnatal depression. In: Neilson J P, Crowther C A, Hodnett E D, Hofmeyr G J, Keirse M J N C (eds) Pregnancy and childbirth module of the Cochrane Database of Systematic Reviews, Issue 3. Cochrane Collaboration. Update Software, Oxford

Reid M, Garcia J 1989 Women's views of care during pregnancy and childbirth. In: Chalmers I, Enkin M, Keirse M J N C (eds) Effective care in pregnancy and childbirth. Oxford University Press, Oxford

Roberts H 1997 Socioeconomic determinants of health: children, inequalities and health. British Medical Journal 314: 1122–5

Robertson C 1988 Health visiting in practice. Longman, Edinburgh

Robinson S 1989 The role of the midwife: opportunities and constraints. In: Chalmers I, Enkin M, Keirse M J N C (eds) Effective care in pregnancy and childbirth. Oxford University Press, Oxford

Romito P 1989 Unhappiness after childbirth. In: Chalmers I, Enkin M, Keirse M J N C (eds) Effective care in pregnancy and childbirth. Oxford University Press, Oxford

Rook K S 1984 The negative side of social interaction: impact on psychological wellbeing. Journal of Personality and Social Psychology 46: 1097–108

Rowley M, Hensley M, Brinsmead M, Wlodarczyk J 1995 Continuity of care by a midwife team versus routine care during pregnancy and birth: a randomised trial. Medical Journal of Australia 163: 289–93

Ruchala P L, Halstead L 1994 The postpartum experience of low-risk women: a time of adjustment and change. Maternal–Child Nursing Journal 22(3): 83–9

Sandall J 1995 Choice, continuity and control: changing midwifery, towards a sociological perspective. Midwifery 11: 201–9

Sandall J 1997 Midwives' burnout and continuity of care. British Journal of Midwifery 5(2): 106–11

Schafer E, Vogel M, Viegas S, Hausafus C 1998 Volunteer peer counselors increase breastfeeding duration among rural low-income women. Birth 25(2): 101–6

Scheper-Hughes N, Lock M 1987 The mindful body. A prolegomenon to future work in medical anthropology. Medical Anthropology Quarterly 1: 6–41

Schumaker S, Brownell A 1984 Towards a theory of social support: closing conceptual gaps. Journal of Social Issues 40(4): 11–36

Shinn M, Lehmann S, Wong N W 1984 Social interaction and social support. Journal of Social Issues 40(4): 55–76

Sikorski J, Wilson J, Clements S, Das S, Smeeton N 1996 The Antenatal Care Project: a randomised controlled trial comparing two schedules of antenatal visits. British Medical Journal 312: 546–53

Sosa R, Kennell J, Klaus M, Robertson S, Urrutia J 1980 The effect of a supportive companion on perinatal problems, length of labour, and mother–infant interaction. New England Journal of Medicine 303: 597–600

Spencer J, Ward R (eds) 1993 Intrapartum fetal surveillance. Royal College of Obstetricians and Gynaecologists, London

Stacey M 1988 The sociology of health and healing. Unwin & Hyman, London

Stamp G, Crowther C A 1994 Women's views of their postnatal care by midwives at an Adelaide women's hospital. Midwifery 10(3): 148–56

Strauss M A 1980 Social stress and marital violence in a national sample of American families. Forensic Psychology and Psychiatry, Annals of the New York Academy of Sciences 347: 229–50

Tarkka M T, Paunonen M 1996 Social support and its impact on mothers' experiences of childbirth. Journal of Advanced Nursing 23: 70–5

Teixeira J, Glover V 1999 Maternal anxiety in pregnancy associated with reduced uterine heart flow. British Medical Journal 318: 153–7

Teixeira J, Fisk N M, Glover V 1999 Association between maternal anxiety in pregnancy and increased uterine artery resistance index: cohort based study. British Medical Journal 318(7177): 153–157

Thacker S, Stroup D 1998 Continuous electronic fetal heart monitoring during labor. Cochrane review, Cochrane library, Update Software, Oxford

Thoits P A 1985 Social support and psychological well-being: theoretical possibilities. In: Sarason I G, Sarason B R (eds) Social support: theory. Martinus Nijhoff, Dordrecht

Tilden V P 1985 Issues of conceptualization and measurement of social support in the construction of nursing theory. Research in Nursing and Health 8: 199–206

Tilden V P, Galyen R D 1987 Cost and conflict: the darker side of social support. Western Journal of Nursing Research 9(1): 9–18

Tilden V P, Stewart B J 1985 Problems in measuring

reciprocity with difference scores. Western Journal of Nursing Research 7: 381–5

Towler J, Bramall J 1986 Midwives in history and society. Croom Helm, Beckenham

Townsend P, Davidson N, Whitehead M 1988 Inequalities in health (the Black Report). Penguin Books, London

Tulman L, Fawcett J, Groblewski L, Silverman L 1990 Changes in functional status after childbirth. Nursing Research 39(2): 70–5

Turnbull D, Holmes A, Shields N 1996 Randomised controlled trial of efficacy of midwife-managed care. Lancet 348: 213–18

Turton P, Orr J 1993 Learning to care in the community, 2nd edn. Edward Arnold, London

Villar J, Farnot U, Barros F et al 1992 A randomized trial of psychosocial support during high-risk pregnancies. New England Journal of Medicine 327: 1266–71

Vincent-Priya J 1992 Birth traditions and modern pregnancy care. Element Books, Dorset

Walker J, Hall S, Thomas M 1995 The experience of labour: a perspective from those receiving care in a midwife-led unit. Midwifery 11(3): 120–9

Wellman B 1981 Applying network analysis to the study of support. In: Gottlieb B H (ed.) Social networks and social support. Sage Publications, Beverley Hills

Wheatley S 1998 Psychosocial support in pregnancy. In: Clement S (ed.) Psychological perspectives on pregnancy and childbirth. Churchill Livingstone, Edinburgh

Whitehead M 1987 The health divide. Inequalities in health in the 1980's: a review. Health Education Authority, London

Wilcox M A, Smith S J, Johnson I R, Maynard P V,

Chilvers C E D 1995 The effect of social deprivation on birthweight, excluding physiological and pathological effects. British Journal of Obstetrics and Gynaecology 102: 918–24

Willmot P 1986 Social networks, informal care and public policy. Policy Studies Institute, London

Wolman W L, Chalmers B, Hofmeyr J, Nikodem V C 1993 Postpartum depression and companionship in the clinical birth environment: a randomised, controlled study. American Journal of Obstetrics and Gynecology 168(5): 1388–93

World Health Organisation 1946 Constitution. World Health Organization, New York

World Health Organization 1986 The Ottawa Charter. World Health Organization, Geneva

World Health Organization 1997 Langer, A., commentary on Hodnett & Roberts, Cochrane Review. WHO Reproductive Health Library. Update Software, Oxford

Wraight A, Ball J, Seccombe I, Stock J 1993 Mapping team midwifery: a report to the Department of Health. IMS Report Series No. 242. Institute of Manpower Studies, Brighton

Young A 1980 The discourse on stress and the reproduction of conventional knowledge. Social Science and Medicine 14(3): 133–46

Young A 1981 The creation of medical knowledge: some problems in interpretation. Social Science and Medicine 15(B) 379–86

Young A 1982 The anthropologies of illness and sickness. Annual Review of Anthropology 11: 257–85

Young M, Willmot P 1957 Family and kinship in East London. Routledge & Kegan Paul, London

USEFUL ADDRESSES

Pals in Pregnancy Tel: Sue Kingswell or Bernadette Fogarty on (01203) 633066 A *Changing Childbirth* project being developed and evaluated in Coventry, UK, aiming to provide peer support to vulnerable pregnant women.

Homestart 2 Salisbury Road, Leicester LE1 7QR Tel: 0116–223 9955 A voluntary organisation that matches volunteer visitors to families needing social support. **Newpin** Tel: 0171–703 6326

13

Dimensions and attributes of caring: women's perceptions

Christine McCourt
Janet Hirst
Lesley Ann Page

When women enter the maternity services, they have a number of expectations, the most fundamental of which is an expectation of good care. Caring is a central characteristic of the midwife's role as it is the responsibility of a practising midwife to provide *care* for a mother and her baby (United Kingdom Central Council for Nursing, Midwifery and Health Visiting 1998). Midwifery care includes interactive activities such as physical measurements and the giving of information and advice. However, there does not appear to be a consensus in the literature regarding a definition of what caring really is. There are well-debated theories surrounding the concept of caring in the context of nursing practice (Morse et al 1991, MacDonald 1993, Leininger 1998; see also Chapter 12). Midwifery is now beginning to develop some theories of care.

For example, Halldorsdottir & Karlsdottir (1996a), in a study of the perceptions of women who have given birth, which took place in Iceland, discuss the need to develop a paradigm of caring for professionals whose role is to help another human being in need. They discuss the need for the psychological as well as the physical presence of the midwife particularly during labour, and the importance of trust in the relationship. The authors work with the metaphor of a journey through labour and birth, describing the importance of the woman's sense of control while having a need for caring and understanding during the birth experience. All the women in their study felt this need for caring and understanding. Included in this was a need for kindness, connection, companionship, assistance and support. Similarly, Swanson, drawing on three phenomenological studies of women's experiences of maternity care, identified five key processes of caring (Swanson 1991, Beck 1995):

1. knowing
2. being with
3. doing for

4. enabling
5. maintaining belief.

These core processes are clearly echoed in the case study that follows below.

Childbearing women need caring, and when they receive appropriate caring, it has a powerful positive effect. However, the opposite, which Halldorsdottir & Karlsdottir (1996b) describe as 'uncaring', may have an even more powerful negative effect. These authors describe caring as empowerment and uncaring as discouragement. There are different dimensions of caring that include the internalized feeling of the care-giver (what it is like to care), the internalized feelings of the recipient (what it is like to be cared for) and the inter-personal interaction (the technical process of care). Within each of these dimensions exist a number of attributes, such as emotions, feelings, love, empathy, trust, helping and sensitivity (Morse et al 1991, MacDonald 1993, Leininger 1988). This means that the process of caring, for example the interaction of giving information or taking a blood pressure measurement, is influenced by emotional attributes such as trust and sensitivity. Support includes listening and giving information, as well as practical support.

Traditional associations of caring with physical care and dependency highlight the importance of defining what we mean by caring. We do not see caring as something that is important only to sick people. On the contrary, caring is important to anyone at any time of life. It is, however, particularly important during times of vulnerability. Childbearing women, although not ill, are often vulnerable. They need support and practical help, and often experience exhaustion, sensory overload and feeling unwell. Caring in midwifery is not intended to produce dependency. Indeed, if dependency is created, this is the very opposite to caring and may meet the care-givers' rather than the woman's need. It will be seen later that effective caring may bolster the woman's self-confidence rather than reduce it.

Other chapters in this volume have examined some of the many facets of caring. Chapter 3, on choices in childbirth, makes it clear that caring does not mean telling women what to do for the best. Caring requires a partnership in which the midwife acts as a facilitator who has expertise but uses this expertise in helping the childbearing woman to make her own decisions. Other chapters offer a discussion of physical care in labour, the power of an established relationship between the woman and her midwife in creating a caring partnership, and the importance of social support in pregnancy and birth.

Caring is manifest in a number of ways, some of them very simple. It may involve giving practical help, for example helping a woman who has had a caesarean birth to lift her baby in the immediate postpartum period and attending to her physical needs. Caring involves understanding how a woman is feeling and the kind of help she needs. It entails sensitivity to the individual needs of women and their families, helping to provide and helping them to get the most beneficial care. This may at times involve challenging routines or organizations that do not work. It may require political activity as well as individual care. Caring requires meeting the needs of individual women and is more likely if the system is geared to this.

EVALUATING 'CARE'

Midwives are concerned with the process of caring and the effect that this has upon women, their families and those who provide the service. However, because caring is difficult to define, it is also difficult to measure within our profession and to know what characteristics of caring we are measured against by others. What we can measure is when we are perceived as caring (by the views of women who receive care) and when we feel we are caring (using the views of the midwives providing care) and the clinical outcomes of the care we give. Evaluations of maternity care over the past decade have provided information about women's views of their care, and we now have good information regarding women's positive and negative experiences (Green et al 1988, Percival 1990, Brown & Lumley 1994, Kempe 1994, Garcia et al 1998, Hirst et al 1998, Proctor 1998). Several of these evaluations of care have found that the organization of care affects the experiences that women have (McCourt & Page 1996, McCourt 1996, Green et al 1998, Hirst et al 1998, McCourt et al 1998). Apart from women's positive and negative experiences of their care, we can identify from these evaluations the dimensions and attributes of caring that are important to women. However, a problem with most maternity care evaluations is that some women, for example women who have a low income, teenagers and, despite our multicultural society, ethnic minority women, are not fairly represented, unless the evaluation focuses upon forms of care only offered to them, such as the evaluation of health advocacy services (Parsons & Day 1992). This chapter gives the opportunity to report the views of ethnic minority women who have received care from two different organizations of midwifery. We will then draw out from their views the dimensions and attributes of caring that are important from this often 'muted' group of women (Bowes & Meehan-Domokos 1996).

It is important to mention that many evaluations of maternity care that have set out to obtain the views of ethnic minority women have been criticized for categorizing participants from different ethnic groups as homogenous, grouping them by social class irrespective of their ethnicity or not designing the study appropriately for culturally different women (Garcia 1994, McIver 1994, Baxter 1996). In particular, women from Pakistan, India and Bangladesh have been consistently classified as Asian despite differences in their culture, language and religion. The women who were recruited for the study reported in this chapter were of particular interest because of their cultural diversity as they represented the community in which the two ways of organizing care were provided. Also, as many midwives provide care for women in culturally diverse communities, we need to know what culturally diverse women have to say.

Some of the women in the study reported here were cared for in an innovative pattern of care – One-to-One midwifery practice – others were cared for in the conventional service that One-to-One replaced. One-to-One was set up to provide care that was responsive to the individual needs of women, respecting their beliefs, religion and values. The interviews on which this report is based were part of the evaluation to determine whether or not these aims had been met.

The report is also used in this chapter as a case study to start to examine what it means to women to be cared for, and the opposite – to be treated disrespectfully, unkindly, without concern and physical help when it is needed.

It seems from this study that both the system of care and the place of care will affect caring behaviour. The system may alienate women from the professionals who are there to support them, preventing the care of individual women. When women, as they do when they enter the maternity service, expect to be cared for and are not, or when staff are perceived as uncaring, there is often an extremely powerful negative effect that counteracts positive care. A lack of care or uncaring encounters may be caused by staff being frantically busy and having to rush from one woman to another (Kitzinger 1998). Sometimes, however, negative care is a simple lack of kindness and concern. This negative care, including negative social interactions and unmet expectations, may have potent harmful effects (Rook 1984).

The key to caring for all women is sensitivity to their individual needs, both social and medical. Each woman will have different dreams, hopes and fears for the birth of her baby. These will, to a large extent, come from her personal background, nationality and ethnicity. However, although expectations and the complexity of pregnancy and birth will differ, it is a time of vulnerability for all women, and there are universal needs for support. We have chosen as a case study this report on a small number of women who are potentially even more vulnerable than others. Most midwives serve women from diverse populations, including women from different classes and ethnic minority groups, and disabled women. They may well care for a number of women who do not speak the same language, who do not read or write and for whom local customs and hospital customs and practices may be difficult to understand. (In fact, hospital practices may be difficult to understand for a number of people!)

The perception of being cared for did not, however, seem to differ greatly between this group and women from the indigenous population. The lessons to be drawn from the study may well apply to all women. However, although personal sensitivity to the needs of individuals will help to provide good care to all women, even the most vulnerable, it is important to take account of the individual cultural background (Le Var 1998) and to know how to do this without creating cultural generalities and thus stereotyping. There are lessons to be learned from New Zealand, where a concept of cultural safety has been instituted in midwife and nurse preparation. Cultural safety goes beyond cultural awareness and sensitivity to a transfer of power from the provider to the consumer (Nursing Council of New Zealand 1996).

This chapter, then, describes the maternity care experiences and perspectives of a small group of minority ethnic women. The interviews on which it is based formed part of a large scale, multidisciplinary evaluation of a new model of maternity care: caseload midwifery. The study took place in a West London NHS Trust with two teaching hospital maternity units:

- one large unit (4000 births per year) that was obstetrically led, with high rates of intervention;
- a smaller unit (1000 births per year) with a more midwifery-orientated ethos.

One-to-One midwifery practice was introduced in this Trust as a pilot project in order to demonstrate and evaluate an approach to the implementation of *Changing Childbirth* principles (Department of Health 1993). The study aimed to evaluate whether the introduction of caseload midwifery was associated with similar or improved standards of care and health outcomes, satisfaction and costs (McCourt & Page 1996, Piercy et al 1996, Beake et al 1998, McCourt 1998, McCourt et al 1998). The study of women's responses to care was a major aspect of the evaluation since the main rationale for making such changes was stated to be consumer choice and interests. In particular, the qualitative aspect of the study sought to explore whether the service met the needs and wishes of women from socially disadvantaged groups, who are often assumed to be less vocal consumers of health services.

THE BACKGROUND TO THE STUDY

One-to-One midwifery was a form of practice modelled on that of independent midwives in the UK. The One-to-One midwives carried a personal caseload, set at 40 women of all 'risks' giving birth per year, working with a partner to provide availability to women and within group practices that provided general support, back-up availability and peer review. The midwives did not work single-handedly with women but provided coordination and most of the care from 'booking' in the pregnancy to postnatal discharge. The term 'One-to-One' was intended to convey the notion of personalized care with a known main carer providing continuity, but it also illustrated the aim of greater autonomy for practising midwives, in a context where services had become highly fragmented and reliant on obstetric technology (Robinson 1989, 1990).

The One-to-One model differed from conventional team midwifery in two main ways: midwives worked across hospital and community boundaries, according to women's needs or choices, and they exercised greater personal control and responsibility with respect to their patterns of work (McCourt 1998). Whereas many midwives, particularly those based in hospitals, work around the needs and rhythms of the service (Kirkham 1989, Pizzini 1992, Thomas 1992), the aim was that One-to-One midwives would work around the needs and rhythms of the women on their caseloads. As a result of this more woman-centred pattern of work, it was hoped that the key stated principles of *Changing Childbirth* (Department of Health 1983) – choice, continuity and control for women – would be achieved.

MINORITY ETHNIC WOMEN AND MATERNITY SERVICES

Although *Changing Childbirth* was developed on the basis of a consensus between different professional and consumer groups, and evidence was gathered on the views of minority ethnic women (Rudat et al 1993), a number of stereotypes of the attitudes, needs and preferences of ethnic minority women using maternity services persist (Phoenix 1990, Woollett et al 1991, Bowler 1993, Bowes and Meehan-Domokos 1996). The MORI study indicated concerns and preferences very

much in line with those of the majority population, with additional concerns about communication and sensitivity of care (Rudat et al 1993). However, it has become common for service providers, since its publication, to describe *Changing Childbirth* as a policy for affluent, white, middle-class women. Green et (1988, 1990), in exploring the stereotypes of the white, middle-class mother as demanding, overoptimistic and more concerned with her fulfilment than the safety of birth – and the poor or working-class mother as ignorant and feckless but helpfully compliant and mainly concerned with the avoidance of pain – found no evidence to support such simplistic views.

THE STUDY OF WOMEN'S EXPERIENCES OF AND RESPONSES TO CARE

The study of women's responses to care involved a large-scale, longitudinal postal questionnaire survey, interviews and focus groups with a smaller sample of women. We felt it important that this study incorporated the perspectives of a wide range of women and were aware of higher rates of responses to postal self-completion questionnaires among (broadly speaking) white, middle-class women. The key motivations for conducting in-depth interviews and focus groups were twofold: first, to ask whether the research concerns addressed in our questionnaire design matched those expressed by women using the service when responding to an open approach; and second, whether women in socially disadvantaged groups, who might be less likely to complete the questionnaires, shared views and experiences similar to those of the overall study group.

The interviews

Altogether, 50 women were interviewed individually, half of whom were receiving the new model of care and half conventional care, as shown in Table 13.1.

In this chapter, the main focus is on the accounts of the 20 minority ethnic women interviewed, our findings from the wider study being reported elsewhere (McCourt et al 1998). The women were identified through the clinical audit of women's hospital records, which generally identify ethnicity (described in the records as 'race') because of the relevance of some screening tests (such as those for sickle cell disease and thalassaemia) to particular groups. Therefore, the ethnic minority categories included for these interviews were black Caribbean and African, South and East Asian and Mediterranean/Middle Eastern. We

Table 13.1 Women interviewed in the study (*N* = 50)

Type of respondent	Type of care	
	One-to-One	Conventional
Had returned questionnaires	10	10
No questionnaires returned		
Minority ethnic group	10	10
Younger mothers	2	2
Somali refugee women	2	4

did not sample women on the basis of socio-economic class since there was no readily available means of identifying this in the notes. Six Somali refugee women were also interviewed, using a different sampling strategy, as part of a small case study (Harper-Bulman & McCourt 1997) since it was felt that such women might have particular needs and concerns, reflecting their recently migrated position, whereas many minority communities in West London are long established and settled.

All the interviews were conducted postnatally, most taking place around 3–6 months following the birth. All women who had not refused consent for the study but who had not returned any questionnaires were identified and cross-checked against date of birth and ethnic coding. They were contacted by letter and, where possible, telephone, to explain this part of the study, to request their participation and, if agreed, to arrange an interview. Although the possible problems of using interpreters for research interviews were recognized, the range of language groups in this part of London precluded the use of bilingual interviewers. Access to interpreting services was arranged prior to contacting women, and all were offered an interpreter if they needed or preferred this. In the event, only one of the women interviewed requested an interpreter. One woman who did not speak fluent English preferred to be interviewed without an interpreter.

Interviews were conducted, where possible, in the women's own homes and using a tape recorder. All but two of the women were happy with this. One woman was initially unsure about being taped but readily agreed after assurance that the tapes were not necessary but simply helped us to get a fuller and more accurate record of what women had to say than was possible with notes. A semi-structured approach was taken, using a brief schedule designed to encourage open responses. The schedule was narrative in style but focused on pregnancy and birth and maternity services rather than taking a broader life-historical approach (Gluck & Patai 1991). We asked women to

describe what happened at different stages of their pregnancy, birth and adjustment to life after the birth and then asked them to think about what was helpful or what could be improved at each stage of maternity care. The schedule was not adhered to rigidly since the intention was to encourage women to describe and comment on their experiences, in their own words and according to their own perspective.

Data analysis

The interviews were transcribed in full and were analysed in two stages. A content analysis was conducted for the purposes of the overall evaluation report, which aimed to highlight the key themes and issues that women raised within the tight time and decision–making schedules of the health service. All codes and themes generated were cross-checked by three members of the research team. Subsequently, a more detailed open text analysis was performed in order to explore and elucidate these themes further.

Analysis was frustrating in many ways since it involved dissecting a series of narratives that were powerful and compelling in their own right, in order to identify patterns and to identify themes that, in the context of the narratives, appeared essentially coherent and inseparable. Teasing them apart was in many ways a denial of what the women themselves had argued about the need for coherence and the avoidance of fragmentation, on the level of the self as well as the level of service provision (Scheper-Hughes & Lock 1987, Jordan 1993) However, the process of analysis proceeds to knitting back together in a patterned way what has been deconstructed in the process of attempting to understand and describe a number of women's experiences.

Response to the study

Response rates to the interview study were good, particularly considering our focus on women who had not returned questionnaires. We were also interested to find that response rates to questionnaires, although there was a slight skew towards white and 'middle-class' women, had been good across a wide range of women, considering the high mobility of the local population. As a result, the number of women we needed to contact for interviews in this 'non-responder' group was small. Few women, of those who were contactable, declined participation, and if they did, this was generally because they were back at work and too busy. Several women commented that they had not wished to complete the questionnaires because they preferred a face-to-face interview. The records of our study database also suggested that women with health problems (in themselves or the baby) had been less likely to return questionnaires, and this was supported by our analysis since a large proportion of the women we interviewed in this group had complicated pregnancy or births.

It is important to note that the women interviewed, although we have described them using terms such as 'minority' or 'socially disadvantaged', were a very varied group in terms of class, ethnic or national origin, religion, social support and personal history or interests. Caution is needed when using sociological categorizations that are in themselves cultural constructs. Categories such as social class and ethnicity are likely to overlap, as well as being fluid and complex rather than rigid or immutable realities (Shore 1998, Wright 1998). Nonetheless, it is possible to argue that this group shared the experience of being in cultural groups that experience structural and individual disadvantage or discrimination.

THE STUDY FINDINGS: KEY THEMES

Choices and knowledge: self- or expert knowledge?

In these and our other interviews, women did not usually use the language of consumer choice. However, most women discussed concerns that we might relate to the concepts of choice and control used in *Changing Childbirth*. A pattern of lack of choice and denial, or ignoring women's personal or embodied knowledge, commenced with their initial visit to the GP. The anthropological concept of 'embodiment' is used to convey the person's experience and sense of his or her own body and to discuss the cultural location of ideas about the body (Martin 1989, Scheper-Hughes & Lock 1987). It is often used by anthropologists as a point of contrast with the separation of mind and body, based on Cartesian theory, which is integral to modern 'Western' epistemologies and fundamental to the way in which biomedicine developed in the 18th and 19th centuries.

What we are referring to here, therefore, is a tendency for maternity services to treat women as though *their own direct knowledge* or embodied knowledge was not important or valid (true). Instead, expert knowledge or, increasingly, external and technological forms of measurement are seen as the most reliable. For example, most women went to their GP either to confirm their pregnancy 'officially' or simply to arrange maternity care. Most were told that they were pregnant,

despite knowing this already, and several were unhappy about being contradicted by their GPs: one woman, for example, was told that her 'dates' were wrong, until it was discovered that she had a multiple pregnancy. Several women had avoided visiting the GP until later in pregnancy because of previous negative experiences of being contradicted or ignored.

Few women were offered information on or a choice of where to give birth, which hospital to book with or the options for care available, and on the whole, like many women in our wider study, they did not question this lack of choice. Those women who did make choices about hospitals wanted to book with the hospital that was easiest to get to or where a previous baby had been born – or, in one case, to avoid this hospital because of an association with the loss of her previous baby. None were offered any choice about systems of care, although several GPs recommended One-to-One care as being nice for the woman. Since it was a pilot scheme, One-to-One care was not self-selected but allocated on a neighbourhood base, and women described being offered choices about care – such as where and with which professional to have most of their visits – at the 'booking' visit with their named midwife. Women in the neighbourhood selected for comparison (which will be referred to as the conventional care group) were allocated to shared or full hospital care on the basis of medical or obstetric 'risk'. The only woman who had 'domino' care arranged this personally with a community midwife she was related to.

This pattern of lack of choice continued throughout conventional care, although several women used antenatal classes as a mean of getting information on and exploring the options surrounding birth. In contrast, women with One-to-One midwives were able to discuss their feelings about birth antenatally with the midwife who was most likely to be there.

The place of care: home or hospital?

All but one of the women in the One-to-One group had most of their antenatal visits at home, only attending hospital as needed for tests or to see an obstetrician. They described home visits as more relaxing and conducive to discussion, as well as more convenient. One woman had all her visits at the hospital, with her midwife, since she felt more comfortable and secure there. Women in the conventional care group had a mixture of GP surgery visits (with the GP or community midwife) and hospital visits at key stages. As with home-based care, they tended to find surgery-based visits more relaxed and felt more able to talk, but this depended very much on the individual GP:

you see your doctor all the time so you could have a chat with the doctor, you could tell her your difficulties you know and she was always there to listen. (s312)

it seemed as though they'd given him the surgery to do, rather than ... I felt better under the community midwives ... I don't think he didn't care, just... (s388)

Hospital visits were the focus of common complaints about difficult journeys, long waiting times, poor organization and generally feeling uncomfortable, but what was more important to the women in conventional care was the manner and quality of these visits, which they described as rushed and inattentive:

and it was just, like you're waiting to be seen, and then when they call you, you're just in and out like anything. (s167)

they'd want to get rid of me but I'd have questions and they'd just look impatient. (s370)

you wait so long for the appointment and before you know it within five minutes they have finished with you so you haven't got time to say or ... you know. (s312)

It was apparent from their accounts that women had expected to receive a high level of care when in hospital, during labour and birth and postnatally, an expectation that was not often met. Several women, as in our wider study, experienced a particular lack of care when they were admitted to an antenatal ward in early labour or for induction. Women with One-to-One midwives exercised more control over when to enter hospital for birth since they were able to call their midwife and receive telephone support or home assessment and care in early labour. This was generally preferred, and they did not experience the problems associated with being admitted to an antenatal ward that are described below. The exception was one women who, because of a rapid labour, felt she had been wrongly advised by her midwife to wait at home for her to visit. As a result, she was admitted very late in the first stage of labour and found her admission to hospital and the birth far more stressful as a result. Women receiving conventional care were only able to exercise such choice if they felt confident enough to stay at home without professional support or assessment, perhaps because of their experience of previous births. One woman had 'lasted my labour out' because, after previous experiences, she preferred to 'be in my own environment' (s167). Although this woman also arrived very late in the first stage of labour, she felt positive about this because she had been able to exercise control over where she laboured.

Most of the women interviewed had a number of criticisms about postnatal care in hospital, which stemmed largely from a dissonance between their expectations of hospital care and the general lack of support, which is discussed below. Postnatal care at home was regarded more positively as it matched up better to women's expectations, and even where visits were from a community midwife they did not know, women at least received more individualized attention.

The focus of care: the woman or the system?

At antenatal hospital visits, as the above quotes illustrate, women receiving conventional care felt that they were being hurried through a system that took little regard of them as a person and offered little real opportunity for discussion. This was sometimes countered by a good relationship with the GP or community midwife. The women wanted to feel special and cared for in their pregnancies (this being especially important for those who did not have good social support), but they felt that the system of care was not responsive to them as individuals. Hospital care in particular was not centred on them: they had to fit into a system that seemed to have little regard for their personal needs or feelings:

I suppose when you are pregnant you want to be, I don't think they pampered me as much as I would have liked. Although you could have 5 children, you still want to be seen to ... maybe they felt I knew everything and it was OK, just to leave me to get on with it. I sensed that anyway. I don't think it is they didn't care, there just wasn't a great urgency – making sense? (s388)

I was never introduced to anybody. Everytime I went I saw three, I saw a different person and one of them was really horrible ... I don't think I had any support at all, well probably only from my GP ... because if I had a problem I just had to talk to him without getting a frowned face or being treated like I was in a cattle market, cause that is what it was. (s370)

Women with One-to-One midwives, because they had a midwife they knew and who coordinated their care, were less exposed to such problems in their hospital visits. The problems women described with hospital-based birth and postnatal care also appeared to relate strongly to the environment and organization or care, women not feeling that it always took sufficient account of them as a person.

Although their criticisms of hospital-based care, particularly postnatally, were often severe, women tended to perceive the midwives and other staff as also being disregarded within this system and often tempered their criticisms with comments about staff difficulties. This woman, for example, felt that services had declined since her previous baby's birth as a result of staff cuts:

they're trying to fight all the way, need more staff, cutting here, there and everywhere. (c116)

Some women, therefore, felt that the service was neither woman-centred (to use *Changing Childbirth* terminology) nor centred on staff needs.

Concepts of care and support

Feeling that you were the focus of care – that people were interested and concerned with you and prepared to treat you as a person – was closely bound up with what the women viewed as good care. Good care was often described as supportive. A small number of women specifically discussed the concepts of care and support because they felt so let down by the service. One described feeling 'on my own until he was born'. She felt that the GP had been the only supportive professional since she always saw different hospital staff, who were rushed and unavailable to talk to.

Women described support in terms similar to those identified by researchers: emotional (feeling supported and cared for), practical and informational support, all three being important, linked components of good care (Wheatley 1998; see also Chapter 12). This woman, like several others in the conventional care group, felt that she had been offered no emotional or social support by maternity professionals:

I was just having a horrible time and I just didn't feel there was anybody there for me to talk to. I literally just didn't know what was going on and I went to my classes but it's that emotional side, there was no support at all. I didn't know what I was doing, I just learnt and I still don't even believe I am a mum. Do you know what I mean? That care could have made that little bit of difference. (s370)

Other women highlighted the value of practical support, which depended on the midwife or GP taking time to listen to what the woman's needs were and to respond appropriately. This need not imply doing everything but might mean finding ways of facilitating more appropriate sources of social support. For example, although the women interviewed were a very varied group, some were without the support of partners or family members. The following woman, who was isolated from family support during a multiple pregnancy, appreciated quite simple but effective forms of support:

The midwife came to my home to give me the injection. I was very worried at this time as my husband was in … [home country] … she gave me nice words, reassuring, it was very important, she was friendly and didn't want to rush you. (c48)

This woman had found her care overall very supportive, both emotionally and practically – coming to her home and writing in support of her husband's visa application so that he could be there with her. Another

woman, also from a refugee community, described the supportive value of the midwife just being 'with' the woman.

The women also saw support as an active rather than a passive concept, as something that should be enabling rather than overbearing or pushed on the person, regardless of her wishes or needs. Good support would enhance rather than undermine confidence. Several women, particularly younger mothers and those with unplanned pregnancies, described ways in which One-to-One midwife care enhanced their confidence. One, for example, described how her midwife's support had enabled her to make a positive decision about her pregnancy rather than letting things happen by default. She felt she had grown up and gained a great deal in the process of becoming a mother and was planning her future with confidence:

reassurement and that, 'cause I was still two minded. It was really nice the way she handled the situation. She kept me going and made me finally decide. (c411)

Support as reassurance

A number of women also talked about the importance of reassurance as support in pregnancy. The way in which reassurance was handled, however, could make a considerable difference in its impact on the woman's feeling of confidence. Women with One-to-One midwives described how knowing that their named midwife, or her partner, was available for queries or problems at any time was very reassuring. Rather than encouraging overdependency on the midwife, and thus undermining confidence, several women described how knowing that help was easily accessible gave them the confidence not to turn to a professional for support too readily.

Knowing that I could like pick the phone up and talk to someone on a one-to-one basis sort of, like really relaxed me and gave me the confidence to carry on. (c717)

she said, do you want me to come and see you? All I needed was reassuring that I would not lose the baby. (c391)

In contrast, several women in the conventional care group described attempts at reassurance that did not relax them because they felt uninformed and fobbed off: the words of reassurance 'not to worry' did not fit with what they were experiencing. Two women, for example, were very worried when their babies did not breathe immediately following birth and required resuscitation. One described how she did not find the professionals' words reassuring:

they said its ok, everything's alright, which wasn't really true. It wasn't alright, but I suppose they need to reassure you, not worry you and stress you. (s388)

Instead, she relied on indirect signs such as observing the staff to gain reassurance. She described how her husband gave her a thumbs up sign when he could see the doctor's face relax. She also commented on how important it had been to her, for reassurance during labour and birth, that the midwife did not leave her alone at all.

Support during labour and birth was particularly highly valued in terms of promoting relaxation and reducing anxiety. Women with One-to-One midwives, in particular, described in detail how the support role of their midwife helped them to relax and cope with the pain and fears they experienced. Their midwives used a combination of talking, touch – especially massage – and guided breathing to help the woman to cope with her labouring. This was supported by the trust and knowledge they had built up antenatally:

She was very calm, very patient. She made me feel very relaxed. She massaged me ... My midwife was very relaxing and I was more relaxed because I was with someone I knew ... and er, talking to her, talking through the birth plan. I'd never had the opportunity before. (c391)

Other women similarly mentioned the importance of staying with the woman, being calm and kind.

Medical versus social support

A number of women in this sample experienced medical or obstetric problems during pregnancy or had had previous obstetric problems that meant they were regarded as 'high risk'. The concept of risk applied in this Trust was defined solely, at least formally, in biomedical terms. Although this meant that women were not subjected to stereotyping as being inherently 'at risk' because of their ethnicity or some concept of social disadvantage, it was apparent from several women's accounts that those defined as medically high risk felt that they had received better care and support than those who might have other, non-biomedically defined, needs for support. The comments of these two women illustrate the contrast in experience neatly. The first, who was admitted with medical problems, experienced good support and communication:

he [the consultant] was round the ward checking that everybody was alright you know, to see that everything was OK so I find it was very useful to talk to them about any problem you had ... I talked to the nurses as well. Some were very helpful, just the way they take care of you, you know, if anything, they asked if anything was bothering you and did I want to talk to anybody about it. (s553)

The second, however, described hoping that someone would ask her how things were at home, giving her permission to tell them about an abusive relationship with her partner:

and I would probably have broke down and let the whole thing out. But they've got a hard job to do as well so I must appreciate that, because there are a lot of women having babies. (s370)

Instead, she found that her need for support was met with 'raised eyes' and clear signals not to bother them or to take up too much time:

because you'd start to say something and they made you feel, oh my god, I'm not going to say any more. (s370)

In general, medically 'high-risk' women also experienced greater continuity of care and support than did other women in conventional care because of their frequent hospital visits; in many ways, their care, in these terms, was closer to that experienced by women with a One-to-One midwife, albeit more medically focused, since with frequent visits to the hospital's fetal care unit or inpatient stays, they were far more likely to get to know and be known by the doctors and midwives caring for them. However, in this system, medical and psychosocial needs are treated as unrelated, so that a consideration of the latter is an incidental rather than a planned or explicit aspect of care. The power of dualistic concepts of body/mind in medical care is illustrated very clearly by the case of one woman who described herself as having had 'special' care as a result of a previous stillbirth:

I was treated extra special because I'd lost a baby ... so I was treated with care and caution. I was explained a lot of things too so I knew where I was from day to day and why they were giving me certain drugs and what to look for. And so I was in tune with them and they were in tune to me because they knew about me and my previous history. (s600)

Yet once the baby was born safely, all the previous concern seemed to dissipate, and she was treated without regard for the impact of her previous loss:

and you know, after what has happened of course I don't want to leave her to go to the loo, but the fact of the matter is she was crying quite badly, obviously she needed a feed but I wanted to go to the toilet too or I would be in trouble later ... and I wheeled her out there, it was a draughty corridor, and I said to the nurse can I just ask you to keep an eye on her 'just leave her, just leave her in there' (dismissive tone) ... I remember wheeling her back to the room with my eyes stinging with water like I wanted to cry, it was stinging me and I wanted to cry but I thought no, I'm not going to let her get to me, I'm not going to let her get to me. I remember patting the baby saying I will be back in a second and I remember turning her on one side in case she cried and choked. (s600)

Such a split may also help to explain the greater dissatisfaction that women generally express about postnatal care in hospital, where they commonly describe little care or concern (Ball 1994; see also Chapters 10 and 12). The impression from the narratives of women in this obstetrically orientated hospital is that birth is regarded within a narrow, medically defined time-frame. The longer-term and more personal transition of becoming a mother is not given prominence, and antenatal care is regarded as important mainly for screening possible medical or birth-related problems rather than for personal preparation for the adjustments of parenthood.

Practical and emotional support

Pregnancy, birth and new parenthood constitute a major social and personal transition for women and their families, and support – both practical and emotional – features as an important component of what they see as good maternity care. We have already seen how women in conventional care received little attention to their emotional or practical support needs, particularly in hospital settings, at all stages of care. The postnatal period was a time in which these needs intertwined and practical support became particularly important. A minority of women were very happy with the levels of support they received. They tended to be women who had been admitted antenatally, so they were familiar with the hospital environment, routines and staff. The majority in both groups felt that support was generally inadequate and often inappropriate, although their experiences also differed according to which midwives were 'on', some being more helpful than others.

This group of women had experienced a greater than average level of pregnancy and birth complications; they were somewhat less likely to be first-time mothers but also less likely to have a supportive partner relationship. Therefore, their needs for support were significant, and this was reflected in a longer than average length of postnatal hospital stay. However, several women who had experienced serious complications felt that, once any emergency was over, basic care was lacking. One woman, for example, had been seriously ill as a result of 'an eclamptic fit' and had an emergency caesarean section:

when you are lying there with all them drips and everything I had my caesarean, the following day my brother came to wash me, the following day I was left for 2 or 3 days never been washed cause you lie there and you have all those tubes and machines and everything and you expect somebody to come and help. (s312)

She felt that the special care for her premature baby had been excellent but was upset and angry that she had often had to wait for a family member to visit and wheel her up to the special care unit. Others felt 'left to get on with it' but that staff would have been willing to help if asked. Several women, all with second or third babies and without medical complications, attributed the low level of support they received to staff assumptions that they did not really need it. They showed ambivalence about this, accepting that they would not require as much support as some women and that they had 'got on with it' themselves, but nonetheless feeling that genuine needs had been overlooked:

yes, with both babies, I think I would have, just a little. I suppose just to see you are OK. How are you doing? Are you alright? Is everything OK? Is the baby OK? Are you feeding alright? I think it is fair if you are ill and the baby is ill to spend more time with you, but the mothers that aren't still make them feel (pause) because you've gone through something traumatic, you know, having a baby is not easy. (s388)

Appropriate support

The way in which help was offered and its degree of congruence with a woman's expectations was also important. Women sometimes felt that when they asked for help, they were simply told what to do rather than being encouraged or helped practically. The following woman's comments on this theme also bring out the degree to which many new mothers can feel exhausted and helpless in the face of the many demands of recovering from birth and caring for a new baby in an unfamiliar environment, without friends or relatives around to help:

S decided that he wanted to go to the toilet and have something to eat at the same time and I was in the ward so I changed him while he was on the bed, but he was screaming the place down and she came into me and said 'feed your baby' and I went mad. I went mad because I had no sleep, I'm still trying to recover from the caesarean, I've got no experience whatsoever with the baby, this is only the second night, I don't know, he's making me sleep, I'm tired, I want to go to sleep. All I want him to do is shut up and he is crying and she is telling me about feeding the baby and I turn round and I said, literally said I've got one pair of hands and you can wait … Not like the old days where you got your rest and be ready for the baby. (s370)

Receiving conflicting advice was not as important an issue as feeling talked down to and told what to do rather than advised and supported. In this context, one woman commented that receiving conflicting advice from staff reassured her about her own abilities, since they could not all be right all of the time. Another woman, who did not speak fluent English, found it difficult to get advice because of the language barrier and said that she felt ashamed at having to ask people to explain things again.

The above quotation also highlights the degree of exhaustion that new mothers experience, which is apparently given little weight in the structures of care. Even after a caesarean, for example, another woman described feeling desperately tired and struggling with her baby but unable to persuade the staff to take her baby overnight until her third night with little sleep. Another described missing a meal since she felt too weak to get out of bed to get to the table. Lack of rest was the major issue that women raised in talking about postnatal support, and several harked back to the days when new mothers could expect more practical support and at least one night of relatively undisturbed sleep, their baby being brought to them by staff for feeding (Woollett & Dosanjh-Matwala 1990).

Women receiving One-to-One care felt less exposed to a lack of postnatal support in hospital since they received daily (or more frequent) visits from their One-to-One midwife, who generally carried out the basic medical checks, helped with feeding and offered general information and a chance to talk about any problems. Although several noted some tensions, or simply a lack of clarity or coordination concerning roles, between the hospital and the One-to-One midwives, their reports of hospital postnatal care were essentially similar to those of women in conventional care.

Support and feeding

Lack of rest and support was also mentioned by a number of women – both in this group and in our wider study – as a problem in establishing breast-feeding. However, in this group, despite more medical complications, rates of breast-feeding were very high. Generally, the women saw breast-feeding as more desirable but more difficult than bottle-feeding. Early problems experienced included pain and fatigue followed by concern, for a few women, that the baby was not satisfied with breast milk. Support from professionals was sometimes inadequate, inappropriate or counterproductive. As with other forms of support, help needed to be appropriate to the woman. Several women described the encouragement of their One-to-One midwife as being very helpful, whereas two control group women complained about professional pressure, one feeling that staff were heartless, just telling her to keep at it, the other saying that the midwife made her feel she would not be a good mother unless she breast-fed. Several women in each group did not need help because they had breast-fed successfully before and their babies settled quickly into feeding.

The general impression from talking to women in this and the wider study group is that health promotion or education efforts by professionals may be ineffective because they misread the issues from the woman's viewpoint. Most women were well aware of the benefits of breast-feeding. Many were strongly motivated to breast-feed, and those who were not were influenced by quite different considerations. Possible cultural and social differences in attitude and in the degree of embodied knowledge that women have before becoming mothers (Hodinott 1999) may have contributed to the particularly high breast-feeding rate in this group. However, the perception that bottle-feeding was easier and less tiring than breast-feeding was often borne out in practice by early difficulties, combined with generally low levels of postnatal support.

Communication and information

Good communication was extremely important to all the women and was seen as integral to good supportive care. In their views, communication should be open and a matter of dialogue: giving and receiving information and responding to it. Having a named midwife appeared to be particularly important in terms of feeling known and understood by professionals, meaning that the concept of knowing your midwife was very much a reciprocal one. As we have noted above, women in the conventional system lacked this type of relationship except with a good GP, or antenatally with a community midwife.

The conditions for and expectations of communication were in many ways set up by the experience of the initial GP visit, where most women said they had received little, if any, information about pregnancy or maternity services and were not encouraged to ask for it. Ironically, it was at this early point, when it might be argued that health education and promotion are most likely to be effective, that women experienced a considerable gap in care since (in terms of the service providers' rationale for care) there was no clinical need for visits. Yet pregnancy is a time when many women are eager for knowledge:

a first time mum who hasn't got a family, who hasn't got a partner should have the support of a midwife from 3 weeks pregnant, whenever she finds out ... the beginning stages are the worst. Nobody tells you anything, not even your GP. You are told to go away and come back ... 12 weeks is a very long time ... without knowing anything. (s370)

As we have noted above, this pattern of inadequate communication, of trying to explain yourself to strangers and feeling it a nuisance to ask questions, was continued at hospital visits and some GP visits. The degree to which the biomedical division between 'real' (i.e. clinical) and 'invalid' (other) concerns in pregnancy is constituted as part of women's care is illustrated in the comments of women who felt able to communicate well with their known midwife, even over 'silly' things:

she was much better in a way because if there was any small problem bothering you, you go to the hospital or the GP, you think oh, should I tell her? this is what was bothering me, whereas a midwife comes to you, you are friendly and you talk to them, you have no fears or anything you can say to them, look there is something bothering me, how small it is. They don't make you feel as if you are wasting their time. (c116)

Women receiving One-to-One care were very happy with the communication with their named midwife, and although they were as critical of communication with some other professionals as were the women receiving conventional care, they were less reliant on them in this respect. Several women emphasized how a continuing relationship with their midwife enabled good communication to take place, partly by building up trust and confidence and partly through the midwife coming to know and understand them and what they wanted and needed. Such a relationship made it less likely for the woman to need to communicate her wishes at stressful points such as labour and birth. Reaching such a relationship of understanding enabled some women to feel that they could confide in their midwife if they wished to do so:

my midwife and myself got on well. She was like my family there. I mean there was no difference between me and her, if I had to say to her, I can say anything and everything. (c116)

This situation contrasts strongly with the account of one woman in conventional care (quoted above) who felt that she could not confide in hospital midwives despite desperately wanting to, so that her needs for support were consequently disregarded.

Good communication was therefore a matter of feeling that information and understanding was being conveyed effectively between the woman and her carers. Most women commented about the importance of this. Some women felt fobbed off in routine hospital visits, where staff appeared very busy and uninterested and sometimes displayed an abrupt, impatient manner with women who wanted to ask questions but perhaps found it difficult to do so:

I think that mothers have the right to ask questions and get proper answers and the doctors and nurses need to have more patience with the member of the public really. (s312, when asked what could be improved about care)

Again, women with complex medical problems seemed to obtain more information and felt less anxious and more supported as a result. They also felt that staff were more interested and better informed about them.

Language and communication

The two women interviewed who did not speak fluent English had particular problems in communication with professionals. Both were receiving conventional care, and neither was offered an interpreter for any of their care, even though an interpreting service was officially available to midwives in this setting. Although they could speak some English, it was apparent that these women received very limited information and had been given few opportunities for discussion. Non-English-speaking women in our case study of Somali refugee women's experiences also felt that a lack of interpretation was a major shortcoming in their care, although those women who had a One-to-One midwife were much happier with their care overall (Harper-Bulman & McCourt 1997). Their problems in communication were particularly severe during labour and birth. Antenatal care had not been used as an opportunity to provide information or to find out what the woman's wishes were. Both complained that they were not offered pain relief despite their requests. One received an epidural later in labour, after a shift change introduced a different, more 'caring' midwife. The other was kept on the antenatal ward for most of her labour, with no support or pain relief, until her cries persuaded a midwife to examine her:

they found out only 30 or 40 minutes before he was born. When one of the midwives came to see me I am crying with pain, she found out the baby was being born ... she took me to the labour ward, she said quickly, the baby is being born. (s319)

Although communication was a major issue here, and it seems probable that the stereotyping of minority ethnic women – such as that 'Asian' women make a fuss and cannot tolerate pain well (Bowler 1993) – was at play, such experiences were described by a number of women in our wider survey who had been admitted to antenatal wards, either for induction, because they were thought not to be in 'established' labour or because the delivery suite was busy. All were subsequently treated as being 'not in labour' regardless of their own experiences of pain or fear, and a number were only transferred to the delivery suite late in the first stage, perhaps because they had laboured far more rapidly than the midwives had anticipated. Such a pattern of not listening to women or of not communicating effectively appeared to respond to what I have suggested above is the focus on the system rather than on the woman. In this case, the woman was not regarded as being in labour, despite her perceptions, because she was not in the appropriate place for labour and perhaps because staff did not perceive her to be in 'real' pain.

This tendency to disregard the women's views and experiences was also reflected in the birth experience of the other non-English speaking woman, whose request for an anterior episiotomy for female genital mutilation was ignored and who consequently blamed her difficulties in giving birth and her third-degree tear on the failure to consider her request. Similarly, she was unhappy that she was not consulted about using a ventouse to deliver the baby, even though she was very happy for this to be done. It was apparent from such accounts, and from other women's general comments about communication, that it was not the reciprocal process that they were seeking, particularly in hospital settings where important antenatal visits and all their births and early postnatal experiences occurred.

Professional attitudes and relationships with women

The women's accounts revealed important contrasts both between midwives and doctors on the one hand, and between One-to-One and hospital-based midwives on the other.

Although there were individual differences between professionals, some being described as extremely caring and attentive, others being seen as offhand and insensitive or even rude, their interactions with women fell into clear patterns. In general, negative contacts with professionals took place in hospital and with professionals whom the women did not know and who seemed too busy to be bothered with them:

I came across quite a few rude doctors and quite a few rude sisters. (s312; prompted to explain further, the woman described visits in detail and demonstrated their offhand manner)

Although the medical care was regarded as good, several women described patronizing or insensitive behaviour by some doctors, and it was clear that such behaviour could come from professionals who were otherwise very 'caring' in giving attention to a problem. Although none of the women ventured a view on whether the doctors' behaviour towards them was racist or discriminatory, it was noticeable, in comparison with our other interviews, that several women experienced medical attempts to control their fertility that, if not conscious or unconscious racism, simply did not trust women to make good, informed decisions. One woman commented that her GP had

attempted to persuade her to have an abortion because she had separated from her partner and already had several children. She felt that it was only her One-to-One midwife who supported her decision to continue with the pregnancy and therefore her confidence in being a good mother. Another described being firmly advised to undergo sterilization after a serious medical problem in her pregnancy and birth, without any information or counselling on other contraceptive options. A third commented that, when medical problems arose in her previous pregnancy, doctors had repeatedly questioned her about whether this baby really had the same father as her previous children. In this pregnancy, she had been deeply upset by one doctor's implication that she was being irresponsible in deciding to go on holiday, even though she had consulted midwives about her plans: she felt the doctor had no understanding of how deeply she cared about not losing her baby.

Women's views of midwives varied according to whether they were hospital-based, community or One-to-One midwives. Antenatally, women were generally happy with their contacts with community or One-to-One midwives, who were perceived as being more informative and more interested in the women as an individual. Hospital midwives were viewed as often being too busy and remote to provide support. Although midwives are the major care providers to women in labour, the lack of detailed comment about midwives in the conventional care group women's accounts of labour and birth is surprising. Views and experiences were very mixed, most women describing 'good' and 'bad' midwives, and most women seeing at least two because of shift changes. Good midwives were kind and sensitive, like family, willing to explain things and to listen, calm and willing to stay with the woman. Bad midwives were abrupt, caused anxiety as a result of their own insecurities, did not explain or ask permission for what they did and refused to acknowledge the woman's feelings. All but one of the women receiving conventional care were attended by midwives they had not met before, although several women were familiar with some hospital doctors and midwives as a result of antenatal admission.

Women receiving One-to-One care gave far more detailed and specific accounts of their midwife's role and used more emphatic terms in describing them, for example 'wonderful, good girls' as opposed to 'nice, kind'. All but one were attended by their named midwife and all by a midwife they knew. An analysis of the pronouns used by the two groups of women to describe midwives revealed an interesting relationship difference that connects with both knowing the midwife and the focus of care. Women with One-to-One midwives used a combination of personal names and possessive pronouns – typically 'my midwife' – whereas women in the conventional care group used impersonal pronouns such as 'they' and 'the midwife'. This use of language seemed to mirror women's comments on whether their care was personal or impersonal, and whether it centred on them or whether they felt they had to fit into a system (see Chapter 6 and Walsh 1998).

Continuity of carer

Women did not generally use the terminology of continuity of care or carer that is so familiar to midwives but talked instead of the value of knowing their carers and why this was important to them. As we have seen above, women's comments about their One-to-One midwives were mostly and often emphatically very positive, and women linked supportive care with knowing the midwife. Women saw their midwives as offering communication, trust, confidence and reassurance in a way that was far more patchy and unpredictable for women in conventional care:

you had that person you knew you could turn to all the time. (c537)

Their comments on knowing and being known were closely tied in with those on communication, attitudes and reassurance since they found hospital visits, with different staff every time, so unsatisfactory in this respect. Although such problems were described partly as staff being rushed, there was also a sense of staff as not being interested, not caring about the woman as a person since they had no chance to get to know her. Some women also felt that professionals were more likely to miss problems or provide contradictory advice in such a system.

One woman had a change of named midwife during her pregnancy. Changes are inevitable at times in such a system since midwives may leave, have babies themselves or take sick leave. This woman's experience suggested that the relationship did not need to be exclusive, with one person, as much as personal and centred on the woman. The new One-to-One midwife was readily able to take up this role:

well I could talk to her about anything and say to her everything, that's how much confidence I had in her. (c116)

When it came to the birth, the woman was less nervous than she had been for her first baby because she knew what to expect and knew the midwife:

whereas the second time, I knew exactly what was going to happen, when and how, that was one bit of it. Another thing

is you knew the person there and she was there only herself, no-one else. (c116)

The women did not have high expectations about continuity of carer at the outset, and it was clear that women receiving conventional care did not necessarily mind not knowing the midwife who attended them in labour as long as she was a good midwife. However, with some exceptions – such as the non-English speaking woman quoted above (s319), who described the midwives who were with her when she was eventually admitted to the delivery suite as being 'like sisters' – positive accounts tended to coincide with being able to get to know the professionals involved. Several women with One-to-One midwives were able to compare this with previous experiences of conventional care and felt that, even where previous care had been good, this was qualitatively quite different. For example, one study group woman compared this birth favourably with her previous experience. She felt that she had rapport with the midwife and was more relaxed with someone she knew; before, it had felt very clinical:

well they do know me, they recognise me, but my midwife, she was part of it, part of the birth, the baby. (c0391)

Another woman described similar feelings of relaxation and emphasized the importance of the midwife knowing her fears and how she felt about her previous birth experience as well as being able to take this into account:

we were talking for some time but because I had bad experience with N and I was scared about this talking but when I go in hospital when I saw [midwife] I was happy. I had confidence in her. I trusted her advice. (c492)

These comments, and those of several other women, also alluded to the importance of privacy, which was more commonly experienced by those with One-to-One midwives. Although a number of these women had birth complications, those with One-to-One midwives saw fewer professionals as well as knowing more of them. In contrast, several women in the conventional care group described being upset and anxious because of the large number of professionals coming into the room. Ironically, when one woman started to 'panic' about this, the midwife sent out the only person she knew, her sister, who had been holding her hand and comforting her.

Confidence and trust

Those women who knew their midwives well demonstrated greater trust and confidence in them and argued that this trust was important for their own sense of reassurance and confidence. Trust in the midwife appeared to engender more open communication but was also a product of feeling able to communicate and feeling listened to, cared for and taken seriously. This was particularly important in labour and birth, and was strongly linked to the feelings of relaxation and reassurance also described by the women.

DISCUSSION

It was clear from all the interviews that women generally hope for support from the maternity services. That support includes information, not just being told things but having an effective exchange of information that can build trust and confidence and help the woman to feel reassured and well prepared for birth and parenthood – practical and emotional or psychological support. The circumstances of these women varied greatly, but all expressed a desire to feel reassured, to feel special and self-confident in mothering. While some women praised the specialized medical care (and attendant support) that the hospitals were able to give, several women also suffered from what may have been very poor care or advice.

None of the women interviewed mentioned a direct experience of racism or discrimination in the services. It is possible that, without any means of comparison, they were simply not in a position to judge whether their treatment was worse than anyone else's (Proctor 1998). It is also possible that, in speaking to white interviewers, the women would not have felt comfortable about speculating on whether the care they received was fair. However, much of the research evidence is that, although there are many experiences of direct racism (Phoenix 1990, Douglas 1992, Neile 1997), much race discrimination arises from stereotyping and patronizing behaviour, which may not be recognized by the professional as such (Bowler 1993). There were several instances of such behaviour in women's accounts. The women did not single out or typify these as racist behaviour, and, owing to the open, narrative approach of the interviews, the researchers did not prompt women to say whether they thought this behaviour was racist or discriminatory. There is a sense in these accounts that the women often felt patronized by the maternity services and did not feel treated as people with their own strengths and problems, ideas, needs and wishes. This was largely in their contact with hospital maternity services, at all stages of care. Although the women valued information and support highly, what was offered was sometimes inadequate and at other times misplaced or inappropriate. Support is only likely to be effective if it

is perceived by the recipient as being acceptable and appropriate, and as not bearing too many other costs (see Chapter 12).

Our research arose partly from a desire to learn whether continuity of carer really mattered to women and whether it would increase their satisfaction with care. As we have noted, there has been some questioning of whether such concepts are important to women as long as they have a good midwife (Lee 1997, Green et al 1998), or of whether they are important to socially disadvantaged women. The women in this study had positive relationships with both traditional community and One-to-One midwives, but in the shared care system, the community midwives were rarely able to follow women through the service and maintain that sort of positive contact with them. Although some of the women clearly felt very strongly about the benefits of continuity of carer for them – including some who did not receive any continuity and felt that it was a major weakness in their care – others simply focused on aspects of care that they found helpful and that seemed somehow to go along with having 'your own' midwife. The term or concept of continuity is not sufficiently broad to capture entirely what these women saw as good about their care, yet it was also extremely difficult in the analysis to 'unpick' different concepts such as support, continuity, reassurance and so on from each other since each seemed to be connected and mutually reinforcing in the women's accounts. These women's accounts suggested that it was possible, but more difficult, to be a 'good' midwife without the sort of relationship entailed in caseload midwifery.

It was also apparent, from other aspects of our evaluation, that the midwives themselves felt a greater sense of personal control in caseload practice. This may facilitate the midwife's ability to provide care that is supportive without being patronizing and that enhances rather than undermines confidence, to learn the needs and wishes of the individuals on their caseload and to work in a more woman-centred way. There are hints in the women's accounts that the care seemed at times to go beyond an ordinary job, yet these midwives showed fewer signs of 'burn-out' and disaffection with their work than did the hospital midwives, despite being at times very tired as a result of calls to women in labour (Sandall 1997, McCourt 1998). For example:

She gave me her number and said I could call her any time and I thought Anytime! She said, you know, don't worry about it, as soon as you go into labour it doesn't matter what time in the morning and I felt she really cared you know. I felt this went beyond a job. I felt that she enjoyed her job. Some people that do it and my job and don't actually enjoy it, that comes across, but she was so caring. (c391)

It is important in research of this type not simply to assume that close relationships or the concept of support from professionals is necessarily or inherently a good thing. Sociological critiques of the concept of patient-centred medicine, for example, have drawn attention to the possibility that discourses of the social may effectively be a means of extending the medical gaze (Silverman 1987, Foucault 1973). There is a danger that taking a more 'holistic' approach could be misused as a means of surveying and intervening further in people's lives. However, pregnancy and birth represent a particular case, from the woman and family's viewpoint, of personal, social and cultural transition, and this was reflected in the way in which this group of women spoke about their desire for support from the maternity services, as long as the support offered was appropriate and responsive.

Women enter maternity care with an expectation of good care, that is, support, practical help and positive communication. Although reasonable, these are not always met. Fiore et al (1983) have argued that unmet expectations of network support and negative input can act as either stressful events or chronic stressors, adding to the individual's stress level. One key example of such 'negative input' found in this study was the tendency of professionals to disregard women's own knowledge and experience. This displacement of the woman's own and self-knowledge is the first step in telling women that they have no expertise or authority in caring for themselves and their child; it is as if they are being told 'You don't know what you are talking about.' This denial of personal authority and capability creates a fundamental problem in involving women in decisions about their care.

CONCLUSION

The aims of this study were twofold: to compare the experiences of women receiving two different models of maternity care, and to understand more fully the views and experiences of those minority ethnic women who were less likely to respond to a written questionnaire survey. Although they were an ethnically and socially varied group in themselves, the women described similar overall hopes and wishes with respect to the service, views that were similar to those in our wider survey and that have been found in a range of consumer studies (Reid and Garcia 1989, 1998, Brown & Lumley 1994, Percival 1994, 1998, Audit Commission 1997, Kitzinger 1998, Proctor 1998). They valued good communication, support and effective reassurance, sensitivity and the feelings of trust and confidence that they associated with knowing and being known by the professionals who care for them. These values were not distinct but connected and embedded in the overall system of care in such a way that any of these values appears to imply or at least to enhance the others.

What these women wanted and valued did not differ fundamentally from that seen in our wider study sample, so that the study did not support the assumption that women in minority or less advantaged groups will not be concerned about the issues raised in the *Changing Childbirth* report. The health professionals working within this context were also a socially and culturally diverse group, but this is not necessarily sufficient in itself to ensure that staff are sensitive to the needs of individual women in their care, as the particularly poor birth experiences of non-English speaking women in conventional care illustrate (Harper-Bulman & McCourt 1997).

Language remains a major barrier to access to good services for non-English speaking women, which is aggravated in a fragmented care system by a professional reliance on stereotypes in the absence of prior knowledge of the individual (Woollett & Dosanjh-Matwala 1990, Bowler 1993). Caseload midwives did not need to rely to the same extent on stereotypes since they had the opportunity to build up a knowledge of and communication with the woman. The degree to which the problems the women described in this study were the result of discrimination by staff should not be assumed, however, since similar themes – such as inadequacy of communication or support – emerged in our wider study (McCourt & Page 1996, McCourt et al 1998). The experience of unequal access is as much a structural one as an individual matter and needs to be addressed on a number of levels.

While they shared similar basic aspirations and values with the women in the wider study sample, this group of women experienced greater dissonance between their expectations and experiences: comparison between the conventional and One-to-One care groups revealed a *greater* divergence of views and experiences according to the system of care in this group of women than in the wider study. Therefore, minority ethnic women in the One-to-One group may have gained more, rather than less, from having 'their own' midwife, either because of greater social stress and a consequent need for socially as well as medically supportive care, or because of the mitigating effect of midwives who knew women personally and were therefore able to support ordinary personal needs, not needing to rely on stereotypes to understand what was required.

Table 13.2 Women's perspectives of the dimensions and attributes of caring: a fundamental framework for midwives

Dimensions	Attributes
Attitude	A friendly presence, i.e. body language, tone of voice, use of language
Respect	For a woman's knowledge of herself; for a woman's need; that she has a right to receive care; that it is the woman's experience that is of most importance; that she is a woman and part of a family
Support	To enable and enhance the woman's experience, i.e. being with her when she needs the midwife psychologically and/or with her physical presence; to offer and provide the amount and type of help she needs rather than what the midwife wants to give
Reassurance	That a woman will know her carers; that she can easily access her carers; that physical and practical care will be provided to a high standard; that she will be treated honestly; by the type of words and language used with appropriate knowledge; by the midwife's presence and attitude
Interest	In her pregnancy; with listening and focusing upon her at that moment
Communication	In particular, the ability to communicate through the choice of words, tone of voice, presence, use of language, listening, interest and focus

IMPLICATIONS FOR PRACTICE

It is clear from reading the study reported in this chapter that the way in which maternity care is organized affects the care that midwives are able to offer. This in turn affects women's perceptions of the care that they receive. The framework shown in Table 13.2 summarizes the six dimensions and attributes of caring that women mentioned frequently in this study. Although Table 13.2 is arranged linearly, the dimensions are interactive and thus support one another; in fact, the dimension of communication relies upon most of the other attributes to be effective.

While we acknowledge that particular ways of organizing midwifery care, such as One-to-One or caseload practice, helps the midwife to adopt these attributes more easily than others, all women have the right to these fundamental dimensions of caring.

Just as in the analysis, where it is frustrating to have to break up women's narratives and unpick coherent stories, in practice being caring and feeling cared for are not discrete actions. Care arises from genuine respect and concern for a woman and her family, and is more likely to occur outside the hospital situation and in situations where there is a relationship between the woman and the professionals caring for her. Nevertheless, although care may be limited by the lack of a relationship, there are a number of simple actions that will at least avoid negative care.

An important principle of *Changing Childbirth* was that the maternity services should be attractive and accessible to all women. One of the strategies foreseen was to move as much care as possible to the community. Having professionals who are part of a woman's community and who have some understanding of her way of life is an important step in creating a climate of care. Equity is important; this does not mean dividing resources up equally but targeting populations with a greater need. Thus, if only a small number of women in a service can receive continuity of care, it would be best to target groups such as those of ethnic minority families.

Practical support is important to childbearing women, but practical support will probably not have a positive effect if it is given with the wrong attitude. Impressions and presence are important to women. In addition, body language says a lot. It is no good going through the motions of caring if your body is saying something different. Sometimes, it is possible to think that you are being helpful, but you may be perceived as looking bored or harassed by those for whom you care.

What women mean by care is not well defined, and we should accept that although the characteristics may be similar, the emphasis may not be the same. We can and have characterized what women in this study

---

Pointers for practice

- Women expect good care from the maternity services.
- What they see as good care is often quite simple.
- Negative care or uncaring (acts of omission or acting in an uncaring way) are powerful negative influences.
- It is important to get to know the woman as an individual and respond to her needs.
- Caring is made easier by knowing women over time and in community settings.
- Care involves practical help, support and empathy.
- Care requires that the midwife acts as a facilitator to help the woman in making decisions.
- Communication is a foundation for good care.
- The fundamental care needs of women across different social and cultural groups are similar but the details will differ: good communication is vital to learning what these are.

meant by caring. This also fits with the results of a number of other studies illuminating the idea of caring (Hallsdottir & Karlsdottir 1996, Percival 1990).

We found that the women in this subgroup did not differ substantially in their perceptions of care from the women in the remainder of the study. One of the most important aspects of care for women is for midwives to be able to get to know them as individuals. This is facilitated by an appropriate system of care. Even if such a system is not available, women need sensitive care that is appropriate to their needs. Midwives should consider their individual practice to assess whether or not they are providing this care. To do so will make a great deal of difference to the experience of childbearing women.

REFERENCES

Audit Commission 1997 First class delivery: improving maternity services in England and Wales. Audit Commission, London

Ball J 1994 Reactions to motherhood: the role of postnatal care. Cambridge University Press, Cambridge

Baxter C 1996 Working from a multi-racial perspective. In: Kroll D (ed.) Midwifery care for the future: meeting the challenge. Baillière Tindall, London

Beake S, McCourt C, Page L 1998 The use of clinical audit in evaluating maternity services reform: a critical reflection. Journal of Clinical Evaluation in Clinical Practice 4(1): 75–83

Beck C T 1995 Perceptions of nurses' caring by mothers experiencing postpartum depression. Journal of Gynaecological and Neonatal Nursing 4(9): 819–25

Bowes A M, Meehan-Domokos T M 1996 Pakistani women and maternity care: raising muted voices. Sociology of Health and Illness 18(1): 45–65

Bowler I 1993 'They're not the same as us': midwives stereotypes of South Asian descent maternity patients. Sociology of Health and Illness 15(2): 157–78

Brown S, Lumley J 1994 Satisfaction with care in labor and birth: a survey of 790 Australian women. Birth 21(1): 4–13

Department of Health. Changing Childbirth. Report of the Expert Maternity Group (Cumberledge report). HMSO, London

Douglas J 1992 Black women's health matters: putting black women on the research agenda. In: Roberts H (ed.) Women's health matters. Routledge, London

Fiore J, Becker J, Coppel D B 1983 Social network interactions: a buffer or a stress. American Journal of Community Psychology 11: 423–40

Foucault M 1973 The birth of the clinic: an archeology of medical perception. Tavistock, London

Garcia J 1994 Assessing the needs and experiences of women using the maternity services who do not speak or write English – report of the meeting. Unpublished document, National Perinatal Epidemiology Unit, Oxford

Garcia J, Redshaw M, Fitzsimons B, Keene J 1998 First class delivery: a national survey of women's views of maternity care. Audit Commission/National Perinatal Epidemiology Unit, Abingdon

Gluck S, Patai D (eds) 1991 Women's words. The feminist practice of oral history. Routledge New York

Green J, Coupland B A, Kitzinger J 1988 Great expectations: a prospective study of women's expectations and experiences of childbirth. Child Care and Development Group, Cambridge

Green J, Kitzinger J, Coupland V 1990 Stereotypes of childbearing women: a look at some evidence. Midwifery 6: 125–32

Green J, Curtis P, Price H, Renfrew M 1998 Continuing to care: the organisation of midwifery services in the UK: a structured review of the evidence. Hochland & Hochland, Hale

Halldorsdottir S, Karlsdottir I 1996a Journeying through labour and delivery: perceptions of women who have given birth. Midwifery 12: 48–61

Halldorsdottir S, Karlsdottir I 1996b Empowerment or discouragement: women's experience of caring and uncaring encounters during childbirth. Health Care for Women International 17: 361–79

Harper-Bulman K, McCourt C 1997 Report on Somali women's experiences of maternity care. Centre for Midwifery Practice, Thames Valley University, London

Hirst J, Hewison J, Kauser Z 1998 Assessing the quality of maternity care for Pakistani and indigenous white women. A report to the Northern and Yorkshire Region. Unpublished document. Northern and Yorkshire Region

Hodinott P, Pill R 1999 Qualitative study of decisions about infant feeding among women in the East End of London. British Medical Journal 318: 30–35

Jordan B 1993 Birth in four cultures. A crosscultural investigation of childbirth in Yucatan, Holland, Sweden and the United States, 4th edn (revised and expanded by R. Davis-Floyd). Waveland Press, Prospect Heights, IL

Kempe A 1994 The quality of maternal and neonatal health services in Yemen, seen through women's eyes. Swedish Save the Children, Radda Barnen

Kirkham M 1989 Midwives and information-giving during labour. In: Thomson S, Robinson A (eds) Midwives, research and childbirth, vol. 1. Chapman & Hall, London

Kitzinger S 1998 Having a baby in the John Radcliffe: some women's experiences. Unpublished document

Lee G 1997 The concept of 'continuity' – what does it mean? In: Kirkham M, Perkins E (eds) Reflections on midwifery. Baillière Tindall, London

Leininger M 1988 Caring, an essential human need. Proceedings of the three national caring conferences. Wayne State University Press, Detroit

Le Var R M H 1998 Improving educational preparation for transcultural health care. Nurse Education Today 18: 519–33

McCourt C 1996 One-to-one midwifery: women's responses. Modern Midwife 6(1): 8–11

McCourt C 1998 Working patterns of caseload midwives: a diary analysis. British Journal of Midwifery 6(9): 580–5

McCourt C, Page L 1996 Report on the evaluation of One-to-One midwifery. Centre for Midwifery Practice. TVU, London

McCourt C, Page L, Hewison J, Vail A 1998 Evaluation of One-to-One midwifery: women's resposes to care. Birth 25(2): 73–80

Martin E 1989 The woman in the body. Open University Press, Milton Keynes

McIver C 1994 Obtaining the views of black users of the Health Services. King's Fund, London

MacDonald J 1993 The caring imperative: a must? Australian Journal of Advanced Nursing 11(1): 26–30

Morse J M, Bottorff J, Neander W, Solberg S 1991 Comparative analysis of conceptualizations and theories of caring 23: 119–27

Neile E 1997 Control for black and ethnic minority women: a meaningless pursuit. In: Kirkham M, Perkins E (eds) Reflections on midwifery. Baillière Tindall, London

Nursing Council of New Zealand 1996 Draft guidelines for the cultural safety component in nursing and midwifery education. Nursing Council of New Zealand, Wellington, NewZealand

Parsons L, Day S 1992 Improving obstetric outcomes in ethnic minorities: an evaluation of health advocacy in Hackney. Journal of Public Health Medicine 14(2): 183–91

Percival P 1990 The relationship between perceived nursing care and maternal adjustment for primipara during the transition to motherhood. PhD thesis, Curtin University of Technology, WA

Percival P 1994 Womens' perceptions of care from community child health practitioners. Primary Health Care (ed) C Cooney 295–312 Prentice Hall, Sydney

Percival P 1998 Research in progress. Edith Cowan University, Perth, Western Australia

Phoenix A 1990 Black women and the maternity services. In: Garcia J, Kilpatrick R, Richards M (eds) The politics of maternity care. Clarendon Press, Oxford

Piercy J, Wilson D, Chapman P 1996 Evaluation of One-to-One midwifery practice. York Health Economic Consortium and Centre for Midwifery Practice, University of York

Pizzini F 1992 Women's time, institutional time. In: Frankenberg R (ed.) Time, health and medicine. Sage, London

Proctor S 1998 What determines quality in maternity care? Comparing the perceptions of childbearing women and midwives. Birth 25(2): 85–93

Reid M, Garcia J 1989 Women's views of care during pregnancy and childbirth. In: Chalmers I, Enkin M, Keirse M J N C (eds) Effective care in pregnancy and childbirth. Oxford University Press, Oxford

Robinson S 1989 The role of the midwife: opportunities and constraints. In: Chalmers I, Enkin M, Keirse M J N C (eds) Effective care in pregnancy and childbirth. Oxford University Press, Oxford

Robinson S 1990 Maintaining the role of the midwife. In: Garcia J, Kilpatrick R, Richards M (eds) The politics of maternity care. Clarendon Press, Oxford

Rook K S 1984 The negative side of social interaction: impact on psychological wellbeing. Journal of Personality and Social Psychology 46: 1097–108

Rudat K, Roberts C, Chowdhury R 1993 Maternity services: a comparative survey of Afro-Caribbean, Asian and white women commissioned by the Expert Maternity Group. MORI Health Research, London

Sandall J 1997 Midwives' burn-out and continuity of care. British Journal of Midwifery 5(2): 106–11

Scheper-Hughes N, Lock M 1987 The mindful body. A prolegomenon to future work in medical anthropology. Medical Anthropology Quarterly 1: 6–41

Shore C 1998 Creating Europeans: politicisation of culture in the European Union. Anthropology in Action 5(1/2): 11–16

Silverman D 1987 Communication and medical practice: social relations in the clinic. Sage, London

Swanson K 1991 Empirical development of a middle range theory of caring. Nursing Research 10: 161–6

Thomas H 1992 Time and the cervix. In: Frankenberg R (ed.) Time, health and medicine. Sage, London

United Kingdom Central Council for Nursing, Midwifery and Health Visiting 1998 Midwives rules and code of practice. UKCC, London

Walsh D 1998 An ethnographic study of women's experience of partnership caseload midwifery practice (the BUMPS scheme). Master's dissertation, Leicester Royal Infirmary NHS Trust

Wheatley S 1998 Psychosocial support in pregnancy. In: Clement S (ed.) Psychological perspectives on pregnancy and childbirth. Churchill Livingstone, Edinburgh

Woollett A, Dosanjh-Matwala N 1990 Postnatal care: the attitudes and experiences of Asian women in east London. Midwifery 6: 178–84

Woollett A, Dosanjh-Matwala N, Hadlow J 1991 Reproductive decision-making: Asian women's ideas about family size, and the gender and spacing of children. Journal of Reproductive and Infant Psychology 9: 237–52

Wright S 1998 The politicization of 'culture'. Anthropology Today 14(1): 7–15

Adaptation and growth in pregnancy, birth and early life

The unicellular sperm and egg come together, and, in the space of 266 days, a multicellular organism has been formed, capable of functioning as an independent being, no longer supported by the placenta and the maternal tissues. The woman is pregnant, bearing within her a new and soon to be separate life. During that 266 days, her body undergoes dramatic physical changes to support the life growing within her. After birth, the newborn adapts to the new extrauterine environment, in most cases without problems. Midwives support women and their babies through this physical adaptation, assessing for problems and providing advice and support for healthy development. In addition, they help to prepare parents for the task of caring for the newborn. This requires an understanding of the physiology and associated experiences for the mother as well as the potential for problems. The following chapters describe in detail genetic, embryonic and fetal development, and newborn life as a basis for midwifery care. The final chapter provides mini sessions to use in teaching parents about the care of the newborn.

14

The beginning of life

Anna Kessling   Di Watt

Genes contain all the instructions for growing and running the human body: a complete instruction manual for building, maintenance and repair – what to do where, when and for how long. Genes are made of DNA, which is contained in chromosomes. There is a complete set of chromosomes in every cell of the body.

THE CELL AS THE CONTAINER OF GENETIC MATERIAL

Every part of the body is made up of cells. Each cell of the body, starting from the first one (the fertilized egg) contains the complete genetic information of the individual in its nucleus, except for circulating red blood cells, which have no nuclei. As a cell divides into two, it makes a copy of the genetic information so that both new cells have identical copies. Ultimately, all the cells of an adult's body contain all the genetic information that was in the original fertilized egg. Since it is not useful to make, for example, heart tissue in brains (or vice versa), the genetic information regulates its own use in order to ensure that, although each nucleus contains *all* the genetic information, only the instructions relevant to any particular cell, tissue, organ and developmental stage are used in any individual cell. Some of the basic maintenance instructions (functions analogous to plumbing, wall maintenance, energy supply and sewerage), are the same for every cell but others are highly specific to different cell types. Thus, heart muscle cells make heart muscle (and not, say, brain or kidney cells), and brain cells make brain rather than heart proteins. Thus, the differences between the organs and tissues of the body arise because they make different proteins at different times in different amounts. In most cases, each gene contains the precise instructions for the body's manufacture of one protein. The genetic information contained within

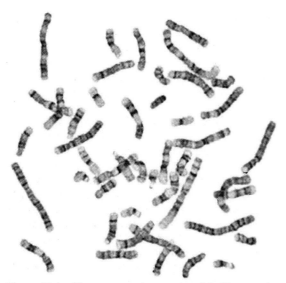

Figure 14.1 Chromosomes in a man's cell that is preparing to divide. (Reproduced with kind permission, copyright © 1995 Department of Pathology, University of Washington, Seattle, from the web site http://www.pathology.edu/Cytogallery)

the nucleus of each cell is the instruction manual for life. This genetic information is conveniently packaged within the nucleus in chromosomes.

CHROMOSOMES

Apart from eggs and sperm, every cell of the human body contains 46 chromosomes (in 23 pairs) (Fig. 14.1). They are given numbers according to their size (chromosome 1 being largest) (Figs 14.2 and 14.3).

Each chromosome contains a 'landmark' called the centromere somewhere along its length. The centromere is involved in cell division (see below). The centromere is never exactly in the middle of the length of the chromosome so each chromosome has a long arm (cytogeneticists call this the q arm) and a short arm (the p arm; see Fig. 14.4). Differences in the relative lengths of the p and q arms and in the size of the chromosomes, together with special staining methods, allow cytogeneticists to distinguish between all the chromosomes in dividing cells by the pattern of bands they show (see the photographs in Fig 14.1 and 14.2 and the schematic diagram in Fig. 14.3 above). Chromosomes in which the centromere is at around the middle of the length (e.g. chromosome 1) are called

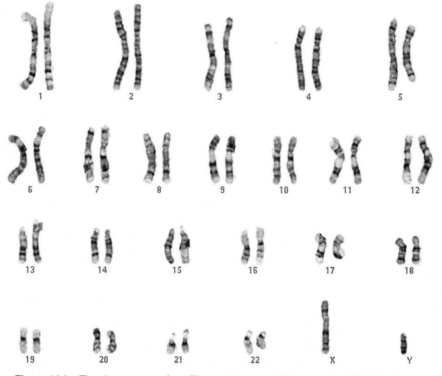

Figure 14.2 The chromosomes from Figure 14.1 arranged in size order. Note that there are two of each chromosome except for X and Y.

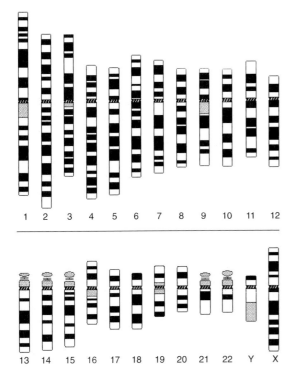

Figure 14.3 numbering:
1 2 3 4 5 6 7 8 9 10 11 12
13 14 15 16 17 18 19 20 21 22 Y X

Figure 14.3 Diagram (called an idiogram) of the banding patterns seen on the chromosomes in Figure 14.2 (only one chromosome of each pair being shown).

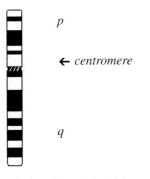

p

← *centromere*

q

Figure 14.4 The long (q) and short (p) arms of a chromosome, and its centromere.

metacentric chromosomes; if the centromere is very near one end, the chromosome is said to be acrocentric (e.g. chromosome 14 or chromosome 21).

The chromosomes form the 23 volumes of the instruction manual, one set of 23 being inherited from the father, the other from the mother. Volumes 1–22 are precisely matched in the two sets; these 22 paired chromosomes are called the *autosomes*. For each of the 23 pairs of chromosomes, one chromosome of the pair

is inherited from the mother and the other from the father. This is achieved because eggs and sperm have only one chromosome from each pair (so the fusion of the egg and sperm reconstitutes a 46-chromosome cell containing all the genetic material needed to make a new person). A person with 46 normal chromosomes is said to be *euploid*.

Chromosomes are like long, thin threads made up of DNA (see below) and protein. The threadlike structures are so fine that they cannot be seen under an ordinary microscope unless a cell is dividing (see Fig. 14.1 above). All the genetic information is contained within the DNA. The order of the genes on the chromosomes is the same in all humans, but the gene order does not relate to the order in which we grow, nor are the instructions for any particular part of the body grouped logically together on the same chromosome. The position of a gene on one chromosome of a pair is precisely matched by the position of a second copy of the same gene on the other chromosome of that pair. However, through the course of evolution, the body has worked out how to interpret all the genetic information and to make sense of sets of instructions concerning the same process but taken from different chromosomal sources. In effect, each cell has two complete sets of the instruction manual in the two sets of chromosomes. The body reads both sets of instructions and follows them both. Since the father inherited his set of chromosomes (volumes of the manual) from all the generations of his ancestors and the mother inherited her set from all the generations of her ancestors, it is no surprise that the passage of time will have resulted in some small differences between the two sets in their child. (Consider what differences there might be between two well-read copies of the same book passed down the generations of different families for hundreds of years.) Genetic disorders result from errors in the instructions (which may be as small as a single-letter typographical error; see the section on DNA below). The body's use of both sets of instructions is a useful failsafe mechanism that may allow normal function despite an error in one set of instructions when there is no corresponding error in the matching set.

Small errors in the genetic instructions are called mutations (see also below).

Sex chromosomes versus autosomes

At the genetic level, all the differences between men and women depend on a single pair of chromosomes: the sex chromosomes. Women have two X chromosomes, while men have a Y chromosome and only one X (see Figs 14.1 and 14.2 above). This is the root cause of all the gender differences. The sex chromosomes make up the twenty-third pair – the '23rd volume' of the instruction manual; the Y chromosome is smaller, so the sex chromosomes are a matched pair in women and a less well-matched pair in men. The Y chromosome is essential to male gender. Since women have no Y chromosomes, they cannot pass them on to their children. Thus, the gender of babies is determined entirely by the contribution from the *father*. Each egg contains one X chromosome but no Y. Each sperm contains either an X or a Y. Each fertilized egg has an X chromosome from the mother and gets either a Y chromosome or an X chromosome from its father (in the fertilizing sperm) to become a boy or a girl respectively.

The genetic instructions on the autosomes pass to children of either gender with equal probability.

CHANGES IN THE CHROMOSOMES

If the chromosomes are damaged or rearranged, or if there is an extra one, the body may turn out differently.

Disorders of chromosome number

(*Aneuploidy* = being 'not euploid')

The body is well adapted to using two sets of genetic instructions. However, if the fertilized egg has a whole extra chromosome (as in trisomy; see below) extra to the usual 46 (or one less), it has more instructions than it needs (or not enough if one chromosome is missing). The body has no mechanism to 'switch off' the 'spare' instructions (or to make up for the absence of a set of instructions). Thus, it over- (or under-) does everything that was controlled by the extra (or absent) chromosome. The importance of this over- or underproduction depends entirely on the nature of the particular tasks being over- (or under-) performed, their timing in development, growth and life, their location within the body and their importance. The importance of a set of genetic instructions, or the task for which it codes, itself depends on timing and location, and also on fail safe 'insurance' mechanisms within the body. The body has more than one way of carrying out some of its functions (like a bypass or an alternative route in travelling), and extra copies of some of its genetic instructions, but, in general, genes on all the autosomes are essential to normal bodily function.

How is it possible to have a fertilized egg with 47 chromosomes? In general, this happens if either the egg or the fertilizing sperm has an extra copy of one chromosome. This, in turn, can arise because of a problem in the specialized form of cell division (called meiosis) that gives rise to eggs or sperm, such that the egg or sperm ends up with 24 chromosomes, including

two copies of a particular chromosome. (Conversely, an egg or sperm that has 'lost' one chromosome may end up with only 22, so that the fertilized egg would have only 45). (See also mosaicism below.) The presence of an extra copy of a chromosome is called trisomy (tri = three). Figure 14.5 shows the chromosomes of a girl with trisomy 21, Down syndrome. It should be noted that three chromosomes 21 instead of two are present.

The relevance of aneuploidy to midwifery

Trisomy has been recorded for all human chromosomes. For most autosomes, trisomy is incompatible with life outside the womb. Trisomy of chromosome 1, the largest chromosome, is very rare and is not compatible with fetal development, perhaps because there are so many genes on chromosome 1. Trisomy of chromosome 19 is also very rare in spontaneous abortions (maybe because some genes crucial to normal development are found on chromosome 19). The most common trisomy at birth is trisomy 21 (Down syndrome); trisomies of chromosomes 13 or 18 are also compatible with survival to birth but have far more severe consequence for the fetus and baby. The trisomy most often found in fetuses is trisomy of chromosome 16. Trisomy of chromosome 21 and the X chromosome, and the presence of an extra copy of the Y chromosome, are all compatible with survival into adulthood, as are aneuploidies with larger numbers of X or Y chromosomes. The lack of one copy of a chromosome is called monosomy for that chromosome. Monosomy of the X chromosome causes Turner syndrome. Children with other complete monosomies do not survive. It is also possible for a fetus to have an extra complete set of chromosomes (polyploidy).

Mosaicism

If a person has a proportion of cells showing one chromosome constitution (for example, a normal one) and the other cells show a different chromosome constitution (for example, missing an X chromosome, or some other aneuploidy or rearrangement), that person is said to show mosaicism. It is as if their cells make up a mosaic of more than one type. The only way to exclude mosaicism definitively in any of us is to study every individual cell in our body. Clearly, this is never practical. Similarly, if mosaicism is found in, say, the white blood cells, this is no guarantee that the whole body will show mosaicism to the same extent, or less, or more. By the same token, it is possible to miss a case of mosaicism in testing a particular tissue that does not show it, or shows it at very low frequency. Thus, it is

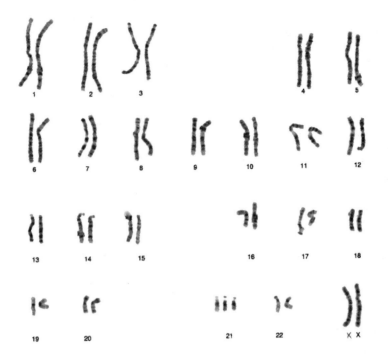

Figure 14.5   Chromosomes of a girl with trisomy 21 (Down syndrome).

possible to find mosaicism in a baby born after amniocentesis has shown normal chromosomes. Mosaicism can occur for all sorts of chromosome disorder. The outcome for the affected child will depend upon which tissues show mosaicism and is not predictable with complete certainty. However, the higher the proportion of mosaicism in the amniotic fluid, the greater the likelihood of some abnormality in the baby. Conversely, a very low level of mosaicism is so common as to be considered normal.

Mosaicism is thought to result from a problem with the sharing out of chromosomes when a cell divides, during the early cell divisions after fertilization. Provided that the new chromosome number is compatible with cell survival, it will pass on through subsequent cell divisions to all the cells and parts of the body eventually produced from the first cell in which the problem arose. Meanwhile, all the other body cells will have the standard chromosome number as they will have arisen from cells that did not have the chromosome-sharing problem.

Chromosome rearrangements

A part of a chromosome may be missing: this is a dele-

tion of part of a chromosome, together with the genetic information it contained. In the instruction manual analogy, if one volume has missing pages, those instructions cannot be followed. If there is a perfect set of those instructions in the matching volume, the body may manage to compensate for the missing parts, but this does not always work as the body sometimes needs 'two lots' of what the instructions say, so 'one lot' may not be enough. If the same pages are missing from both volumes of a pair, the body has no instructions to work on so it cannot carry out the tasks specified in the missing parts. The consequences for the body depend on the importance of the task for which the instructions are lost.

The most common type of chromosome rearrangement is an inversion, in which a small piece of an individual chromosome appears to have been removed, turned upside down and replaced. All the genetic material is there, but rearranged. If this happened in a volume of our instruction manual, we might still manage to follow the instructions by turning the book upside down to read the inverted section. The body also seems to cope with some inversions, so much so that some of them are considered by cytogeneticists to be simply a part of normal variability.

Some chromosome rearrangements in parents may cause problems in pregnancy. That most often encountered is a translocation, in which parts of two different chromosomes are broken off and joined back together in a new arrangement. The most common type of translocation is one in which two acrocentric chromosomes (with particularly short 'short arms') are joined together through their centromeres, losing the short arm material from both. The loss of this genetic information has no known effect on the body. (Perhaps there are spare copies on other acrocentric chromosomes, or were these missing pages of the manual blank?) This type of translocation is known as a Robertsonian translocation. Balanced chromosome rearrangements (see below) are found in around 1 in 500 newborn babies and unbalanced rearrangements in about 1 in 200 newborn babies (Evans 1977) if pregnancies are allowed to go to term.

If two different chromosomes both break and each broken end then rejoins to the main part of the other chromosome – in other words, the chromosomes 'swap' part of their material – the consequences for the body will depend on where the break was; this is called reciprocal translocation.

Imagine ripping the last 30 pages from each of two volumes of a manual and sticking them back into the wrong volume. It might not matter at all if the rip happened neatly between self-contained sets of instructions for separate functions of the body. A person with normal body function who has a chromosome rearrangement without loss of genetic material is said to have a balanced translocation. All the right instructions are intact, and the body is able to manage, even though the instructions are on a different chromosome. Balanced translocation may become important for future pregnancies. Rearrangements are not, however, always so neat. Mending the ripped manual could create major problems if the tears were in the middle of sets of instructions but the repaired pages seemed to read smoothly through, resulting in, for example, the loss of instructions for when to stop a particular function. (Consider the consequences if this happened with, say, the building of a brick wall.) Another example might be if, for example, instructions for puberty were interrupted and continued as instructions for a little toe joint (consider half a garage being built in an upstairs bedroom). If this type of translocation arises, depending on the importance to the body of the particular instructions interrupted, it may result in disease, malformation or non-viability, which might present as spontaneous abortion or as loss of a pregnancy so early that it had not yet been detected.

Translocations in midwifery

Translocations inherited from the parent or arising anew in the fetus (*de novo* translocations) impinge on midwifery because they may lead to spontaneous abortion, fetal abnormality or congenital malformation.

The proportion of healthy people with a balanced translocation is 0.8% (roughly 1 in 200 people possessing a Robertsonian translocation and 1 in 500 a reciprocal translocation). The consequences in pregnancy depend on the nature of the translocation and the precision of the mechanisms of egg and sperm formation. Consider a person who has a Robertsonian translocation between two chromosomes from two different pairs (e.g. 14 and 21). Each cell in that person also has a normal chromosome 14 and a normal chromosome 21. Only one chromosome from each pair is meant to go into an egg or sperm. If both normal chromosomes go into the egg or sperm, there is no problem. If the translocated chromosome goes into the egg or sperm and neither normal chromosome accompanies it, there is no problem for a fetus formed from the union of that egg or sperm with a normal sperm or egg, respectively. However, the egg or sperm production mechanisms may not recognize the translocated chromosome as being both chromosome 14 and chromosome 21, and may add the normal version of one or other chromosome, resulting in a disorder of the amount of chromosome material, equivalent to a disorder of chromosome number (see below). In the case of a 14:21 translocation, the presence of extra chromosome 14 material would cause spontaneous abortion; the presence of extra chromosome 21 material would result in a pregnancy with Down syndrome. Here, see Figure 14.6; if the grey chromosome were chromosome 14 and the black chromosome were chromosome 21, part F shows how a translocation between chromosomes 14 and 21 could give rise to trisomy 21, and parts C and D show two ways in which a parent with such a translocation can have a child who does not have Down syndrome. Using the same principle, consider what would happen if a translocation in a healthy person involved both copies of the same chromosome (e.g. between both chromosomes 21). Then any egg or sperm formed in that person and containing any material from that chromosome would necessarily contain material from both copies (the translocation) and would thus result, again with the addition of the chromosomes from a regular sperm or egg, in a fetus with an extra copy of the chromosome 21 material and Down syndrome.

Consider also the situation with respect to the formation of an egg or sperm in someone who has a balanced

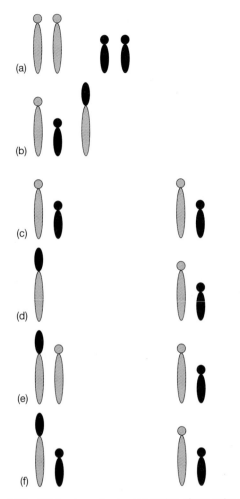

reciprocal translocation. If pieces of chromosome material have been 'swapped' between two chromosomes from different pairs, and both rearranged chromosomes enter the egg or sperm (with neither of the normal, matching 'partner' chromosomes from either pair), the child will also carry the balanced translocation and will develop normally. However, if either of the rearranged chromosomes ends up in an egg or sperm with a non-rearranged 'partner', that egg or sperm will have an extra copy (partial trisomy) of the genetic information shared by the non-rearranged partner and the 'swapped' part of the rearranged chromosome. This situation is an extension of that shown schematically in Figure 14.6. This will have consequences for the fetus and child, the severity of which will depend on the size of the region of partial trisomy and the importance of the genes it contains.

The importance of chromosome rearrangements in midwifery

More than half of all spontaneously aborted fetuses have a chromosomal abnormality. Professor Pat Jacobs' work (with colleagues) has informed much of current knowledge on this subject; over 8% of all clinically recognized pregnancies have some chromosomal abnormality (Hassold & Jacobs 1984). The same study commented that increasing maternal age is probably a risk factor for all trisomies (at least when the extra chromosome comes from the mother), but the pattern of increase of frequency with age is not the same for all

Figure 14.6 (**A**) A schematic representation of two pairs of chromosomes (one black and one grey), both acrocentrics. (**B**) The result of a Robertsonian translocation between two chromosomes, one for each pair. The short arms are 'lost' and the chromosomes joined through the centromere. A person with this kind of translocation usually shows no ill-effects but is said to be a translocation carrier. (**C–F**) These consider the theoretical consequences of a person with this type of chromosome rearrangement having children. In each of C–F, the two chromosomes on the right of the figure represent those contributed to a potential child by the partner after the translocation carrier (i.e. one chromosome from each pair), and the chromosomes to the left of each section of the figures represent the different combinations of genetic material that could be contributed by the translocation carrier. All the chromosomes in each of the sections C–F would be found together in the fertilized egg. The translocation carrier's cells may contribute chromosomal material to the egg or sperm in a number of different ways.

If the chromosomes passed on are as in **C**, the future child will have the same normal two pairs of these particular chromosomes as anyone else (one of each pair from each parent). If the chromosomes passed on are as in **D**, the child will have the chromosome constitution of the carrier parent.

In both **C** and **D**, the egg or sperm formed contains only the normal amount of genetic material (apart from the missing acrocentric short arms, which it can usually manage without). Thus, the body can be assumed to have 'recognized' that the right amount of genetic material was going into the egg or sperm. This does not always work as smoothly. E shows (on the left) the combination of genetic material that may be found in the carrier's egg or sperm if the body should happen to treat the translocated chromosome as if it represented only the genetic material from the black chromosome. Thus, the body recognizes the translocated chromosome as though it contains only the black chromosome's genetic material, and supplies an entire grey chromosome to the egg or sperm. In E, the resulting fetus would be trisomic for the genetic material on the long arm of the grey chromosome.

F shows the consequences if only the genetic material from the grey chromosome is 'counted' by the body. Thus, the body recognizes the translocated chromosome as though it contains only the grey chromosome's genetic material, and supplies an entire black chromosome to the egg or sperm. In F, the resulting fetus would be trisomic for the genetic material on the long arm of the black chromosome.

chromosomes. Note that even in very young mothers, a fetus can have Down syndrome. Indeed, the chance of having a child with Down syndrome (around 1 in 1500) is higher than the chance of having a child with cystic fibrosis (around 1 in 2000 for Northern Europeans), for example. Most chromosomal abnormalities in spontaneously aborted fetuses are trisomies and do not reflect any parental chromosomal abnormality. Although 50% of spontaneous abortions are caused by a chromosomal abnormality in the fetus only, and because spontaneous abortion is so common, most genetics centres do not look for parental chromosome abnormality until a couple have had three spontaneous abortions.

More subtle chromosome rearrangements are also possible. Some of these have been described only a few times or never before. These rearrangements vary from the adding in (insertion) or removal (deletion) of a tiny piece of chromosome from within a particular band (cytogeneticists being able to detect rearrangements virtually invisible to the untrained eye) to a bigger duplication in which a part of the chromosome is 'repeated'. An example of this would be if the heading of this section read 'The importance of chromosome rearrangements in midwifery': the letters are all there, but the order is different. The importance of these kinds of rearrangement may be related to the size of the rearranged chromosomal material and to the specific genes (if any) interrupted in the rearrangement. A duplication is likely to render a person partially trisomic for genes in the duplicated region. The consequences for the person depend on the nature and importance of the genes in the duplicated segment.

The cytogenetics service laboratories will usually search the published literature from all over the world to see whether there has been a previous report of a particular chromosome rearrangement that happens to be new to them, in order to give the most complete information possible about the probable consequences for the person with that rearrangement. If a fetus is found to have such a rearrangement, the cytogeneticists will often ask to test the parents' blood too because if a parent has the same rearrangement without ill-effects, the child may be equally unscathed. Some rearrangements are always accompanied by the same types of consequences for the child; others vary from one child to the next – again, the cytogenetics service laboratory will usually try to give the fullest possible information on the particular rearrangement found.

Detecting chromosome rearrangements

Many chromosome rearrangements are detectable on microscopy as alterations in the banding pattern of the chromosomes. To identify or exclude a particular rearrangement (because of, for example the family history or the characteristics found in a fetus or child) or one or a few particular types of trisomy (in amniocentesis, for instance), cytogeneticists may use a more recent technique known as FISH (fluorescent in-situ hybridization). This allows them to use commercially available material (which has been prepared from a particular chromosome or chromosome region and labelled with a fluorescent dye) as a 'probe' to find and identify matching chromosomes or regions in a cell. These matching regions will fluoresce or 'light up' in a cell whose chromosomes are visible under the microscope because it is in the process of dividing (metaphase FISH), or even in a cell in which the chromosomes themselves cannot be seen because it is not in the process of dividing (interphase FISH). A chromosome region present in the normal matching places on a pair of chromosomes will give two fluorescent dots on matching chromosomes in metaphase FISH or two dots (without the chromosomes being visible) on interphase FISH. If one copy of the region is, for example, deleted, only one dot will appear in either case. FISH with a fluorescent probe for a part of chromosome 21 will give three dots in a cell from someone with Down syndrome (trisomy 21). FISH for the whole of a chromosome can be used to detect when part of that chromosome has become rearranged, whether by translocation or by insertion within another chromosome.

Fetal cells in maternal circulation　The occasional cell from a fetus can make its way into the mother's bloodstream. A great deal of research effort is going into the search for ways in which efficiently to identify these cells and test them for specific genetic problems. This may become feasible using FISH or gene tests on the DNA.

Limitations of cytogenetics.　Cytogenetic techniques can detect only those changes big enough for cytogeneticists to see, although they can see better and more sharply as time goes on, given the refinements in technique available to them. However, they cannot examine every cell in a person's body, nor can they detect small rearrangements – individual spelling mistakes in the genetic instructions – or even whole missing genes, where the amount of material missing is not enough to change the appearance of a chromosome under the microscope. Many genetic changes cannot (yet) be detected by cytogenetics.

Detailed cytogenetic investigation relies on the presence of a sufficient number of dividing cells to study, among those examined under the microscope. In most cases, this means that the cells taken in the sample for cytogenetics have to be allowed or encouraged to divide in the laboratory, which takes a few days, and the cells then have to be treated and stained so that the cytogeneticists can see the banding pattern. This means that chromosome tests cannot be carried out instantly. Laboratories can usually check the chromosomes on an urgent blood sample within 2–3 days, but the average reporting time for amniocentesis samples is 14–15 days (because there are fewer cells and they grow more slowly). Some centres are able to give a faster result using different techniques. In future, techniques for single-cell analysis may shorten the reporting time, but, with current detection technologies, faster tests tend to be more limited in scope: quick tests on single cells will be unlikely to detect subtle chromosome abnormalities unless a major technological breakthrough happens first.

GENES AND DNA

All our genetic information (all the instructions) are stored inside the chromosomes. The information is stored as a sequence of chemicals joined together end to end in a molecule called DNA (deoxyribonucleic acid). DNA is rather like a long ladder in that it is made of two long strands (the 'backbone', like the uprights of the ladder), each joined to the other at regular intervals (these links being like rungs of the ladder; see Fig. 14.7). The chemicals that store the genetic information are the rungs of the ladder. There are only four sorts of chemical making up these 'rungs', and the whole of the genetic information (and thus the instruction manual for the whole of human life) is written using a chemical language with an alphabet of only four letters. The four chemicals are abbreviated to A, T, C and G. A (adenine) and G (guanine) are similar to each other in structure, being members of a group of chemicals called purines, and are bigger than the other two, C (cytosine) and T (thymine), which are part of a group of chemicals called pyrimidines. To keep the ladder straight, the chemicals pair up across the rungs in such a way that each rung has a big and a small chemical; thus, overall, each rung is the same length. To lend stability to the DNA as a whole and to each individual rung, the pairing is even more sophisticated. A pairs only with T, and G with C, because this is how they fit together best. A and T fit together like jigsaw pieces with two 'prongs' and 'holes' each; G and C are like jigsaw pieces with three prongs and three holes; thus they fit together best in the pairs as stated and represented in the diagram in Figure 14.8. Each A, T, C or G is tightly attached to the upright of the ladder

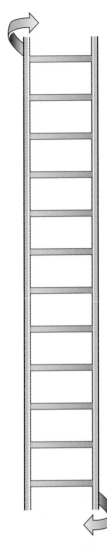

Figure 14.7 DNA is like a ladder. The uprights are twisted around each other, as indicated by the arrows.

and more loosely to its pair from the other upright. The whole of the ladder arrangement is twisted around itself, like the strands that make up a piece of wool or string, to form the characteristic double helix shape (represented in Fig. 14.9).

There are 3000 million of these chemical 'letter' pairs contained in the human DNA instructions. All the genetic information is contained within the DNA and is 'written' in, or coded by, the order of these four chemicals in the DNA molecule. All the instructions for making and maintaining people are written in this DNA code. Some parts are organized into genes.

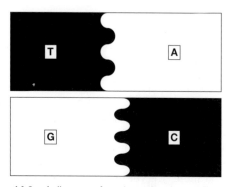

Figure 14.8 A diagram of two 'rungs', or base pairs of DNA. Each base pair is of the same length, and they fit together only as G with C or A with T.

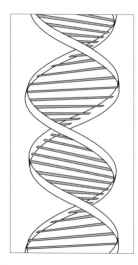

Figure 14.9 Diagram to represent the DNA 'ladder' after it has been twisted into the double helix shape. The rungs are all the same length in this three-dimensional structure. Each 'turn' contains 10 'rungs' of base pairs (see text).

A gene is a piece of DNA that directs and organizes the formation of a protein. DNA is stored in the nucleus of the cell, and proteins are made outside the nucleus, in the cytoplasm. The instructions on the DNA have to be moved into the cytoplasm so that these proteins can be made. The DNA is too big (and too important to the nucleus) to move. What happens is that the DNA strands (each upright and its half of each rung) separate, and the DNA code of one strand is then rewritten (transcribed) into RNA: ribonucleic acid. RNA is similar to DNA in its backbone and its chemicals, except for two major differences. First, it is (usually) single stranded; second, T is replaced by U (uracil). Thus, in making RNA from a DNA strand, the body adds a G to the RNA for every C in the DNA, a C for every G, an A for every

T and a U for every A. This is done very precisely in order to correspond to the DNA molecule. Encoded within the DNA molecule are special signals for the start and stop of the rewriting process (transcription).

The newly made RNA strand then moves out of the nucleus into the cytoplasm, where the body has a protein-manufacturing system. Here, the order of chemicals on the new RNA strand is 'read' in words of three chemical letters. Each three-letter word signals the protein-manufacturing system to add a specific amino acid (the building blocks of proteins) to the protein. The order of the three-letter words determines the order of the amino acids. Thus, the RNA chemical letter sequence is translated into the order of amino acids in a protein. Since it was the DNA sequence that determined the RNA sequence, it is the DNA sequence that encodes the protein.

As the proteins are encoded by 'words' of three chemical letters, typographical errors in the DNA can have minor or devastating effects on the proteins produced, and thus on any body function to which those proteins may be essential. Consider a simple example in English. 'The cat can eat cod' makes sense, and a reader might still understand 'tha cat can eat cod' or 'the rat can eat cod': neither is right, but they are still comprehensible. In the same sort of way, some chemical errors in the DNA are still compatible with a nearly normal protein being made. Not all mutations, which is what the 'typographical errors' in the DNA sequence are, cause disease. If a letter is added or removed while retaining the three-letter word rule, the result is nonsense. Consider 'tha eca tca nea tco d' or 'thc atc ane atc od'. The body has as much difficulty making sense of garbled messages as we do. This is the simplest way in which mutations in the DNA cause altered proteins that cause genetic disease. Other genetic diseases may arise because a large piece of a gene is missing (a deletion) or because of mutations involving non-coding regions of the DNA.

Since most proteins in the body are not needed in most cells of the body for most of the time, parts of the DNA 'letter' sequence also code for instructions specifying when, where and how much protein is to be made. These regulatory sequences usually lie outside the main 'coding' part of the gene. Mutations involving regulatory sequences can also cause genetic disease if protein manufacture then takes place at the wrong time in development and growth or in the wrong tissue or organ. The DNA also contains a very large number of sequences, still made up of A, T, G and C, that have functions not yet known or understood. Some of these sequences, called introns, are interspersed within the coding regions of genes. One source of their importance to genetic disease is that they need to be removed before a protein is made, otherwise non-coding bits of DNA will be made into 'nonsense' protein. The full functioning of introns is poorly understood at present. Other species may even have whole genes within the introns of other genes, although this has not yet been shown in humans. The size or DNA sequence of the introns may be crucial to the proper functioning of genes.

The A-T and C-G pairs fit together so predictably that the sequence of one strand of the DNA completely determines the sequence of the matching strand. The body uses this remarkable property to ensure that the genetic information is passed intact from cell to cell. When a cell is going to divide, forming two cells, the whole of the genetic information must be passed on to both of them. To ensure that this is done accurately, the body copies both strands of the DNA molecule. The DNA molecule separates (between the pairs of chemicals forming the 'rungs'), and new As, Ts, Cs and Gs are added alongside each of the long single strands, in order to reconstitute two new double-stranded molecules from the original one. Each new molecule is an exact replica of the original. This is called semi-conservative replication as the original DNA molecule is 'half conserved' in each of the new ones. When chromosomes are visualized in a dividing cell, their DNA has already replicated, but the two copies stay joined together at the centromere until the cell is ready to divide, when they separate through the centromere, one copy going into each of the two new cells formed. As this happens for every chromosome in every pair, each new cell receives the complete set of genetic instructions intact.

The A-T and C-G pairs fit together so well that if a DNA molecule is taken apart between the pairs of chemicals (through the 'rungs'), the two strands will find each other again and pair up. It also means that if the precise DNA sequence of a particular gene region is known or available to scientists, that region can be 'found' in the whole of the human DNA by a complementary DNA sequence. This is useful because identifying one base pair change among 3000 million possible sites would be difficult without some means of focusing effort on a particular gene of interest. The complementarity of the DNA strands is the whole basis of DNA diagnostic techniques.

DNA diagnostic tests are currently based on two main techniques. The first, useful in searching for a known mutation in a limited gene region, is the polymerase chain reaction (PCR). It is based on semi-conservative replication and in the laboratory generates a very large number (millions) of copies of a very small DNA region. A single cell may contain enough DNA to start the reaction. The PCR reaction makes enough DNA to be able to see (with appropriate staining) and investigate. PCR is quick and can be carried out within a day, but each PCR reaction investigates only a finite DNA region; thus, a very big gene might need a number of reactions to cover it.

The second main technique (called Southern blotting, after its inventor) is slower but allows any part of the DNA to be studied. DNA is extracted (usually) from white blood cells and cut into manageable pieces using enzymes that recognize particular sequences of bases and cut at those. The cut pieces are then separated by size by loading them into thin oblong 'wells' in one end of a flat gel (which looks like a square about 20×20 cm of grey jelly with a row of long, thin wells parallel to one end) and driving an electric current through the gel. The smallest fragments move through most quickly, the largest fragments most slowly, so if the DNA from one person is put into one well, all that person's genetic material becomes spread across the gel in a lane (like a runner's lane on an athletics track, only straight) on the gel. The current is turned off and the gel is blotted onto a matching square of a special nylon membrane. The DNA comes out of the gel and becomes 'stuck' to a supporting membrane. The scientists then use a separated, single strand from a natural or synthetic DNA molecule containing a sequence of interest, label it with a chemical stain or radioactivity and then use the single strand as a 'probe' against the blot. The parts of the blot containing DNA matching that in the probe will be detectable by the stain or the radioactivity as a line (or 'band') across the part of the blot corresponding to the lane. If the person has a few hundred bases deleted from the band in question, for example, the band corresponding to the probe sequence will be smaller in that person than in others whose DNA lies in parallel lanes on the blot. Everyone's DNA moves at the same rate through these gels, so a band of the same size will always be at the same level on the blot. It takes about a week to get a result from this technique. A complex or new mutation may need many reactions or blots and studies of affected family members before it can be detected.

There are thousands of small differences between people's DNA sequences. These determine all the variability among us of normal functions as well as the uniqueness of the individual.

MODES OF INHERITANCE: HOW GENETIC DISEASE IS INHERITED

While women have two X chromosomes and thus two sets of instructions for those body functions controlled by the X chromosome, men have only one. If there is a mutation in the genetic instructions on a boy's X chromosome, his body will make a corresponding mistake in carrying out those instructions. Although the boy inherited his X chromosome from his mother, she had another X, which is likely to have 'masked' the mutation in her. Thus, in general, when there are mutations in genetic instructions on the X chromosome, the following can be said:

- These mutations are carried and passed on to their children by females.
- Males inherit mutations on the X chromosome from their mothers and are affected.
- Affected males (provided that the condition does not interfere with their fertility) can pass mutations on the X chromosome on to their daughters.
- The daughters of affected males become carriers.
- The daughter of a carrier mother can become a carrier by inheriting the X chromosome with the mistaken instructions.
- The daughter of a carrier mother can become a non-carrier (unaffected) by inheriting the mother's other, unaffected chromosome.

This is called sex-linked inheritance. (Like most things in biology, however, this rule has occasional exceptions.)

Errors in the genetic instructions on the autosomes pass to either gender with equal probability. Some mutations on the autosomes can be severe enough to cause a disorder if they are present in only one copy, that is, if the instructions on the other chromosome are intact. Thus, everyone who has this type of mutation will be expected to have the corresponding disorder, and everyone who inherits the chromosome with the gene with the mutation will get the disorder too … but since each child inherits only one chromosome (and one copy of the gene) from the affected parent's particular pair:

- children have an equal chance of inheriting the disorder (or not);
- on average, one in two children of an affected person will be affected;
- the risk of being affected is the same for each child, in the same way as a tossed coin can land as 'heads' or as 'tails' with equal probability each time it is tossed.

This is called autosomal dominant inheritance.

Again there are exceptions as, in some cases, it is possible to inherit and pass on the mutation for a dominant disorder without being affected oneself. This is called partial penetrance, and is usually stated as a percentage: 100% penetrance means that everyone who gets the gene with the mutation will also get the disease; 80% penetrance means that 80% of people who get the gene with the mutation will get the disease, and 20% will not, but they can still pass the mutation on to their children. Geneticists do not yet understand the causes of variable penetrance.

A person who has one copy of an autosomal dominant mutation and a normal copy of the same gene is said to be heterozygous (hetero meaning different).

Other errors on the autosomes do not cause any disorder unless both matching sets of genetic instructions on a pair of chromosomes carry the same, or similar, errors. Thus, a person can have a chromosome that carries this type of error without being affected. This type of person is called a heterozygous carrier. The carrier has two different versions of the gene. If two heterozygous carriers of the same genetic disorder (the same error or mutation in the genetic instructions) have children, each of the children can inherit either a gene with the mutation or one without it, from either parent, again with one chance in two of getting either chromosome – the one with or the one without the mutation in that gene – from either parent. So any child of such parents can end up with:

- two chromosomes with no mutation in the particular gene on either;
- one chromosome with a gene with a mutation and one without (heterozygous carrier);
- two chromosomes with genes with the mutation (homozygous affected), 'homo' meaning 'the same'.

When the egg and sperm come together to initiate development of a new individual, all the genetic information stored in them is passed on to the growing embryo, thus laying down his or her unique genetic blueprint.

The development of the human is a remarkable event. It starts with the coming together of the unicellular sperm and egg, yet, in the space of 266 days, a multicellular organism has formed, one capable of functioning as an independent being no longer supported by the placenta and the maternal tissues.

GETTING STARTED

It is during sexual intercourse that the sperm and egg, or male and female gametes, normally first encounter each other. With the development of *in vitro* fertilization (IVF) of course, such events need not take place within the female genital tract. The coming together of the two gametes is the signal to initiate the onset of development and the consequent formation of the new individual. The gametes are very complex cells that have a long life history of their own. They begin their sojourn in life within the testis and ovaries of the fetus when the latter is developing within the mother's uterus. Thus, during our fetal lives, we produce the cells necessary to enable us to reproduce, the maturation of these cells not occurring until we ourselves reach puberty.

Fertilization, be it within the female genital tract or in the artificial environs of the test tube, is the event that brings together the genetic information of the father and mother, thereby setting the 'blueprint' for the new individual with his or her own unique set of characteristics, or phenotype. Prior to fertilization, the female gamete is called a secondary oocyte, its final maturation and the completion of the second meiotic division being triggered by fertilization, with the resultant production of the ovum or egg containing the 23 chromosomes contributed by the mother. During fertilization, the sperm penetrates the outer coats surrounding the ovum, passing through the outer protective clear membrane, or zona pellucida, and gaining access to the plasma membrane of the egg. Fusion of the membrane of the egg with that of the sperm head allows the genetic material present in the nucleus of the sperm to pass into the substance of the egg. This results in a fertilized ovum or zygote containing the genetic material of both the mother and the father, and hence all the genetic information needed for the new individual.

The zygote divides by mitotic division to form two cells or blastomeres, around which the zona pellucida persists (Fig. 14.10). Mitosis continues until a multicellular structure, or morula, is formed, each cell of the morula containing a complete set of 46 chromosomes. Division to the multicellular state occurs while the zygote journeys down the fallopian tube to the fundus of the uterus, where implantation of the developing embryo into the uterine wall (endometrium) will take place.

IMPLANTATION – A MUTUAL EVENT

At approximately 7 days post-fertilization, the conceptus implants into the uterine wall, the normal site of implantation being high up in the posterior wall of the uterus. Abnormal sites of implantation can occur, leading to an ectopic pregnancy. The fallopian tube is the most common site of an ectopic pregnancy, less common being abdominal and ovarian pregnancies. Implantation may not always occur in the most favourable site. In the condition known as placenta

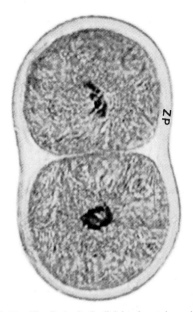

Figure 14.10   The first mitotic division has taken place in this hamster zygote to form the two-cell stage of development. The two blastomeres are clearly seen, still surrounded by the zona pellucida (ZP). In normal development, the zona pellucida protects and nourishes the developing embryo as it migrates through the fallopian tube.

praevia, the placenta wholly or partially covers the cervical canal. Here, detachment of the placenta prior to term could result in haemorrhage during the later stages of pregnancy, the consequence being fetal or even maternal death.

Implantation takes place during the blastocyst stage of development. The multicellular morula changes its structure to consist of an outer layer of cells – the trophoblast – and inner cells – the inner cell mass – the rest of the space within the blastocyst being occupied by a cavity (Fig. 14.11). The trophoblast is predestined to give rise to the chorion, a membrane that will be elaborated into finger-like projections or villi, this structure forming the basic unit of exchange in the placenta. The embryo itself will develop from the inner cell mass. Thus, as the embryo develops, it is separated from the maternal tissue by the chorion and is therefore said to develop within a chorionic sac (Fig. 14.12). As development proceeds, cells are laid down between the trophoblast and the inner cell mass. Although these cells, called extraembryonic mesodermal cells, form a solid continuum between the inner cell mass and the trophoblast, they eventually thin down to give rise to cells that cover the membranes supporting the embryo and also to cells that line the trophoblast.

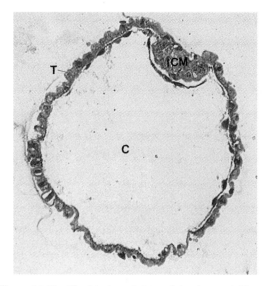

Figure 14.11   The blastocyst stage of development. The inner mass (ICM) will give rise to the embryonic tissues, whereas the outer trophoblast (T) cells will elaborate the chorion. The large blastocyst cavity (C) allows room for the developing embryo to grow.

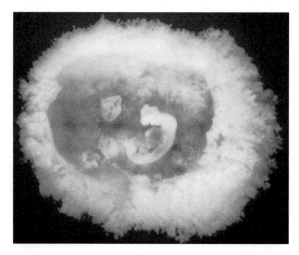

Figure 14.12   A human embryo at approximately 35 days post-fertilization developing within the chorionic sac. The chorionic villi, forming the basic unit of the placenta, are seen around the chorion as frond-like projections. In this picture, the villi and chorion have been dissected from one side of the chorionic sac to reveal the developing embryo. Chorionic villi extend into the maternal endometrium, and gaseous and nutrient exchange occurs by diffusion between the pools of maternal blood within the intervillus spaces and the fetal blood contained within the fetal blood vessels that differentiate from mesoderm formed within each villus.

PLACENTAL DEVELOPMENT

Prior to implantation, the developing embryo has shed the zona pellucida, enabling the sticky trophoblast cells overlying the inner cell mass to adhere to the endometrial surface. Implantation is a two-way process, the maternal endometrium being receptive to the blastocyst and capable of providing a supportive environment for it. At the area of trophoblast contact with the endometrium, the trophoblastic cells lose their cell boundaries and form a multinucleate tissue or syncytium. Syncytiotrophoblasts insinuate themselves between the epithelial cells of the endometrium, forming the placental villi that penetrate into the endometrial stroma. This stroma is rich in blood vessels and glands, and will supply nutritional support to the embryo prior to the establishment of the placenta. In response to the invading syncytiotrophoblast, a reaction known as the decidual reaction occurs within the endometrium. The endometrial cells accumulate glycogen and lipids, and form a barrier of tightly adherent cells around the developing embryo. This reaction is thought to be an adaptation to prevent rejection of the 'foreign' embryo by the maternal tissue. The syncytiotrophoblast is so invasive that it erodes the walls of endometrial blood vessels, resulting in maternal blood oozing into the spaces between the syncytiotrophoblastic villi. Gaseous and nutritional exchange will take place between the fetal blood vessels that subsequently develop within the syncytial villi and the maternal blood within the spaces. Not all of the trophoblasts become syncytial, however. Those which retain their cell boundaries – the cytotrophoblast – proliferate and form a core of cells in each of the villi. The cytotrophoblast cells penetrate through the tip of each villus and mushroom out to join up with each other, forming a cytotrophoblastic shell.

The villi now consist of a core of cytotrophoblast that has emanated from the tips of the villi and an outer covering of syncytium. They are described as anchoring villi as they attach the developing chorionic sac to the maternal tissue. Towards the end of the 3rd week, the mesodermal cells lining the trophoblast also proliferate and form a core of cells within the villi, and it is from these cells that the fetal blood vessels of the placenta develop. All these developments establish the basic structural unit of the placenta – the tertiary villus containing the fetal blood vessels (Fig. 14.13A).

During the early stages of placental development, villi project from the entire circumference of the embryonic disc. As development progresses, the villi regress from all around the chorion save in the area overlying the inner cell mass, which is in turn rapidly

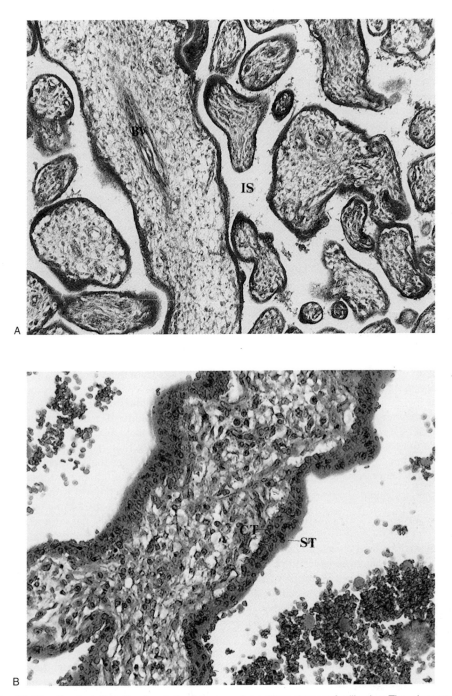

Figure 14.13   (**A**) Site of implantation of a developing human embryo 16 weeks post-fertilization. The micrograph shows an area through the placental villi. Some of the villi are seen in longitudinal section and others in transverse section. Trophoblastic cells are confined to the periphery of each villus whereas the core consists of mesoderm and fetal blood vessels (BV). Intervillus spaces (IS) between the villi are filled with maternal blood. (**B**) In this micrograph of a section cut from a human placenta 2 months after fertilization, examination of the villi at higher magnification reveals each to be surrounded by two layers of cells. The inner layer is the cytotrophoblast (CT) and the outer layer the syncytiotrophoblast (ST). The cytotrophoblast regresses from most of the villi around the fourth month of pregnancy, thinning down the placental barrier and allowing a greater diffusion of oxygen and nutrients between maternal and fetal blood.

differentiating to establish the basic layers of the embryonic body. With regression of the rest of the villi and the continued growth and differentiation of those overlying the embryo, the discoidal placenta is formed. In order to cope with the increasing demand for fetal–maternal exchange, the remaining villi branch and sub-branch. Each increasingly smaller sub-branch receives a smaller fetal blood vessel, resulting in a greater surface area for exchange to occur between the fetal and maternal blood. It should be stressed, however, that there is no mixing of maternal and fetal blood; there is merely an exchange of oxygen and nutrients that occurs by diffusion between the two blood streams.

The placental barrier between maternal and fetal blood thus consists of the syncytiotrophoblast, the cytotrophoblast, mesodermal cells and the endothelium of the fetal blood vessels. Figure 14.13B shows a villus at higher magnification. At this stage of placental development, both cytotrophoblastic and syncytiotrophoblastic cells are present around the villi. As pregnancy continues, the fetal growth rate increases, the demand for nutrients and oxygen increases, and there is in turn a need for the placental barrier to thin down to allow for an even greater exchange between the two circulatory systems. This is achieved by a breaking down of the cytotrophoblastic layer within the villi and a disappearance of the mesodermal cells in the core of the villi. During weeks 6–9 of development, it is possible to take samples from the villi. By undertaking such chorionic villus sampling, screening for chromosomal and hence fetal abnormalities can take place.

THE EMBRYO ITSELF

It is obviously essential for the placenta to be formed at an early stage of development in order to nourish and support the developing embryo. As implantation is taking place, changes are also occurring within the inner cell mass to establish both the basic tissue plan of the embryo and some of its supporting membranes. The cells nearest to the blastocyst cavity flatten and give rise to a single layer – the hypoblast or primitive endoderm. These cells will eventually form the embryonic gut and its associated glands. The rest of the inner cell mass forms the epiblast or primitive ectoderm. The amnion becomes evident approximately 7 days post-fertilization, although in human development it is unclear exactly how this structure arises. It is thought that a cavity arises in the primitive ectoderm to give rise to the amniotic cavity and the cells that form the roof of the cavity give rise to the amnion.

Approximately 10 days post-fertilization, cells from the primitive endoderm migrate to line the blastocyst cavity. The cavity so enclosed is called the yolk sac (Fig. 14.14).

At this stage of development, there is no clue to which end of the embryo will form the head end and which the more caudal structures. The axis of the embryo is established by the appearance of the primitive streak (Fig. 14.15A) approximately 13 days post-fertilization. This is formed by a thickening of the primitive ectodermal cells that converge to the central area of the disc. A groove appears within the streak, the cells arriving at the streak migrating into the groove and flowing out laterally, thus establishing layers of cells below the ectoderm but above the endoderm. By taking a transverse section through the developing embryonic disc as indicated by the line XY in Figure 14.15A, the way in which the third layer of the embryo is developed can be visualized, and the cross-sectional diagram represented in Figure 14.15B shows this process occurring. The cells that have migrated via the primitive streak give rise to the embryonic mesoderm layer, and some of these cells also contribute to the endoderm, although the latter is also derived from the hypoblast.

The earliest cells to pass through the primitive streak migrate the furthest laterally to form the extra-embryonic mesoderm, which lies between the developing embryonic disc and the trophoblast. The mesoderm cells that remain between the ectoderm and endoderm form the intra-embryonic mesoderm (Fig. 14.15C). Although the extra-embryonic mesoderm is initially very thick, it thins down to line the trophoblast and cover the amnion and yolk sac, leaving a well-defined cavity, the extra-embryonic coelom, between the developing embryo and the trophoblast, in all but one area (Fig. 14.15C). The cavity allows for growth of the embryonic disc. The area where the extra-embryonic mesoderm remains solid is the body stalk (Fig. 14.15c), which represents the forerunner of the umbilical cord.

At the cranial end of the primitive streak, a small accumulation or 'node' of cells also occurs; these migrate below the ectoderm but this time in a cranial and midline rather than a lateral direction. These cells are of great significance because they establish the notochord (Fig. 14.15A). Cells in the notochord are capable of signalling to undifferentiated tissues present in the newly formed embryo, directing them to differentiate and develop into the definitive tissues and organs of the body. In particular, notochordal cells signal to certain areas of the ectoderm, inducing them to form the rudiments of the nervous system.

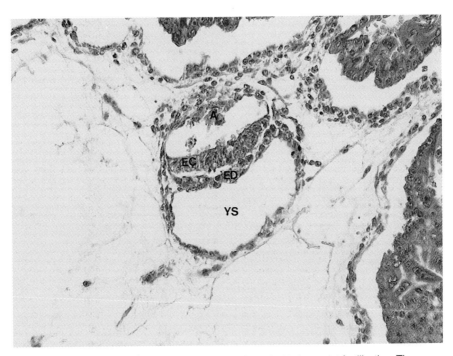

Figure 14.14 Developing human embryo approximately 12 days post-fertilization. The primitive ectoderm (EC) and endoderm (ED) are visible. Roofing the ectoderm are the cells that will give rise to the amnion (A), and below the endoderm the yolk sac (YS) is visible.

The embryo now consists of three germ layers:

1. *ectoderm:* responsible for the development of the nervous system and the epidermis of the skin;
2. *mesoderm:* giving rise to cartilage and bones, the muscles of the body wall, blood vessels and the heart, the urogenital system, the limbs and the membranes lining the body cavities;
3. *endoderm:* forming the alimentary system and its associated glands.

Mesoderm insinuates itself between the ectoderm and endoderm in all areas of the embryonic disc apart from the region of the prochordal plate, which is situated towards the cranial end of the embryo, and an area at the caudal end of the embryo, which will eventually give rise to the anal membrane (Fig. 14.15A). The prochordal plate is the first indication of the future development of the mouth. Up until this stage, the embryo is represented as a flat disc. With the development of the nervous system at approximately 17–18 days post-fertilization, the head and tail folds are established, which together with the lateral folding results in the formation of a cylindrical embryonic body with a rudimentary brain, spinal cord and gut tube.

FOLDING OF THE EMBRYONIC DISC

Induced by the underlying notochord, the ectoderm along the embryonic axis thickens to give rise to a neural plate. In surface view, this is seen as a thickened area of cells broader at the head end and narrowing towards the caudal end (Fig. 14.16A). A cross-section through this region, as represented by line XY on Figure 14.16A, shows the changes that occur in the neural plate with the resulting formation of the neural tube.

As a result of changes of cell shape in this neural plate (Fig. 14.16B), it begins to fold, and as each fold meets the other, the neural tube so formed detaches itself from the overlying ectoderm (Figs 14.16C and 16D). The cranial end of the neural tube rapidly grows to establish the future brain as distinct from the more caudally placed spinal cord. The growth of the tube results in the head end of the embryo folding in such a way that the most anterior parts of the embryonic disc are carried to a more ventral position. This is also true of the caudal end of the disc, where the development of a tail fold also results in the more caudal region of the disc taking up a more ventral position (Fig. 14.17).

The consequence of this is that the prochordal plate

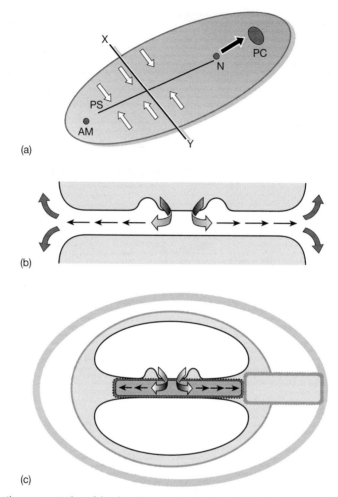

(a)

(b)

(c)

Figure 14.15 Diagrammatic representation of the developing embryonic disc. (**A**) Surface view of the disc, indicating the position of the primitive streak (black line) and the position of the cells that are the precursors of the notochord. The latter cells are first identified at the anterior end of the streak (N) and migrate forward below the ectoderm, maintaining a position in the midline region of the disc. Notochordal cells can migrate as far forward as the prochordal plate (PC). Migration of epiblast cells from both sides of the disc (thick arrows) to its centre result in the appearance of the primitive streak (PS). (**B**) In transverse section (i.e. through line XY in Fig. 14.15A), the primitive streak can be represented as a building up of cells on either side of the centre of the disc with the resultant formation of a groove between the two regions of cells. Cells from the primitive streak migrate round the edges of the groove, as indicated by the arrows, and insinuate themselves between the primitive ectoderm and primitive endoderm. These cells flow out laterally between the ectoderm and endoderm, establishing the third germ layer or mesodermal layer of the embryonic body.

The direction of the arrows in Figures 14.15 A and B indicate the movement of the embryonic mesoderm, between the ectoderm and endoderm. These cells insinuate themselves between ectoderm and endoderm in all parts of the embryonic disc, save for the region of the prochordal plate (PC) and the prospective anal membrane (AM). (**C**) Diagrammatic representation of developing embryo sitting within the chorionic sac. The sac has been diagrammatically sectioned to show the early developing embryo and its relation to the surrounding chorionic sac (compare with Fig. 14.12 above). Mesodermal cells that remain within the embryonic body form the intra-embryonic mesoderm (IEM). Those which migrate beyond the margins of the disc form the extra-embryonic mesoderm (light stippling). Although initially occupying all the space between the developing embryo and the trophoblast, this extra-embryonic mesoderm thins down considerably to cover only the developing amnion enclosing the amniotic cavity (AC), the membrane enclosing the yolk sac (YS). In addition, the extra-embryonic mesoderm lines inner aspect of the trophoblast, these two layers thereby constituting the chorion. The space between the developing embryo and the chorion is the extra-embryonic coelom (EEC). This develops in all areas apart from at the future tail end of the embryo, where the mesoderm remains 'solid' and forms the body stalk (BS), which is the progenitor of the umbilical cord.

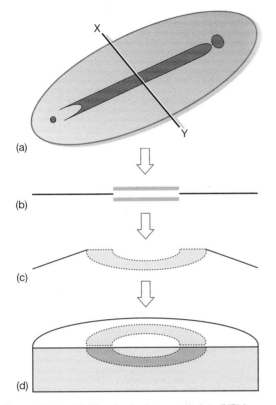

(a)

(b)

(c)

(d)

Figure 14.16 **(A)** The developing neural plate (NP) is thicker at its anterior end than posteriorly. **(B)** A cross-section of the disc through the line XY diagrammatically shows the cells forming the neural plate become more elongated or 'columnar' than those either side of it. **(C)** This results in a folding of the plate in the direction of the arrows, subsequently forming a tube, as seen in **(D)**. The tube sinks down from the overlying ectoderm, thus establishing the neural tube along the dorsal surface of the embryo below the developing ectoderm, the latter contributing to development of the skin.

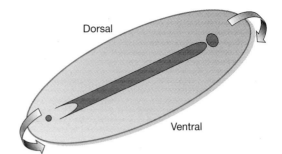

Dorsal

Ventral

Figure 14.17 The embryonic disc undergoes folding by the most anterior part of the disc folding in the direction of the arrow to take up a more ventral position. This is governed by the excessive growth of the neural plate in the most anterior part of the disc as the tube in this region grows to form the large anterior end of the neural tube, thus establishing the brain of the embryo. Similar folding occurs at the posterior end of the disc, again in a ventral direction, as indicated by the arrow, thus establishing the tail fold. Lateral folds will also occur on either side so that the lateral edges of the disc take up a more ventral position. The three types of fold – head fold, tail fold and lateral folds – provide a cylindrical body shape to the embryonic body.

SEGMENTAL ARRANGEMENT OF THE HUMAN BODY

The human body displays a segmental arrangement, reflected in the adult by, for example, segmentation of the vertebral column and the presence of a pair of spinal segmental nerves at each level. The embryological basis of this is segmentation of the intra-embryonic mesoderm. Soon after its formation, this mesoderm divides itself into three distinct regions: paraxial mesoderm, intermediate mesoderm and lateral plate mesoderm (Figs 14.19A and 14.19B).

Paraxial mesoderm segments to give rise to 42–44 blocks of tissue, or somites (Fig. 14.19C), flanking the developing neural tube. Each pair of somites demarcates out a future segment of the body. Components of somites form the axial skeleton, the skeletal muscle of the body walls and the limbs, and the dermis of the skin. They are clearly visible in the embryo from day 15 post-fertilization, first seen at the cranial end of the embryo and continuing their development to complete the 42–44 pairs by day 30–32 (Fig. 14.20). The intermediate mesoderm forms a large part of the urogenital system, contributing to both the kidney and the ureter.

In cross-section (see Fig. 14.19C), it can be seen that the lateral plate mesoderm develops a large cavity within it. As this mesoderm extends around the anterior end of the disc, the cavity or intra-embryonic coelom is horseshoe in shape. This is more easily iden-

and the future anal membrane are now more ventrally placed and, because of this movement, the endoderm, which is strongly adherent to ectoderm at both these points, is pulled into the embryonic body, establishing the endoderm as a tubular structure – the precursor to the adult gut (Fig. 14.18A–C). A further consequence of the tail fold is that the body stalk is also carried to a more ventral position. In addition, the sides of the embryonic disc are also involved in a lateral folding of each side of the disc so that, by a 'purse-string' effect, the head, tail and lateral folds, together with a detachment of the yolk sac from the gut tube, give rise to a cylindrical embryonic body, the folds meeting at the future umbilical region where the body stalk, destined to become the umbilical cord, is attached.

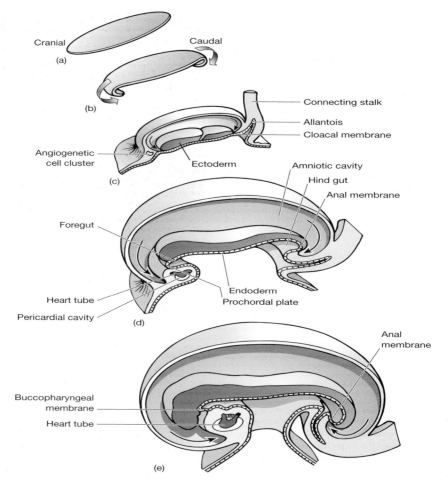

Figure 14.18 The process of folding results in the embryonic disc becoming a cylindrical structure and laying down the future body plan. The most prominent fold is the head fold, seen at the cranial end of the disc, and a similar fold occurs at the caudal end of the disc, known as the tail fold. The direction of each fold is depicted by arrows in Figure 14.18(b). The consequence of the head fold is that the most anterior part of the intra-embryonic coelom is carried ventrally and a cluster of angiogenetic cells develops close to this. The repositioning of this part of the intra-embryonic coelom marks the development of the pericardial cavity and the angiogenetic cells are the first sign of the developing heart. The development of the tail fold shifts the body stalk to a more ventral position (Fig. 14.18(c)) and this structure will elongate to give rise to the umbilical cord which is now positioned ventrally in the future umbilical region of the embryo. Because the prochordal plate and anal membrane are two fixed points where endoderm and ectoderm firmly adhere to each other, the result of folding is also that the endoderm begins to be pulled into the forming cylindrical body of the embryo (Fig. 14.18(d)). This results in a tube of endoderm being formed, which is the forerunner of the embryonic gut. The connection between the gut tube and the yolk sac below becomes more and more attenuated until the connection between the two, normally, closes off to complete the development of the gut tube itself. However, during development, part of the gut remains outside the embryonic body as it lengthens; this mid-gut loop returns to the body cavity when growth of the gut is complete. The prochordal plate becomes the buccopharyngeal membrane (Fig. 14.18(e)). When this membrane breaks down, as occurs in all regions of the embryonic body where endoderm and ectoderm are in apposition, the opening of the alimentary canal at the cranial end of the embryo will be established, giving rise to the mouth. Similarly, when the anal membrane breaks down, the anus is established. Lateral folding of the embryo also occurs to bring the right and left sides of the embryonic disc together. The head fold, tail fold and two lateral folds (right and left) all come together at the umbilicus rather like a purse-string effect to close off the anterior abdominal wall and complete the cylindrical shape of the body. Of course, *in utero* the umbilical cord attaches at this point but after birth, in normal development, with the regression of the umbilical cord stalk, the abdominal wall is complete.

tified when the disc is viewed in surface view (see Fig. 14.19D). The cavity is of course within the mesoderm, and Figure 14.19D is only a diagrammatic representation of the position of the intra-embryonic coelom

as the ectodermal layer lies on top of the mesodermal layer. As described above (see also Figs 14.18A–C), the head fold results in the most anterior part of the coelom being carried to a ventral position, behind

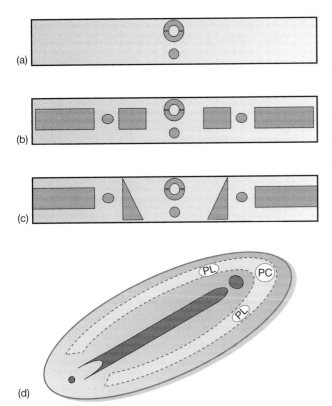

(a)

(b)

(c)

(d)

Figure 14.19 (**A**) After the formation of the intra-embryonic mesoderm, this third layer of the embryonic disc first appears as a diffuse layer. (**B**) The mesoderm begins to condense into three distinct regions: the paraxial mesoderm (P), the intermediate mesoderm (IM) and the lateral plate mesoderm (LPM) on either side of the neural tube. (**C**) The paraxial mesoderm further develops into pairs of somites that flank the neural tube on the dorsal surface of the embryo. The lateral plate mesoderm develops a cavity that will form the intra-embryonic coelom and develop into the various cavities of the body. (**D**) The intra-embryonic cavity is horseshoe shaped and develops within the lateral plate mesoderm on both sides of the developing neural tube. In addition, because of the migration of the intra-embryonic mesoderm to the anterior of the disc, this cavity also develops anterior to the prochordal plate and notochord. The most anterior region of the intra-embryonic coelom is the progenitor of the pericardial cavity (pc), which will take up its final ventral position once the head fold has developed. The region of the coelom marked pl will later form the pleural cavities, and the rest of the coelom will eventually develop into a single peritoneal cavity.

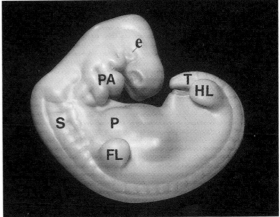

Figure 14.20 Model of an embryo at the 4-week stage of development, indicating the external features visible at this stage. The segmental arrangement of the somites (S) are seen along the dorsal aspect of the embryo. The developing eye (e) is present, and the pharyngeal arches (PA) dominate the region of the future neck. The forelimbs (FL) are evident level with the pericardial bulge (P), and the early hindlimbs (HL) are located close to the embryonic tail (T).

ties on each side forms the future pleural cavities (see Fig 14.19D), into which the developing lungs will invaginate.

EMBRYONIC DEVELOPMENT IN RELATION TO STAGES OF PREGNANCY

The embryonic period begins at the beginning of the 4th week of pregnancy, the first 3 weeks being termed the pre-embryonic period. It continues until the end of week 8 of pregnancy, and during this period, the embryo grows approximately 1 mm per day. By the end of week 4, the embryonic body contains all the rudiments of the organ systems, although the urogenital system is at a very early stage of its genesis. During this period, the embryo is very susceptible to damage by environmental agents, which can cause abnormalities in the organs that are forming at this time. Although the individual events in organ development are not discussed here, examples of their abnormal development are illustrated at the end of the chapter.

At the beginning of week 4, the embryo measures only approximately 4 mm when measured from crown to rump (the crown–rump or CR length). It has a characteristic 'C' shape because of the folding it has undergone, and its pairs of somites are prominent along its dorsal surface, flanking each side of the neural tube. The rudiments of the eyes, developed from the forebrain, are making an appearance underneath the ectoderm (see Fig. 14.20). The eye develops as a vesicle

the prochordal plate. This part of the cavity is the future pericardial cavity (see Fig. 14.19D), where the heart will differentiate from the lateral plate mesoderm bounding this area of the cavity (see Fig. 14.18C). Similarly, with the advent of the lateral folds, the more caudally positioned intra-embryonic coelom is placed round the developing gut, thereby giving rise to the future peritoneal cavity. The region of coelom between the pericardial and peritoneal cavi-

that grows out from the forebrain towards the ectoderm overlying this part of the brain. This vesicle invaginates and gives rise to the optic cup, which forms the neural structures of the eye. However, the lens of the eye is formed from a 'placode' of ectoderm overlying the forebrain eye vesicle thickening and detaching from the ectodermal tissue.

At this stage, the otic vesicle, responsible for the formation of the inner ear, will also be making its appearance, derived from the ectoderm overlying the hindbrain. The otic vesicle differs from the optic vesicle in that it actually develops from surface ectoderm, which sinks internally to form the utricle, saccule, cochlea and semi-circular canals of the organ of hearing. These structures therefore originate from surface ectoderm, which moves inwards from the surface of the embryo.

The limbs are just visible projecting from the sides of the embryo. Level with the pericardial bulge, where the embryonic heart is developing, the forelimbs are further on in their development than the hindlimbs, which are visible near the tail region of the embryo. The limbs form as a result of the mesoderm underlying the ectoderm in these regions, pushing forward to result in the formation of small flattened buds of mesoderm covered by ectoderm.

The embryo does not yet resemble a human. There is little definition to the face. The prominent feature in the future cervical region is the presence of pharyngeal arches, which will later be involved in development of the face and structures pertaining to the pharynx and foregut (see Fig. 14.20 above). The pericardium and developing liver project as a prominent bulge on the ventral aspect of the embryo, and the area of attachment of the body stalk is also large.

By this stage, the embryonic heart is functioning as a two-chamber structure. Fetal blood vessels from individual villi in the placenta form an umbilical vein on each side of the body, carrying oxygenated blood to the fetal heart. Two other venous systems also enter the venous end of the heart: the common cardinal veins on each side, formed by the anterior cardinal vein draining blood from the cranial end of the embryo and the posterior cardinal vein draining from the caudal end; and a right and left vitelline vein returning blood from a plexus of venules covering the yolk sac (Fig. 14.21). Blood from the venous end of the heart flows into the arterial end and flows out through two ventral aortae, first to the head and brain, ensuring a good supply of highly oxygenated blood to the latter, but also around the system of aortic arch arteries surrounding the pharynx to enter two unfused dorsal aortae before being returned to the placenta for oxygenation via two umbilical arteries (Fig. 14.21).

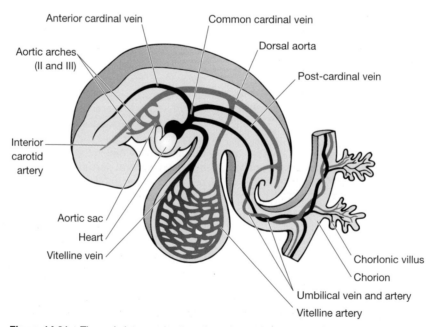

Figure 14.21 The main intra- and extraembryonic arteries and veins in a 4-mm embryo (end of the 4th week). Only the vessels on the left side of the embryo are represented.

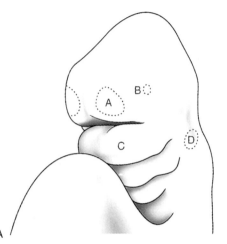

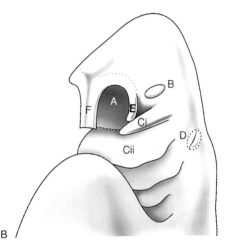

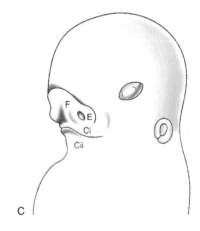

Figure 14.22   (**A**) Between 4 and 5 weeks of development, various structures begin to make their appearance on the future head region of the embryo. The diagram indicates the future positions of the olfactory placode, which will give rise to the olfactory epithelium of the nose (A), the optic vesicle, the forerunner of eye development (B) and the otic vesicle, which will contribute to the development of the ear (D). Dominating the future neck region of the embryo are the pharyngeal arches (C), some of which are involved in the development of the future face. (**B**) Facial development is marked by the growth and fusion of several processes. From the region of the future forehead, a process grows downwards and forwards, overgrowing the olfactory placodes (A). This process divides to give rise to medial processes (F) and two lateral processes, only one of which is seen on the diagram. The lateral process (E) fuses with a process that has arisen from the first pharyngeal arch (Ci). E represents the lateral nasal process, which will fuse with Ci, the maxillary process, to form the lateral aspect of the nose and part of the upper lip. Cii, the remaining part of the first pharyngeal arch, will contribute to formation of the lower jaw or mandible. (**C**) The maxillary process (Ci) fuses not only with the lateral nasal process, but also with the medial nasal process (F). This occurs on both sides of the face. By the fusion of Ci, E and F, the nose and upper lip are formed. The remainder of the first arch, Cii, is involved in the formation of the lower jaw.

Marked changes take place in the embryo during the second month, and at this time, it begins to resemble a human. The growth of the pharyngeal arches is now very pronounced (Fig. 14.22A) A pair of maxillary processes begin to make their appearance and grow upwards and forwards from the first arch (Fig. 14.22A). The olfactory placodes, the forerunner of the sensory epithelium of the nose, are also beginning to appear. In addition to this, the mesoderm underlying the ectoderm in the central region of the face proliferates and surrounds the nasal placodes, forming two lateral and two medial folds around the placodes, which now lie in a depression (Fig. 14.22B). Between the 11 and 14 mm crown–rump stage of development, the maxillary processes fuse first with the lateral nasal processes and then with the medial nasal processes (Figs 14.22B and 14.22.C), establishing the nose and upper lip of the embryo in such a way that the embryonic face now possesses human qualities. Malfusion of these processes can result in the conditions of cleft lip and/or cleft palate depending on the processes involved. By this time, the embryo is approximately 40 days of age.

The limb buds rapidly change their shape from paddle-shaped structures and begin to differentiate into structures in which definite joints are apparent, demarcating out arm, forearm and hand, and thigh, leg and foot, regions in the fore- and hindlimbs respectively. The hand is the first to display digital rays:

areas where the cells undergo programmed cell death, resulting in their degeneration to allow for the formation of digits. Failure to do so results in syndactyly, in which the fingers, or at a later stage of development the toes, are webbed.

By the 46th day of development, the embryo has developed a neck region and become less curved. At this stage, the head is very large in relation to the rest of the body. With the appearance of the neck at this stage, the developing embryo becomes less curved. By the end of the 8th week, the embryo is definitely a miniature human and ready to embark upon its fetal stage of development.

THE FETAL PERIOD

From 9 weeks gestation until birth is the fetal period, when the fetus grows approximately 1.5 mm per day. At the beginning of this time, the fetus has a crown–rump length of 30 mm, and by birth this length is approximately 300–330 mm. The fetal period is therefore characterized by an immense time of growth of the new individual. At the start of this period, all the organ rudiments have been formed so this is a time when the tissues mature to a functional state. Bone is laid down, and the central nervous system is rapidly undergoing maturation. Any environmental damage at this stage could have severe consequences for the development of normal function in the nervous system. Functional maturation is therefore the hallmark of the fetal period as it is imperative that, at term, the neonate is well equipped to survive in the external world as a being independent of the placenta and the support of the maternal tissues.

CAUSES OF ABNORMAL DEVELOPMENT

Development usually results in a normal healthy neonate being born. However, approximately 2–3% of live births result in abnormal development. Although genetic factors cause defects in development, as discussed above, environmental factors are also linked to birth defects. Gross structural abnormalities are termed congenital abnormalities.

As the organ systems are being laid down, each of them is susceptible to agents that can result in disruption of the normal developmental pattern. These periods are known as critical periods of development. This is the time when structural abnormalities will therefore arise. Functional abnormalities or abnormalities in the growth of the fetus are more likely to occur after the third month of development. During the first

3 weeks of intrauterine life, agents acting on the embryo are unlikely to result in abnormal development but are more likely to cause death of the embryo at this early stage. The major teratogenic agents that cause abnormality act at different periods of development and therefore act on the organ system during its critical stage of development.

Although animal studies have indicated certain agents to be the cause of abnormal development within the species studied, it is difficult definitively to correlate substances directly to abnormal development in humans. It is also clear, from the tragedy of the drug thalidomide, that certain agents that are teratogenic in humans appear not to cause abnormality in other species, thus making testing for potential teratogens in humans extremely difficult. The major known human teratogens fall into several categories. These include chemical agents, infectious agents, hormones, drugs and alcohol. In addition to these agents, physical factors such as ionizing radiation can cause severe defects in the developing fetus. The number of agents and factors that cause abnormal development are too numerous to discuss here, but the effects of some of these agents on the development of the fetus are outlined below.

Thalidomide

The drug thalidomide was prescribed to pregnant mothers during the latter part of the 1950s. This drug caused abnormalities in multiple systems of the body, the one that is most noted being the total or partial absence of the limbs (amelia or meromelia).

Aminopterin

The drug aminopterin is a folic acid antagonist. In the past, this agent was used to induce therapeutic abortion. However, in some cases abortion did not ensue, and the surviving fetus was grossly malformed. The defects affected many of the organ systems, including the nervous system and the development of the face and palate.

One cannot discuss folic acid antagonists without mentioning folic acid itself. There is some evidence that dietary levels of folic acid can protect against the malformation spina bifida. This abnormality is the result of a failure of closure of the neural arches. In some forms of the defect, the neural tissue and/or the membranes, or meninges, surrounding the neural tissue are also involved. In cases of spina bifida occulta, only the neural arches fail to close, and neural impairment does not occur. This is also the case where only the meninges protrude from the open arch to form a cyst below the skin. However, if the neural tissue is also involved in cyst formation, neurological deficits in the lower limbs occur together with urinary bladder and rectal incontinence. In the most severe form of the condition the neural tube itself fails to close and lies exposed in the lumbosacral region, with resulting lower limb paralysis.

It is possible to screen for spina bifida. The levels of the protein alpha fetoprotein are raised in cases where the neural tube remains open. Increased levels can be detected in the maternal blood. If levels are higher than would be expected for the gestational age of the fetus, amniocentesis may then be indicated, where the levels of the protein are subsequently measured within the amniotic fluid.

Viruses

Certain viruses are capable of crossing the placental barrier and causing abnormal development, the nature of which depends on the time of the infection during development. Examples of viruses that cross the placenta and cause fetal abnormality are rubella virus cytomegalovirus and HIV. Rubella infection during the embryonic period can induce cataract formation, deafness and cardiac abnormalities. Cytomegalovirus infection is often embryolethal, but it can result in abnormalities such as microcephaly, in which the development of the brain is grossly retarded, or microphthalmia, in which the globe of the eye is very much reduced in size.

Ionizing radiation

Ionizing radiation causes abnormalities within DNA, particularly strand breaks. Although the amount of irradiation delivered by diagnostic X-ray procedures is very low and should not cause any risk to the mother and developing fetus, pregnant women should not be exposed to such treatment.

Disturbed pattern of organ or tissue formation

In discussing abnormal development, it should also be noted that defects in development can arise not only as the result of an external environmental agent, but also because of a disturbance in the pattern of formation of an organ or tissue structure. Examples here are numerous and fall into different categories.

In inductive interactions, one tissue induces the development of a second structure during the formation of organs and tissues. If this inductive interaction fails to occur, the second structure is often not formed or is malformed. An example of this is seen in the development of the kidneys. The kidney is formed from the intermediate mesoderm (see Fig. 14.19A–C above), but the intermediate mesoderm is only induced to develop into a kidney when a small bud grows up from the region of the hind gut to contact the mesoderm. This small bud eventually gives rise to the ureter and, under its inductive influence, the kidney develops. If the ureter fails to form and contact the intermediate mesoderm, the kidney fails to develop, and the condition of renal agenesis occurs. Although the fetus is not reliant on its kidneys *in utero*, bilateral agenesis will result in death of the neonate soon after birth.

In its early stages of development, the heart consists of a common atrium and common ventricle. Both structures develop septa to divide them into right and left atria and ventricles respectively. The septation of the atrium is a complex affair as it involves the growth of two septa that form in such a way that they do not quite overlap each other, the result being a communication between the right and left atria in the fetal heart. This communication or foramen – the foramen ovale – is an adaptation to fetal life. The majority of blood entering the developing right atrium is high in oxygen as it has reached the venous part of the heart from the umbilical vein, which in the fetus carries oxygenated blood returning from the placenta to the fetal heart (Figs 14.21 and 14.23). The oxygenated blood is carried directly from the right atrium to the left atrium via the foramen ovale. From the left atrium, the oxygenated blood enters the left ventricle and is transported round the fetal body, first being distributed to the head, where the brain is rapidly developing. The consequence of this is that the right ventricle is bypassed, an adaptation to fetal life as blood entering the right ventricle would transport the highly oxygenated blood to the fetal lungs, which are not yet required because gaseous exchange is carried out via the placenta. At birth, the foramen ovale rapidly closes, establishing the normal anatomy of the heart and resulting four chambers, blood flowing to the lungs to be reoxygenated. In some cases, however, there is insufficient growth of one of the atrial septa, which fails to close against the other septum, resulting in a patent foramen ovale or 'hole in the heart'. The result is a blue or cyanosed baby as there is a mixing of oxygenated and deoxygenated blood within the circulatory system.

The human small intestine is approximately 6 m long. During its development, there is a stage where a loop of gut – the midgut loop – protrudes out of the embryonic body in the region of the umbilicus. In

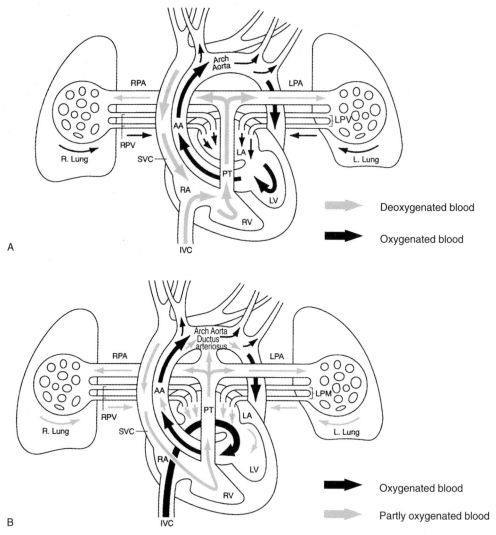

A

Deoxygenated blood

Oxygenated blood

B

Oxygenated blood

Partly oxygenated blood

Figure 14.23 (**A**) The normal circulation pattern in the human following birth. Deoxygenated blood returns from the tissues of the body via both the superior vena cava (SVC) and inferior vena cava (IVC), entering the right atrium (RA) of the heart. The deoxygenated blood then passes to the right ventricle (RV) and into the pulmonary trunk (PT), to be carried via the right and left pulmonary arteries (RPA and LPA respectively) to the lungs. Here, the blood is reoxygenated and flows back via the right and left pulmonary veins (RPV and LPV) into the left atrium of the heart (LA), into the left ventricle (LV) and into the ascending aorta (AA) and arch of the aorta, where branches of the arch take the highly oxygenated blood to the head, neck and brain to supply these tissues of the body with oxygen. The rest of the blood flows into the descending aorta, oxygen reaching the rest of the body tissues. In this way, the systemic and pulmonary systems are separate, and there is no mixing of deoxygenated and oxygenated blood. (**B**) There are many distinctions to be made between the fetal and adult circulation. In the fetus, the IVC carries oxygenated blood back from the placenta via the umbilical vein. This highly oxygenated blood enters the right atrium but, because of the existence of a foramen in the interatrial septum – the foramen ovale – the blood flows directly into the left atrium and then the left ventricle. From here, the highly oxygenated blood enters the arch of the aorta to supply highly oxygenated blood first to the tissues of the head, neck and brain, and eventually to other developing body tissues. In this way, the lungs are bypassed as no oxygenation of blood occurs here, this being the function of the placenta. The blood returning from the fetus's brain is now less well oxygenated, but it returns to the SVC and enters the right atrium. This stream of blood is directed in a more anterior stream in relation to the oxygenated blood coming from the placenta via the developing IVC, thus keeping these two streams of blood separate and ensuring that the most highly oxygenated blood is first directed to the head and neck, where the developing brain requires a high level of oxygen. Blood returning via the fetal SVC and entering the right atrium is only partially deoxygenated and flows into the pulmonary trunk. A special adaptation, known as the ductus arteriosus, joins the pulmonary trunk to the arch of the aorta during fetal life. Instead of the blood in this vessel travelling to the lungs,

Figure 14.23   (*Cont'd*) which are not required for oxygenation in fetal life, this blood passes into the ductus arteriosus and hence into the arch of the aorta and descending aorta. Thus, in the fetus, there is mixing of the blood from the pulmonary trunk with that which has come from the aorta. At birth, however, the foramen ovale closes off so that the right ventricle and pulmonary trunk cannot be bypassed, and the ductus arteriosus also closes. The consequence of this is that the pulmonary and systemic circulations are separated, thus setting up the adult circulatory pattern.

normal development, the loop returns to the peritoneal cavity, and the anterior abdominal wall musculature develops to close off the umbilical region and establish the anterior abdominal wall. In some cases, maldevelopment occurs in this region. If the anterior wall musculature fails to grow adequately, parts of the gut may protrude through the unclosed umbilicus, giving rise to a congenital umbilical hernia, although the protruding gut is normally covered in skin in this form of abnormality. In contrast to this, a condition known as omphalocele is the result of failure of the midgut loop to re-enter the abdominal cavity at the appropriate stage of development. In such cases, the loops of gut remain as a large membrane-bound cyst external to the embryonic body.

The causes of abnormal development are therefore extremely varied and depend not only on the nature of

---

Pointers for practice

- Translocations inherited from the parent or arising anew in the fetus may lead to spontaneous abortion, fetal abnormality or congenital malformation.
- More than 50% of all spontaneously aborted fetuses have a chromosomal abnormality; the majority are trisomies and do not reflect any parental chromosomal abnormality. Most genetic centres do not look for parental chromosomal abnormality until a couple have had three spontaneous abortions.
- Development usually results in a normal healthy neonate being born. However, approximately 2–3% of live births result in abnormal development.
- Both genetic and environmental factors are linked to birth defects.
- There are critical periods of development, and major teratogenic agents may act at different stages of development.
- Major known teratogens include chemical agents, infectious agents, hormones, drugs, alcohol and ionizing radiation.

---

the agent or factor causing the perturbation of normal development, but also on the time at which such factors act. Nevertheless, in the majority of cases, conception leads to the development of a perfect human infant carrying its own unique and individual genetic code.

REFERENCE

Hassold T, Jacobs P A 1984 Trisomy in man. Annual Review of Genetics 18: 69

FURTHER READING

Acosta A A 1994 Processes of fertilisation in the human and its abnormalities; diagnostic and therapeutic possibilities. Obstetric and Gynecologic Survey 49: 567.

Allen M I Van, Fraser F C, Dallaire L et al 1993 Recommendations on the use of folic acid supplementation to prevent the recurrence of neural tube defects. Canadian Medical Association Journal 149: 1239

Aplin J D 1991 Implantation, trophoblast differentiation and hemochorial placentation: mechanistic evidence *in vivo* and *in vitro*. Journal of Cell Science 99: 681

Bellairs R, Sanders E J, Lash J W 1992 Formation and differentiation of early embryonic mesoderm. Plenum Press, New York

Beller F K, Zlatnick G P 1995 The beginning of human life. Journal of Assisted Reproduction and Genetics 12: 477

Brent R I, Holmes L B 1988 Clinical and basic science from the thalidomide tragedy; what have we learned about the causes of limb defects? Teratology 43: 241

Di Maria H, Courpotin C, Rouzioux C et al 1986 Transplacental transmission of human immunodeficient virus. Lancet 2: 215

Edwards R G, Brody S A 1995 Principles and practice on assisted human reproduction. WB Saunders, Philadelphia

Evans H J 1977 Chromosomal anomalies among livebirths. Journal of Medical Genetics 14: 309

Hadlock F P 1994 Fetal growth. In: Callen P W (ed.)

Ultrasonography in obstetrics and gynecology, 3rd edn. WB Saunders, Philadelphia

Hinrichsen K 1985 The early development of morphology and patterns of the face in the human embryo. Advances in Anatomy, Embryology and Cell Biology 98: 1

Johnstone F D 1996 HIV in pregnancy. British Journal of Obstetrics and Gynaecology 103: 1184

Morris G K, Hampton J 1985 Congenital heart lesions – an introduction. Medicine International 18: 745

Persaud T V N 1990 Environmental causes of human birth defects. Charles C Thomas, Springfield, IL

Sansoucie D A, Cavaliere T A 1997 Transition from fetal to extrauterine circulation. Neonatal Network 16: 5

Sheoenwolf G G, Smith J L 1990 Mechanisms of neurulation: traditional viewpoint and recent advances. Development 109: 243

Sarwark J L 1996 Spina bifida. Pediatric Clinics of North America 43: 1151

Skandalakis J E, Gray S W 1994 The embryological basis for the treatment of congenital defects. Williams & Watkins, Baltimore

Wolpert L 1991 The triumph of the embryo. Oxford University Press, Oxford

15

Physical adaptations to pregnancy

Joanna C. Girling

COPING WITH PREGNANCY

Although for many women pregnancy is an enjoyable and exciting period, for the majority it can also be uncomfortable, frightening or exhausting. Many of the so-called 'minor symptoms and signs of pregnancy' are the result of the physiological changes that occur during normal pregnancy as the maternal adaptation to support and protect the growing baby. The aim of this chapter is to elucidate these changes and thereby to offer an explanation for the symptoms that are so troublesome for women. It is probable that if women have a good understanding of why they have, for example, backache, urinary frequency, varicose veins, palpitations and heartburn, they may be able to tolerate them better and act in such a way as to ameliorate them; as health care professionals, an increased awareness of the underlying processes should make us more sympathetic and our advice more constructive. The chapter will also describe the physiological processes that are pertinent in the development of some of the major medical complications of pregnancy. Finally, the complex subject of the initiation of labour will be outlined.

Each section will follow a similar theme, dealing with a particular system of the body, considering the normal physiology and the physiological changes that occur in normal pregnancy and the 'problems' to which these may give rise.

Cardiovascular system

The changes in the cardiovascular system, circulating volume and blood pressure are closely intertwined and quite dramatic. A full understanding is required in order to ensure that normal changes are not misconstrued and that abnormal features are not overlooked. A good knowledge of these changes is also helpful for the management of important pregnancy complications such as pre-eclampsia, thromboembolism and haemorrhage.

Stroke volume (SV) is the amount of blood leaving the left (or right) ventricle each time it contracts; cardiac output (CO) is the amount of blood leaving the heart per minute and is calculated as SV multiplied by heart rate (HR). Blood pressure (BP) depends upon CO and peripheral resistance (PR):

$$BP = CO \times PR;$$

$$CO = SV \times HR$$

Changes in all of these parameters occur in normal pregnancy.

The synchronicity of the heart is controlled by specialized conducting tissue, which ensures that contraction of the left and right atria occurs together and is followed by left and right ventricular contraction. Electrical activity commences in the sino-atrial node in the right atrium and spreads to the atrioventricular node, also in the right atrium. From there, specialized conducting tissue called the bundle of His conducts the impulse to the left and right ventricles (Fig. 15.1). Heart rate depends upon the rate of discharge of the sino-atrial node, which is directly controlled by the autonomic nervous system: sympathetic neurones (via the vasomotor centre in the medulla) causing tachycardia, and parasympathetic nerves (via the cardio-inhibitory centre, also in the medulla) slowing down the heart. At rest, the latter predominates, its action being mediated via the vagus nerve. The sino-atrial node, and therefore the heart rate, is also directly influenced by thyroxine, extremes of temperature and changes in beta-adrenergic activity (increases in each of these increasing the heart rate, and vice versa).

Systole refers to the emptying phase of a chamber and diastole to its filling phase, reference usually being, by convention, to the ventricles unless otherwise specified. Systole is relatively fixed in duration, but changes in heart rate usually influence the length of diastole. During diastole, the mitral valve is open and the ventricle fills. This is initially rapid and 'passive', as atrial pressure exceeds ventricular pressure at this point, but in the last third of diastole, atrial contraction (atrial systole) occurs. Shortly after the beginning of ventricular systole, both the aortic and mitral valves are closed since ventricular pressure is lower than that in the aorta and higher than that in the atrium respectively. This is the period of isovolumetric contraction. However, as ventricular contraction continued, left ventricular pressure exceeds that of the aorta and the aortic valve opens. Blood is ejected from the ventricle, and this continues until the ventricle relaxes and the forward kinetic pressure of blood flow wanes. At this point, left ventricular pressure is at a nadir. Consequently, the aortic valve closes, and, shortly after (when atrial pressure is at a maximum), the mitral

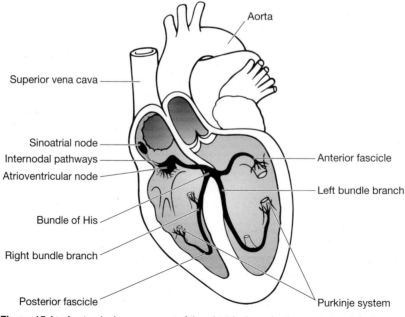

Figure 15.1 Anatomical arrangement of the electrical conducting systems of the heart. (Reproduced from Ganong 1989.)

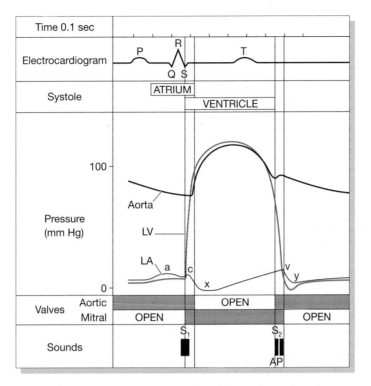

| Time 0.1 sec | | | | |

Figure 15.2   Haemodynamic correlations of the cardiac cycle pressure. (Reproduced from *Companion in Medical Studies*, Blackwell Scientific.)

valve opens, thus recommencing the cycle (Fig. 15.2). In health, valve closure causes heart sounds, but valve opening does not. Thus, on auscultation, the first heart sound is caused by the closure of the mitral valve at the beginning of systole, and the second heart sound is the closure of the aortic valve at the end of systole. Although right heart activity is coordinated with that of the left heart, right ventricular systole is slightly later than left ventricular systole. As a consequence, the second heart sound is often split into two components, the latter being caused by pulmonary valve closure; this difference is exacerbated during deep inspiration, since this delays right ventricular ejection even further, and in normal pregnancy.

As stated above, cardiac output depends upon heart rate and stroke volume. Starling's law of the heart states that the force of contraction is proportional to the initial length of the cardiac muscle fibre, which in turn depends upon how dilated the ventricle is at the end of diastole. The force of contraction increases with increasing end-diastolic volume until, at a certain point, the heart fails and contractility decreases despite (or because of) increasing ventricular volume. The end-diastolic volume is also referred to as the preload and is

controlled by factors influencing the effective circulating volume; in practice, this means the venous return. Venous return is increased by the pumping action of leg muscles, which overcomes the gravity-related pooling of blood that occurs on standing still, and decreased by lower venous tone – peripheral vasodilatation. High intrathoracic pressure and high intrapericardial pressure both reduce ventricular filling. Stroke volume is also influenced by the contractility of the myocardium. For a given preload, ventricular performance improves with increased sympathetic and beta-adrenergic stimulation, and decreases if the afterload (that is, the systemic arterial blood pressure or systemic resistance) is too high, or in the presence of hypoxia, acidosis or damaged myocardial tissue.

The details of the physiological changes of normal pregnancy are still debated, in part because of the difficulties of performing reliable and safe measurements. The studies by Robson et al (1987, 1989, 1991) provide the most robust data. Pregnancy has a number of effects on the haemodynamic *status quo*. The placenta creates a low-resistance circulation, vasodilatation occurs peripherally, and circulating volume increases. Increased heart rate, myocardial contractility and preload, and reduced afterload all influence cardiac performance in pregnancy, by improving cardiac output.

Heart rate increases from about 75 beats per minute to almost 90 beats per minute from early in the first trimester. Stroke volume increases significantly, from 65 ml to 85 ml, in the first trimester, reaching a peak at 20 weeks that is maintained until term. Cardiac output changes over a similar time span, from 5 L/min to 7 L/min. This is also maintained until term and probably does not decrease in the third trimester: older studies that suggested a fall at the end of pregnancy were probably inaccurate, being confounded by use of the supine position, and because of changes in pulmonary vasculature and aortic dilatation for which older techniques could not account. Serial (that is, longitudinal) echocardiography with Doppler measurement of blood flow at the pulmonary, mitral and aortic valves and in the ascending aorta using women as their own non-pregnant controls seems to be the most accurate assessment currently available (Robson et al 1989, 1991).

Peripheral vascular resistance falls, by almost 50% in early pregnancy, before the low-resistance placental circulation has a major effect. It is probably one of the major reasons for the increase in cardiac output that occurs during pregnancy. The underlying aetiology of this is uncertain, but oestrogen, prostaglandins, nitric oxide, relaxin and calcitonin gene-related peptide have all been suggested. Increases in left atrial and left ventricular end-diastolic volume (preload) occur in the second and third trimesters, reflecting the increase in venous return (Robson et al 1987). This combination of increased venous return and reduced peripheral vascular resistance is achieved by a marked increase in blood volume (by 50%) and a relatively smaller increase in erythrocyte count (by 20–40%) such that there is a reduction in blood viscosity.

Diastolic, and to a lesser extent systolic, blood pressure falls during normal pregnancy. Blood pressure depends upon cardiac output and peripheral resistance: in pregnancy, the increase in the former is less than the decrease in the latter, so that overall blood pressure falls. The nadir is reached at 12–16 weeks' gestation, systolic blood pressure falling by 0–9 mmHg and diastolic pressure by 12–17 mmHg (MacGillivray et al 1969, Wilson et al 1980). In the late second and third trimesters, blood pressure increases towards levels found in the non-pregnant woman (Fig. 15.3). There are considerable problems in measuring blood pressure in pregnancy, including:

- compression of the inferior vena cava by the gravid uterus;
- white coat hypertension, a stress response to an environment, typically a hospital or the presence of a doctor, either because these are stressful in themselves or because the woman associates them with circumstances in which management decisions might be made;

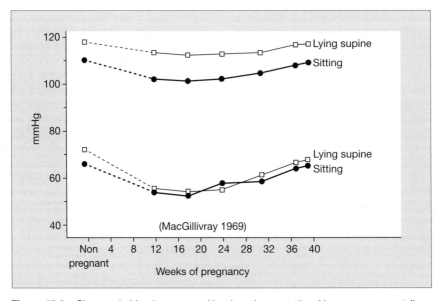

Figure 15.3 Changes in blood pressure with advancing gestation. Upper curves, systolic pressure; lower curves, diastolic. (Reproduced with permission from I. MacGillivray, G. A. Rose and B. Rowe 1969 Clinical Science 37:395–407. © Biochemical Society and the Medical Research Society.)

- observer error;
- threshold avoidance: the individual measuring the blood pressure avoids recording a diastolic blood pressure of 90 mmHg because he feels that the blood pressure is normal;
- equipment inaccuracies;
- uncertainty about which Korotkoff sound to use. Evidence is now accumulating that Korotkoff sound V is more appropriate than sound IV for use in pregnancy (Shennan et al 1996).

During labour, cardiac output increases by a further 15–20%, in part because of 'autotransfusion' from the contracting uterus. Sympathetic nervous system stimulation by maternal pain or anxiety results in a further increase in heart rate and possibly an increase in blood pressure.

Feeling hot and sweaty

Cardiac output increases during pregnancy by 2 L/min. A substantial portion of this goes to the uterus, kidneys and gut. However, a considerable amount is distributed to the breasts and skin, which, in combination with peripheral vasodilatation, accounts for the warm peripheries that pregnant women so often notice. In the hands, the combination of increased blood flow, peripheral vasodilatation and a fast, bounding pulse may give rise to the sensation of burning throbbing skin, also called palmar erythema. This resolves after delivery, although intractable cases may be helped by a beta-blocker before delivery.

Funny turns

Dizziness and fainting are relatively common in pregnancy. Hot, crowded situations, standing for prolonged periods and lying supine are frequent causes so pregnant women should avoid luxurious baths, supermarket queues and various forms of public transport. Additional peripheral vasodilatation resulting in pooling of the blood in the legs, and compression of the inferior vena cava by the gravid uterus, conspire to reduce venous return, cardiac output and blood pressure, resulting in dizziness and possibly syncope. It follows that blood pressure should not be recorded in the supine position.

Hypertension

The first trimester physiological fall in blood pressure may mask chronic hypertension; thus, prepregnancy records of blood pressure should be sought, often from the GP or family planning clinic, in cases of doubt. For women known to have hypertension, this physiological fall may allow a reduction or cessation of therapy, particularly at the beginning of pregnancy when there may be concerns about teratogenesis. Vigilance is also required in the second half of pregnancy when increasing levels will be expected. It is usual for antihypertensive medication therapy to be reintroduced or increased in the third trimester.

There are a number of definitions of pre-eclampsia but all include hypertension. The cut-off points for the latter are not related to the duration of pregnancy, despite the gestation-related changes in normal blood pressure. Over 20% of women have a blood pressure recording greater than or equal to 140/90 prior to delivery, which far exceeds the incidence of pre-eclampsia (Redman 1995). Thus, the interpretation of blood pressure measurement should take into account not only other maternal and fetal factors, but also the gestational age.

Physiological anaemia

The changes seen in blood volume and erythrocyte number have been explained. The total red cell mass in fact increases so the oxygen-carrying capacity of the blood increases. Therefore, assuming that there is an adequate dietary intake of iron (and in the absence of other chronic causes of anaemia such as malaria, worm infestation, malnutrition and malabsorption), the resulting physiological fall in haemoglobin concentration does not necessarily require treatment. In fact, the consequent reduction in haematocrit is one factor helping to counterbalance the prothrombotic tendency of pregnancy; it is possible that routine iron supplementation may increase blood viscosity and impair uteroplacental circulation (Koller 1982). In addition, many women suffer minor side-effects, for example constipation or diarrhoea, when taking iron treatment (*British National Formulary* 1999).

There is controversy over how low the haemoglobin concentration may fall in normal pregnancy without recourse to iron supplementation. On balance, most authorities believe that haemoglobin concentrations below either 10.0 or 10.5 g/dl require treatment (Letsky 1995). However, in generally healthy populations, there is no convincing evidence that routine iron supplementation is advantageous to either the mother or the baby; neither are there data to confirm that it is safe (Mahomed 1998). The only proven value of routine iron supplementation is a reduction in the incidence of low haemoglobin level, but it is probable that regular estimations of haemoglobin concentration and selective iron supplementation could have a similar effect.

Other markers of iron deficiency may be useful when there is doubt surrounding the diagnosis of iron deficiency, if compliance with therapy is incomplete or if additional causes of anaemia may be involved. The mean cell volume (MCV) of red blood cells is shown on most automated full blood count reports. An early effect of iron deficiency is the appearance of small red blood cells, that is, a low MCV reading. However, thalassaemia trait is also associated with a low MCV, and folate or vitamin B12 deficiency and alcohol abuse result in large red blood cells (a high MCV), which may mask the iron deficiency. Ferritin level is a measure of iron stores, which are reduced in iron deficiency anaemia. The acceptable range of ferritin level for pregnancy is debated, since iron stores have not so much been 'lost' as transferred to the increased number of red cells. Nonetheless, a low serum ferritin is suggestive of iron deficiency.

Therefore, for healthy women in the UK, there is no clear consensus either for or against routine iron supplementation (Mahomed 1998). Many units choose to offer supplementation only for women in whom the haemoglobin concentration falls below a certain threshold, usually either 10.0 or 10.5 g/dl.

Tiredness in pregnancy

Many pregnant women feel more tired than usual. This is undoubtedly multifactorial, contributed to by:

- poor sleep (see below)
- increased body mass
- anaemia.

However, tiredness may be particularly prominent in the first trimester before most of these factors are active. It may be a direct effect of the considerable hormonal changes or result from the extra energy required for the additional cardiac work and renal and uteroplacental activity. On a teleological basis, its purpose may be to encourage the mother to rest, thereby initiating the 'nesting phenomenon'.

Varicose veins and haemorrhoids

Varicose veins are distended tortuous superficial veins, usually of the leg but also of the vulva or vagina. Haemorrhoids are distended tortuous veins of the inferior haemorrhoidal complex occurring in the anal canal. Both varicose veins and haemorrhoids are common in pregnancy. They result from a combination of peripheral vasodilatation and pressure from the gravid uterus on the pelvic veins, together causing there to be more blood in the venous bed. These veins have one-way valves ensuring that blood flows only in one direction (that is, towards the heart). The valves may be damaged by the additional pressure, and this can result in worsening of the condition.

The action of gravity worsens varicose veins in the leg, and standing still for any length of time should be avoided. Walking does not exacerbate the condition as the muscles of the calf act as a pump to maintain the circulation of the blood. Most women with varicose veins complain that they are unsightly and uncomfortable. They should be advised to minimize the amount of blood pooling in the legs by:

- resting as often as possible in a left lateral position, with the legs elevated;
- not standing still for any length of time, and if this is unavoidable, by 'walking on the spot';
- by wearing a full leg support stocking.

Whenever possible, more specific, surgical treatment is avoided until childbearing is complete.

Piles are made worse by constipation and prolonged 'bearing down' at delivery. As well as avoiding these, sufferers may find it helpful to use ice packs or cream containing local anaesthetic, and to replace the haemorrhoids into the anal canal quickly if prolapse occurs. They usually resolve in the puerperium, and rarely require surgical treatment unless thrombosis of the pile occurs, which is extremely painful.

Epistaxis

Epistaxis (nosebleeds) is more common in pregnancy and generally benign. The nasal passages are lined by a profuse network of veins, which become engorged as a consequence of the vasodilatation of pregnancy. Minor trauma readily results in bleeding, or it may occur spontaneously, especially in warm environments, when there is even further vasodilatation. The increased blood supply results in the production of additional mucus; thus, many pregnant women suffer from nasal congestion. This, of course, increases the probability that a woman will blow her nose more frequently and perhaps more forcefully.

Thromboembolism

Thromboembolism (also referred to as TED) is the leading cause of maternal death in the UK, occurring approximately equally in the antepartum and postpartum periods, the former being mostly in the first trimester (Department of Health 1998). The most common event is deep vein thrombosis in the left femoral vein; the most serious event is pulmonary embolism. Thromboembolism is also a frequent cause of morbidity, both physical and emotional, and in the long term may complicate further pregnancies or cause chronic deep venous insufficiency. It behoves us to consider the diagnosis in any pregnant woman with chest symptoms.

The risk of thromboembolism is increased sixfold in pregnancy as the result of a combination of various physiological changes:

- increased coagulation factors and decreased natural anticoagulants;
- decreased venous return secondary to compression of the pelvic veins by the gravid uterus;
- increased peripheral vasodilatation.

It is further increased in obese women, those subjected to bed rest or undergoing a caesarean section, women aged over 35 years, those who smoke and possibly women of increased parity. Women who have a personal history of previous thromboembolism are believed to have a particularly increased risk, especially if they have an inherited or acquired thrombophilia, or a family history of thromboembolism (itself suggestive of a thrombophilia).

Every woman must be specifically asked at the booking appointment about a personal history of thromboembolism. Women who give a positive response must be seen as soon as possible by an obstetrician with the appropriate expertise so that appropriate investigations and prophylactic measures can be initiated. These may include support stockings; low-dose aspirin, heparin for labour and the puerperium, and heparin for the whole pregnancy plus the puerperium (Royal College of Obstetricians and Gynaecologists 1995). Each unit should have a protocol for thromboprophylaxis, such as that suggested by the Royal College of Obstetricians and Gynaecologists (1995), which must be adhered to (Table 15.1).

Health care workers looking after pregnant women must be aware throughout the whole pregnancy and the puerperium of the importance of this condition and have a low threshold for seeking appropriate advice if symptoms suggestive of thromboembolism arise. In the majority of women who died from thromboembolism the diagnosis had not been considered (Department of Health 1998); none of those who died post-caesarean section had received appropriate thromboprophylaxis (Department of Health 1998). These are sombre thoughts in the late 1990s. A recurring theme is that staff thought that chest X-ray or ventilation–perfusion scans were contraindicated in

Table 15.1 Recommendations for thromboprophylaxis at caesarean section. (Reproduced from Royal College of Obstetricians and Gynaecologists 1995 with permission.)

Risk category	Definition	Management
Low	• Elective LSCS • Uncomplicated pregnancy • No other risk factors	Early mobilization Good hydration
Moderate	• Age >35 years • Obese >80 kg • Gross varicose veins • Current infection • Pre eclampsia • Immobilization prior to LSCS >4 days • Major current illness, e.g. heart or lung disease, inflammatory bowel disease, nephrotic syndrome, diabetes • Emergency LSCS in labour	TED stockings **or** Subcutaneous heparin
High	• 3 or more moderate risk factors • Extended abdominal or pelvic surgery, e.g. caesarean hysterectomy • Personal or family history of TED • Antiphospholipid syndrome • Paralysis of lower limbs	TED stockings **plus** Subcutaneous heparin (commencing during LSCS and continuing until day 5)

LSCS, lower segment caesarean section; TED, thromboembolic disease.

pregnancy. This is absolutely incorrect, any exposure of the fetus, who should of course be shielded anyway, being trivial in comparison with the seriousness of the diagnosis (Donaldson 1995) (Fig. 15.4).

Haemorrhage

Antepartum and post-partum haemorrhage are relatively common in pregnancy. In their most severe forms, they cause considerable maternal morbidity and mortality: in the UK, approximately four women each year die as a result of obstetric haemorrhage, and in two-thirds of cases care is said to be substandard (Department of Health 1998).

The healthy pregnant woman has a degree of physiological protection against haemorrhage, which allows her to compensate for considerably greater blood loss than would be possible outside pregnancy. The most important factors are the increased circulating volume and the increased level of coagulation factors. 'Early' blood loss accounting for one-quarter of a pregnant woman's blood volume may not be

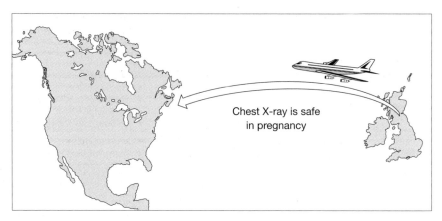

Figure 15.4 A chest X-ray should be used in pregnancy if clinically indicated. The radiation exposure to the fetus from a chest X-ray is the same as that from a one-way transatlantic flight.

recognized if monitoring of blood pressure alone is relied upon to make the assessment (Table 15.2). Tachycardia is an important sign of hypovolaemia: it should not be assumed to be caused by excitement, pain, fear or heat until it is certain that blood loss has been accurately assessed. Similarly, nausea and vomiting may result from both hypoxia and hypovolaemia, and should not be considered to be an important warning sign of significant haemorrhage.

If appropriate replacement fluid is not given and bleeding is not stopped, maternal cardiovascular collapse may be rapid and catastrophic, and the subsequent management complicated by the development of end-organ damage and failure, including adult respiratory distress syndrome, disseminated intravascular coagulation and renal failure. The early and active management of blood loss which needs to involve the multidisciplinary team, is imperative.

Oedema

Oedema occurs in the majority (over 80%) of normal pregnancies (Robertson 1971) and is therefore no longer considered to be a part of the diagnosis of pre-eclampsia; it should also be noted that 15% of women with pre-eclampsia may not have oedema. As health care workers, it is important to appreciate this point since many pregnant women will be convinced that they have pre-eclampsia as soon as they develop oedema, and for the majority, firm reassurance is the appropriate measure.

Oedema is most prominent in the legs during the day and the hands overnight. If in doubt, it is most readily demonstrated by exerting firm, sustained pressure with the thumb on the skin of the lower leg, compressing it against the lower tibia: a temporary indentation confirms the diagnosis. Its aetiology is multifactorial:

Table 15.2 Blood loss and shock in pregnancy

Blood loss (ml)	% Circulating volume lost	Systolic blood pressure (mmHg)	Symptoms/signs	Shock
500–1000	10–15	Normal	Palpitations Dizziness Tachycardia	Compensated
1000–1500	15–25	Slight fall	Weakness Sweating Vomiting	Mild
1500–2000	25–30	80	Restlessness Palor Oliguria	Moderate
2000–3000	33–50	50–70	Collapse Air hunger Anuria	Severe

- obstruction of venous return by the gravid uterus;
- peripheral vasodilatation;
- increased plasma volume;
- decreased colloid osmotic pressure (as a result of haemodilution rather than altered protein production);
- increased vascular permeability.

Although oedema is generally quite uncomfortable and unsightly, the pregnant woman can be reassured that it will begin to resolve after delivery. In the interim, it may be relieved by wearing 'comfortable' shoes, and full leg compression stockings if the symptoms are sufficiently severe, and by elevating the legs when resting. The latter may, however, exacerbate heartburn (see below)! If oedema in the fingers persists throughout the day, as is common in later pregnancy, the woman would be sensible to remove her rings before this becomes impossible and they have to be cut off.

The oedema of pre-eclampsia is often only different from that of normal pregnancy with the assistance of hindsight. Very aggressive or rapid-onset oedema in the mid-second trimester, especially if it involves the face, may suggest pre-eclampsia. The findings of normal blood pressure and a lack of proteinuria are usually sufficient to exclude the diagnosis.

Respiratory system

Respiration incorporates the processes of taking in oxygen and expelling carbon dioxide. Outside pregnancy, the oxygen consumption is 250 ml/min at rest, and this increases during pregnancy by about 20%, to around 300 ml/min, mostly to maintain the additional metabolic requirements of pregnancy: the uteroplacental circulation and the additional 'work' of the maternal circulation. However, there is a greater – 40% – increase in ventilation (the exchange of gases), such that the partial pressure of oxygen is unchanged (i.e. more oxygen is consumed but more is acquired), remaining at about 100 mmHg. The partial pressure of carbon dioxide is considerably reduced, from 40 mmHg to about 30 mmHg.

This increase in ventilation is achieved by increasing the tidal volume – the volume of air moved during a normal inspiration or expiration – from 500 to 700 ml, the 'driving force' of this being progesterone, which

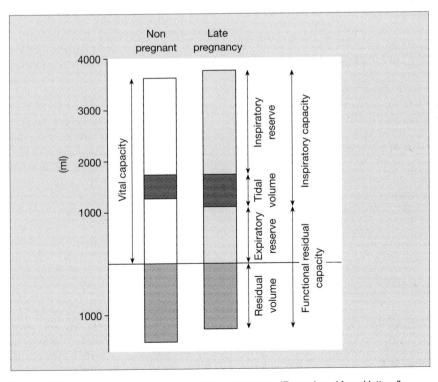

Figure 15.5 Changes in lung volumes during pregnancy. (Reproduced from Hytten & Chamberlain 1980, with permission.)

stimulates the respiratory centre directly and increases sensitivity to carbon dioxide. This is achieved at the expense of the inspiratory and expiratory reserve volumes, the consensus being that the vital capacity, the volume that can be inhaled from forced expiration, is unchanged. The expanding uterus decreases the residual volume – the volume of air remaining in the lungs at the end of forced expiration – and therefore the total lung capacity too, thereby reducing the 'dilution' effect of inspired air and consequently further improving ventilation in the alveoli (Fig. 15.5).

There is no change in the respiratory rate, peak expiratory flow rate (as used in the assessment of asthma) or forced expiratory volume in 1 second (a measure used in the assessment of chronic, restrictive lung conditions such as cystic fibrosis). In the case of peak expiratory flow rate, this is because the bronchodilator and bronchoconstrictor effects of pregnancy are equal.

Clinical consequences

Pregnancy represents a relatively small stress on the respiratory system compared with the maximum changes that the body is capable of achieving during, for example, exercise. This contrasts with the cardiovascular system, to which pregnancy presents a relatively tough challenge (Table 15.3).

Subjective breathlessness

Many pregnant women have a sensation of being unable to 'catch their breath', as if they were lacking oxygen. The mechanism of this is unclear, but it is certainly not due to any changes in the respiratory rate. It may be related to the extra work resulting from the increased ventilation of pregnancy. Alternatively, or in addition, it may be caused by a change in the shape of the thorax, the ribs becoming more horizontal and therefore at a potential mechanical disadvantage. The timing of ventilatory changes and anatomical changes are both in keeping with the onset of this sensation in first trimester.

In a woman complaining of breathlessness, exclusion of disease is usually possible if the history and examination fail to reveal any features of cardiac or pulmonary disease and the transcutaneous (non-invasive) oxygen saturation (obtained using a pulse oximeter) is normal, that is, approaching 100%. Further investigation is required if any of these factors suggest cardiopulmonary disease or if the oxygen saturation falls below 95% during exercise; for example, ask the woman to run up a flight of stairs and then repeat the measurement of oxygen saturation.

Unexpected hypoxia

In the supine position, the gravid uterus may compress the inferior vena cava, and a functional reduction in the residual capacity and closing volume (the volume at which the airways in the dependent parts of the lung close) can occur; together, these result in hypoxia in the supine position. Thus, whenever arterial blood gas measurements are made, the woman should be in the upright position. It also means that a pregnant woman is particularly vulnerable to hypoxia during apnoea: the reduced residual volume means that there is less oxygen remaining in the lungs at the end of expiration. On a more practical level, she may notice that she feels dizzy when standing after lying supine. When lying supine, sufficient oxygen usually reaches the brain despite the inferior vena caval compression; on standing, the additional effect of gravity prevents sufficient oxygen reaching the brain until autoregulation has 'caught up'.

Pregnancy at altitude

It is accepted that women who live at extreme altitude are relatively hypoxic compared with their sea-level compatriots, and this is associated with intrauterine growth restriction. Commercial long-haul aeroplane flights, in which the cabin is pressurized to the equivalent of 2500 m, are not apparently associated with any untoward effects for the mother and fetus. Altitude is also associated with a further fall in the partial pressure of carbon dioxide in the blood – to 24 mmHg – compared with normal pregnancy, hyperventilation being part of the compensatory mechanisms for hypoxia.

Table 15.3 Comparative changes in the respiratory and cardiovascular systems in normal pregnancy and with exercise

	Respiratory system minute ventilation (L/min)	Cardiovascular system cardiac output (L/min)
Non-pregnant	7.5	4.5
Pregnant	10	6
Exercise	80	12
% Increase in pregnancy	33	33
Increase in pregnancy, as % of maximum possible in exercise	12.5	50

Thromboembolism

See cardiovascular system above.

Asthma

Asthma is a common complaint, affecting more than 3% of young women. In general, pregnancy has no effect on asthma, and asthma no effect on pregnancy unless the disease is unusually severe: sustained hypoxia secondary to severe asthma may occasionally result in intrauterine growth restriction. In some studies, exacerbations of asthma have seemed more frequent than expected, but in the majority of cases this was the result of a reduction in the use of medication. Pregnant women should be encouraged not to alter their treatment without seeking medical advice: all commonly prescribed treatments for asthma are safe throughout pregnancy and breast-feeding.

Pregnancy is an ideal time for a general review of a woman's asthma, which may, in many cases, have been ignored for years but might be improved by a simple modification of treatment. Women using inhaled beta-sympathomimetics (e.g. Ventolin) more than once a week should use prophylactic inhaled steroids (British Thoracic Society et al 1997); a GP or an obstetrician with an interest in the subject is an ideal person to make these changes. The relative hypocapnia of pregnancy must be remembered in the management of acute asthma in pregnancy, as a partial pressure of carbon dioxide of around 35 mmHg would in fact represent carbon dioxide retention and therefore severe disease.

Exercise

Anecdotal evidence suggests that women have undertaken prolonged and strenuous exercise in pregnancy, such as running a marathon, without apparent detriment to themselves or the baby. Scientific evidence is harder to ascertain, not least because the pregnancy-induced increase in maternal weight influences weight-bearing exercise. Exercise lasting more than 20 minutes is associated with an increase in fetal heart rate but no other changes (Clapp 1985).

Renal tract

The renal tract undergoes marked anatomical changes during normal pregnancy. The kidney itself increases in length by 1 cm, and the renal calyces, renal pelvis and ureter all dilate. This is more marked on the right than the left because of the uterine tendency to dextro-rotation. However, the aetiology is more complex since these changes begin in the first trimester before significant pressure effects are relevant and persist for up to 3 months postnatally. It is thought that smooth muscle relaxation, under the influence of factors such as progesterone, is important.

Essentially, the kidney filters substances out of blood at the glomerulus, the concentrations of some substances being altered as they pass through the proximal and distal tubules before finally reaching the ureter. Glomerular filtration is dependent upon the blood flow through the glomerulus (renal blood flow), the filtering capacity of the barrier (the glomerular basement membrane) and the physical forces acting across it (the hydrostatic and oncotic pressures on each side).

In clinical practice, creatinine concentration is used as a marker of glomerular function. This is because its clearance by the kidney is dependent only on glomerular action and is not, to any substantial degree, affected by tubular function. Most other substances that are excreted from the body by the kidney are subject to filtration out of the blood by the glomerulus and then to various combinations of tubular reabsorption into the blood, re-excretion into the urine and further reabsorption into the blood, processes that may be passive – depending on gradients – or require active transport.

Renal function changes dramatically in pregnancy. Renal blood flow increases, one consequence of this being a 50% increase in glomerular filtration by the end of the first trimester. The filtered load therefore increases, this being paralleled by increments in tubular reabsorption.

Interpretation of blood results relating to renal function

The increase in glomerular filtration rate is reflected in clinical practice by a rise in creatinine clearance. As a consequence of this, the serum creatinine level falls early in the first trimester, reaching a nadir in the second trimester and then increasing slightly towards term. For the second half of pregnancy, the upper limit of normal is around 85 μmol/L, considerably less than the laboratory upper limit of around 120 μmol/L (Girling 1999). This is a simple but important fact, the appreciation of which is essential for the correct interpretation of blood results: levels that are normal outside pregnancy may in pregnancy represent a significant impairment of renal function.

Glycosuria

Glycosuria occurs commonly in pregnancy and does

not necessarily warrant further investigation. Glucose enters the urine following filtration by the glomerulus. As 'urine' passes through the proximal tubule, the glucose is reabsorbed by active transport into the blood. Glucose remains in the urine if the load is too great for the active transport system of the proximal tubule. This occurs in a women with undiagnosed or inadequately treated diabetes mellitus. However, in pregnancy, it is usually a consequence of the increased glomerular filtration rate. This may be so efficient that the increased amount of glucose passing into the urine saturates the active transport system, which is consequently unable to remove it all. This is particularly probable if there has been a significant carbohydrate load.

In general, occasional or slight glycosuria does not need investigation unless there are other more significant factors suggesting diabetes. Undiagnosed diabetes usually causes persistent and marked glycosuria, which does need to be examined further.

Uric acid, pre-eclampsia and the kidney

Uric acid is also freely filtered by the glomerulus and actively reabsorbed by the proximal tubule, the net consequence in pregnancy being a fall in the circulating level. The tubular handling of urate is complex, involving active secretion (into the urine) and further reabsorption (from the urine). Changes in renal function in the first trimester include increased glomerular filtration and, importantly, an increase in the fractional urate excretion (that is, the proportion of filtered urate that appears in the urine), so that plasma urate concentrations are approximately 25% lower than outside pregnancy. As pregnancy progresses, tubular function changes, net excretion by the tubules falling, and plasma levels consequently increase towards their non-pregnant values in the third trimester. In pre-eclampsia, urate levels are increased compared with normal pregnancy. This often occurs early in the course of the disease and is the result of impaired tubular function. Later in pre-eclampsia, glomerular function may be altered, resulting in an increase in creatinine level. Thus, the interpretation of the result in relation to normal values for pregnancy is critical.

Proteinuria

In normal circumstances, there is virtually no protein in urine. Around 12 kg protein is filtered into the tubules each day, most of which is reabsorbed. The passage of proteins through the glomerulus depends upon their size, electrochemical and physical proper-

ties, and these same features in the 'holes' (fenestra) in the glomerular basement membrane. In normal pregnancy, it is disputed whether there is an increment in proteinuria beyond the non-pregnant limit of 150 mg/24 hours (Sturgis et al 1994), although most accept an upper limit of 300 mg/24 hours (Kuo et al 1992). This may reflect the increased glomerular filtration rate, changes in the glomerular basement membrane or altered tubular function.

In pre-eclampsia, proteinuria may be quite marked, values commonly reaching 3 g/24 hours, 10 times higher than in normal pregnancy. This is due to glomerular damage by the process of pre-eclampsia and usually occurs after an increase in uric acid level.

Urinary frequency and nocturia

In normal pregnancy, urinary frequency is a common and early complaint. This occurs, at least in part, because of pressure from the expanding uterus on the bladder, restricting its maximum volume. At night, increased frequency of micturition may occur because of broken sleep or may cause broken sleep. It may, of course, also be a symptom of a urinary tract infection.

Urinary tract infection

Urinary tract infections are more common in pregnant women than their non-pregnant counterparts. This is largely secondary to the stasis of pooled urine in the dilated renal tract. Further consequences of this are that asymptomatic bacteriuria more frequently develops into a symptomatic urinary tract infection, and urinary tract infections more readily ascend to become acute pyelonephritis. Clinically, the differentiation of urinary frequency caused by infection or by pregnancy pressure effects may be difficult; there should be a low threshold for sending a midstream urine sample since the former may be associated with preterm labour.

Gastrointestinal tract

The causes of the extensive physiological changes in the gastrointestinal tract in pregnancy are controversial. Hormonal effects including smooth muscle relaxation and pressure effects from the gravid uterus are likely to be important.

Gastro-oesophageal reflux

'Heartburn' is a common symptom in pregnancy, affecting up to 80% of women, especially in the second and third trimesters. Its aetiology is complex. Changes in oestrogen and progesterone result in a fall in pressure at the lower oesophageal sphincter, and, in combination with the slowing of peristaltic waves in the lower oesophagus, it is 'easier' for stomach contents to reflux into the oesophagus (Depue et al 1987, Baron et al 1993). There is also a small increase in intragastric pressure from early in pregnancy, which plays only a minor role in the causation of heartburn, except for during late pregnancy. The pH of gastric contents and the production of gastric acid are unchanged in pregnancy. However, the contractile response to exogenous stimuli is impaired in pregnancy; for example, protein-rich foods stimulate a lesser production of gastrin in pregnancy, resulting in decreased gastric emptying.

Ptyalism

Ptyalism, or excess salivation, is a distressing feature of some pregnancies: the woman is unable to swallow her own saliva and usually carries with her a small pot or a copious supply of handkerchiefs, into which she spits frequently. The aetiology of the condition is unclear, but it may be a consequence of altered autonomic innervation of the salivary glands.

For some women, nausea may be so severe that they are unable to swallow their (normal volume) saliva for fear of vomiting. This may be in part because the saliva has an unpleasant taste. Spitting may sometimes persist after the nausea has settled, presumably because, psychologically, it may reinitiate the vomiting cycle.

Nausea and vomiting

Nausea is so common in the first trimester that it may be considered to be a diagnostic feature of pregnancy. Although it is commonly referred to as 'morning' sickness, almost one-third of pregnant women regularly suffer in the afternoon or evening (Chamberlain 1994). Up to one-half of pregnant women will vomit at some stage (Klebanoff et al 1985). Nausea usually settles by the end of the first trimester, although in about 20% of women, it may continue into the second or even third trimester.

The aetiology of pregnancy-induced nausea and vomiting is unclear. Hormonal changes have been widely implicated, although without any consensus. Abnormalities of gastric motility have also been suggested. Oestrogen was originally thought to be the guilty party, but this has not been confirmed. Similarly, the roles of progesterone and cortisol (which are increased in normal pregnancy) as well as thyroxine (which is unchanged in the first trimester of normal pregnancy) are unclear.

Hyperemesis gravidarum

Hyperemesis gravidarum is an extreme form of vomiting in pregnancy, associated with dehydration, weight loss, ketonuria, electrolyte disturbances and eventually malnutrition. Its aetiology is unclear, but binding of placentally derived endorphins to opiate receptors in the hypothalamic vomiting centre and human chorionic gonadotrophin (HCG) are thought to play a role. HCG was initially suggested when the association between molar pregnancy, high HCG titre and marked nausea was noted. However, it is now clear that there is no direct correlation between hormone levels and symptoms, and it is likely that a variety of other factors are involved (Mori et al 1988). Aberrant forms of HCG, for example glycosylated and 'nicked' forms, may produce more nausea than normal HCG. However, as most commonly used assays do not differentiate the various forms of HCG, or may not even detect the abnormal types, measuring hormone levels is not helpful.

Biochemical hepatitis and thyrotoxicosis occur in over one-half of cases of hyperemesis gravidarum and are used as markers of the severity of the disease (Goodwin et al 1992). HCG and thyroid stimulating hormone share identical alpha subunits and receptors, and HCG therefore has a mild thyrotropic effect; it is likely that the abnormal forms of HCG have increased thyrotropic activity. This biochemical abnormality does not need specific treatment and will resolve as the hyperemesis settles. It should be noted, however, that thyrotoxicosis may rarely present with vomiting, so if there are any unusual symptoms or signs to suggest Graves disease, confirmation of this diagnosis should be sought.

The treatment of hyperemesis gravidarum is supportive, fluid, electrolyte and vitamin replacement being essential. Antiemetic agents are not, in general, teratogenic and should be prescribed regularly and by a route that is acceptable to the woman. Wernicke's encephalopathy is a rare but serious neurological complication, involving diplopia, ataxia and confusion, consequent upon thiamine deficiency; thus, oral or parenteral thiamine must be given regularly to women with hyperemesis gravidarum. Rehydration should be with normal saline or Hartmann's solution only: 5% dextrose and dextrose saline contain insufficient sodium, and there is a real risk of hyponatraemia and central pontine myelinolysis (Bergin & Harvey 1992).

Changes in appetite

An increase in appetite at some stage in the pregnancy is almost universal. The increased work of 'growing the baby' makes a major metabolic demand on the woman, and an increase in calorie intake is required.

As well as feeling more hungry, many women will develop either cravings for or aversions to certain foodstuffs. In the case of cravings, these may sometimes be for non-food items such as chalk, coal and soil. Although this has been ascribed to a defence mechanism to counteract mineral and vitamin deficiency, there is no scientific evidence to support this. A dislike of certain foods is often caused by their ability to worsen nausea, vomiting or gastro-oesophageal reflux.

Constipation

Constipation is common in pregnancy, affecting over one-third of women, particularly in the third trimester (West et al 1992). It is caused by a combination of factors. Reduced small and large bowel motility prolongs gastrointestinal transit time (Lawson et al 1985) and allows an increased absorption of fluid, contributing to the passage of a harder stool less regularly. The underlying mechanism is likely to involve the effect of progesterone on the smooth muscle of the bowel wall. Oral iron supplements may exacerbate this tendency. It may also be worsened, in a vicious cycle, by haemorrhoids (see above), which may be a painful deterrent from defaecation.

A high-fibre, low-sugar diet containing plenty of fluid is helpful. Fibre supplements or mild laxatives may also be required, but purgatives are not generally recommended.

Weight gain

Weight gain is variable in pregnancy, being on average around 12 kg. This derives mostly from the developing fetoplacental unit, with significant contributions from increases in maternal circulating volume, enlarging breasts and the deposition of fat and oedema. In the woman who is neither obese nor malnourished and who does not have a chronic illness such as diabetes or cystic fibrosis, it is highly debatable whether serial measurements of weight are of any value in pregnancy, and it is quite possible that they cause undue maternal distress (Dawes & Grudzinskas 1991).

Musculoskeletal system

A number of changes occur in the musculoskeletal system in pregnancy as a response to the increase in maternal weight and the change in the maternal 'shape', and because of hormonal changes that facilitate the 'preparation' for delivery.

Backache

Backache is common in pregnancy (LaBan et al 1983). It is predominantly caused by an increased lumbar lordosis as a compensatory mechanism to stop the pregnant woman toppling forward under the influence of her expanding uterus. Backache may be relieved by improving posture when sitting and lying, wearing shoes with flat heels, lifting heavy items with bent knees and a straight back (rather than vice versa) or delegating the task to someone else, and ensuring that the mattress is firm. Backache will certainly resolve after delivery, although care should be taken when lifting the baby to ensure that it is not exacerbated. Simple analgesia and localized heat may also relieve the pain, although non-steroidal anti-inflammatory drugs should be avoided in the second half of pregnancy. Sciatica may develop from pressure on a nerve root in the lumbar region as it leaves the spinal column, resulting in shooting pains in the leg in its distribution, most commonly the back of the thigh. This condition may be the result of movement of a lumbar disc or oedema in it.

'Backache' may also be caused by increased movement in the pelvic joints, which are usually fixed. This may affect the sacroiliac joints and the pubic symphysis, and is probably the result of hormonal changes, including an increased secretion of relaxin. It is part of the preparatory process for labour. The discomfort may be relieved by a well-fitted supportive girdle or orthopaedic belt. Advice should be given to protect the pelvis, including the avoidance of movements that involve opening the legs (laterally, as in getting out of bed). Bed rest may occasionally be recommended for unusually severe cases.

Cramp

Leg cramp is a common occurrence in pregnancy, affecting the foot, calf or thigh in almost one-third of women, most frequently at night (Hammar et al 1981). There is no proven remedy, partly at least because the physiological process underlying the cramps is unclear. Increased fluids and extra warmth at night may be helpful for some women, but there are no randomized studies to support either this view or the use of a wide range of recommended treatments. Strong massage of the afflicted area should relieve the acute spasm.

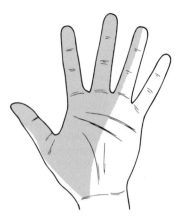

Figure 15.6 Sensory distribution of the median nerve on the palmar surface of the hand.

Carpal tunnel syndrome

Carpal tunnel syndrome is a common problem in pregnancy, affecting one-third of women and becoming more frequent as pregnancy progresses (McLeannan et al 1987). It arises because of oedema around the median nerve as it passes through the carpal tunnel within the lateral part of the wrist; the condition is often bilateral. The main symptoms are of tingling and numbness in the hand in the distribution of the median nerve (Fig. 15.6), that is the thumb, the first and middle fingers and the adjacent palm; weakness of the abductor pollicis brevis (shown when lifting the thumb perpendicularly above the palm against resistance) is a rare and late symptom in pregnancy. This may initially be worse in the morning, presumably because of the collection of fluid in the carpal tunnel after lying down overnight. However, paraesthesia may later be constant, resulting in a decreased ability to pick up or hold things securely. The syndrome usually resolves postnatally but may take several weeks to do so.

For the majority of women, an explanation of the cause of the symptoms and reassurance that it usually resolves after delivery is all that is required. However, for severe cases, the use of wrist splints at night may be beneficial. Rarely, corticosteroid injection of the carpal tunnel is required, but surgical decompression is only indicated for the atypical case that has not resolved many months after delivery.

Central nervous system

There are no specific changes in the central nervous system in relation to pregnancy. In particular, lumbar puncture is permissible, and the results are no different from those in non-pregnant women.

Headache

Most headaches are benign but a considerable nuisance. However, headache may be a presenting feature of a wide range of more sinister diagnoses, including, in pregnancy, pre-eclampsia and cerebral vein thrombosis, or it may be related to ENT problems such as sinusitis or toothache. A careful history and examination should help to establish whether there is a need for further investigation.

Headache occurs commonly in pregnancy. The majority are muscle contraction headaches, precipitated as a response to stress or 'depression', although the majority of women will not have recognized this in themselves. It may be a relatively simple stress such as poor sleep or a more complex one in relation to the changing physical and emotional states and responsibilities of pregnancy. Treatment should, of course, be avoidance of the precipitating factor whenever possible. In addition, simple analgesia such as paracetamol plus massage of the affected muscles is beneficial.

Migraine headache. Migraines may be precipitated by the hormonal changes of pregnancy, especially in the first trimester. Treatment includes resting in a darkened room, analgesia and antiemetics. If migraines occur frequently, prophylactic measures may be taken. The simplest is low-dose aspirin, 75 mg daily; this is known to be safe in pregnancy (CLASP Collaboratory Group 1994) and is (anecdotally) very effective. Other options that may be considered are propranolol and tricyclic antidepressants (Rubin 1995).

Epilepsy

Women who suffer from epilepsy need specific advice relating to the effects of their condition and its treatment on the pregnancy and the effect of the pregnancy on the epilepsy. In general, a woman who has few fits before she conceives is unlikely to have more fits during pregnancy. However, if her epilepsy is poorly controlled – for example, more than one fit per month – there is a high chance of the frequency increasing. The most common reasons for fitting are an ill-advised reduction in antiepileptic medication, the increased metabolism or haemodilution of medication, tiredness or stress, or, in labour, malabsorption or hyperventilation. Appropriate planning, which is beyond the scope of this article, should enable these factors to be avoided.

A first fit in pregnancy will most commonly be caused by eclampsia. It must be recalled that half the cases of eclampsia occurs postnatally and that in only 57% of cases are both hypertension and proteinuria present at the time (Douglas & Redman 1994). There are a large number of other conditions, related to or coincidental to the pregnancy, which can cause fitting, and these must be considered in atypical cases, they include hypotension, amniotic fluid embolus, cerebral vein thrombosis and stroke.

Stroke

During pregnancy, stroke does not occur more frequently than expected for an age-matched group of women. However, in the puerperium, there is a great increase in both haemorrhagic and ischaemic events, the former more markedly than the latter, the relative risks being 9 and 28 respectively (Kittner et al 1996). Transient ischaemic attacks may be a 'warning' sign of an impending stroke and should not be treated lightly.

Skin

Physiological changes in the skin occur in pregnancy, probably under hormonal control. Women who expect their skin to 'bloom' in pregnancy may be disappointed when it is clouded by acne, striae, hyperpigmentation and hypertrichosis.

Palmar erythema and spider naevi

Palmar erythema refers to hot, throbbing palms that are either diffusely mottled or red (see page 333). Spider naevi are small superficial blood vessels with a central arteriole and radiating telangiectasia, which blanch on pressure and refill from the centre. Both are common in pregnancy, more so in light-skinned than dark-skinned women, probably reflecting the ease with which they can be seen. Outside pregnancy, these two conditions are associated with liver dysfunction, including chronic alcohol abuse, because the damaged liver is unable to break down circulating oestrogens efficiently. In pregnancy, it is assumed that these changes reflect the increased circulating oestrogen levels. Palmar erythema may be worsened by peripheral vasodilatation and increased blood flow to the hands. Both features resolve after delivery, although up to one-quarter of spider naevi may persist, and others may recur in the same site in subsequent pregnancies.

Striae

Striae gravidarum are common, occurring on the abdomen, thighs and breasts. They develop perpendicularly to tension lines in the skin and progress from pink wrinkles to white atrophic lines. Their exact aetiology is uncertain, and there is no clear understanding as to why some women do not develop any yet others

have extensive and disfiguring striae. There seems to be a link with local stretching of skin, and there is an association with multiple pregnancy, large-for-dates babies and obesity (Davey 1972). Striae may be caused by the weakness and subsequent rupture of elastic and collagen fibres, which may be familial (Liu 1974). Others have suggested that oestrogen and relaxin alter skin mucopolysaccharides so that stretching results in an easier disruption of collagen. There are no scientifically proven prophylactic measures or remedies.

Pigmentation

Oestrogen and progesterone have marked melanogenic stimulation properties and may be the sole cause of the changes in pigmentation that occur in normal pregnancy. Normal pregnancy is also associated with increased melanocyte stimulating hormone concentrations, although it is not clear that the levels are high enough to account for the pregnancy-associated changes in pigmentation (Thody et al 1974).

Increased pigmentation is common in pregnancy, usually affecting the nipples, areolae, perineum and vulval and perianal regions. The linea alba, which runs on the anterior abdominal wall from the pubic symphysis to the umbilicus or even the xiphisternum, changes from being the colour of normal skin to being more pigmented; it is then called the linea nigra. Irregular pigmentation of the face, called melasma, occurs in three-quarters of women in the third trimester. Although these changes may fade after delivery, they rarely disappear completely.

Pruritus gravidarum

Generalized pruritus is a common feature of pregnancy and, when it occurs in the absence of a rash or other precipitating factors, is termed pruritus gravidarum. However, it should be recalled that there is a long list of causes of pruritus, and other conditions could be important, for example drugs, infestations, urticaria, eczema and systemic disease (such as diabetes, severe iron deficiency anaemia, malignancy and liver disease). In particular, obstetric cholestasis (or intrahepatic cholestasis of pregnancy) must be considered to be a possible diagnosis in every case of pruritus in pregnancy unless the pruritus can definitely be attributed to another cause. The main importance of obstetric cholestasis is the increased risk of intrauterine death, the latter varying from 2% to 10% (Raine-Fenning & Kilby 1997). Liver function tests should be performed on every pregnant woman with unexplained pruritus only if they are normal can intrahepatic cholestasis be excluded. As with so many other parameters in pregnancy, it is essential to compare the results with accurate and pregnancy-specific reference ranges: liver function tests are significantly different in pregnancy (Girling et al 1997).

If pruritus is localized to the vulval area (pruritus vulvae), candidiasis and trichomoniasis should be excluded. It is most likely to be caused by increased sweating in association with weight gain and the more profuse vaginal discharge of pregnancy. It resolves quickly postpartum.

Sweating and acne

Sweating increases in pregnancy and accounts for the occurrence of intertrigo (particularly under the breasts, which have also increased in size) and mila (obstructed sweat glands). Activity in the sebaceous glands increases, and acne may occur, although it is not common. On the areolae, hypertrophy of the sebaceous glands results in Montgomery's tubercles, which are important for local antisepsis.

INITIATION OF LABOUR

Labour is a remarkable event. The uterus changes from a relaxed, quiescent structure to one with considerable rhythmic power. Similarly, the cervix changes from being rigid, long and closed to being soft and dilated. Together, these changes allow the expulsion of the baby and the placenta. In the majority of cases, this occurs at term when the baby is mature.

As the human uterus, fetus and placenta are largely inaccessible to research, much of the early work on the initiation of labour was performed on sheep, in which the placenta maintains the pregnancy. In the sheep, maturation of the fetal pituitary–adrenal axis and a subsequent increase in fetal cortisol seem to initiate the onset of labour. In humans, however, it is probable that the fetal pituitary–adrenal axis plays a smaller part, involved mainly in the fine-tuning of the onset of labour. Evidence for this comes from large studies of babies with anencephaly in whom the pituitary gland is absent or abnormal and the adrenal glands hypoplastic. Honnebier & Swaab (1973) showed that babies with anencephaly and normal liquor volume deliver preterm, term or post-term in equal numbers.

Prostaglandins

In human labour, it is probable that prostaglandins play an important role and that an increased production in the uterus is essential for the onset of labour. The primary stimulus for this increase is unknown:

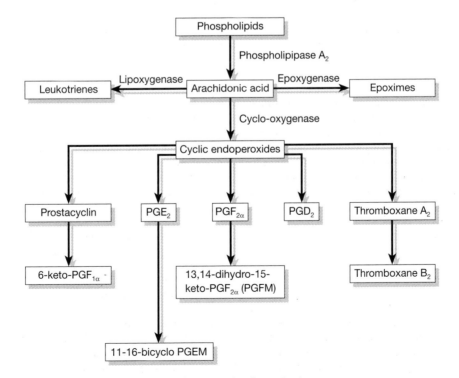

Figure 15.7   Metabolic pathways for prostaglandin synthesis.

amniotic fluid may possibly have a reduced ability to inhibit prostaglandin synthesis (Saeed et al 1982), or the fetus may produce a stimulatory factor to increase its production (Strickland et al 1983). It is also unclear where precisely it is made.

One of the major problems of studying prostaglandins is that they probably exert a mainly paracrine effect, that is, a local action, within the cell or only in adjacent cells (as opposed to an endocrine effect, in which the hormone circulates in the blood and is more accessible for research). Prostaglandins are made from arachidonic acid (Fig. 15.7), which is in rich supply in the amnion. However, to reach its target tissues (that is, the cervix, myometrium and decidua), prostaglandin must cross the chorion, which has a rich supply of prostaglandin dehydrogenases (enzymes important for the degradation of prostaglandin). Nonetheless, it does seem that at least some of the amnion-derived prostaglandin reaches the chorion. Others have suggested that the prostaglandin is derived from the decidua. Prostaglandin F2α and several of its metabolites cause myometrial contraction, in both the upper and lower uterine segments. Prostaglandin E2 is a less potent oxytocic agent, causing contraction of the upper uterus and relaxation of the lower uterus and cervix. Prostaglandin levels are increased by amniotomy and vaginal examination (Sellers et al 1980).

Cyclo-oxygenase (COX) is an important enzyme in the production of prostaglandins. COX has a short half-life, and any increase in the production of prostaglandin must therefore be accompanied by an increase in COX concentration. This has been shown to occur in amnion at the onset of labour (Smeija et al 1993). Two COX enzymes are known COX I, which occurs in tissues that make prostaglandin continuously (e.g. the fetus and the maternal gastrointestinal tract), and COX II, which is found in tissues making prostaglandin only in response to an external signal (Slater et al 1994). Ongoing trials of the use of selective COX II inhibitors (e.g. Nimesulide) in the prevention of preterm labour hope to show that the fetal side-effects of oliguria and premature closure of the ductus arteriosus that occur when COX I is also inhibited (e.g. when using indomethacin) can be avoided.

Substrate availability is also increased. This is brought about by an increase in concentration of a specific phospholipase A2.

Progesterone and oestrogen

Until recently, data concerning the roles of oestrogen and progesterone have been conflicting. It seems that a high level of progesterone is needed to maintain pregnancy and that when it falls, labour can begin. Evidence to support this view comes from the ability of RU486, a progesterone antagonist, to induce labour. In vitro, it also enhances prostaglandin synthesis and decreases prostaglandin dehydrogenase activity. Furthermore, at the time of labour, the ratio of progesterone to oestrogen synthesis in fetal membranes falls, although this is not apparent systemically (Chibbar et al 1986). This change of ratio promotes the synthesis of oxytocin and the expression of its receptor (see below). It also increases gap junction formation (Garfield et al 1980), myometrial gap junctions being areas of rapid communication between adjacent cells, at which intermembranous proteins span the gap between the membranes of apposing cells; these increase in number at the onset of spontaneous labour.

Oxytocin

Oxytocin is made in the posterior pituitary, the ovary, the decidua and the fetal pituitary. Although it is

---

Pointers for practice

- The pregnant woman may suffer a number of very unpleasant symptoms as a result of the physiological changes that occur in the adaptation to support and protect the growing baby. These include oedema in 80% of women, nausea and vomiting in 50%, heartburn in 80%, varicose veins, constipation, frequency of micturition, backache, feeling hot and sweaty, and dizzy spells.
- If midwives understand the basis of these changes, they will be able to give advice regarding amelioration and help the woman to understand what is happening.
- A number of physiological alterations occur including increased cardiac output, a fall in the diastolic pressure in the first two trimesters of pregnancy, respiratory changes, and changes in the musculoskeletal system.
- Generally speaking, slight or occasional glycosuria does not need investigation.
- Thromboembolism is the most common cause of maternal death in the UK. If there is a personal history of this, prophylaxis should be given. The diagnosis should be considered if any pregnant woman has chest symptoms.
- Pregnant women should not adopt a supine position because the gravid uterus may compress the inferior vena cava, which may lead to hypoxia.
- Urinary tract infections are more common in pregnancy and may be associated with premature labour; thus, symptoms must be investigated.

able to stimulate myometrial contraction, its importance in the initiation of labour is in doubt. It does not increase in concentration in the circulation (Vasicka et al 1977), although in normal labour, the frequency and duration of oxytocin pulses is increased (Fuchs et al 1991). It may have a paracrine effect. As previously stated, changes in the oestrogen-to-progesterone ratio result in an increase in the synthesis of oxytocin (Richard & Zingg 1990) and its myometrial (Maggi et al 1992), decidual and fetal membrane (Takemura et al 1994) receptors. The binding of oxytocin to these receptors results in an increased synthesis and release of prostaglandins, which itself completes a positive feedback loop to increase further oxytocin release.

The local synthesis of oxytocin is also increased by inflammatory factors such as cytokines, which may be relevant in preterm labour secondary to chorioamnionitis. The oxytocin antagonist Atosiban has been shown to inhibit preterm labour, suggesting that, at least in premature labour, oxytocin does play an important role (Goodwin et al 1994).

Corticotrophin releasing hormone

The concentrations of corticotrophin releasing hormone increase towards term. It does not directly affect myometrial contractility but seems to enhance the myometrial response to oxytocin (Quartero et al 1992) and to increase the oxytocin-driven production of prostaglandin by the fetus (Jones & Challis 1989). In addition, the affinity of its myometrial receptor increases and that of its binding protein decreases with increasing gestation, so that binding to the myometrium increases markedly at term.

Relaxin

The role of relaxin may be to promote connective tissue remodelling, inhibit myometrial activity in early pregnancy and promote cervical ripening at term. Relaxin is produced by the chorionic cytotrophoblast cells and is thus not found in non-pregnant women or in men. In pregnancy, its concentration falls with each trimester (MacLennan et al 1986).

REFERENCES

Baron T H, Ramirez B, Richter J E 1993 Gastrointestinal motility disorders during pregnancy. Annals of Internal Medicine 118: 366–75

Bergin P S, Harvey P 1992 Wernicke's encephalopathy and central pontine myelinolysis associated with hyperemesis gravidarum. British Medical Journal 305: 517–18

British National Formulary 1999 British National Formulary 7: 400–403

British Thoracic Society, National Asthma Campaign, Royal College of Physicians of London et al 1997 The British guidelines on asthma management, 1995 review and position statement. Thorax 52 (suppl. 1): S1–S21

Chamberlain G 1994 Antenatal care. In: Turnbull A, Chamberlain G (eds) Obstetrics, 2nd edn. Churchill Livingstone, New York

Chibbar R, Hobkirk R, Mitchell B F 1986 Sulfohydrolase activity for estrone sulfate and dehydroepiandrosterone sulfate in human fetal membranes and decidua around the time of parturition. Journal of Clinical Endocrinology and Metabolism 62: 90–4

Clapp J F 1985 Fetal heart rate response to running in mid pregnancy and late pregnancy. American Journal of Obstetrics and Gynecology 153: 251–2

CLASP Collaboratory Group 1994 CLASP: a randomised trial of low-dose aspirin for the prevention and treatment of pre-eclampsia amongst 9368 pregnant women. Lancet 343: 619–29

Davey C M H 1972 Factors associated with occurrence of striae gravidarum. Journal of Obstetrics and Gynaecology of the British Commonwealth 79: 113

Dawes M G, Grudzinskas J G 1991 Repeated measurement of maternal weight during pregnancy. Is this a useful practice? British Journal of Obstetrics and Gynaecology 98: 189–94

Department of Health 1998 Report on confidential enquiries into maternal deaths in the UK 1991–1993. Norwich, HMSO

Depue R H, Berstein L, Ross R K et al 1987 Hyperemesis gravidarum in relation to oestradiol levels, pregnancy outcome and other maternal factors: a seroepidemiologic study. American Journal of Obstetrics and Gynecology 156: 1137–41

Donaldson J O 1995 Neurological disorders. In: de Swiet M (ed.) Medical disorders in obstetric practice, 3rd edn. Blackwell Science, Oxford

Douglas K, Redman C 1994 Eclampsia in the United Kingdom. British Medical Journal 309: 1395–1400

Fuchs A R, Romero R, Keefe D, Parra M, Oyarzun E, Behnke E 1991 Oxytocin secretion and human parturition: pulse frequency and duration increase in spontaneous labor in women. American Journal of Obstetrics and Gynecology 165: 1515–23

Ganong W F (ed.) 1989 Review of medical physiology, 14th edn. Lange, California

Garfield R E, Kannan M S, Daniel E 1980 Gap junction formation in myometrium; control by oestrogens, progesterone and prostaglandins. American Journal of Physiology 238: C81–C89

Girling J C 1999 Renal function in normal pregnancy (in press)

Girling J C, Dow E, Smith J H 1997 Liver function tests in pre-eclampsia: the importance of comparison with a reference range derived for normal pregnancy. British Journal of Obstetrics and Gynaecology 104: 246–50

Goodwin T M, Montero M, Mestman J H 1992 Transient

hyperthyroidism and hyperemesis gravidarum: clinical aspects. American Journal of Obstetrics and Gynecology 167: 648–52

Goodwin T M, Paul R, Silver H 1994 The effect of the oxytocin antagonist atosiban on preterm uterine activity in the human. American Journal of Obstetrics and Gynecology 170: 474–8

Hammar M, Larson L, Tegler L 1981 Calcium treatment of leg cramps in pregnancy. Acta Obstetrica et Gynaecologica Scandinavica 60: 345–7

Honnebier W I, Swaab D F 1973 The influence of anencephaly upon intrauterine growth of fetus and placenta and upon gestation length. Journal of Obstetrics and Gynaecology of the British Commonwealth 80: 577–88

Hytten F E, Chamberlain G (eds) 1980 Clinical physiology in obstetrics. Blackwell Scientific Publications, Oxford

Jones S A, Challis J R G 1989 Local stimulation of prostaglandin production by corticotrophin releasing hormone in fetal membranes and placenta. Biochemical and Biophysical Research Communications 159: 964–70

Kittner S J, Stern B J, Feeser B R et al 1996 Pregnancy and the risk of stroke. New England Journal of Medicine 335: 768–74

Klebanoff M A, Koslowe P A, Kaslow R et al 1985 Epidemiology of vomiting in early pregnancy. Obstetrics and Gynecology 312: 1616–19

Koller O 1982 The clinical significance of haemodilution during pregnancy. Obstetrical and Gynecological Survey 37: 649–52

Kuo V S, Koumantakis G, Gallery E D M 1992 Proteinuria and its assessment in normal and hypertensive pregnancy. American Journal of Obstetrics and Gynecology 167: 723–8

LaBan M M, Perrin J C S, Latimer F 1983 Pregnancy and the herniated lumbar disc. Archives of Physical Medicine and Rehabilitation 64: 319–21

Lawson M, Kern F, Everson G T 1985 Gastrointestinal transit time in human pregnancy: prolongation in the second and third trimesters followed by postpartum normalization. Gastroenterology 89: 996–9

Letsky E A 1995 Blood volume, haematinics and anaemia. In: de Swiet M (ed.) Medical disorders in obstetric practice, 3rd edn. Blackwell Science, Oxford

Liu D T Y 1974 Striae gravidarum. Lancet i: 625

MacGillivray I, Rose G A, Rowe B 1969 Blood pressure survey in pregnancy. Clinical Science 37: 395–407

McLeannan H G, Oats J N, Walstab J E 1987 Survey of hand symptoms in pregnancy. Medical Journal of Australia 147: 542–4

MacLennan A H, Nicholson R, Green R C 1986 Serum relaxin in pregnancy. Lancet ii: 241–3

Maggi M, Magini A, Fiscella A et al 1992 Sex steroid modulation of neurohypophyseal hormone receptors in human nonpregnant myometrium. Journal of Clinical Endocrinology and Metabolism 74: 385–92

Mahomed K 1998 Routine iron supplementation during pregnancy. In Neilson J P, Crowther C A, Hodnett E D, Hofmeyr G J (eds) Pregnancy and childbirth module of the Cochrane Database of Systematic Reviews. Cochrane Collection, Issue I. Update Software, Oxford

Mori M, Amino N, Tamaki H, Miyai K, Tanizawa O 1988 Morning sickness and thyroid function in normal pregnancy. Obstetrics and Gynecology 72: 355–9

Quartero H W P, Srivatsa G, Gillham B 1992 Role for cyclic adenosine monophosphate in the synergistic interaction between oxytocin and corticotrophin releasing factor in

isolated human gestational myometrium. Journal of Clinical Endocrinology 36: 141–5

Raine-Fenning N & Kilby M 1997 Obstetric cholestasis. Fetal and Maternal Medicine Review 9: 1–17

Redman C W G 1995 Hypertension. In: de Swiet M (ed.) Medical disorders in obstetric practice, 3rd edn. Blackwell Science, Oxford

Royal College of Obstetricians and Gynaecologists 1995 Report of the Royal College of Obstetricians and Gynaecologists working party on prophylaxis against thromboembolism in gynaecology and obstetrics. Chameleon Press, London

Richard Z, Zingg H H 1990 The human oxytocin gene promoter is regulated by estrogens. Journal of the Biological Sciences 265: 6098–103

Robertson E 1971 The natural history of oedema during pregnancy. Journal of Obstetrics and Gynaecology of the British Commonwealth 78: 520–9

Robson S C, Hunter S, Moore M et al 1987 Haemodynamic changes in the puerperium: a Doppler and M mode echocardiography study. British Journal of Obstetrics and Gynaecology 94: 1028–39

Robson S C, Hunter S, Boys R J, Dunlop W 1989 Serial study of factors influencing changes in cardiac output during human pregnancy. American Journal of Physiology 256: 1060–65

Robson S C, Hunter S, Boys R J, Dunlop W 1991 Serial changes in pulmonary haemodynamics during human pregnancy: a non-invasive study using Doppler echocardiography. Clinical Science 80: 113–17

Rubin P 1995 Prescribing in pregnancy, 2nd edn. BMJ Publishing Group, London

Saeed SA, Strickland D M, Young D C, Dang A, Mitchell M D 1982 Inhibition of prostaglandin synthesis by human amniotic fluid: acute reduction in labor. Journal of Clinical Endocrinology and Metabolism 55: 801–5

Sellers S, Mitchell M D, Bibby J, Anderson A B M, Turnbull A C 1980 Prostaglandin serum levels following vaginal examination or artificial rupture of membranes. British Journal of Obstetrics and Gynaecology 87: 43–6

Shennan A H, Gupta M, Halligan A, Taylor D J, de Swiet M 1996 Lack of reproducibility in pregnancy of Korotkoff phase IV as measured by mercury sphygmomanometry. Lancet 347: 139–42

Slater D, Berger L, Newton R, Moore G E, Bennett P R 1994 The relative abundance of type I and type II cyclo-oxygenase mRNA in human amnion at term. Biochemical and Biophysical Research Communications 198: 304–8

Smeija Z, Zakar T, Walton J, Olson P 1993 Prostaglandin endoperoxide synthase kinetics in human amnion before and after labor at term and following preterm labour. Placenta 14: 163–75

Strickland D M, Saeed S A, Casey M L, Mitchell M D 1983 Stimulation of prostaglandin synthesis by urine of human fetus may serve as a trigger for human parturition. Science 220: 521–3

Sturgis S N, Dunlop W, Davison J M 1994 Renal haemodynamics and tubular function in pregnancy. Baillière's Clinical Obstetrics and Gynaecology 8: 209–33

Takemura M, Kimura T, Nomura S et al 1994 Expression and localisation of human oxytocin receptor mRNA and its protein in chorion and decidua during parturition. Journal of Clinical Investigation 93: 2319–23

Thody A J, Plummer N A, Burton J L et al 1974 Plasma beta-melanocyte stimulating hormone levels in pregnancy. Journal of Obstetrics and Gynaecology of the British Commonwealth 81: 875–7

Vasicka A, Kumarsan P, Han G S, Kumaresan M 1977 Plasma oxytocin in the initiation of labor. American Journal of Obstetrics and Gynecology 130: 263–73

West L, Warren J, Butts T 1992 Diagnosis and management of irritable bowel syndrome, constipation and diarrhoea in pregnancy. Gastroenterology Clinics of North America 21: 793–815

Wilson M, Morganti A A, Zervuodakis I et al 1980 Blood pressure, the renin angiotensin system and sex steroids throughout normal pregnancy. American Journal of Medicine 68: 97–104

16

The newborn

Wolfgang Müller   David Harvey

DEVELOPMENT OF NEONATOLOGY

Neonatology is a fast developing specialty and has shown dramatic changes over the past few decades (Tarlow 1991). A new knowledge and understanding of fetal and neonatal physiology and pathology have led to breakthroughs in the management of the most vulnerable babies. In the 1960s, only a few specialized neonatal intensive care units existed. Great advances have been made since then in ventilatory support, surfactant therapy, the prevention of haemorrhagic disease, the management of major congenital abnormalities and total parenteral nutrition. One of the most important advances has been in effective resuscitation.

The improvements have, however, gone beyond the pure technical support of the neonate. A further understanding of the parent–infant relationship, new concepts in counselling and new methods of parental education and support have taken great strides since the early days of neonatology.

Assisted ventilation

There is a record of mouth-to-mouth resuscitation from the time of the Old Testament, and Hippocrates reported on his experience with tracheal intubation (Goldsmith & Karotkin 1981). However, it took 2000 years for it to be rediscovered. Flagg (1928) and Blaikley & Gibberd at Guy's Hospital (1935) recommended intubation and positive-pressure ventilation for neonatal resuscitation. In the 1950s, Ian Donald and his colleagues were one of the first teams to use positive-pressure, patient-cycled respirators in the newborn (Walker 1989). Ventilation was then only used in moribund infants, and the majority of efforts to save the infant's life were therefore futile. At that time, ventilators had the reputation of being death machines as most infants never came off them. It gradually became obvious that starting assisted ventilation earlier during the disease produced a much better outcome. Since then, ventilation has improved immensely, and different methods, such as nasal continuous positive airway pressure and patient-triggered, synchronized and high-frequency oscillatory ventilation, have been developed (Chetcuti 1997). This has contributed to the enormous increase in the survival rate of preterm babies over the past decades (Gultom et al 1997).

Surfactant therapy

Outcome in the treatment of respiratory distress syndrome (RDS) of the neonate has improved dramatically over the past few years not only because of better methods of assisted ventilation but also as a result of surfactant therapy. Over 30 randomized controlled trials undertaken during the 1980s have shown that the use of surfactant in RDS reduces the risk of death by 40% and pneumothorax by about 50% (Halliday 1992, Soll & McQueen 1992). Many other trials have subsequently shown that early and multiple doses of surfactant in the treatment of RDS reduce the mortality and risk of pneumothorax even further (Osiris Collaborative Group 1992, Speer et al 1992). These additional survivors do not seem to have a worse developmental outcome (Gerdes et al 1995). These encouraging results in the early treatment of RDS have led to the speculation that surfactant might also be helpful in the management of other lung diseases (Robertson 1996), but this needs further evaluation.

Vitamin K

At the beginning of the 20th century, physicians were searching for methods of preventing spontaneous bleeding in breast-fed babies. Salomonsen (1940) described how adding extra vitamin K in the form of cow's milk in the first few days could prevent haemorrhagic disease of the newborn (HDN). Many maternity units started using vitamin K routinely in breast-fed babies. Large doses up to 50 mg of the water-soluble vitamin K_3 (Synkavit) were commonly used at that time. Initially enthusiastic claims of the virtual disappearance of HDN (Dam et al 1952) were overshadowed by the fact that Synkavit was associated with severe jaundice and kernicterus (Meyer & Angus 1956). This led to the use of fat-soluble vitamin K_1 given intramuscularly. HDN received new attention in the early 1960s after Craig published his observations on bleeding in 345 infants (Craig 1961). However, the routine use of vitamin K_1 as prophylaxis for all newborns was never universally accepted because of the occurrence of kernicterus. Tripp & McNinch (1987) suggested using the oral route in well babies and reserving the intramuscular or intravenous route for infants at special risk of HDN. This seemed even more acceptable after the suggestion of a possible link between cancer and intramuscular vitamin K in newborns (Golding et al 1990). This link has now been disproved in a number of studies (Ekelund et al 1993, Klebanoff et al 1993), but new doubts about its carcinogenicity have been raised (Parker et al 1998). The oral administration of vitamin K bears its risks as poor compliance with repeated doses is a problem (Croucher & Azzopardi 1994). Furthermore, there is a risk of inadequate plasma concentration because of vomiting or malabsorption. However, in the late 1990s, the discussion surrounding vitamin K remains open (von Kries 1998).

PHYSIOLOGICAL ADAPTATIONS TO EXTRAUTERINE LIFE

The adaptation to extrauterine life is a complex and gradual process in response to the dramatic changes that occur immediately after delivery. The amniotic sac and uterus protect the fetus and keep it warm. The maternal circulation supplies the fetus with oxygen and nutrition as well as removing waste products. After birth, the newborn becomes independent, surrounded by air and depending on his own breathing and feeding. In between, there is a series of events enabling a smooth transition from one state in the vast majority of cases, to the other. The complexity of this transitional period makes this phase vulnerable, but nature usually achieves the correct end result without any problem.

The following section describes the transition from fetal to neonatal circulation and the establishment of normal respiration and thermoregulation after birth.

Transition from fetal to neonatal circulation

Blood flow undergoes major changes from a fetal circulation through a transitional to a permanent circulation. The changes in circulation go hand in hand with the development of normal respiration. Four important mechanisms contribute directly after birth to the fast adaptation to the new demands:

1. the loss of the low-resistance placental circulation;
2. a decrease in pulmonary vascular resistance and functional closure of the ductus arteriosus;
3. the end of the production of pulmonary fluid and the reabsorption of any fluid present;
4. the release and production of surfactant.

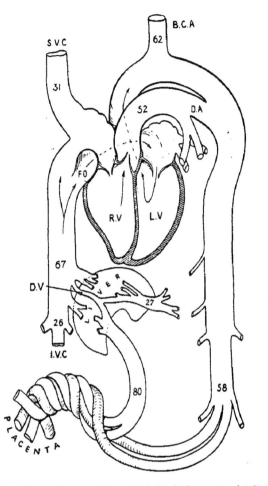

Figure 16.1   Diagram of the circulation in the mature fetal lamb. The numerals indicate the mean oxygen saturation (%) in the great vessels of six lambs. R.V. = right ventricle; L.V. = left ventricle; S.V.C. = superior vena cava; IVC = inferior vena cava; B.C.A = brachiocephalic artery; FO = foramen ovale; D.A = ductus arteriosus; D.V. = ductus venosus (Reproduced with kind permission from Cold Spring Harbor Laboratory Press from Born et al 1954, Fig. 1, p. 103.)

Fetal circulation

The main difference between the fetal (Fig. 16.1) and permanent circulations consists of the unique shunts within and outside the heart that enable the right and left circulations to run almost parallel rather than in series (Freed 1992). Shunting in the fetal circulation occurs through the ductus arteriosus, foramen ovale and ductus venosus. A closure of these shunts takes place during the transition to the permanent circulation.

Highly oxygenated blood flows from the placenta via one umbilical vein into the portal venous system;

40–60% of the blood flow bypasses the liver through the ductus venosus, going into the inferior vena cava (Ho et al 1990). Well-oxygenated blood enters the right atrium via the inferior vena cava, while less well-oxygenated blood enters the right atrium via the superior vena cava. The shape of the patent foramen ovale allows mainly well-oxygenated blood from the inferior vena cava to enter the left atrium. From there, it leaves the heart via the left ventricle and delivers oxygen to heart, brain and upper part of the fetal body. Most of the blood that returns from the upper part of the fetal body passes through the right atrium and enters the right ventricle and pulmonary artery. The high resistance in the pulmonary vascular system facilitates the shunting of 90–95% of the blood entering the pulmonary circulation through the ductus arteriosus into the descending aorta, bypassing the pulmonary capillaries. This blood is low in oxygen and enters the aorta distally to the branches of the carotid and subclavian arteries, which supply the upper part of the fetal body. The descending aorta delivers mixed oxygenated blood to the lower fetal body. Some of this blood returns via the two umbilical arteries to the placenta, where the exchange of oxygen, carbon dioxide, metabolites and nutrients takes place. The vascular resistance in the placental circulation is low. Approximately two-thirds of the combined ventricular output originates from the right ventricle (Haworth 1990), hence the predominance of the right ventricle in the fetus.

Transitional circulation

After clamping the cord, the low-resistance placental circulation ceases. Approximately a quarter of the circulating blood volume remains in the placenta (Wardrop & Holland 1995).

The high pulmonary vascular resistance seen during fetal life falls rapidly after the first few breaths. Physical expansion of the pulmonary vessels, an increase in pulmonary blood flow, a rise in oxygen tension and the release of substances such as bradykinin are important for the changing pulmonary resistance. The pulmonary vasculature of the newborn is much more reactive to oxygen and vasoactive substances compared with the adult pulmonary vasculature (Haworth 1990). This explains why adequate oxygenation plays such an important role in neonatal resuscitation.

Shunting through a patent ductus arteriosus and to some degree a patent foramen ovale characteristically occurs during the transitional circulation. The right-to-left shunt through the ductus arteriosus initially persists until the pressure in the pulmonary circulation has fallen below that on the left. This is followed by a bidirectional shunt when pressures are equalizing and reverses when systemic pressure exceeds pulmonary pressure. Transition to the permanent circulation is virtually complete within the first days of life.

Permanent circulation

The wall of the ductus arteriosus is highly responsive to oxygen, and layers of smooth muscle cause constriction and functional closure within several hours of life (Freed 1992). Permanent closure may take weeks (Freed 1992) but will definitely have occurred by the end of the first year of life; failure of closure beyond this age is considered to be permanent (Cassels 1973). The ductus arteriosus is sensitive to the dilatory effect of endogenous prostaglandin E (Coceani & Olley 1973), so an infusion of synthetic prostaglandin may keep it open for weeks after birth. The inhibition of endogenous prostaglandin synthesis with indomethacin is used in the drug therapy of patent ductus arteriosus. Studies have shown that this is effective in about 80% of preterm infants weighing less than 2 kg (Gersony et al 1983).

Pulmonary adaptation

The first breath is a unique physiological experience for each newborn. As mentioned above, apart from changes in pulmonary blood flow, rapid resorption of the pulmonary fluid and the release and production of surfactant take place soon after birth.

The fetal lung produces fluid, which it secretes into the alveoli. This production is slowed down and eventually stops completely during the changes in labour. The thoracic squeeze during birth results in a partial expression of the pulmonary fluid from the lungs. The remaining fluid is absorbed by the alveolar cells. Babies born by vaginal delivery are subjected to a more prolonged squeeze of the chest than are babies born by caesarean section (Vyas et al 1981). Filling the lungs with air after birth is an active process (Saunders & Milner 1978). The mean inspiratory pressure during the first breaths after birth of a healthy newborn is around 50 cmH$_2$O below atmospheric pressure, but pressures of more than 80 cmH$_2$O have been recorded (Milner 1991). The mean inspiratory volume is approximately 40 ml, a proportion of which will remain in the lungs. The remaining air forms the functional residual capacity after the first breath, comprising about 15 ml (Vyas et al 1986).

The second important step is the release of surfactant. The production of surfactant in type 2 pneumatocytes starts around the 24th week of gestation.

Surfactant is a complex mixture of phospholipids, neutral lipids and proteins. Phospholipids form the major component; among others, dipalmitoylphosphatidylcholine (lecithin) and sphingomyelin are important. They are characterized by a water-soluble end and a lipid-soluble end to each molecule. The phospholipids are able to form monolayers, their main function being to splint the alveoli by decreasing the surface tension.

The majority of full-term neonates master this complex transition from intrauterine oxygenation via placental blood flow to breathing air within minutes of delivery. Only a small number will need help with initial expansion and oxygenation. In a large Swedish study of nearly 100 000 live births fewer than 2% of babies had an Apgar score of less than 3 at 1 minute and less than 6 at 5 minutes (Palme-Kilander 1992). Bag and mask ventilation was sufficient for 80% of these infants.

Surfactant release and production are commonly a problem in premature infants. Premature lungs release most of the stored surfactant at birth, but pneumatocytes are subsequently unable to produce adequate amounts. This results in an initial honeymoon period and typically a worsening of respiratory function within the first hours of life. Large trials have demonstrated that steroids given to mothers before delivery reduce the occurrence of respiratory distress syndrome in preterm babies (Crowley et al 1990). Steroids have their greatest effect between 24 hours and 7 days after the first dose but provide some response even outside this range (Crowley et al 1990). The effect of thyroxine releasing hormone administered antenatally is currently under evaluation, and it may play an important role in the prevention of respiratory distress syndrome.

Thermoregulation

Temperature regulation is one of the challenging tasks that all newborn babies face after delivery. Cold stress increases morbidity and mortality in the newborn and diminishes their rate of growth.

Thermal neutrality and normal temperature

Thermal neutrality is the range of temperature over which the infant's heat production and loss are at a minimum (Hey 1975).

The normal rectal temperature lies between 36.5°C and 37.5°C and the axillary temperature between 35.6°C and 37.3°C (Rutter 1992) regardless of the weight and length of gestation of the infant.

It is, however, important to realize that a normal

body temperature does not necessarily mean that the environmental temperature is satisfactory. A baby subjected to marked cold stress might be just maintaining a normal temperature by a maximal heat production and utilization of oxygen and energy. This compromises the newborn's natural defence against other problems following birth. Furthermore, any sick infant shows impaired heat regulation.

This section outlines the physical principles of heat loss and heat production, and thermoregulation in the newborn.

Heat production

The main heat production in a newborn infant results from non-shivering thermogenesis. This is achieved by increased metabolic activity in the brown adipose tissue, which is unique to the infant. The main stores of brown fat are at the back and in the mediastinum (Rutter 1992). The heat production in relation to body mass of a well term baby is similar to that of an adult, but in relation to body surface, it is almost half the adult value. The ratio becomes even lower for preterm infants.

Heat loss

There are four principal routes of losing heat in a neonate:

1. radiation
2. convection
3. evaporation of water
4. heat loss through respiration (Davies et al 1995).

Evaporation. Heat losses via evaporation are important whenever the newborn's skin becomes wet. Evaporation results in a loss of the latent heat of vaporization of moisture, the latent heat of vaporization being that heat required to change liquid to vapour. This is the most important way of losing heat in a newborn infant covered in amniotic fluid. Heat loss through evaporation is also likely to occur through urine, in skin sterilization with excessive disinfectant or during surgical procedures. Physiological heat loss through evaporation occurs in response to hyperthermia in the form of sweating.

Radiation. This is an important mechanism of heat loss and may account for up to 50% of the heat loss from a dry body. The heat loss occurs from radiation over a spectrum of wavelengths, predominately in the infrared region. The radiating object thereby transmits energy onto the absorbing object.

In a clinical environment, the surrounding walls and windows are usually cooler than the body of an infant and can absorb large amounts of heat. The radiating body thereby loses heat from emitting energy. This is important for an infant who is nursed in a room with large, cool surfaces. Clothing and the double glazing of incubators reduce the loss of temperature through radiation.

Convection. Heat loss via convection results when the body warms up the surrounding air. This warm air rises and causes cooler air to follow. Convection results from the ensuing current of air that carries heat away from the body. The presence of air movement (e.g. a draft or air-conditioning) increases the speed of heat exchange and results in a faster cooling of the body. The area of the exposed surface also plays an important role in heat loss via convection. A healthy term infant usually adapts a well-flexed and curled up position and therefore minimizes his exposed surface. The preterm or sick infant commonly lies flat or in the typical frog-like position and exposes far more skin to the environment.

Both preterm and term infants expose a great proportion of their body surface through their relatively large head so covering the head considerably reduces the heat loss. However, overheating should be avoided because of the risk of cot death.

Heat loss through respiration. The respiratory tract loses heat by two mechanisms. One is through evaporation in the process of increasing the humidity of inhaled air to 100%. The other is through warming of the inhaled air by the upper respiratory tract. Highly vascularized nasal conchae pre-warm the inspired air before it reaches the lungs.

The loss of body temperature via the respiratory tract is important in ventilated or oxygen-dependent neonates. Oxygen is stored under pressure without any humidity and cools after expansion. A high respiratory rate adds to the significant heat loss. It is now standard to humidify and preheat oxygen for ventilation.

Environmental exchange of temperature

Thermal exchange. As described above, there are different modes of losing heat from a newborn infant. Thermal exchange between the neonate and the environment depends on air temperature, radiant surface temperature, relative humidity and wind velocity (Scopes & Ahmed 1966).

Draught and humidity. Absolute air temperature is therefore only adequate to assess a thermal environment if the other variables are known. In order to control the temperature in a healthy term newborn, relative humidity and wind velocity are kept fairly constant. Rooms are preferred to have no or only a little draught as well as a humidity of around 50%. The radiant surface temperature is much more difficult to control but depends on, among other factors, outside temperature and insulation.

Ambient air temperature. As mentioned above, ambient air temperature *alone* is a poor indicator of a neutral thermal environment. Figure 16.2 shows the change of optimal environmental temperature for newborn babies in the first few days of life.

Natural environment. In summary, it is important to keep newborns dry, covered, free of draughts and in a warm environment. Close contact with a human body results in an adequate heat exchange. Moderately hypothermic newborn infants rewarm well with pure skin-to-skin contact after delivery (Karlsson 1996).

Temperature measurement

Different methods are used in the assessment of the core temperature of newborn infants. Measurements of rectal, axillary and between skin and mattress temperature are commonly used. Mayfield et al (1984) compared these three methods with deep rectal temperature and found a close agreement between all of them providing they were carefully obtained. Mercury in glass thermometers require 3–5 minutes to adjust accurately to the surrounding temperature. Obtaining measurements in fewer than 5 minutes is thus not recommended. If a rectal temperature is obtained, the thermometer should be inserted carefully about 3 cm in term babies (Young 1965).

NEONATAL RESUSCITATION

Fortunately, the majority of newborns will establish spontaneous respiration and maintain their normal heart rate with little or no support. Out of 3.5 million births per year in the USA, only 6% of all newborns require life support at birth (Emergency Cardiac Care Committee and Subcommittees, AHA 1992). In one recent study of low-risk pregnancies in the UK, about 5% of offspring received assisted ventilation after delivery (Arya et al 1996). At least one person attending deliveries should be able to perform basic resuscitation (Emergency Cardiac Care Committee and Subcommittees, AHA 1992).

Everyone experienced in neonatal resuscitation will realize that effective resuscitation starts well before the management of ABC – airway, breathing and circulation – the golden rule of resuscitation. Prevention of the need to resuscitate in the first place, anticipation of when resuscitation is likely to be needed and preparation for resuscitation should have occurred long before helping new arrivals with their first breaths.

Guidelines for resuscitation are under constant review, and recent recommendations have been made by the Royal College of Paediatrics and Child Health and the Royal College of Obstetricians and Gynaecologists (1997).

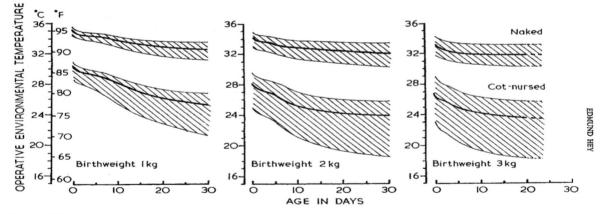

Figure 16.2 Diagram summarizing the changes in optimum environmental temperature that occur with age in babies weighing 1, 2 or 3 kg at birth. The dark line indicates the 'optimum' temperature (at the lower limit of the neutral environmental temperature range), and the shaded area the range of temperature within which a baby can be expected to maintain a normal baby temperature without increasing either heat production or evaporative water loss more than 25%. The higher temperatures appropriate for a baby being nursed naked in a draught-free environment of moderate humidity (50% saturation), and the lower temperatures are appropriate for a baby clothed and well wrapped up in a cot in a similar environment. It must be remembered that environmental temperature in a single-walled incubator can, however, be estimated by subtracting 1°C from the air temperature for each 7°C by which the incubator air temperature exceeds room temperature. (Adapted from Hey 1971, with permission.)

Prevention

However important the latest achievements in resuscitation and intensive care may be, the greatest achievement has to be the effective prevention of the need for resuscitation in the first place. The medical and midwifery profession are involved not only in acute diagnosis and treatment plans, but also in disease prevention, risk and behaviour modification and counselling (Cefalo et al 1995). The medical profession is, however, still faced with many unsolved problems of antenatal care. Fiscella (1995) critically reviewed the current evidence on whether prenatal care has improved outcomes and came to the disappointing conclusion that the differences are not significant. A multicentre randomized, controlled trial of a preterm prevention programme also failed to show reliable benefits (Collaborative Group on Preterm Birth Prevention 1993). This clearly shows the need for further intensive efforts to understand the physiology and adaptations that occur throughout pregnancy and labour.

Anticipation

The aim to be one step ahead of potential disasters makes it important to pay particular attention to mothers with high-risk pregnancies and their newborns.

Box 16.1 lists the antepartum and intrapartum factors that are likely to increase the need for resuscitation of the newborn. Many hospitals adopt the policy that a paediatrician should attend these deliveries. Whether elective caesarean sections routinely require the presence of a paediatrician is debated. There is little evidence that caesarean section performed under regional anaesthesia with no signs of fetal heart rate abnormality increases the risk of active resuscitation after birth (Jacob & Pfenninger 1997).

Antenatal details might be completely unavailable after the unexpected arrival of a pregnant woman well progressed in labour and likely to deliver imminently. The person in charge of the resuscitation should focus on the most important factors and assess the following as soon as possible:

- the presumed gestation of the baby;
- the number of expected babies;
- the presence of meconium;
- known abnormalities.

Any of these factors may directly influence the strategy of resuscitation.

Preparation

Neonatal resuscitation equipment including an

Box 16.1 Maternal factors associated with an increased risk for neonatal resuscitation

Antepartum factors
Diabetes mellitus
Haemorrhage
Previous fetal or neonatal death
Lack of antenatal care
Chronic or pregnancy-induced hypertension
Anaemia or alloimmunization
Multiple pregnancy
Post-term fetus
Preterm labour
Premature rupture of membranes
Substance abuse
Drug therapy:
- magnesium
- adrenergic blocking drugs
- lithium carbonate
Maternal illness:
- cardiovascular
- thyroid
- neurological
Immature pulmonary studies
Oligohydramnios
Diminished fetal activity
Fetal malformation identified by ultrasound

Maternal or fetal intrapartum factors
Breech or abnormal presentation
Infection
Prolonged labour
Prolapsed cord
Maternal sedation
Prolonged rupture of membranes
Operative delivery
Meconium-stained amniotic fluid associated with abnormal
    fetal heart rate patterns
Fetal distress

oxygen supply should be checked for completeness and functioning on a daily basis. Box 16.2 lists basic equipment that should be available (Emergency Cardiac Care Committee and Subcommittees, AHA 1992, American Heart Association 1994).

Box 16.2 Equipment for neonatal resuscitation

Gloves
Towels
Stopwatch
Heat source: radiant warmer or heating lamps
Neonatal stethoscope
Suction with manometer
Bulb syringe
Meconium aspirator
Oxygen source with flowmeter and tubing
Suction catheters: 5F or 6F, 8F, 10F
Neonatal resuscitation bag, pressure limited
Face mask: premature, newborn and infant sizes
Oral airways: premature and newborn sizes
Endotracheal tubes: (2.0), 2.5, 3.0, 3.5, (4.0) mm; two of each
Endotracheal tube stylets
Two laryngoscopes with spare batteries and bulbs
Straight laryngoscope blades: size 0, 1
Umbilical catheters: size 3.5F, 5F
Three-way taps (stopcocks)
Sterile umbilical catheterization tray
Nasogastric tubes: 8F, 10F
Needles: size 21G, 23G, 25G
Syringes 1, 2, 5, 10, 20 ml
Intravenous catheters: 22G, 24G
Alcohol wipes
Medications:
- epinephrine (adrenaline) 1:10 000
- naloxone hydrochloride   1 mg/ml or 0.4 mg/ml
- volume expander
  - albumin solution 4.5% or 5%
  - normal saline
- sodium bicarbonate: 0.5 mEq/ml–4.2% solution*

*Premade sodium bicarbonate 4.2% solution or sodium bicarbonate 8.4% solution should be diluted 1:1 with sterile water for injection.

Just prior to the delivery and while waiting for the arrival of the newborn, a quick check of the resuscitation equipment should be performed by the person intending to use it. This usually starts with checking that the overhead radiant heater is switched on and the oxygen supply is plugged in or turned on. In case oxygen from a cylinder is used, there should be enough gas for the entire resuscitation. The blow-off valve of the bag and mask device needs to be checked carefully. One easy way of doing this is by pressing the mask against the palm of the hand, creating an airtight seal, while compressing the bag. The reservoir bag should fill with oxygen and not leak. The mask should have a good seal and be appropriate for the expected size of the baby. Larger and smaller masks should also be present. The pressure relief valve should move freely. There is a danger from old secretions causing the valve to stick, and inadvertently high pressures might be applied through a non-functioning valve. A further uncommon but completely unnecessary mishap is that the blow-off valve is missing, resulting in a constant air leak and a failure to create any pressure. An alternative oxygen source and ventilation device should be readily available. The suction device should be checked and pressures should not exceed –100 mmHg (–136 cmH$_2$O). The stop watch should be wound up and working. Laryngoscopes with straight blades of sizes 0 and 1, and endotracheal tubes of different sizes, should also be working and readily accessible. Drugs should be checked for completeness; as drugs are infrequently used in neonatal resuscitation, it is not uncommon for them to expire before they have been used.

Resuscitation

As emphasized earlier, most babies are delivered in good condition and do not require any further resuscitation (American Heart Association 1994, Arya et al 1996). However all babies need help to maintain their body temperature (Hey 1974). A loss of body heat has a detrimental effect on newborn resuscitation (Adamsons et al 1965, Scopes & Ahmed 1966). Temperature management therefore has top priority before attending to airway, breathing and circulation in the newborn. Resuscitation after meconium staining of the liquor is different from normal resuscitation and is discussed separately below.

Heat loss

The mechanism of heat loss is discussed above.

After delivery, the baby should be wrapped in warm towels and gently rubbed dry. It is then important to remove all the wet towels and to cover the newborn again in warm blankets. This should take not longer than 20 seconds. This is the ideal time to hand a well baby to one of the parents to be cuddled and warmed. Ideally, the baby is placed skin to skin on his mother's chest (Karlsson 1996). Only if it is necessary should the baby be placed under an overhead radiant heater for further assessment. It is easy to forget to switch the radiant heater of the resuscitaire on, something often noticed only once the baby is obviously cool. This

Table 16.1 Normal values for temperature, heart rate and respiratory rate in term newborns (first 12 hours of life)

	Lower limit	Upper limit	Reference
Rectal temperature	36.5°C	37.5°C	Rutter (1992)
Heart rate	100	180	Hazinski (1992)
Respiratory rate	30	60	Hazinski (1992)

Table 16.2 Scoring system proposed by Virginia Apgar in 1953

Sign/points scored	0	1	2
Skin colour	Blue or pale	Pink body with blue extremities	Completely pink
Heart rate per minute	Absent	Less than 100	Greater than 100
Respiratory effort	Absent	Slow, irregular	Good, crying
Reflex irritability	No response	Grimacing	Cough or sneeze
Muscle tone	Limp	Some flexion	Active motion

means that important ground has already been lost, and it sometimes takes hours for the newborn to regain his normal temperature. For the normal range of temperature, see Table 16.1.

Alternatives to radiant warmers are heating lamps, heated intravenous fluid bags and latex gloves filled with warm water (the latter two items being wrapped in towels). Particular care must be taken to ensure that the distance between heating lamps is correct to avoid burning the skin by lamps being too close. When fluid-filled bags are used, they should never be overheated or placed directly on the baby's skin, to avoid burns and the spillage of hot fluid. The risk of thermal burns may occur from an external heat source when the surface skin or tissue reaches 45°C or more (Davies et al 1995).

Assessment of the newborn

The basic evaluation of the newborn baby includes the assessment of the airway, breathing and circulation – the ABC of resuscitation. The patency of the airway needs to be ascertained and supported if necessary. Once it has been ensured that the upper airway is clear, respiratory effort should be assessed. It is important to establish whether any effort at all is being made and whether or not it is sufficient. If breathing is ineffective or absent, support should not be delayed. The circulation is best assessed by feeling the cord stump for pulsation. An adequate heart rate in a newborn infant is above 100 (Table 1.1). An undetectable heart rate may result from severe bradycardia with long gaps between two beats, or from true asystole. Most babies with undetectable heart rate at birth who respond more or less quickly to adequate oxygenation have profound bradycardia rather than true asystole.

Resuscitation does not however, end here, and the mnemonic for it can be extended to ABCDEF by including:

- drugs
- evaluation of progress
- family support.

Checking airway, breathing and circulation is the only way to assess whether the newborn requires resuscitation. However, an additional assessment of skin colour, heart rate, respiratory effort, reflex irritability and muscular tone is recorded, which is commonly summarized as the Apgar score.

Apgar score. This score was first introduced by Virginia Apgar in 1953. It provides a quick and systematic assessment of the condition of the newborn at birth. The newborn is scored for:

- skin colour
- heart rate
- respiratory effort
- reflex irritability
- muscular tone.

Zero, 1 or 2 points are given for each sign and added up to achieve the final score. This results in a minimum Apgar score of zero and a maximum score of 10 (Table 16.2). The newborn is routinely assessed at 1 and 5 minutes. Thereafter, further scores are given every 5 minutes up until 20 minutes if the Apgar score remains below 7.

It has been shown that the Apgar score may vary considerably between observers. It should preferably be obtained by someone attending the delivery who is not the person delivering the infant (Apgar 1966). The correct timing is crucial because estimating 1, 5 or 10 minutes is almost impossible while dealing with other tasks.

It is important to realize that the Apgar score does not indicate the need for resuscitation as a newborn with a high Apgar score may need resuscitation. The need for resuscitation is assessed by checking airway, breathing and circulation. Furthermore, the correlation between a low Apgar score and long-term neurological outcome is controversial (Bryce et al 1985). The length of time over which a newborn has a low Apgar score may be more significant for the severity of birth asphyxia. Of the three different times, a low Apgar score at 10 minutes is the most sensitive for predicting adverse outcome (Levene et al 1986).

Virginia Apgar has reported that the assessment of skin colour is the least satisfactory sign of the five criteria. Peripheral cyanosis is a common observation in newborn infants, and observation of the trunk or tongue correlates better with the state of oxygenation of the neonate. Subsequent studies have confirmed the poor correlation of the colour with umbilical arterial pH, partial pressure of carbon dioxide and base excess at birth (Crawford et al 1973). Some studies use a modified Apgar score without the assessment of the skin colour.

Airway

Positioning. The newborn can be placed on his back or side to resuscitate him. A newborn that needs his airway clearing or supporting is best placed on his back. The correct positioning of the newborn's head is achieved by a neutral position of the neck. Placing a towel under the infant's shoulders prevents the prominent occiput causing flexion of the neck. Overextension of the neck should be avoided.

Suction. Routine suction is not required in well, crying infants, and it has to be borne in mind that deep suctioning may cause vagovasal stimulation and bradycardia, transforming an otherwise healthy newborn into one who needs resuscitation (Cordero & Hon 1971). The anterior oropharynx should be suctioned before the nose, and the maximum negative pressure should not exceed $-100\,mmHg$ ($-136\,cmH_2O$). Each suctioning should take less than 5 seconds, and the infant should be allowed to breathe in between. The heart rate needs to be monitored carefully throughout suctioning. It has to be re-emphasized that resuscitation in cases of meconium staining of the liquor differs from routine resuscitation, and suctioning, if indicated, has first priority.

Breathing

Stimulation. Drying and rubbing with towels and gentle suctioning (if indicated) will provide enough stimulation for the majority of babies. Lifting newborn babies by their feet and slapping their bottoms in the head-down position has long been banned in neonatal resuscitation: gentle flicking of the soles of the feet or rubbing the back is adequate for further stimulation. Gentle stimulation should result in spontaneous and effective respiratory effort within 5–10 seconds.

Ventilatory support. The quality of respiratory effort is assessed as soon as possible; this is usually carried out simultaneously with drying and stimulation of the newborn. Facial oxygen is only helpful if breathing is shallow or slow but not adequate if the respiratory effort is ineffective or even absent. Positive-pressure ventilation with a bag and mask is indicated in these cases. The face mask is placed tightly after positioning the head and clearing the airway. The mask should cover the mouth and nose, sparing the eyes. The initial pressure required is between 20 and $30\,cmH_2O$ but may be up to $50\,cmH_2O$. A respiratory rate of 40–60 breaths per minute is commonly used. The best way to judge adequate ventilation is the movement of the chest. This should result in a prompt improvement of heart rate and colour.

Some of the air will fill the stomach and cause abdominal distension. This can compromise ventilation and spontaneous respiration. If the length of bag and mask ventilation exceeds 2 minutes, a size 8 or 10 F nasogastric tube should be placed and intermittently aspirated to empty the stomach.

The majority of newborns will not need tracheal intubation (Palme-Kilander 1992). Intubation by inexperienced staff can cause an unnecessary delay in oxygenation and be detrimental if attempted for longer than 30 seconds at a time. Indications for the intubation of a newborn are:

1. if positive-pressure ventilation is necessary for a prolonged period or may be needed during transport;
2. if meconium aspiration is likely;
3. if a diaphragmatic hernia is suspected.

Ineffective bag and mask ventilation is often considered as a further indication for intubation, but this should not happen if the technique is adequate.

Oxygen. It has always been assumed that 100% oxygen is best for the acute resuscitation of an asphyxiated newborn, although it is known that oxygen toxicity occurs with its long-term use (Saugstad 1996). Some recent studies have compared the efficacy and safety of room air versus 100% oxygen in the resuscitation of newborn. The results indicate that room air may be as effective as 100% oxygen (Ramji et al 1993). Further studies will be required to confirm these findings and assess the effect and/or toxicity of various oxygen concentrations between 21% and 100%.

Equipment failure. Even after careful checking, equipment failure can never be completely eliminated. As pointed out above, effective resuscitation is possible even in the absence of oxygen. In cases of failure of the bag and mask device, mouth-to-mask resuscitation has been shown to be adequate (Massawe et al 1996).

Circulation

Assessment of the circulation is best carried out by palpating the umbilical cord and can easily be assigned to an assistant. Less reliable is palpation of the apex beat. Auscultation is another way of assessing the heart rate. Cardiac massage should be commenced if the heart rate is (a) less than 60, or (b) less than 80 during adequate positive-pressure ventilation with 100% oxygen.

Different methods of cardiac massage have been described. One method is compressing the chest with two fingers placed one finger breadth below the level of the nipples. Thaler & Stobie (1963) recommend encircling the chest with both hands using four fingers, and compressing the chest with both thumbs at the same level as described above. This method has been shown to produce better cardiac output (David 1988). The ratio between compression and ventilation is 3:1, with approximately 120 events (90 compressions and 30 breaths) per minute (Todres & Rodgers 1975).

Drug resuscitation

Very rarely, the above-mentioned measures fail to result in adequate ventilation and circulation. 'D' for drugs is often added to the ABC of resuscitation, this being part of advanced resuscitation and thus beyond the capacity of this chapter. The two most commonly used drugs in neonatal resuscitation are naloxone and adrenaline (Epinephrine).

Naloxone hydrochloride.

Indication. Respiratory depression of the neonate resulting from maternal analgesia with opioids within 4 hours of delivery.

Dosage and route.
- Dose: 100 μg/kg or 200 μg stat
- Route: intramuscular.

Practical points. Even after the administration of opioids to the labouring mother, the majority of infants with inadequate respiration after birth will respond well to oxygen alone and the administration of naloxone should never delay the adequate ventilatory support of these newborns. If the heart rate remains less than 100 beats per minute despite adequate respiratory support, naloxone is not indicated. Other causes of respiratory distress may co-exist and should always be considered. Naloxone reverses the respiratory depression caused by opioids but not by other drugs that may be used in general anaesthesia. All babies who receive naloxone should be carefully observed for the recurrence of respiratory symptoms as the half-life of naloxone is shorter than the half-life of most commonly used opioids. Naloxone should not be used if the mother is a known drug abuser as it can cause a severe withdrawal syndrome in the newborn.

Adrenaline (Epinephrine).

Indication. Persistent bradycardia (less than 60 beats per minute) despite adequate positive-pressure ventilation with 100% oxygen, or complete asystole.

Dosage and route.
- First dose: 10 μg/kg (0.1 ml/kg of 1 in 10 000) intratracheal administration or via an umbilical catheter.
- further doses: 10 μg/kg (0.1 ml/kg of 1 in 10 000) up to 100 μg/kg (0.1 ml/kg of 1 in 1000) via an umbilical catheter

Practical points. As mentioned for the administration of naloxone, effective and prompt oxygenation should not be delayed or interrupted in the attempt to administer any drug. Different routes are used for the administration of adrenaline, with varying reliability; the effectiveness of the intratracheal route is questioned (Quinton et al 1987).

Meconium-stained liquor

Meconium staining of the liquor occurs in about 9–12% of deliveries (Gregory et al 1974, Wiswell et al 1990). If aspirated by the newborn, it may be associated with severe respiratory compromise. The resuscitation of neonates differs fundamentally when meconium is present at birth. Whereas rubbing and drying have first priority in a newborn in the absence of meconium, in the presence of meconium clearance of the airway is most important. Suctioning of the mouth should be dore immediately after the delivery of the head. Once the baby is born the vocal cords are inspected and, if necessary, meconium is sucked from the trachea (Gregory et al 1974). This should be performed through a large-bore endotracheal tube or directly with the largest possible suction catheter. The tube may require frequent changing if thick meconium is present. During this process, the newborn should be wrapped in towels, but the stimulation of spontaneous respiration through rubbing is delayed. The heart rate and condition of the newborn have to be monitored closely. However, ventilation has eventually to be started even if meconium is aspirated from the lungs, and it should be initiated if neonatal bradycardia persists at 1 minute. A nasogastric tube should be passed after stabilizing the baby and removing meconium from the stomach. Laryngoscopy may not be performed at all if there is only light meconium staining or the neonate is crying vigorously at birth (Halliday 1997).

Rarely, green liquor occurs in listeria chorioamnionitis and may be confused with meconium staining of the liquor.

Transport

Transport to the neonatal unit for either observation or further management may become necessary following resuscitation in the delivery suite. This should be done after the baby has been stabilized as much as possible and with adequate equipment and personnel. An elevator should never be used for a sick neonate *without* full resuscitation equipment in case of sudden deterioration of the newborn or a breakdown of the elevator.

Post-resuscitation care

Any infant requires careful observation following resuscitation. Temperature, colour, respiratory rate and heart rate should be frequently assessed. Symptoms such as nasal flaring, grunting, the presence of intercostal or subcostal recession, a tachypnoea of over 60 breaths per minute and cyanosis indicate respiratory distress.

Parental support

The anxiety of parents during and after resuscitation is usually great. Even after delivering a healthy newborn baby, a few words with the parents are appreciated. This is even more true after stressful moments of waiting when resuscitation is required. Parents are commonly present during the resuscitation and may overestimate the severity of the condition of their newborn child. It is, therefore, good practice to spend a few moments talking to them during resuscitation and give them a full explanation of events at the end. This should be as reassuring as possible until the full extent of any problem is known.

THE FIRST WEEKS AFTER BIRTH

Parent–infant relationship

There is a natural development of an intimate relationship between the parents and the newborn. It is uncertain when the mother–infant relationship begins to form, but habituation of the fetus to maternal heart beat and voice may occur long before delivery. The maternal attachment to the fetus may also be influenced by fetal activity and movement during pregnancy.

At the end of the 19th century, the French neonatologist and obstetrician Pierre Budin recognized that separation of the mother and infant after birth had a devastating effect on the mothering process. This was, however, unfortunately the practice for most of the 20th century in maternity units until the pioneering studies of Klaus et al (1972) and Kennell et al (1974) in the early 1970s suggested that mother–infant contact immediately postpartum played an important role in bonding. This encouraged fundamental changes in early postnatal care. It is now standard practice to leave newborns with their parents after birth to encourage rooming-in, early breast-feeding and the early involvement of fathers. Although early and prolonged mother–infant contact has been extensively studied (O'Conner et al 1980, Siegel et al 1980, Ainsfield & Lipper 1983), it has proved difficult to demonstrate a long-term effect on the parent–child relationship (Lamb 1982, 1983, Lamb et al 1983, Ainsfield et al 1983, Klaus & Kennell 1983). However, it has been demonstrated that the prolonged absence of intensive contact between parents and infants, which commonly occurs after the deliveries of premature babies, carries a higher risk for future emotional relationships and later child abuse (Powell 1974). The parent–infant relationship seems to be a progressive process in the early days following the delivery. Minde et al (1978) demonstrated a correlation between the amount of time that mothers spent with their infants after birth and the amount of stimulation they gave at home: mothers who were observed to stimulate their babies a lot after birth tended to continue doing so at home and vice versa. A positive effect of extra stimulation on the development of low birth weight infants was demonstrated in a study by Powell (1974). Among other factors that positively influence the development of a relationship, skin-to-skin contact, eye contact, breast-feeding and mimicry play an important role. A failure of bonding has been reported in infants with neuromuscular disease and decreased facial expression (Lynch et al 1979).

In practice, efforts must be made to provide a nonclinical atmosphere for labour and delivery and to enable the maximum time for parents and infants to develop an intimate relationship.

Feeding

Feeding is a further challenge that a newborn infant has to master soon after delivery. Sucking starts to develop around 32 weeks gestation and is well developed at term. After birth, the infant should be encouraged to feed early regardless whether feeding with breast milk or formula milk is planned.

What is best?

Worries are frequently expressed about pesticides and lipophilic chemicals accumulating in the lactating breast, but recent recommendations (Wise 1997) emphasize that the maxim 'Breast is best' still applies. Breast-feeding not only supplies the infant with nutrition, but also facilitates his adaptation to extrauterine nutrition, provides immunological protection from antimicrobial agents and supplies the newborn with hormones, growth factors and digestive enzymes such as milk lipase. It is also a natural way of stimulating the maternal–infant relationship. Breast-feeding is also known to provide some postpartum protection from conception. On average, the first ovulation is observed between 30 and 40 days after delivery in breast-feeding mothers. However, this shows considerable variation and may be an unreliable method for any given individual.

The maternal intake of medication, drugs or alcohol during lactation sometimes causes concerns about breast-feeding. It has been suggested that even small amounts of alcohol per day in the first 3 months of breast-feeding may result in decreased motor development at 1 year (Little et al 1989).

Certain infections are transmitted via breast milk, some maternal infections being regarded as contraindications to breast-feeding in certain circumstances.

Contraindications to breast-feeding

There are only a few definite contraindications to breast-feeding.

Some metabolic diseases of the newborn such as galactosaemia and alactasia are absolute contraindications. In others such as phenylketonuria, breast-feeding might be managed with skilled dietetic assistance.

Maternal drug treatment rarely constitutes an absolute contraindication, but cytotoxic drugs are usually not compatible with breast-feeding.

Breast-feeding increases the risk of transmission of the human immunodeficiency virus (HIV) and human T-cell lymphotropic viruses I and II (HTLV-I and HTLV-II) from mother to infant. It is therefore no longer recommended in industrialized countries that mothers who are infected with these viruses should breast-feed (Ruff 1994). However, in areas where infants who are not breast-fed are at a higher risk of dying from infectious diseases or malnutrition, the World Health Organization recommends breast-

feeding regardless the infectious status of the mother (Weekly Epidemiology Record 1992).

Cleft palate in a newborn is often considered to be a contraindication. These newborns require assistance with any kind of feeding, but breast-feeding *per se* is not contraindicated.

Growth

Weight, body length and head circumference at birth are commonly obtained. However, growth is a continuous process from conception to adulthood, and any assessment of it requires serial observations. These observations, taken in comparison with those of the general population, allow an assessment of the individual. Weight, height and head circumference are commonly plotted on centile charts. Growth charts based on UK cross-sectional data (Freeman et al 1995) have recently replaced previous versions such as the widely used Tanner & Whitehouse (1976) growth charts. Measurements between certain standard deviations are regarded as normal, but all growth charts need to be considered individually. By definition, 4% of all individuals will be either below the 2nd or above the 98th centile. Furthermore, an infant on the 30th centile who was until recently growing along the 80th centile may be failing to thrive and warrant investigation.

Physiological weight loss after birth

Babies lose some of their birth weight postnatally before they put on weight. The average bottle-fed infant loses 2–6% of his birth weight, whereas the average weight loss for breast-fed babies is slightly higher, lying around the 5–10% mark. Thereafter, the weight starts increasing at around 1 week of age. The weight loss does not usually exceed 10% of the birth weight, and it is regained within 10 days after birth.

Normal weight gain after birth

After the birth weight has been regained, a normal infant grows quickly. The growth velocity after birth is greater than at any other time in life: even during puberty it does not reach similar levels. As a rule of thumb, the growth of an infant can be divided into four quarters during the first year. The average weight gain is approximately 30 g per day during the first 3 months. It then falls to 20 g and then 15 g and 10 g per day for the following quarters. Most term newborns double their birth weight at 6 months of age and triple it by 1 year. However, growth-retarded infants may show a catch-up growth after the cause of poor growth has been treated. Similarly, big infants may gradually lose weight after birth until they establish steady growth along a certain centile.

Jaundice

Jaundice occurs in about 50% of newborn infants. The challenge facing care-givers is that of differentiating between physiological and pathological jaundice in a neonate. Early postnatal discharge means that a high proportion of babies will develop their jaundice at home. It is therefore crucial for hospital medical personnel to identify those at increased risk of significant jaundice and for health professionals in the community to be alert to features that may indicate an underlying problem. Good communication between all involved is essential, and easy access to paediatric units will optimize the management of the jaundiced newborn.

Bilirubin metabolism

Bilirubin is a metabolite of haemoglobin and is transported in its unconjugated non-water-soluble form (indirect bilirubin) in the bloodstream. It reaches the liver in a complex with serum albumin. In the liver, it is conjugated to a water-soluble form (direct bilirubin) that is excreted via the gallbladder. Conjugation requires the enzyme bilirubin-UDP glucuronyl transferase. Only unconjugated (indirect) bilirubin is thought to pass the blood–brain barrier (Clark et al 1976). The main importance of large amounts of non-water-soluble (indirect) bilirubin passing the blood–brain barrier is the danger of kernicterus and hearing impairment. Conjugated (direct) bilirubin is only elevated in the serum if it leaks from the liver cells back into the bloodstream. This occurs in liver cell damage (e.g. hepatitis and sepsis) or obstruction of the bile flow (e.g. biliary atresia).

Hyperbilirubinaemia

Clinically, infants appear jaundiced once the serum bilirubin level rises above 80–90 μmol/L. Discolouration of the skin spreads from the face to the trunk and then to the limbs in a cephalocaudal progression (Kramer 1969).

Hyperbilirubinaemia occurs when the serum bilirubin level exceeds a certain level or rate of rise. What is considered to be an abnormal level of bilirubin depends on the gestation and age of the infant. It is very important, however, to understand that it is not only the absolute level of serum bilirubin that should alert the

health care professional to a problem: the potential danger of hyperbilirubinaemia depends also very much on the underlying course of the condition, the speed of the increase and the condition of the newborn. For example, a rising level of bilirubin in a term newborn with rhesus incompatibility should be treated promptly even before it reaches abnormal levels for a healthy term baby. Between 3% and 6% of healthy term newborns develop hyperbilirubinaemia (a serum bilirubin level of over 200–200 μmol/L) by day 3 (Suckling et al 1995, Dai et al 1997). The feared complications of hyperbilirubinaemia are kernicterus and hearing impairment. The term 'kernicterus' is used to describe damage of the basal ganglia by bilirubin deposition. Kernicterus can theoretically occur in term newborns with serum bilirubin levels exceeding 250 μmol/L but is rare at levels of less than 340 μmol/L in healthy full-term babies.

Newborns with an increased bilirubin level often appear uninterested and less alert than those with a lower level. However, it has been demonstrated that milk consumption in moderately jaundiced term infants (a serum unconjugated bilirubin level of 233–332 μmol/L) does not differ significantly from that in their healthy counterparts (Alexander & Roberts 1988), although their gastric emptying seems to be slightly delayed (Costalos et al 1984).

More recent follow-up studies of newborns with transitory neonatal hyperbilirubinaemia without evidence of bilirubin encephalopathy have not demonstrated any long-term effect on their intelligence quotient (Newman et al 1994) or ability to hear (Thoma et al 1986). Recent studies indicate that bilirubin may have a protective effect in the metabolism of the newborn. In particular, the role of bilirubin in protection from free oxygen radicals needs to be further investigated (Bervoets et al 1994).

It is generally accepted that the aggressive treatment of mild-to-moderate jaundice in a well term infant is unnecessary; treatment should also interfere with the mother–infant relationship as little as possible (Paludetto et al 1986). The discontinuation of breast-feeding in healthy newborn is generally not necessary (Oski 1994) as controlled trials have shown that phototherapy reduces bilirubin levels adequately despite the continuation of breast-feeding (Martinez et al 1993).

Those infants who develop pathological jaundice still need full attention and prompt management.

Methods of measurement

Studies show that the use of transcutaneous bilirubin

estimation is an effective and reliable screening method when correctly performed (Merritt & Coulter 1994). It is obtained by portable instruments that use reflectance measurements from the skin to determine transcutaneous bilirubin level. They do not, however, accurately predict the serum bilirubin level and are only used as screening devices. Factors that influence the reading of these devices are gestational age (Yamauchi & Yamanouchi 1991a), birth weight, phototherapy, skin pigmentation (Linder et al 1994), site of measurement (Yamauchi & Yamanouchi 1991a) and daylight (Yamauchi & Yamanouch 1991b). If there is any abnormal level or a suspicion of a falsely low reading, the serum bilirubin should always be measured. However, in a well-baby nursery, the use of a jaundice meter can reduce the need for blood sampling by 20% and increase the efficacy of screening for significant hyperbilirubinaemia by 5% (Dai et al 1996).

Physiological jaundice

Most healthy infants show a rise in serum bilirubin level after birth, some becoming clinically jaundiced. The serum bilirubin level is determined by the production and excretion of bilirubin as well as the ability of proteins to retain the bilirubin in the plasma. The production of bilirubin in a newborn is increased because of a shortened lifespan of the erythrocytes. The hepatic excretion is slowed by a decreased uptake into the liver cells and glucuronyl transferase activity. Most physiological jaundice is mild and shows a peak around the third day of life that usually does not exceed 220 µmol/L (Ives 1997). A number of common conditions may exacerbate physiological jaundice, for example polycythaemia, extravasated or swallowed blood, dehydration, a decreased calorie intake, breastfeeding and the delayed passage of meconium.

Indications for investigation

Those babies who are likely to have an underlying abnormal cause for jaundice should be investigated further. Indications for investigation include the following:

- a suspected pathological cause ascertained from the history;
- the time of onset of the jaundice (early jaundice), that is, within first day of life;
- the rate of rise of serum bilirubin level;
- an abnormal serum bilirubin level;
- the duration of the jaundice (term babies still being jaundiced at 14 days, and pre term infants still jaundiced at 21 days)

Management of jaundice

A careful history should be taken in any infant who appears jaundiced. A family history or a report of previously affected infants sometimes gives a clue to a severe underlying problem. Any jaundice in the first 24 hours of life requires prompt action and investigation, and is regarded as pathological until proven otherwise. Haemolysis, sepsis and severe bruising at birth are common causes for early jaundice. Less mature infants are at higher risk of developing jaundice, and lower serum bilirubin levels are potentially dangerous. They thus need careful observation for a longer period than term infants.

Treatment of jaundice

Rehydration. Dehydration causes haemoconcentration and thus a relative increase in the levels of all substances in the blood. In jaundiced babies, this results in a further elevation of serum bilirubin level. Adequate hydration therefore avoids an unnecessary concentration of unconjugated bilirubin and is particularly important in a poorly feeding or sick, jaundiced infant. In such ill infants, intravenous albumin can be useful because it acts as binding protein for free bilirubin.

Phototherapy. Phototherapy uses the ability of blue-green light (wavelength 420–550 nm) to convert lipid-soluble (unconjugated) bilirubin to water-soluble photoisomers (lumirubin and photobilirubin), which are excreted by the kidneys. This allows bilirubin to bypass the liver and therefore less bilirubin is metabolized by the liver enzymes. It does not, however, treat the cause and may, conversely, mask early signs of illness.

Overhead lamps or phototherapy blankets may be used. Effective phototherapy relies on the dose of light as well as the amount of exposed skin. Therefore, as much of the newborn's skin as possible, including the nappy area and the head, should be exposed. Phototherapy does not work as prophylaxis and seems to be effective only once the serum bilirubin level exceeds 80 µmol/L. In mild-to-moderate jaundice, intermittent phototherapy may be as effective as a continuous application (Ives 1997).

Neonates undergoing phototherapy require careful observation.

Hydration. The hydration of the infant needs to be carefully assessed. Overhead lamps warm up and radiate heat on to the infant and may increase his insensible water loss. Phototherapy blankets operate with a separate light source connected through a glass fibre cable with the blanket. They are 'cold lights' and do not heat up the infant.

Temperature. Body temperature also needs careful monitoring as an exposed infant can easily lose heat and become cool (see above). On the other hand, overhead lamps in addition to an incubator may overheat an infant. The correct distance of the phototherapy light is essential.

Eye protection. Eye protection is necessary as phototherapy light is very bright and may cause damage to the retina (Abramov et al 1985), but sufficient data on human infants are lacking. Head box shields, goggles and gauze are widely used, all having their advantages and disadvantages.

The response to phototherapy is also important: a failure to respond may indicate a severe underlying problem, inadequate phototherapy or equipment failure.

Separation from the mother is one of the major disadvantages of phototherapy. Fibreoptic blankets have the advantage that phototherapy can be continued while the infant is being cuddled or fed. Even if these devices are not available, enough time should be allowed in the well newborn with mild-to-moderate hyperbilirubinaemia for close contact with the parents and feeding.

Exchange transfusion. The underlying cause of neonatal jaundice is occasionally so severe that the above measures are not adequate and the newborn requires an exchange transfusion in order to reduce the bilirubin level. This requires intensive care facilities and skilled personnel.

Ten golden rules

Ten golden rules in the management of neonatal jaundice are summarized by Maisels (1995):

1. Remember to take a careful history.
2. Jaundice in the first 24 hours is abnormal until proven otherwise.
3. Do not treat 35–37-week gestation infants as if they were full-term infants.
4. Document your assessment, especially if the infant is discharged early.
5. A late-rising bilirubin is typical of glucose-to-phosphate dehydrogenase deficiency.
6. Do not use homeopathic doses of phototherapy.
7. Do not ignore a failure of response to phototherapy.
8. Provide timely follow-up.
9. Do not ignore prolonged jaundice.
10. Do not ignore severe jaundice.

Vitamin K

Vitamin K is required in hepatocytes for the synthesis of certain clotting factors. It is transferred across the placenta from mother to fetus. Like other fat-soluble vitamins, the postnatal store of vitamin K does not reach the same level as that of water-soluble vitamins (Malone 1975). The only source of vitamin K after birth is milk.

A lack of vitamin K may result in early or late HDN. Early HDN is characterized by spontaneous bleeding occurring in newborn infant within the first week of life. Late HDN occurs months after birth and commonly involves bleeding into the gastrointestinal tract. Breast milk has lower levels of vitamin K_1 (15 µg/L) than formula milk (60 µg/L), and additional vitamin K is given to decrease the risk of HDN. As mentioned above, the use of vitamin K in the newborn has changed over the past few decades. Different routes of administration have been used, the intramuscular route currently being favoured. Alternatives are the oral and intravenous routes. Potential problems with the oral route are less reliable absorption and the need to repeat the administration to prevent late HDN (Croucher & Azzopardi 1994).

Care of the umbilical cord

Two important issues arise in the care of the umbilical cord. One concerns clamping after birth, which needs to be secure as the clamp must not come off accidentally. Unnoticed bleeding from the cord can be severe and lead to considerable blood loss that could be fatal. Commercial cord clamps are usually used. Furthermore, the umbilical cord is an important port of entry for infections during the postnatal period. In developing countries, contamination with soil and dung is known to cause neonatal tetanus. In the past, powder containing hexachlorophane has been used to sterilize the umbilical cord, but this is no longer generally recommended. However, the cord stump should be kept dry and clean. The Wharton's jelly usually becomes black and falls off before 10–14 days of age. Signs of localized infection include an offensive smell, a discharge, pus and oozing. Infections are treated with oral or intravenous antibiotics, which should cover infections by *Staphylococcus*. A swab from the umbilicus is often helpful in determining the correct antibiotics.

Urine output after birth

Infants normally void urine in the first 24 hours; many babies pass their first urine at or shortly after birth. This, however, sometimes goes unnoticed. In well babies, especially breast-feeding babies, urine may not be passed thereafter for a day.

Bowel activity

The first stool a neonate passes is a mixture of secretions, shed mucosal cells, swallowed amniotic debris and bile, and is called meconium. It is dark greenish-black and sticky. If not passed during delivery or at birth, meconium is usually passed in the first 24–48 hours. A delayed passage of the first meconium until after 48 hours may indicate an underlying problem such as Hirschsprung's disease. On day 2 and 3, a mixture of meconium and yellow stools forms the so-called changing stool, which gradually turns into the typical mustard-yellow stool. Breast-feeding stools are often softer, and there is a considerable variation in their frequency, from with every feed to once weekly.

Immunization in the first months of life

BCG. Infants born in populations with a higher prevalence of tuberculosis should be immunized with BCG at birth or within the first 2 months of life (Jenner 1996a).

Hepatitis B. All babies whose mothers are either chronic carriers of the hepatitis B virus or have had hepatitis B during pregnancy (Jenner 1996b) should receive immunization against hepatitis B at birth.

Polio, diphtheria, pertussis, tetanus and *Haemophilus influenza* type B. In the UK, children should receive primary immunization against poliomyelitis, diphtheria, pertussis, tetanus and meningitis with *Haemophilus infuenzae* type B at 2, 3 and 4 months of age unless it is contraindicated. The primary course of vaccination should be completed by 6 months.

Problems in the newborn period

The majority of babies are born at term and in good condition, and there is only little or no need to interfere with the natural course of childbirth and development. However, the list of possible problems in the neonatal period is vast, descriptions filling whole textbooks. Infection, transient tachypnoea of the newborn, birth asphyxia, congenital abnormalities and prematurity are among the more common problems.

Infection

Universal precautions should be routine in handling any child. Particular care must be taken in the delivery room, where contact with blood and body fluids is impossible to avoid. The use of gloves and gown should be standard. The routine wearing of goggles is not commonly practised, but HIV infections have occurred after splashes to the eye (Berry 1995).

> **Box 16.3** Features that may indicate sepsis in a newborn infant
>
> - Tachypnoea, apnoea and grunting
> - Tachycardia or bradycardia
> - Lethargy or irritability
> - Feeding intolerance
> - Abdominal distension
> - Vomiting and/or diarrhoea
> - Jaundice
> - Pyrexia or hypothermia
> - Hyperglycaemia or hypoglycaemia

Suspected sepsis and true neonatal infection are common reasons for admission to the neonatal unit (Philip 1994). Early symptoms and signs of sepsis may be very subtle or even misleading. The infection may present with signs of shock such as poor peripheral circulation, abnormal heart rate and cyanosis, or neurological signs such as fitting, arching of the back and a bulging fontanelle. However, it is equally important to recognize early signs of infection, which vary considerably and are particularly challenging in making a correct diagnosis. Box 16.3 lists signs and findings that may indicate sepsis. It can cause instability of almost any autoregulatory mechanism in the newborn, which may result in either an increase or a decrease of its function. It can thus mimic many other conditions, for example respiratory distress in hyaline membrane disease or transient tachypnoea of the newborn, heart failure in congenital heart disease, and bilious vomiting in bowel obstruction.

The site of entry for systemic infections is often unknown but may be through the placental circulation before the time of birth, and the birth canal during birth. At birth, colonization with pathogens may occur and lead to sepsis in the first days of life. Later on, an infected umbilical cord, wound or intravenous catheter may serve as a port of entry.

The empirical treatment of sepsis is started if sepsis is suspected or cannot be excluded, often before a pathogen is isolated, and sometimes continued even without confirmation from culture. A full or partial septic screen is usually performed before antibiotics are commenced. A septic screen includes at least a full blood count, C-reactive protein, blood culture and urine culture. Further cultures are frequently taken from surface swabs, ear swabs or lumbar puncture fluid. Different pathogens can cause neonatal sepsis, their spectrum changing over the first few days of life. Early-onset sepsis (within 24–48 hours of birth) is often caused by *Escherichia coli*, group B streptococci or *Listeria monocytogenes*, whereas late-onset sepsis (after 24–48 hours) may be caused by *Staphylococcus* spec. or coliforms. Thus, the choice of first-line antibiotics changes in the first few days, and different regimens are commonly used for the treatment of early and late sepsis.

Transient tachypnoea of the newborn

This condition is also known as 'wet lungs' and commonly occurs in newborns after caesarean section. It is thought that thoracic compression during vaginal delivery decreases the amount of pulmonary fluid, which speeds up its absorption. After caesarean section, this thoracic squeeze is shorter and may result in temporary respiratory distress, which can result in an increase of respiratory and heart rate, grunting, laboured breathing or cyanosis. The condition is self-limiting, resolving within a few days, during which the newborn usually requires support with breathing and feeding.

Birth asphyxia

Asphyxia refers to a lack of sufficient oxygen supply (hypoxia) and a lack of elimination of waste products. It is the most common cause of major brain damage following birth and occurs in between 3 and 9 babies per 1000 live births (Levene et al 1985). Asphyxia can occur before, during or after birth. Compression of the cord, placental abruption, a prolonged second stage of labour and inadequate or depressed respiration after birth may cause birth asphyxia. Hypoxia may occur over several hours or even days before birth. This initially results in a depletion of high-energy phosphates in cells. Failure of the energy metabolism subsequently follows after several hours (Edwards & Mehmet 1996). Organs with a high oxygen dependency such as the brain are typically affected most. A severely damaged cell may switch on genetically programmed self-destruction leading to cell death known as apoptosis (Kerr et al 1972). Studies have demonstrated that lowering tissue temperature before secondary damage has occurred slows down cell metabolism and reduces brain injury (Sirimanne et al 1996), and trials on asphyxiated newborns are being planned. Hypoxic-ischaemic encephalopathy is the pathophysiological consequence of an hypoxic insult to the brain around birth. It may manifest itself in increased irritability or lethargy, increased or decreased muscular tone, abnormalities or asymmetry of posture, convulsions, an absent or incomplete Moro reflex or poor sucking and feeding.

Table 16.3 Congenital malformations and their frequencies. (Data from different countries from Pschyrembel 1998)

Malformation	Frequency (%)
Overall	1–2
Anencephaly	0.6–4.6
Spina bifida	0.2–4.1
Hydrocephalus	0.5–1.8
Congenital heart abnormalities	1.0–9.0
Talipes	0.6–2.4
Polydactyly	0.6–2.4
Congenital dislocation of hip	0.7–3.4
Cleft lip and/or palate	0.8–3.0

Table 16.4 Approximate risk per live births of giving birth to a child with Down syndrome, according to maternal age

Maternal age (years)	Risk of Down syndrome
Overall	1.2–1.5 per 1000
30	1 per 1000
35	1 per 375
40	1 per 100
45	1 per 50

Congenital malformation

Malformations are common in newborns, but most are minor (Table 16.3). Minor malformations do not cause any medical or cosmetic problems, but this may well vary from individual to individual. The prevalence at birth of minor congenital malformations is around 14–20% and that of major malformations 1–2%. Only a quarter of major malformations are apparent at birth (Venter et al 1995). Their frequency varies considerably with ethnic and other differences. Table 16.3 summarizes common major malformations and their approximate frequency.

Chromosomal abnormalities

The most common chromosomal abnormality is trisomy 21, also known as Down syndrome. Other less frequent trisomies are trisomy 18 (Edward's syndrome) and 13 (Patau syndrome).

Down syndrome. The incidence of Down syndrome increases with maternal age. Its overall incidence is declining as a result of amniocentesis, now accounting for approximately 1.2–1.5 per 1000 live births. Table 16.4 summarizes the risks with increasing maternal age.

Newborns with Down syndrome have a characteristic appearance, but none of the clinical features are pathognomonic. The only way to confirm the diagnosis is a chromosomal analysis, which will demonstrate either three chromosomes 21 or an unbalanced translocation of a chromosome 21. In an unbalanced translocation, a third copy of a part or a whole chromosome is attached to another chromosome, resulting in trisomy. Antenatal screening is possible and is offered to older mothers.

Several features of newborns are frequently associated with Down syndrome, but as mentioned above, none of them is unique or invariably present. Among the more common characteristics are upwardly slanting palpebral fissures, epicanthic folds, a separated sagittal suture, a third fontanelle, an open mouth with a protruding tongue, increased neck tissue, a single palmar crease, and a wide space and/or plantar crease between the first and second toes. Infants with Down syndrome are also frequently floppy at birth.

Children with Down syndrome have delayed or limited development but, like any other child, show great variation; the final intellectual ability depends to some extent on the amount of stimulation and tuition they receive. Overall, children with Down syndrome are strikingly good tempered and of a cheerful nature. Intelligence quotients tend to decrease in later adulthood as there is an increased risk of developing Alzheimer's disease. This is unfortunately not the only association with other diseases, and overall morbidity is increased, Down syndrome also being associated with congenital heart disease, Hirschsprung's disease, intestinal atresias, leukaemias, hypothyroidism and other conditions.

Because of the increased awareness of their special needs, local and national family support groups exist for these children and their parents.

Prematurity

Infants born before 37 completed weeks of pregnancy are referred to as preterm. The incidence of preterm labour in low-risk singleton pregnancies is around 50 in 1000 (Harlow et al 1996), although seasonal variations are known (Cooperstock & Wolfe 1986). Over the last few decades, the rate of intact survival of premature infants has changed dramatically (Gultom et al 1997). The limit of viability has gradually changed, currently lying between 22 and 26 weeks of gestation. However, the chance of intact survival for these extremely preterm infants is slim (Table 16.5).

A number of predisposing factors have been identified for preterm labour, but in almost half of prematurely labouring women, no reason is apparent. First live births and male infants have a higher risk of being born prematurely. Intra-amniotic infections play an important role, organisms such as *Escherichia coli* and *Listeria monocytogenes* being among the causative agents. Sadly, medical care has made only little impact on the prevention of preterm labour (Collaborative Group on Preterm Birth Prevention 1993). Once preterm labour is established, the management is complex and depends on the underlying factor. Antibiotics, tocolysis and antenatal steroid therapy are important. Steroids given to mothers before delivery reduce the occurrence of respiratory distress syndrome in preterm babies. They are most effective when given between 1 and 7 days before delivery (Crowley et al 1990). Neonatal resuscitation requires skilled personnel, adequate equipment (see above) and a neonatal intensive care unit.

Premature birth brings with it a variety of problems for the whole family and is a very stressful time for everybody involved. There may also be severe maternal illness before, during or after delivery. Additionally, the premature infant may face major problems after delivery and may require intensive care for many months. This period is often characterized by frequent ups and downs, the fear of losing someone very close and/or the fear of permanent handicap. Parents commonly compare this time with a ride on a roller-coaster. In addition, some parents feel grief over a lost normal pregnancy or suffer from the loss of the 'normal' postnatal period, which is often taken for granted.

SCREENING AND HEALTH CHECKS

Health checks

A routine examination of all children should be performed at birth, before discharge home and at 6–8 weeks, 7–9 months, 18–24 months, 36–42 months and 4.5 years of age. During early life, it is particularly important to establish whether malformations or abnormalities are present, while later in life, development and progress become more important. Growth has to be monitored carefully throughout, and a reason for any failure to grow must be sought.

Table 16.5 Summary of survival rates at 23+0 and 26+6 weeks gestation from 1980 to 1994. (Modified from Morrison & Rennie 1997)

Gestation (weeks)	23	24	25	26
Total survivors (%)	17	39	50	61
Handicapped survivors/total survivors (%)	65	34	31	26

Health checks after birth

The first examination is usually carried out immediately after birth and is therefore often performed by the midwife. In this examination, one should concentrate on checking that the infant looks well and that there are no major abnormalities, such as cleft lip or palate, spina bifida, anal atresia or ambiguous genitalia. A long, detailed examination looking for minor abnormalities at this stage will only delay the first contact between parents and infant. A thorough examination should then be made in the first days of life. It does not matter what order the examination is performed in as long as it is complete. As with any other physical examination, it is best to develop a personal routine to avoid forgetting important items. The health check is also a perfect opportunity for parents to learn about their baby and answer questions about their health and other issues. It should thus always be carried out in the presence of one or preferably both parents. This is the perfect opportunity to explain what you are checking for and to describe the capabilities of the newborn baby.

Whatever personal order one develops for the examination, there are some crucial points.

First, before examination it is important to gain information about the past medical, obstetric and social history of the mother, the birth and resuscitation, and any important family history.

Second, the examination requires time and a warm, draught-free room.

Third, before starting, the examiner should introduce him or herself and explain the intention. This is also a good opportunity to ask for the baby's given name.

Every examination should begin with a simple observation of the newborn and his interaction with his parents. Vital information can be gathered about the state of the newborn, the posture, the colour, the spontaneous movements, the proportions of the infant, the features of the exposed parts of the body, the breathing pattern and the symmetry of the face (especially when crying). It is also sometimes possible to get an idea of the parents' confidence in handling their new child. All this can be assessed before touching the infant or even separating the newborn from his parents.

The fourth point is that important examinations that require a quiet infant should be made whenever there is a good opportunity. Auscultation of the heart with a prewarmed stethoscope can occur soon after inspection. At some stage during the examination, most babies wake up and open their eyes so it is wise to have an ophthalmoscope handy at all times to capitalize on this opportunity. The worst scenario is to attempt to visualize the red reflex in a crying infant with both his eyes tightly closed. An abdominal examination is exceedingly difficult in a crying infant who has tense abdominal wall muscles. All the examinations are best performed in a quiet infant, but most children will show some form of displeasure at some stage.

Fifth, in order to keep the infant quiet as long as possible, any unpleasant parts of the examination, for example testing the Moro response, or the hips for stability and dislocation, should be kept until the end. Examination of the hips requires an initially peaceful infant, although it often results in a loud protest. Some experts claim that a correct examination of the hips will not result in a screaming newborn, but it is certainly true that dislocatable hips are easily missed in a screaming and kicking newborn.

Sixth, every part of the infant should be completely undressed at some stage. In a warm environment, all clothes are best taken off at the same time, the baby being wrapped in a towel, which can be easily removed for inspection and examination.

Seventh, a systematic approach to the examination of the rest of the body makes forgetting some important items less likely. One approach is to place the undressed infant on his back and gradually work one's way from the top to the feet. Some time should be spent in merely observing the undressed infant before touching him. After a complete examination, the infant is then turned on his front. During turning, the extensor tone can be tested in ventral suspension by supporting the thorax on the palm with head and arms hanging down on one side and the legs on the other. In the prone position, the systematic examination again runs from top to toe.

It must also be remembered that each step of the examination should be explained and the opportunity should be given for the parents to ask questions. Some of the explanations are best given beforehand: parents generally appreciate a warning before extending the infant's head to elicit the Moro reflex, for example.

Last but not least, it has to be appreciated that there is an immense number of normal variations and minor deviations.

Table 16.6 summarizes the important items of an examination of the afterbirth.

Counselling parents

After examination of the newborn, even an experienced examiner might not be entirely sure of the significance of certain findings: there might have been a click when testing the hips of a neonate, or a soft systolic murmur or even just unusual features that might

Table 16.6   Items that should be included in a routine newborn examination soon after birth

General features	Head/neck	Thorax	Upper limbs	Abdomen	Lower limbs/spine

Birth weight	Skull
	  size, shape
	  swellings
	  sutures
		Size and shape
		Nipples
		  number
		  position
		  spacing
			Spontaneous
			  movements
			  tone
			  shape and size
			  posture
			  number of digits
			  palmar creases
				Umbilicus
				  number of vessels
				  signs of infection
				  smell
				  oozing, bleeding
					Spontaneous
					  movements
					  tone
					  shape and size
					  posture
					  number of
					  plantar digits
					  creases

Head circumference					
Body length					

Nutritional state	Fontanelle
	  anterior, posterior,
	  third
		Lungs
		  respiratory rate
		  auxiliary muscle
		  inter/subcostal
		  retraction
				Abdomen
				  organomegaly
				  distension
				  bilious vomiting
				  herniae	

Spontaneous
  movements
					Hip stability and
					  location

Symmetry	Eyes
	  palpebral fissure
	  iris
	  sclera
	  retina (red reflex)
	  conjunctiva
		Cardiovascular
		  apex beat
		  pulses
		  auscultation
				Kidney
				  time of first voiding
				  flow of urine in male
				  infants (poor stream
				  with posterior
				  urethral valve)
					Spine
					  deformities
					  sacral dimple
					  hairy naevus
					  over lower
					  spine

Tone					
Unusual/dysmorphic features					

Cry	Ears
	  shape and size
	  external auditory
	  canal
	  preauricular sinus,
	  skin tag
	  placement – low
	  set, rotated
				Anus
				  patency	

Skin
  colour
  • pink, plethoric,
  • pale, jaundiced,
  • cyanosed,
  meconium staining
  maturity
  birth marks
  defects
  naevi
  rash
				Bowels
				  time of first passage
				  of meconium	

	Nose				

	Mouth, lips, tongue
	  shape and size
	  cyanosis
				Genitalia
				  gender
				  meatus
				  testicles
				  hydrocele
				  discharge
				  vaginal bleeding	

	Palate
	  inspect and palpate
	  with little finger				

	Cysts				
	Clavicles				

be entirely normal. This creates an even greater problem for an inexperienced examiner. On the other hand, there might be a clearly abnormal finding that either is or is not obvious to the parents. The difficulty then arises of what to do and how. Parents may be made unnecessarily anxious after one's doubts are mentioned when it may turn out to be a false alarm. Is it better to walk away and get someone else to check without mentioning any of the doubtful findings? And how does one tell the parents if there is something definitely abnormal?

Each case will be different, needing an individual approach. However, from our own experience, most parents are very careful observers when their baby is examined. They frequently notice any hesitation on the part of the examiner or extra time spent on a certain examination. They certainly suspect that something is wrong when their baby is the only one in the entire room who has been examined by three different

people. Uncertainty often creates more fear, and the worst rather than the best is sometimes expected. An open and honest approach from the start is the optimum, and it is good practice to mention if a second person is needed to assess a certain finding. The approach is obviously far more difficult when something definitely abnormal is found. The handling of this situation depends on the severity of the finding and the consequence it bears. Major problems should be discussed with both parents present, together with the midwife involved in the delivery and the most senior paediatrician available. If a diagnosis has not yet been confirmed, this should also be made clear. Parents can usually only take in small quantities of new information at a time. The first meeting is commonly used to say as much as necessary but as little as possible. This is particularly true if the family's entire life will be turned upside down in a single day. Frequent further meetings will be required, and the

Pointers for practice

- The period immediately after birth encompasses some of the most dramatic changes as the neonate adapts to extrauterine life. These include the transition from the fetal to neonatal circulation, and the establishment of normal respiration and thermoregulation.
- The majority of babies are born without problems.
- The basic initial assessment of the newborn includes an assessment of airway, breathing and circulation (ABC).
- It is important to keep the newborn dry, covered, free of draughts and in a warm environment. Close contact to a human body provides an adequate heat exchange.
- At least one person attending a birth should be able to perform basic resuscitation.
- Bag and mask resuscitation is adequate in the majority of cases.
- Breast-feeding is the best method and has a number of advantages over artificial breast milk and bottle-feeding. There are few contraindications to breast-feeding.
- Weight loss and jaundice are usually physiological but need to be differentiated from pathological causes.
- Most newborns are healthy, the most common problems being infection, transient tachypnoea of the newborn, birth asphyxia and prematurity.
- All newborns should receive regular and systematic health checks, and the parents should be advised regarding vaccination.

full range of implications will be approached step by step, sometimes spanning the entire childhood.

Guthrie test

In 1963, Robert Guthrie proposed a screening method in newborn infants for phenylketonuria using dried blood spots on filter paper (Guthrie 1996). This subsequently became known as the Guthrie test. Dried blood on filter paper can also be used for screening for many other diseases, including congenital hypothyroidism, galactosaemia, maple syrup urine disease, valinaemia, sickle cell disease and medium-chain acyl-CoA reductase deficiency (MCAD). MCAD has been investigated as a possible underlying cause of sudden infant death syndrome. At present in the UK, routine screening has been established for phenylketonuria and congenital hypothyroidism. This is performed at 6–7 days of age when most term infants have established feeding.

Screening for sickle cell disease is routinely included for some groups of people with an increased prevalence of carriers.

OUTLOOK

As mentioned at the start of this chapter, paediatrics has seen dramatic changes in the past, and it is not surprising that the near future will bring further alterations in the understanding, diagnosis and management of diseases in the newborn period. Communication systems have linked the entire world at the push of a button, and a rapid exchange of experience has been enabled through computer technology. New methods of non-invasive imaging such as magnetic resonance spectroscopy enable the observation of metabolism in the body. Understanding mechanisms on the level of molecular genetics gives us an insight into the pathogenesis of diseases as well as opening up new approaches to therapy. New concepts of ventilation, for example liquid ventilation, may reveal entirely different long-term outcomes in infants who are premature.

Whatever promising approaches the future might bring, the greatest impact on the health of newborns will, however, be made by preventing these conditions in the first place.

REFERENCES

Abramov I, Hainline L, Lemerise E, Brown A K 1985 Changes in visual functions of children exposed as infants to prolonged illumination. Journal of the American Optometric Association 56(8): 614–9

Adamsons K Jr, Gandy G M, James L S 1965 The influence of thermal factors upon oxygen consumption of newborn human infants. Journal of Pediatrics 66: 495–508

Ainsfield E, Lipper E 1983 Early contact, social support, and mother–infant bonding. Pediatrics 72: 79–83

Ainsfield E, Curry M A, Hales D J et al 1983 Maternal–infant bonding: a joint rebuttal. Pediatrics 72: 569–72

Alexander G S, Roberts S A 1988 Sucking behaviour and milk intake in jaundiced neonates. Early Human Development 16(1): 73–84

American Heart Association 1994 Newborn resuscitation. In Chameides L, Hazinski M F (ed.) Pediatric Advanced Life Support. Scientific Publishing American Heart Association, Dallas

Apgar V 1953 A proposal for a new method of evaluation of the newborn infant. Anesthesia and Analgesia 32: 260–7

Apgar V 1966 The newborn (Apgar) scoring system.

Reflection and advice. Pediatric Clinics of North America 10: 645–50

Arya R, Pethen T, Johanson R B, Spencer S A 1996 Outcome in low risk pregnancies. Archives of Diseases in Childhood Fetal Neonatal Edition 75(2): F97–F102

Berry K 1995 Reducing the risk of eye contamination. Nursing Standard 9(51): 27–9

Bervoets K, Schlenzig J S, Bohles H 1994 Bilirubin in the early neonatal period. Is there a positive aspect of hyperbilirubinaemia? – a medical hypothesis. Fortschritte der Medizin 112(13): 192–4

Blaikley L B, Gibberd G F 1935 Asphyxia neonatorum. Lancet i: 736–9

Born G V R, Dawes G S, Mott J C, Widdicombe J G 1954 Changes in the heart and lungs at birth. Cold Spring Harbor Symposia on Quantitative Biology 19: 102–8

Bryce R L, Halperin M E, Sinclair J C 1985 Association between indicators of perinatal asphyxia and adverse outcome in the term infant: a methodological review. Neuroepidemiology 4(1): 24–38

Cassels D E 1973 The ductus arteriosus. Charles C Thomas, Springfield, IL

Cefalo R C, Bowes W A Jr, Moos M K 1995 Preconception care: a means of prevention. Baillière's Clinical Obstetrics and Gynaecology 9(3): 403–16

Chetcuti P A J 1997 New techniques for neonatal respiratory support. Current Paediatrics 7: 78–84

Clark C F, Torii S, Hamamoto Z, Kaito H 1976 The 'bronze baby' syndrome: postmortem data. Journal of Pediatrics 88(3): 461–4

Coceani F, Olley P M 1973 The response of the ductus arteriosus to prostaglandins. Canadian Journal of Physiology and Pharmacology 51: 220–5

Collaborative Group on Preterm Birth Prevention 1993 Multicenter randomized, controlled trial of a preterm birth prevention program. American Journal of Obstetrics and Gynecology 169 (part 1): 352–66

Cooperstock M, Wolfe R A 1986 Seasonality of preterm birth in the Collaborative Perinatal Project: demographic factors. American Journal of Epidemiology 124(2): 234–41

Cordero L Jr, Hon E H 1971 Neonatal bradycardia following nasopharyngeal stimulation. Journal of Pediatrics 78: 441–7

Costalos C, Russell G, Bistarakis L, Pangali A, Philippidou A 1984 Effects of jaundice and phototherapy on gastric emptying in the newborn. Biology of the Neonate 46(2): 57–60

Craig W S 1961 On real and apparent bleeding in the newborn. Archives of Diseases in Childhood 36: 575–86

Crawford J S, Davies P, Pearson J F 1973 Significance of the individual components of the Apgar score. British Journal of Anaesthesia 45: 148–58

Croucher C, Azzopardi D 1994 Compliance with recommendations for giving vitamin K to newborn infants. British Medical Journal 308 (6933): 894–5

Crowley P, Chalmers I, Keirse M 1990 The effects of corticosteroid administration before preterm delivery: an overview of the evidence from controlled trials. British Journal of Obstetrics and Gynaecology 97: 11–25

Dai J, Krahn J, Parry D M 1996 Clinical impact of transcutaneous bilirubinometry as an adjunctive screen for hyperbilirubinaemia. Clinical Biochemistry 29(6): 581–6

Dai J, Parry D M, Krahn J 1997 Transcutaneous bilirubinometry: its role in the assessment of neonatal jaundice. Clinical Biochemistry 30(1): 1–9 (review)

Dam H, Dyggve H, Hjalmar L, Plum P 1952 The relation of vitamin K deficiency to haemorrhagic disease of the newborn. Advances in Pediatrics 5: 129–53

David R 1988 Closed chest cardiac massage in the newborn infant. Pediatrics 81: 552–4

Davies P D, Parbrook G D, Kenny G N C 1995 Temperature. In Davies P D (ed.) Basic physics and measurements in anaesthesia, 4th edn. Butterworth-Heinemann, Oxford

Edwards A D, Mehmet H 1996 Apoptosis in perinatal hypoxic-ischemic cerebral damage. Neuropathology and Applied Neurobiology 22(6): 494–8

Ekelund H, Finnström O, Gunnarskog J, Källén B, Larsson Y 1993 Administration of vitamin K to newborn infants and childhood cancer. British Medical Journal 307: 89–91

Emergency Cardiac Care Committee and Subcommittees, AHA 1992 Guidelines for cardiopulmonary resuscitation and emergency cardiac care. VII: Neonatal resuscitation. Journal of the American Medical Association 268(16): 2276–81

Fiscella K 1995 Does prenatal care improve birth outcomes? A critical review. Obstetrics and Gynecology 85(3): 468–79

Flagg P J 1928 The treatment of asphyxia in the newborn. Journal of the American Medical Association 91: 788–91

Freed M D 1992 Normal circulatory physiology: fetal and transitional circulation. In Fyler D C (ed.) Nadas' Pediatric cardiology. Hanley & Belfus, Philadelphia

Freeman J V, Cole T J, Chinn S, Jones P R, White E M, Preece M A 1995 Cross sectional stature and weight reference curves for the UK, 1990. Archives of Disease in Childhood 73(1): 17–24

Gerdes J, Gerdes M, Beaumont E et al 1995 Health and neurodevelopmental outcome at 1-year adjusted age in 508 infants weighing 700 to 1100 grams who received prophylaxis with one versus three doses of synthetic surfactant. Journal of Pediatrics 126(5 part 2): S26–S32

Gersony W M, Peckham G J, Ellison R C, Miettinen O S, Nadas S 1983 Effects of indomethacin in premature infants with patent ductus arteriosus: results of a national collaborative study. Journal of Pediatrics 102(6): 895–906

Golding J, Paterson M, Kinlen L J 1990 Factors associated with childhood cancer in a national cohort study. British Journal of Cancer 62: 304–8

Goldsmith J P, Karotkin E H 1981 Introduction to assisted ventilation. In Goldsmith J P, Karotkin E H (eds) Assisted ventilation of the newborn. WB Saunders, London

Gregory G A, Gooding C A, Phibbs R H, Tooley W H 1974 Meconium aspiration in infants – a prospective study. Journal of Paediatrics 85(6): 848–52

Gultom E, Doyle L W, Davis P, Dharmalingam A, Bowman E 1997 Changes over time in attitudes to treatment and survival rates for extremely preterm infants (23–27 weeks' gestational age). Australian and New Zealand Journal of Obstetrics and Gynaecology 37(1): 56–8

Guthrie R 1996 The introduction of newborn screening for phenylketonuria: a personal history. European Journal of Pediatrics 155 (suppl. 1): S4–S5

Halliday H L 1992 Other acute lung disorders. In Sinclair J C, Bracken M B (ed.) Effective care of the newborn. Oxford University Press, Oxford

Halliday H L 1997 Endotracheal intubation at birth in vigorous term meconium-stained babies. In Sinclair J C, Bracken M B, Soll R F, Horbar J D (ed.) The neonatal module of the Cochrane Database of Systematic Reviews [updated 1 September 1997] Cochrane Collaboration; Issue 4. Update Software, Oxford

Harlow B L, Frigoletto F D, Cramer D W et al 1996 Determinants of preterm delivery in low-risk pregnancies. The RADIUS study group. Journal of Clinical Epidemiology 49(4): 441–8

Haworth S G 1990 Pulmonary vascular development. In Long W A (ed.) Fetal and neonatal cardiology. WB Saunders, Philadelphia

Hazinski M F 1992 Children are different. In Hazinski M F (ed.) Nursing care of the critically ill child, 2nd edn. Mosby Year Book, St Louis

Hey E 1971 The care of babies in incubators. In Gairdner D, Hull D (ed.) Recent advances in pediatrics, 4th ed. J & A Churchill, London

Hey E 1974 Keeping babies warm. Nursing Mirror 139: 62–4

Hey E 1975 Thermal neutrality. British Medical Bulletin 31(1): 69–74

Ho S Y, Angelini A, Moscoso G 1990 Developmental cardiac anatomy. In Long W A (ed.) Fetal and neonatal cardiology. WB Saunders, Philadelphia

Ives N K 1997 Neonatal jaundice. Current Paediatrics 7: 67–72

Jacob J, Pfenninger J 1997 Cesarean deliveries: when is a pediatrician necessary? Obstetrics and Gynecology 89(2): 217–20

Jenner E 1996a Tuberculosis: BCG immunisation. In Salisbury D M, Begg N T (eds) Immunisation against infectious diseases. HMSO, London

Jenner E 1996b Hepatitis B. In Salisbury D M, Begg N T (eds) Immunisation against infectious diseases. HMSO, London

Karlsson H 1996 Skin to skin care: heat balance. Archives of Diseases in Childhood Fetal Neonatal Edition 75: F130–F132

Kennell J H, Jerauld R, Wolfe H et al 1974 Maternal behavior one year after early and extended postpartum contact. Developmental Medicine and Child Neurology 16: 172–9

Kerr J F, Wyllie A H, Currie A R 1972 Apoptosis: a basic biological phenomenon with wide-ranging implications in human tissue kinetics. British Journal of Cancer 26(4): 239–57 (review)

Klaus M H, Kennell J H 1983 Parent to infant bonding: setting the record straight. Journal of Pediatrics 102(4): 575–6

Klaus M H, Jerauld R, Kreger N C, McAlpine W, Steffa M, Kennell J H 1972 Maternal attachment: importance of the first postpartum days. New England Journal of Medicine 286(9): 460–3

Klebanoff M A, Read J S, Mills J L, Shiono P H 1993 The risk of childhood cancer after neonatal exposure to vitamin K. New English Journal of Medicine 329(13): 905–8

Kramer L I 1969 Advancement of dermal icterus in the jaundiced newborn. American Journal of Diseases of Childhood 118: 454–8

Lamb M E 1982 The bonding phenomenon: misinterpretations and their implications. Journal of Pediatrics 101(4): 555–7

Lamb M E 1983 More on infant–maternal bonding. Journal of Pediatrics 103(5): 829–30

Lamb M E, Campos J J, Hwang C P, Leiderman P H, Sagi A, Sveijda M 1983 Joint Reply to 'Maternal–infant bonding: a joint rebuttal'. Pediatrics 72: 574–5

Levene M I, Kornberg J, Williams T H C 1985 The incidence and severity of post-asphyxial encephalopathy in full term infants. Early Human Development 11: 21–26

Levene M I, Sands C, Grindulis H, Moore J R 1986

Comparison of two methods of predicting outcome in perinatal asphyxia. Lancet i: 67–71

Linder N, Regev A, Gazit G 1994 Noninvasive determination of neonatal hyperbilirubinaemia: standardization for variation in skin colour. American Journal of Perinatology 11(3): 223–5

Little R E, Anderson K W, Ervin C H, Worthington-Roberts B, Clarren S K 1989 Maternal alcohol use during breast-feeding and infant mental and motor development at one year. New England Journal of Medicine 321(7): 425–35

Lynch M A, Roberts J, Ounsted C 1979 Myotonic dystrophy and bonding failure. Archives of Diseases in Childhood 54: 807–8 (letter)

Maisels M J 1995 Clinical rounds in the well-baby nursery: treating jaundiced newborns. Pediatric Annals 25(10): 547–52

Malone J I 1975 Vitamin passage across the placenta. Clinics in Perinatology 2(2): 295–307 (review)

Martinez J C, Maisels M J, Otheguy L et al 1993 Hyperbilirubinaemia in the breast-fed newborn: a controlled trial of four interventions. Pediatrics 91: 470–3

Massawe A, Kilewo C, Irani S 1996 Assessment of mouth-to-mask ventilation in resuscitation of asphyxic newborn babies. A pilot study. Tropical Medicine and International Health 1(6): 865–73

Mayfield S R, Bhatia J, Nakamura K T, Rios G R, Bell E F 1984 Temperature measurement in term and preterm neonates. Journal of Pediatrics 104(2): 271–5

Merritt K A, Coulter D M 1994 Application of the Gosset icterometer to screen for clinically significant hyperbilirubinaemia in premature infants. Journal of Perinatology 14(1): 58–65

Meyer T C, Angus J 1956 The effect of large doses of 'Synkavit' in the newborn. Archives of Diseases in Childhood 31: 212–15

Milner A D 1991 Resuscitation of the newborn. Archives of Diseases in Childhood 66: 66–9

Minde K, Trehub S, Corter C, Boukydis C, Celhoffer L, Marton P 1978 Mother–child relationships in the premature nursery: an observational study. Pediatrics 61: 373–9

Morrison J J, Rennie J M 1997 Clinical, scientific and ethical aspects of fetal and neonatal care at extremely preterm periods of gestation. British Journal of Obstetrics and Gynaecology 104: 1341–50

Newman T B, Klebanoff M A 1994 Neonatal hyperbilirubinaemia and long-term outcome: another look at the Collaborative Perinatal Project. Pediatrics 92: 651–7

O'Conner S, Vietze P M, Sherrod K B, Sandler H M, Altmeier W A III 1980 Reduced incidence of parenting inadequacy following rooming-in. Pediatrics 66: 176–82

Osiris Collaborative Group 1992 Early versus delayed neonatal administration of a synthetic surfactant – the judgement of OSIRIS. Lancet 340: 1363–9

Oski F A 1994 Infant nutrition, physical growth, breastfeeding, and general nutrition. Current Opinion in Pediatrics 6(3): 361–4 (review)

Palme-Kilander C 1992 Methods of resuscitation in low-Apgar-score newborn infants – a national survey. Acta Paediatrica 81: 739–44

Paludetto R, Mansi G, Rinaldi P, Ariola P, Cascioli C F 1986 Moderate hyperbilirubinaemia does not influence the behavior of jaundiced infants. Biology of the Neonate 50(1): 43–7

Parker L, Cole M, Craft A W, Hey E N 1998 Neonatal vitamin

K administration and childhood cancer in the north of England: retrospective case–control study. British Medical Journal 316(7126): 189–93

Philip A G 1994 The changing face of neonatal infection. Experience at a regional medical center. Paeiatric Infections Disease Journal 13(12): 1098–102

Powell L F 1974 The effect of extra stimulation and maternal involvement on the development of low-birth-weight infants and on maternal behavior. Child Development 45: 106–113

Pschyrembel W 1998 Kongenitale Fehlbildungen. In Pschyrembel W (ed.) Pschyrembel Klinisches Wörterbuch. Walter de Gruyter, Berlin

Quinton D N, O'Byrne G, Aitkenhead A R 1987 Comparison of endotracheal and peripheral intravenous adrenaline in cardiac arrest. Lancet (Apr 11): 828–9

Ramji S, Ahuja S, Thirupuram S, Rootwelt T, Rooth G, Saugstad O D 1993 Resuscitation of asphyxic newborn infants with room air or 100% oxygen. Pediatric Research 34(6): 809–12

Robertson B 1996 New targets for surfactant replacement therapy: experimental and clinical aspects. Archives of Diseases in Childhood Fetal Neonatal Edition 75(1): F1–F3

Royal College of Paediatrics and Child Health/Royal College of Obstetricians and Gynaecologists 1997 In BMJ Publishing Group, Resuscitation of babies at birth. BMJ Publishing Group, London

Ruff A J 1994 Breastmilk, breastfeeding and transmission of the virus to the neonate. Seminars in Perinatology 18(6): 510–16

Rutter N 1992 Temperature control and its disorders. In Roberton N R C (ed.) Textbook of neonatology. Churchill Livingstone, London

Salomonsen L 1940 On the prevention of haemorrhagic disease of the newborn by the administration of cow's milk during the first two days of life. Acta Paediatrica Scandinavica 28: 1–7

Saugstad O D 1996 Review article: Oxygen toxicity in the neonatal period. Acta Paediatrica Scandinavia 79: 881–92

Saunders R A, Milner A D 1978 Pulmonary pressure/volume relationships during the last phase of delivery and the first postnatal breaths in the human subjects. Journal of Paediatrics 93(4): 667

Scopes J W, Ahmed I 1966 Range of critical temperatures in sick and premature newborn babies. Archives of Diseases in Childhood 41: 417–19

Siegel E, Bauman K E, Schaefer E S, Saunders M M, Ingram D D 1980 Hospital and home support during infancy: impact on maternal attachment, child abuse and neglect, and health care utilization. Pediatrics 66: 183–90

Sirimanne E S, Blumberg R M, Bossano D 1996 The effect of prolonged modification of cerebral temperature on outcome after hypoxic–ischemic brain injury in the infant rat. Pediatric Research 39(4): 591–7

Soll R F, McQueen M C 1992 Respiratory distress syndrome. In Sinclair J C, Bracken M B (ed.) Effective care of the newborn. Oxford University Press, Oxford

Speer C P, Robertson B, Curstedt T 1992 Randomized European multicenter trial of surfactant replacement therapy for severe neonatal respiratory distress syndrome: single versus multiple doses of Curosurf. Pediatrics 89: 13–20

Suckling R J, Laing I A, Kirk J M 1995 Transcutaneous bilirubinometry as screening tool for neonatal jaundice. Scottish Medical Journal 40(1): 14–15

Tanner J M, Whitehouse R H 1976 Clinical longitudinal standards for height, weight, height velocity, weight velocity and stages of puberty. Archives of Diseases in Childhood 51: 170–9

Tarlow M 1991 25 years of paediatrics. British Journal of Hospital Medicine 46(4): 255–6

Thaler M M, Stobie G H 1963 An improved technique of external cardiac compression in infants and young children. New England Journal of Medicine 269(12): 606–10

Thoma J, Gerull G, Mrowinski D 1986 A long-term study of hearing in children following neonatal hyperbilirubin-aemia. Archives of Oto-Rhino-Laryngology 243(2): 133–7

Todres I D, Rodgers M C 1975 Methods of external cardiac massage in the newborn infant. Journal of Pediatrics 86(5): 781–2

Tripp J H, McNinch A W 1987 Haemorrhagic disease and vitamin K. Archives of Diseases in Childhood 62: 436–7

Venter P A, Christianson A L, Hutamo C M, Makhura M P, Gericke G S 1995 Congenital anomalies in rural black South African neonates – a silent epidemic? South African Medical Journal 85(1): 15–20

von Kries R 1998 Neonatal vitamin K prophylaxis: the Gordian knot still awaits untying. British Medical Journal 316(7126): 161–2

Vyas H, Milner A D, Hopkin I E 1981 Intrathoracic pressure and volume changes during the spontaneous onset of respiration in babies born by cesarean section and by vaginal delivery. Journal of Pediatrics 99(5): 787–91

Vyas H, Field D, Milner A D, Hopkin I E 1986 Determinants of the first inspiratory volume and functional residual capacity at birth. Pediatric Pulmonology 2: 189–93

Walker C M H 1989 Neonatology – then and now: assisted ventilation in the newborn 1964 Archives of Diseases in Childhood 64: 629

Wardrop C A J, Holland B M 1995 The roles and vital importance of placental blood to the newborn infant. Journal of Perinatal Medicine 23: 139–43

Weekly Epidemiology Record 1992 Global programme on AIDS. Consensus statement from the WHO-UNICEF consultation on HIV transmission and breast feeding. Weekly Epidemiology Record 67(24): 177–9 review

Wise J 1997 News: High amounts of chemicals found in breast milk. British Medical Journal 314(7093): 1505

Wiswell T E, Tuggle J M, Turner B S 1990 Meconium aspiration syndrome: have we made a difference? Pediatrics 85: 715–21

Yamauchi Y, Yamanouchi I 1991a Transcutaneous bilirubinometry: effect of postnatal age. Acta Pediatrica Japonica 33(5): 663–7

Yamauchi Y, Yamanouchi I 1991b Factors affecting transcutaneous bilirubin measurement: effect of daylight. Acta Paediatrica Japonica 33(5): 658–62

Young D G 1965 'Spontaneous' rupture of the rectum. Proceedings of the Royal Society of Medicine 58: 615–16

17

Caring for the baby

Patricia Percival

In this chapter, mini sessions are presented on breast-feeding, infant crying, infant sleeping, infant activity states and sudden infant death syndrome (SIDS). These topics have been included because they are the areas that are of most concern to many parents during the first few months after the birth. The overall purpose of these sessions is to provide midwives with information that will be useful to new parents during the first 2 months following the birth of their infant, a time that is especially stressful for women (Mercer 1986a, 1986b, Barclay et al 1997).

Knowing the normal

Mothers and fathers knowing what is normal

This chapter is important in that it provides information about what babies' normal behaviour is during the first 6 months of life.

In my own clinical work helping parents with breast-feeding, crying and sleep, I have found that parents often feel inadequate or guilty because their babies do not behave as they think they 'should do'. This 'should do' is usually based on inaccurate information of infant behaviour and an unrealistic expectation of babies' capabilities. I therefore feel that one of the most important things midwives can do for new parents is to give them facts about normal infant behaviour.

Parents will be better equipped to accept their infant's behaviour if they know that it is normal for new babies to feed 2-hourly (rather than 4-hourly), that it is normal for babies to cry for more than 2 hours a day (rather than 15 minutes) and that it is normal for babies to sleep only 15 (and not 22 h) hours a day. Parents are more likely to be able to accept their baby as he or she is and resign themselves to a few hectic months. They are also less likely to blame themselves if their baby feeds frequently, cries frequently and wakes frequently.

In addition, if parents do have a baby that falls outside the norm for feeding, crying or sleeping, it is critical that midwives tell them that *it is not their fault*. Removing the guilt from parents enables them to look more objectively at their infant's behaviour and see it for what it is: a reflection of their infant's own individual temperament and not of poor parenting skills.

Midwives knowing what is normal

Although this chapter is relevant both for midwives and health visitors (community/child health nurses or public health nurses), midwives are the health professionals who have most to do with women before the birth and for the first month after the birth. Indeed, Forsyth & Fowlie (1995) have argued that parents are a captive audience during the postnatal period. What midwives tell mothers about 'what is normal' with respect to breast-feeding, excessive crying or infant sleep is, therefore, important. Midwives also need to initiate early referral to the health visitor if there are problems.

However, with respect to infant feeding, sleeping and crying patterns, some researchers have found that there are marked differences in what individual health professionals view as normal. The midwife or health visitor, instead of basing her advice on normative data, may base it on her own perception of normal behaviour. This has enormous implications for the women in her care; when babies fail to conform to these patterns, professionals may well perceive what is normal actually to be a problem (Coles 1983, Carter & Mason 1989).

The power of information

Obtaining accurate information about infant behaviour is one way in which parents can gain control of an uncertain situation (McKim et al 1995), and feeling in control is related to parental feelings of emotional well-being (Green et al 1990). Such information also enables parents to make decisions about their new baby (Kennedy 1995) and may facilitate maternal role attainment (Koniak-Griffin 1993).

Moreover, Houston et al (1983) found in their research that advice from health professionals actually altered the outcome of breast-feeding. One woman who was feeding every 2 hours was advised that this was normal and was encouraged to continue. A second mother feeding every 3 hours was advised to give complementary feeds. This mother stopped breast-feeding at 5 weeks.

Not being offered informational support can also be seen as stressful and negative (Percival 1990, McKim et al 1995) and may make some women feel powerless (Stamp & Crowther 1994). In my own (1990) research, some mothers commented that midwives were reluctant to volunteer information or help unless asked. These women felt that staff needed to anticipate the needs of new mothers in their care:

> Generally staff were helpful but if you did not ask then you did not find anything out.
>
> I always had to ask if I wanted any information about the baby, yet I have never had a baby before so I didn't know what to ask.

Becoming a parent

As we discussed in Chapter 10, the transition to parenthood has been described as a major life transition or crisis. Childbirth and the early weeks of parenting require major changes as parents alter their lifestyle to accommodate a new family member. For women, the postpartum period has been identified as a time of complex physiological and psychological changes, resulting in considerable stress as well as considerable pleasure. The early weeks after the birth are particularly stressful, a critical time during which women benefit from help as they recuperate physically and learn to respond to their infants' cues (Mercer 1986a, 1986b, Barclay et al 1997).

Learning how to be a parent

As early as 1968, Rossi argued that most American mothers approached maternity with limited previous childcare experience. In 1970, Toffler referred to parenthood as 'the greatest single preserve of the amateur', and in 1975, Rubin argued that the American view of motherhood was 'once the baby is born everyone lives happily ever after'.

Since that time, there has been a significant increase in the number of formal antenatal education courses. However, despite this increase in education, Toffler's assertion of parenthood as 'the greatest single preserve of the amateur' remains true. In countries such as the UK, USA, Canada and Australia, many 1990s parents lack the practical knowledge and skills needed to care for their baby. In addition (as we discussed in Chapter 10), parents may not only lack competence and confidence, but also have little knowledge of the personal adjustments related to role change. Many parents simply do not recognize how childbirth will affect their lives (Ladden & Damato 1992, Astbury et al 1994, Ruchala & Halstead 1994, Sethi 1995, Barclay et al 1997). To quote Barnett (1991): 'In our culture, parenting expertise is supposed to arrive with the baby, especially if you are the mother.'

Moreover, parenthood arrives abruptly. Unlike most work roles, the birth of a child is not followed by a gradual period of learning or taking on of responsibility (Rossi 1968). With increasingly shorter hospital stays, parents must often assume full responsibility for the care of their child while the mother is still recovering physically and emotionally from the birth. It is often not until the baby is born that parents realize how much they need information and practical assistance. For example, a survey by the Health Department of Western Australia (1991) found that, after the birth, 79% of new mothers wanted classes to help them to deal with the reality of caring for their infant and coping with role change.

Before the birth, most parents, then, will have had few opportunities to develop the practical skills required to handle a new baby. In addition, antenatal education courses may also place a greater emphasis on the labour and birth than on the preparation for parenthood. In expressing their concern about this lack of emphasis on parenting, the NSW Women's Consultative Committee (1994, p. 27) stated: 'There should be much more emphasis in antenatal classes on what to do after the baby is born. Let's face it – labour lasts a day, babies go on and on.'

Furthermore, the postnatal period has been described as the 'Cinderella' of the Maternity Services (Ball 1984). A great deal of attention has been paid to 'demedicalizing' the labour and birth process. However, less thought has been given to the postnatal period. Researchers and clinicians have placed less emphasis on this early time than on other phases of the childbearing cycle (Ball 1984, Field 1985, Rider 1985, Samual & Balch 1985, Taylor 1986, Moss et al 1987).

The importance of midwives helping the mother to have a good birth cannot be overemphasized, and I am certainly not suggesting that resources be reduced. It is, however, also vital to emphasize the time 'after the birth is over'. After all, it is during the postnatal period that new parents must learn to care for and largely establish the pattern of their relationship with their baby. It is also the time when the mother is most helped or hindered in her adjustment to her new role and responsibilities (Ball 1987).

The mini sessions

In this chapter, mini sessions are presented on breast-feeding, infant crying, infant sleeping, infant activity states and SIDS. As well as practical information and help on infant care, the sessions can also be used to offer emotional support and feedback to new parents as they adjust to their new role. The sessions also provide an ideal opportunity for midwives to dispel some of the myths surrounding parenthood. In a group setting, they will also encourage mothers to get together and learn from each other's experiences.

As with the teaching sessions in Chapter 10, most of the mini sessions in this chapter can be taught before or after the birth and to individual women or groups. The 'when and how' of using the mini sessions is limited only by the midwife's initiative. For example, they can be used:

- as antenatal classes or group sessions in a hospital or community setting;
- as sessions with women individually after the birth;
- as antenatal group sessions followed by individual postnatal reinforcement;
- as postnatal group sessions (possibly in mothers' homes or a community setting in the early weeks, or in hospital in countries that have longer stays).

The mini sessions are not meant to be rigidly prescriptive. Instead, the package is intended to provide background information, research and strategies that can be used by the midwife or health visitor. The sessions are intended to be brief, so in most cases each topic has been broken up into 'bite-sized snacks' rather than being given as 'full meals'. The number of snacks or courses consumed at any one time is entirely up to the midwife.

Given budgetary constraints, health professionals, including midwives, are being required to provide increasing care with decreasing resources. Informal and formal group teaching by midwives and community nurses is a cost-effective way of increasing family support. Many of the mini sessions could be taught during the antenatal period and then reinforced as needed after the birth. The advantages of group teaching are discussed in more detail in Chapter 10.

BREAST-FEEDING

With respect to infant feeding, this chapter will attempt to answer the following questions about breast-feeding:

- Why is it important that midwives teach families?
- When could midwives teach families?
- How can midwives teach families?
- What could midwives teach families?

WHY IS IT IMPORTANT THAT MIDWIVES TEACH FAMILIES?

Introduction and rationale

It is important for midwives to teach families about breast-feeding for several reasons, some of which I will discuss in this first section. In many developed countries, breast-feeding rates remain lower than those recommended by the World Health Organization (WHO) and the United Nations Children's Fund (UNICEF), and women have increasingly fewer opportunities to learn by observing other women breast-feed. Most midwives would agree that parents have an unequivocal right to be informed of the many benefits of breast-feeding so that they can make an informed choice. Finally, some of the things that influence the duration of breast-feeding are things that you (as a midwife) can do something about. In fact, you are the ideal person to provide breast-feeding information and practical support.

Support for breast-feeding

The WHO believes that 97% of women are physiologically capable of breast-feeding their babies successfully. The WHO and UNICEF (1989) recommend complete breast-feeding until 4 months of age, while the National Health and Medical Research Council (NHMRC) of Australia (1987) suggest that all infants should be exclusively breast-fed for the first 4–6 months of life.

Falling breast-feeding rates

In recent years in the UK, however, the proportion of women who actually start breast-feeding their baby declined from 70% in 1977 to 66% in 1988 and 62% in 1992 (Martin & White 1988, Office of Population Censuses and Surveys 1992). Similarly, in the USA, there is a decrease in the rate of initiation of breast-feeding (Rassin et al 1994). In Australia, however, the number of women who start breast-feeding is stable at 90% (Scott & Binns 1995). Despite these higher commencement rates in Australia, overall only 50% of mothers in developed countries continue to breast-feed to 6 weeks after the birth (McNatt & Freston 1992, Redman et al 1995).

Decreased learning opportunities

Breast-feeding is natural but not instinctive; instead, it is a skill that must be learnt. For many women, establishing breast-feeding requires access to a great deal of information and practical help before and after the birth. In some cultures, breast-feeding skills and information are acquired through the almost daily observation of babies at the breast and from the support of other mothers after the birth (Inch 1990). However, in Western societies, women have limited opportunities to learn and acquire skills through the observation of babies being breastfed. Therefore, women often rely on learning these skills from health professionals. This is where you, the midwife, come in. You are the ideal person to provide breast-feeding information and practical support.

The right of informed choice

Parents have the right to make an informed decision about whether or not to breast-feed their baby. In the next section, I have outlined the basic information that parents need in order to make such a decision. I believe that midwives have both a moral and a legal obligation to inform parents of the many benefits of breast-feeding, both verbally and in writing.

Parents also have a right to be given the help that they need to establish and maintain breast-feeding. I am sure that most midwives feel it unacceptable to tell parents how wonderful breast-feeding is and then not find ways of providing information and practical assistance. The following prepared mini sessions will be a valuable aid to busy midwives where time is limited, particularly if both group and individual teaching methods are used.

It is also very, very important not to criticize or judge parents if they make the informed decision to use artificial methods to feed their baby. It is quite likely that they may already feel ill at ease if they chose not to breast-feed once they are aware of the many benefits. The critical thing is that they make an *informed* decision based on up-to-date information and research.

The benefits of breast-feeding

Breast-feeding is important for a number of reasons. The recommendations of the WHO, UNICEF, NHMRC and other organizations reflect the importance of breast-feeding and are based on the fact that numerous researchers have found this feeding method to provide many benefits for women and their babies.

Physical benefits for the baby

These benefits include:

- positive effects on the infant's growth, development and health (Hartmann & Kent 1988). Research has shown that breast milk contains hormones, growth factors and enzymes that may influence the physiological growth and development of the infant (Hamosh et al 1985, Morriss 1985, Koldovsky et al 1987);

- a decreased risk of the infant developing allergies (Hanson et al 1988);
- immunological protection (Victora et al 1989, Cunningham & Jelliffe 1991);
- less gastrointestinal illness and a reduced incidence of hospital admission for this condition (Howie et al 1990);
- protection against upper respiratory tract infection (Cunningham 1979, Klein 1982) and otitis media (Saarinen 1982, Duncan et al 1993, Pukander et al 1993, Aniansson et al 1994, Sassen et al 1994);
- a reduced likelihood of obesity (Kramer et al 1985, Dewey et al 1993);
- possibly higher IQ scores in breast-fed than bottle-fed babies (Jacobson & Jacobson 1992, Lucas et al 1992).

Physical benefits for the mother

These benefits include:

- more rapid involution of the uterus. The suckling infant stimulates the pituitary gland to release oxytocin, which affects the oxytocin receptors in the uterus, increasing uterine contraction; this diminishes the placental site and minimizes blood loss and the potential for infection, as well as assisting the uterus to return to its pre-pregnant size (Royal College of Midwives 1989);
- a reduced risk of premenopausal breast cancer (Layde et al 1989, Newcomb et al 1994, United Kingdom National Case-Control Study Group 1993) and ovarian cancer (Hartge et al 1989);
- a decreased risk of hip fracture in later life (Cummings & Klineberg 1993);
- a lower risk of osteoporosis (Aloia et al 1985);
- the prevention of pregnancy by suppression of the woman's fertility (Howie 1985, Family Health International 1988, Thapa et al 1988, Lewis et al 1991);
- significantly more rapid postpartum weight loss and lower-body fat loss when used with a low-fat diet and exercise (Hammer et al 1996).

The importance of breast-feeding

As well as having numerous physical benefits, breast-feeding is important because of the psychological or emotional benefits it confers. Indeed, for some women, infant feeding may well be one of the critical elements in their transition to the maternal role, as the following pieces of evidence show.

Successful breast-feeding may equate with successful mothering ability: success at breast-feeding enables some women to perceive themselves as good mothers (Rubin 1967a, 1967b, Mercer 1986a, Virden 1988, Lawson & Tulloch 1995, Cooke 1996).

Breastfeeding is closely allied to mothering and demonstrates a woman's ability to nurture her baby (Rubin 1968, Laufer 1990). Some women feel satisfaction in observing the growth of the infant because this growth is through the gift of breast milk (Bottorff 1990). Furthermore, breast milk is a special gift that only a mother can give (Hauck & Reinbold 1996).

Successful breastfeeding may be the beginning of a woman's adaptation to the maternal role (Laufer 1990). Virden (1988) concluded that there was a relationship between breast feeding at 1 month postpartum and increased adjustment to the maternal role.

Some women view breast-feeding as an innate part of motherhood (Beck 1989) and as an important element in attainment of the maternal role (Leff et al 1994). The ability to give of themselves through their breast milk is, for some women, an important factor in maternal adaptation (Hauck & Reinbold 1996).

Maternal confidence may be increased by the intimacy and physical contact of breast feeding as it provides increased opportunities for enhancing maternal role attainment (Virden 1988).

Breast-feeding emphasizes the closeness and communication between the mother and infant, and has the potential to increase bonding and enhance the mother–infant relationship (Rubin 1967a, Virden 1988, Beck 1989, Renfrew et al 1990, Driscoll 1992, Locklin & Naber 1993, Leff et al 1994). Driscoll (1992) described breast-feeding as a dynamic two-way communication and connection between the mother–infant dyad, while Virden (1988) found that breast-feeding mothers had greater mother–infant mutuality than bottle-feeding mothers.

Virden (1988) reported how breast-feeding mothers perceived feeding time as satisfying, while mothers who bottle-fed viewed feeding as a mundane task.

The satisfaction with and enjoyment of motherhood is enhanced by successful breast-feeding (Hauck & Reinbold 1996).

Some women gain a sense of achievement and accomplishment from successful breast-feeding (Lawson & Tulloch 1995).

Breast-feeding may be emotionally satisfying (Ellis 1983, Virden 1988) and profoundly gratifying (Leff et al 1994). Hauck & Reinbold (1996) found that the signs that their infant was thriving intensified the mother's satisfaction.

Successful breast-feeding may also empower women (Locklin & Naber 1993).

A failure of breast-feeding may be seen as personal failure, decreasing self-confidence (Laufer 1990) and self-esteem (Lawson & Tulloch 1995), as well as negatively affecting maternal identity (Cooke 1996).

Decreased maternal confidence in coping with the infant may also result from breast-feeding failure (Fahy & Holschier 1988).

The emphasis placed on infant feeding in my own research (Percival 1990, 1998, Percival & Duffy 1998) supports the previous conclusions on the importance of infant feeding. In the 1990 research, infant feeding was also the aspect of care that drew the most negative comments, a large number of these concerning conflicting advice. The importance to some women of being able to breast-feed successfully is reflected in the following comment: 'I cried for several days when I realised that I couldn't breastfeed. The emphasis is so strongly in favour of breastfeeding that it makes it very hard if you can't breastfeed your baby.'

Several mothers who had succeeded with breast-feeding their infants mentioned how good this made them feel, as if they had really achieved something: 'To begin with I didn't care whether I breast-fed or gave him the bottle, but now that we've been successful at breastfeeding, I feel really pleased with myself.'

Those women who received encouragement and help that enabled them to continue breast-feeding were extremely grateful for the attention given to them by health professionals:

The midwives always advised me to persevere with breastfeeding. They were very positive and encouraging and understanding of the problems associated with feeding.

The clinic sister continually encouraged me to persevere with breastfeeding until all of the problems settled down. I am so grateful she did.

Moreover, infant feeding remains one of the most frequently identified concerns of new mothers during the first few weeks after the birth (Percival 1990, 1998, Lawson & Tulloch 1995, Cooke 1996). Given the many benefits of breast-feeding, its low rates are of concern for all health professionals. The challenge for each midwife is in encouraging and helping women to successfully start and continue breast-feeding. There is also a need to help women who give up breast-feeding in the early weeks after the birth who may have wanted to continue. The infants of these mothers are deprived of the many benefits associated with breast-

feeding, while the mother herself may be deprived of a positive breast-feeding experience.

Factors influencing the duration of breast-feeding

Researchers have found that breast-feeding success is related to a number of factors. These include:

- higher socio-economic status, which is usually associated with women continuing to breast-feed for longer (Bailey & Sheriff 1992, Peterson & Da Vanzo 1992, Maxwell & Burnmaster 1993, Quarles et al 1994, Hartmann 1995);
- the partner's positive attitude towards breast-feeding, which is important in the mother starting and continuing to breast-feed (Freed & Fraley 1993; Libbus & Kolostov 1994; Littman et al 1994; Anderson 1996);
- professional support and education for the breast-feeding mother, and support within the mother's social network (Raphael 1981, Bottorff 1990, Becker 1992, Freed et al 1992, Rajan 1993, Isabella & Isabella 1994);
- early feeding following the birth of the baby (Widstrom et al 1987, Righard & Alade 1990, Harris 1994);
- good positioning and attachment of the baby on the breast (Fisher 1983, 1994, 1995, Weber et al 1986, Woolridge 1986a, Glover 1997);
- unrestricted frequency and duration of breast-feeds (Thomsen et al 1979, De Chateau 1980, L'Esperance 1980, Houston et al 1983, Johnson 1986, Woolridge 1990).

Other factors related to shorter breast-feeding duration include:

- analgesia and anaesthesia
- inconsistent advice
- complementary feeds from a bottle
- the early introduction of solid foods
- some contraceptive pills.

(Minchin 1989a, Walker 1989, Houston & Field 1991, Bono 1992, Frank 1994, Newman 1994, Redman et al 1995, Pugh et al 1996).

Some of the factors that influence breast-feeding success and duration, for example socio-economic status, are beyond the control of midwives. However, there are other areas in which the midwife has an important role, for example in providing consistent information and practical help, and in preventing nipple pain and trauma by teaching the mother how to position and attach her baby optimally.

Why women say they stop breast-feeding

While many factors contribute to women discontinuing breast-feeding, the most common reasons given by women are nipple pain and trauma, and 'insufficient milk' (Percival 1990, 1998, Bailey & Sherriff 1992, Cox & Turnbull 1994, Lowe, 1994, Fetherston 1995, Fisher 1995, Lawson & Tulloch 1995, Redman et al 1995). Researchers have found that there is a relationship between nipple pain and trauma and inadequate milk supply (Woolridge 1986a, Fisher 1995).

Conflicting advice

Inch (1990) argued that midwives have a responsibility to refrain from deliberate acts that interfere with the establishment of breast-feeding. However, conflicting advice from hospital staff is mentioned by women in most research on postnatal care, for example Ball (1982, 1984, 1987), Field (1987), Murphy-Black (1987, 1990), Percival (1990, 1998), Percival & Duffy (1998) and Stamp & Crowther (1994). This conflicting advice is most often related to breast-feeding. The findings of several studies have demonstrated that conflicting advice from hospital midwives has a negative effect on women. In my (1990) research, 72% of participants felt confused by conflicting advice on infant feeding.

Moreover, in Ball's (1987) study, conflicting advice was a complaint expressed by 37% of all mothers. However, 49% of the distressed mothers mentioned it, in contrast to only 25% of the satisfied mothers. According to Ball (1987), mothers in the satisfied group appeared to have sufficient confidence in themselves to dismiss or ignore conflicting advice and were only irritated by it. Conversely, the mothers in the distressed group who complained about conflicting advice tended to blame themselves for not understanding, and mentioned being 'told off' by one midwife for doing what another had advised. Conflicting advice from midwives was linked with low self-esteem, while being 'told off' created feelings of inadequacy for new mothers.

For this reason, I am perhaps overemphasizing the importance of the midwife giving consistent advice to women. Obviously, different things have to be tried at times. I have found that the important thing is not to present alternatives as being 'right' or 'wrong', but as a list of different things that may be needed because each baby is different. Written protocols based on research findings are essential, and these should, as far as possible, be followed.

Learning to breast-feed

As early as 1984, Flint argued that the midwife's role in breast-feeding is to support and educate the new mother. Flint also felt that the establishment of breast-feeding depended on the mother's confidence in herself before and after the birth. Hauck & Dimmock (1994) found that breast-feeding knowledge increased the new mother's confidence and helped her to reach her intended goal for breast-feeding duration.

Certainly, in Australia, most first-time mothers attend antenatal education classes (Health Department of Western Australia 1995). During these antenatal education classes, general breast-feeding information is usually taught, a breast-feeding video may be used, and the benefits of breast-feeding are presented. However, they do not usually include more specific aspects such as a practical 'hands-on' demonstration of positioning and attachment of the baby to the breast. Women have also commented that antenatal classes do not provide them with the initial skills needed to care for their infants (McIntosh 1993, O'Meara 1993).

At the present time, many antenatal classes may simply not be specific enough to meet the new mothers' learning needs. Groups may be large and lack opportunities for women to be given practical demonstrations of, for example, the positioning and attachment of the baby on the breast.

WHEN COULD MIDWIVES TEACH FAMILIES ABOUT BREAST-FEEDING?

Breast-feeding support and education are usually given during both the antenatal and postnatal periods, most of the education on the positioning and attachment of the baby at the breast being given in the first few days after the birth (Minchin 1985, Woolridge 1986a, 1986b). However, new mothers may not be receptive to education, in particular new information, at this time (Rubin 1967a, 1967b, Gay et al 1988, Martell et al 1989, Smith 1989).

Rubin (1967a) describes these first days as the 'taking-in stage', when women themselves need mothering and are mostly concerned with their own needs. New mothers may also experience fatigue, sensory overload, a reduced attention span and difficulty concentrating on new breast-feeding information after the birth (Martell et al 1989). The 'taking-hold' phase described by Rubin (1967a) is usually present by the third postpartum day. During this 'taking-hold stage', the mother is usually more able to show interest in the infant's care and feel capable of independent action.

It could well be that the best time initially to educate

new mothers on the practical skills of breast-feeding (such as the positioning and attachment of the baby on the breast) is during the antenatal period. This breast-feeding information can then be reviewed and re-inforced by the midwife after the birth. Such practical antenatal breast-feeding education gives mothers sufficient practical skills to begin breast-feeding after the birth without being overloaded with new informa-tion. It may also give mothers the knowledge and confidence to deal with conflicting advice and may reduce the effects of staff shortages.

HOW COULD MIDWIVES TEACH FAMILIES ABOUT BREAST-FEEDING?

The key issues in the following mini sessions can be taught before or after the birth and to individual women or groups. When planning how to teach women, it may also be helpful to look at some of the different interventions that have been employed to increase breast-feeding duration. These interventions have had varying success rates; they include informa-tion sessions, lactation counselling, hospital and home visits, telephone follow-up and breast-feeding infor-mation leaflets.

A recent Australian pilot study of 70 first-time mothers investigated the effects of an antenatal group teaching session on nipple pain and trauma, and breast-feeding duration. In addition to their usual pre-natal education, the experimental group had a practical education session conducted by a lactation consultant in the month before the birth. In small groups of six women, a doll was used to demonstrate the positioning and attachment of the baby to the breast. The control group continued with the usual prenatal education. Six weeks after the birth, 92% of the experimental group and 29% of the control group were breast-feed-ing (Duffy et al 1997). Minchin (1989b) also found that using a doll to teach the positioning and attachment of the baby at the breast was very effective.

In England, Jenner (1988) measured the impact of an information package, pre- and postnatal home visits, and in-hospital visits on breast-feeding success among lower socio-economic group women. Sixty-eight per cent of the experimental group, compared with only 21% of the control group, were breast-feeding at 3 months.

However, other studies have found no difference in breast-feeding duration between women who received extra help and those who did not. In America, Hill (1987) provided women with extra breast-feeding education (a slide presentation, lecture and booklet) in the prenatal period. No difference was found in breast-feeding duration or in the mother's perceptions of success between the control and experimental groups. More recently, an American study of 150 mothers examined the effects of in-hospital breast-feeding edu-cation (Schy et al 1996). The experimental group had access to education from a lactation consultant within 24 hours of childbirth, while the control group received standard care. No significant difference in breast-feeding duration was found between the two groups.

In Australia, Hauck & Dimmock (1994) provided extra help in the form of a breast-feeding information booklet to 75 mothers in the postnatal period. Again, breast-feeding duration was not significantly different between the mothers in the experimental and the con-trol groups. Similarly, in another Australian study of 245 primiparas, Redman et al (1995) found no significant difference in breast-feeding duration between the con-trol and experimental groups. In their study, the experi-mental group had a teaching session at 24–28 weeks gestation, a postnatal hospital visit, and a home visit and follow-up telephone calls at 2–3 weeks and 6–8 weeks, while the control group received the usual prenatal and postnatal education.

WHAT COULD MIDWIVES TEACH FAMILIES ABOUT BREAST-FEEDING?

While the results of these different breast-feeding interventions are mixed, there are several key issues that are important in encouraging successful breast-feeding. Some of these are included in the following mini sessions. When teaching new mothers how to feed their baby, the midwife may chose to discuss some of these. They can be taught before or after the birth (or both) and to individual women or groups.

As I have previously emphasized, midwives are in an ideal position to teach families about breast-feeding both before and after the birth. The care they give to breast-feeding mothers is a critical part of a positive breast-feeding experience. This is even more impor-tant when the mother is experiencing difficulties (Bragg 1991, McNatt & Freston 1992).

Key issues in encouraging successful breast-feeding include the important factors of:

- parents making informed decisions about breast-feeding that are based on up-to-date information and research;
- an early first feed;
- the benefits of correct infant attachment to the breast during feeding;
- allowing the infant to determine the frequency and duration of feeds;

- support and continuous encouragement while the mother is breast-feeding;
- knowing about and being able to access community resources.

MINI SESSION: BENEFITS OF BREAST-FEEDING

Objective

- The prospective parents will be able to make informed decisions about breast-feeding that are based on up-to-date research.

Important teaching points

- These cover physical and psychological advantages of breast-feeding for the mother and baby.

Midwives' teaching notes

The earlier section on physical and psychological advantages of breast-feeding will be useful for midwives both before and after the birth.

MINI SESSION: AN EARLY FIRST BREAST-FEED

Objective

- The parents will understand the importance of an early first breast-feed in establishing good feeding practice.

Important teaching point

- It is important to feed the baby in the labour ward after the birth as the baby's instinct to suck is heightened during the first hour after the birth.

Midwives' teaching notes

A number of researchers have found that the initiation of breast-feeding within the first 2 hours of birth promotes successful breast-feeding (Houston et al 1983, Salariya et al 1987).

The baby's instinct to suck is heightened during the first hour after the birth (Widstrom et al 1987, Righard & Alade 1990, Harris 1994), and gratification of this first instinct to suck helps the development of optimal sucking patterns in the infant (Royal College of Midwives 1991). Researchers have reported the behaviour of babies born to mothers who had received no drugs in labour (Widstrom et al 1987, Righard & Alade

1990). Spontaneous sucking, a rooting reflex and rooting movements occurred between 5 and 15 minutes after the birth and spontaneous sucking after an average of 40–55 minutes. It is essential for midwives and mothers to be aware that analgesia and anaesthesia during labour may be associated with problems in establishing breast-feeding (Righard & Alade 1990, Rajan 1994) so that extra assistance and support can be provided.

MINI SESSION: GOOD INFANT POSITION AND ATTACHMENT

Objective

- The new mother will understand the benefits of good infant position and attachment during breast-feeding for both herself and her baby.

Important teaching points

- Discuss the significant differences in the sucking mechanisms of bottle- and breast-feeding infants.
- Emphasize the importance of ensuring the best possible position and attachment of the baby on the breast.
- Stress that good attachment will increase the milk supply and reduce breast-feeding problems such as sore nipples and engorged breasts, and that poor attachment will decrease the milk supply and increase breast-feeding problems such as sore nipples and engorged breasts.
- Refer women to pictures that show good attachment. The pamphlet 'The key to successful breast-feeding' (Glover 1997) is a valuable aid to this mini session as it is written for mothers and can be kept by them for future reference (see reference list for contact details).
- Discuss, and where appropriate demonstrate, and show pictures of comfortable feeding positions that favour good attachment.

Midwives' teaching notes

Sucking mechanisms

There are significant differences in the sucking mechanisms of bottle- and breast-feeding infants. When feeding from a bottle, the baby uses a sucking motion to extract milk with the tongue thrust upward and forward to control milk flow. A breast-feeding infant, however, *suckles* the breast; this suckling mechanism involves the lips, gums, tongue, cheeks and hard and soft palates (Drewett & Woolridge 1981a, 1981b, Weber

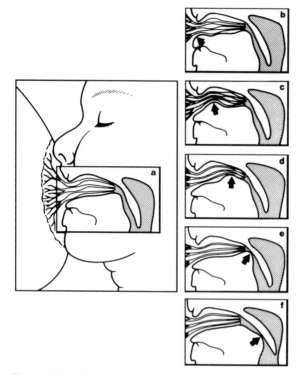

Figure 17.1 Suck cycle. (Reproduced from Woolridge 1986b, with permission.)

et al 1986, Woolridge 1986b). A complete suck cycle is shown in Figure 17.1.

Good attachment during breast-feeding ensures that the baby is able to *suckle* rather than just *suck* at the breast. During suckling, the baby's tongue ripples in a rhythmic, wave-like motion from the front of the mouth toward the back, so that the areola and nipple are pressed progressively upward against the upper gum, the hard palate, and the soft palate at the back of the mouth. This action, together with the alternative compression and release of the gums, moves the milk through the collecting sinuses and out the nipple to the back of the baby's mouth. The tongue's wave-like motion, in combination with the tension of the cheek muscles, creates the negative pressure for suction.

A normal breast-fed baby sucks in a rhythm that corresponds inversely to the amount of milk available. High rates of milk flow result in slower sucking rates of about one suck per second. As the milk is removed, sucking rates increase until they reach about two sucks per second when milk removal is minimal.

At the breast, the cycle begins with rapid sucking until milk let-down occurs. As the baby swallows, his pace slows. He returns to more rapid sucking for stim-

ulation, and then slower sucking as milk is released. This pattern continues until the decreased milk reserve results in non-nutritive sucking. When the baby is switched to the second breast, he resumes the same pattern (Drewett & Woolridge 1981a, 1981b, Fisher 1983, 1984, Minchin 1985, Woolridge 1986a, 1986b, Royal College of Midwives 1989, Lauwers & Woessner 1990, Glover 1997).

Good position and attachment

Enabling women to 'attach baby in the best possible way' is critical to successful breast-feeding (Glover 1997). Good positioning and attachment of the baby on the breast allow the baby to use the tongue to draw the nipple and areola into the mouth to form a cone-shaped extension of the nipple. The mother's nipple then extends back as far as the baby's soft palate, reducing nipple pain and trauma, and increasing breast emptying. As the breast is drained, more milk is produced by the lactiferous sinuses; prolactin levels increase as the breast is emptied, stimulating milk production (Fisher 1983, Glover 1997). Positioning baby is shown in Figure 17.2.

Indicators of good attachment include:

- a contented baby, gaining weight and usually satisfied after a feed;
- no pain or soreness of the nipples;
- the infant's chin being pushed well into the breast,
- the infant's mouth being wide open with the lips curled back and the tip of the tongue under the bottom lip;
- full cheeks with no clicking;
- a normal feeding rhythm of several rapid shallow sucks followed by several long deep sucks and swallows, and a pause;
- the whole breast moving in relation to the pressure from the infant's mouth;
- suction having to be broken in taking the baby off the breast because of the good vacuum seal.

Attachment technique is shown in Figure 17.3.

Poor position and attachment

Poor attachment of the baby on the breast has a number of consequences for both the mother and baby:

- The baby cannot form an efficient teat from the breast tissue. This results in frictional damage to the nipple and sore and cracked nipples.
- The baby is unable to obtain milk efficiently.
- Inadequate emptying of the breasts as a result of

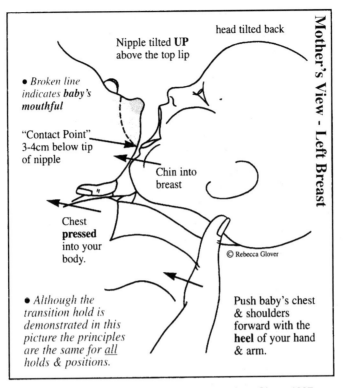

head tilted back

Nipple tilted **UP**
above the top lip

● *Broken line
indicates **baby's
mouthful***

"Contact Point".
3-4cm below tip
of nipple

Chin into
breast

Chest
pressed
into your
body.

© Rebecca Glover

● *Although the
transition hold is
demonstrated in this
picture the principles
are the same for <u>all</u>
holds & positions.*

Push baby's chest
& shoulders
forward with the
heel of your hand
& arm.

Mother's View - Left Breast

Figure 17.2   Positioning the baby. (Reproduced from Glover 1997,
with permission.)

poor attachment can cause breast engorgement. In
turn, engorgement is related to nipple trauma and
mastitis.

● The production of milk declines as, after the first
week, milk production depends on milk removal
from the breast rather than high prolactin levels.
Insufficient milk is one of the most common reason
mothers give for abandoning breast-feeding.

(Drewlett & Woolridge 1981b, Fisher 1983, 1994, 1995,
Minchin 1985, 1989b, Weber et al 1986, Woolridge 1986a,
Bono 1992, Dahlen 1993, Rajan 1993, Jensen et al 1994,
Fetherston 1995, Glover 1997).
Indicators of poor attachment can include:

● an unsatisfied infant or one with a poor weight
gain;
● a cross or fussy baby;
● the infant refusing the breast or falling asleep while
feeding;
● sore, painful or cracked nipples;
● the baby's lips being pursed around the nipple;
● hollow cheeks and clicking because the breast
nipple teat is not filling the oral cavity;
● an incorrect sucking rhythm in which the infant

sucks in a short, rapid flutter or sucks only the
nipple;
● the whole breast not moving in relation to the
pressure from the baby's mouth;
● the breast moving in and out of the mouth, or milk
leaking and the nipple falling easily out of the
mouth.

Factors that can hinder optimal attachment.   Maternal
factors can include:

● a lack of knowledge, confidence or practice at
breast-feeding;
● physical pain or discomfort following the birth;
● the position of the body and the breast: for
example, the breast may fall backwards or be
inhibited by clothing or a bra;
● clothing preventing close contact with the baby or
resulting in the baby being positioned with the chin
down and the nose forward;
● the breast being held too close to the nipple; this
may push the breast tissue away and prevent the
baby grasping an adequate amount of breast and
nipple because the mother's fingers are in the
way;

Attachment Technique

With baby's **chin pointing at the breast and your nipple pointing at baby's nose,** tease baby's bottom lip and chin with the puffy underside of your breast.

Watch and wait for baby to respond with a **wide open** mouth and the tongue down.

Immediately push baby's shoulders forward bringing baby **quickly and firmly onto the underside of your breast.**

Plant baby's bottom lip on the contact point and **push baby's chin into the breast.**

Your nipple will brush or fold under the top lip and roll back to the junction of the hard and soft palate.

This places baby's tongue well under the breast, baby will form the vacuum and begin feeding.

(When necessary use your thumb or finger to help tuck the nipple under the top lip and gum.)

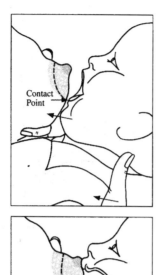
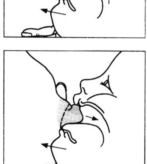
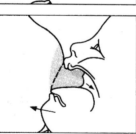
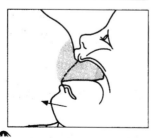

Figure 17.3   Attachment technique. (Reproduced from Glover 1997, with permission.)

- the mother's fingers impinging on the areola when offering the breast;
- the size and the shape of the nipple and/or breast.

Factors in the baby can include:

- a sleepy or disinterested baby;
- the baby lying on his back and not facing the mother so that his head has to be turned to grasp the nipple;
- the baby's head being pushed forward so that the nose is buried in the breast;
- the mouth not being directly opposite the nipple before attachment is attempted;
- too much clothing on the baby, preventing close contact;
- the size and shape of the baby's mouth, tongue and palate.

(Drewett & Woolridge 1981a, 1981b, Minchin 1981, 1985, 1989b, Fisher 1983, 1995, Weber et al 1986, Woolridge 1986a, 1986b, Royal College of Midwives 1989, Lauwers & Woessner 1990, Bono 1992, Rajan 1993, Jensen et al 1994).

Postures that encourage good attachment

It is important for women to be aware of comfortable and relaxed breast-feeding positions that ensure good attachment. Good attachment can be achieved while the mother adopts a number of comfortable relaxed postures, including sitting or lying on her side.

Some women may initially be more comfortable feeding their baby lying on a bed or couch, particularly if they have a sore perineum or caesarean incision. The comfortable lying position shown in Figure 17.4 takes the weight off the spine and perineum. While learning to breast-feed in the early days after the birth, it is best if the woman, when feeding in an upright position, sits in a chair, as shown in Figure 17.5. This ensures that the mother's back is upright and at a right angle to her lap. It also allows her legs to be supported and gives room to move the baby into the best position for good attachment.

Figures 17.6 and 17.7 show alternative ways of supporting the baby's head while feeding in a sitting position. Once the mother and baby have achieved the best possible attachment, the mother can be encouraged to experiment with different postures to find what is most comfortable and convenient for her and the baby.

Sore nipples

The two most common reasons given by breast-

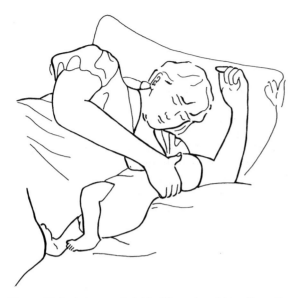

Figure 17.4 Lying comfortably. (Reproduced from Bennett & Brown 1999, with permission.)

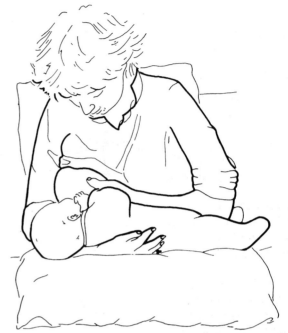

Figure 17.6 Supporting the baby with the forearm. (Reproduced from Bennett & Brown 1999, with permission.)

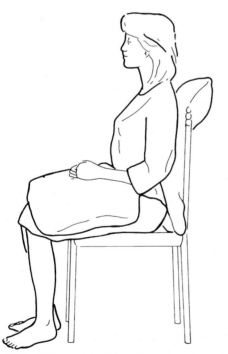

Figure 17.5 Sitting upright. (Reproduced from Bennett & Brown 1999, with permission.)

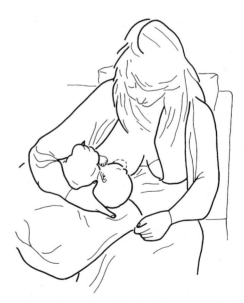

Figure 17.7 Supporting the baby with extended fingers. (Reproduced from Bennett & Brown 1999, with permission.)

feeding mothers for stopping breastfeeding are insufficient milk and nipple pain (Percival 1990, 1998, Fisher 1995, Hartmann 1995, Duffy et al 1997). These two factors correlate positively and significantly with one another and with nipple trauma (Woolridge 1986a, Inch 1990, Fisher 1995).

If inadequate amounts of breast tissue are presented to the baby, insufficient tissue will be formed into a teat. If the nipple is not drawn into the mouth back to the soft palate, the baby may have difficulty feeding and fail to gain weight. In addition, such an inadequate teat does not extend well into the mouth but is instead repeatedly drawn in and out of the mouth between the tongue and gums, causing frictional damage to the nipple (Woolridge 1986a, 1986b).

Although the causes of painful breast-feeding are well documented, a 1995 Australian study of mothers in a private maternity hospital found that nipple pain and trauma were still common among breast-feeding mothers, 71% of mothers experiencing nipple pain and 35% reporting nipple trauma (Fetherston 1995). Similarly, in America, Ziemer & Pigeon (1993) found that 96% of breast-feeding mothers experienced nipple pain and 65% had visible nipple damage. These authors concluded that the nipple skin change resulted from suction damage during normal infant suckling. However, other researchers have found no relationship between sucking strength and nipple pain. Buchko et al (1994) found that high levels of sucking strength did not lead to increased pain intensity or nipple soreness on any of the first 7 postpartum days. Woolridge (1986a) also argued that correct attachment should only be presumed when the mother feels *no pain*.

Over the years, numerous interventions have been used to 'cure' nipple pain and trauma. Inch (1990), in reviewing 10 studies of potential treatments aimed at alleviating nipple pain and trauma, concluded that no treatment or application had been shown to be of any discernible benefit in protecting the nipple from damage.

In 1987, Garcia et al found 32 different treatments being offered to mothers in England. Only three of these treatments had been evaluated by means of a randomized controlled trial: 'resting and expressing', the use of a nipple shield, and repositioning and improved attachment of the baby on the breast. Only the latter – repositioning and improved attachment of the baby on the breast – showed any statistical difference in nipple-healing during the 48-hour period when the three treatments were compared. Moreover, 'resting and expressing' and the use of a nipple shield were significantly less acceptable to the mother. These two treatments can also gradually suppress lactation (Houston et al 1983, Howie 1985).

More recently, Pugh et al (1996) compared the effectiveness of three topical agents (USP modified lanolin, warm water compresses and expressed milk with air drying) in alleviating nipple pain. Although raw sores supported the use of warm water compresses, there was no significant difference between the three groups for pain intensity, pain affect or breast-feeding duration.

If sore nipples are present, poor positioning causing poor attachment must always be considered as the most likely source of the problem. Nipple pain during breast-feeding usually alerts the midwife that the feeding technique needs to be improved because the baby is damaging the nipple. The ideal solution is not to restrict the number of feeds or to remove the baby from the breast, but instead to prevent the trauma by ensuring the best possible position and attachment of the baby on the breast. Removing the infant from the breast may help the nipple to heal but will not correct the underlying cause of the damage. However, if a nipple has been severely damaged, it may be necessary to rest it (Woolridge 1986a, Inch 1990, Fisher 1995).

MINI SESSION: FREQUENCY AND DURATION OF FEEDS

Objective

- Women will appreciate the advantages of an infant-regulated (baby-led) frequency and duration of feeds.

Important teaching points

- Discuss the importance of the infant regulating the *frequency* of feeds.
- Clarify that when feeding is infant led, babies gain more weight and breast-feeding continues for longer.
- Explain the importance of the infant regulating the *duration* of feeds.
- Emphasize that infants vary in the time they need to receive sufficient milk.
- Encourage women to allow the baby to complete feeding from the first breast before offering the second, allowing the infant to obtain both foremilk and hindmilk.
- If appropriate, discuss the sucking needs of infants and how these vary.

Midwives' teaching notes

Unrestricted frequency and duration of feeds

In the early weeks of breast-feeding, it is common for the baby to sleep for short periods and require frequent feeding. Observational studies have revealed that, during the first few weeks, the intervals between feeds may be completely random, ranging between 1 and 8 hours (Royal College of Midwives 1989). Some research based on mothers' records has shown that there is a tendency for breast-fed infants to feed more often than their bottle-fed counterparts (Wenner & Barnard 1980). The number of feeds per day gradually decreases, so that by 12 months of age, it is typical that most infants are having four meals a day.

For most of the 20th century, mothers have been erroneously advised to limit the baby's sucking time at the breast, particularly during the early days after the birth (King 1913, Nash 1913, Inch 1990). Limiting the baby's sucking time at the breast has no effect on nipple pain or trauma. However, it contributes to women stopping breast-feeding by 6 weeks after the birth.

Advantages of unrestricted feeding include (Thomsen et al 1979, De Chateau 1980, L'Esperance 1980, Houston et al 1983, Johnson 1986):

- the early establishment of lactation as frequent stimulation increases milk supply;
- frequent emptying of the breasts reducing engorgement;
- a more contented baby who cries less frequently;
- a greater weight gain than if feeding frequency is limited;
- the continuation of breast-feeding for a longer period of time.

The findings of a Western Australian study that measured the storage capacity of breast-feeding mothers' breasts shows the need for flexible breast-feeding. Hartmann (1995) found that the storage capacity for milk varied but that mothers were still able to produce the same amount of milk for their babies; mothers with smaller storage capacities simply fed their babies more often.

In addition, a great deal of variation exists in the amount of sucking time that infants require to obtain sufficient food to meet their needs. In early research by Woolridge et al (1982):

- one baby fed for 4 minutes on only one breast, achieving a total milk intake of 67 g;
- eight babies fed on both breasts for a period of 22 minutes and achieved a final intake of 68 g;
- feeding time for other babies in the study sample varied between 4 minutes and 22 minutes before they had received sufficient milk for their needs.

These findings suggest that feeding time is not an accurate indication of the actual intake of milk, that is, a baby feeding for a short time cannot be assumed to be taking only a small amount of milk.

In addition, the composition of breast milk changes throughout the feed from the high-lactose, low-calorie foremilk to the higher fat-containing hindmilk (Drewett & Woolridge 1981a, Hartmann & Prosser 1984, Saint et al 1986, Woolridge et al 1990).

These findings of a variation in feeding time and a changing composition of breast milk suggest that a flexible approach to infant feeding be adopted. Restricting the duration of infant feeds may be harmful in that the infant may receive a larger quantity of low-calorie foremilk but may be deprived of the higher fat-containing hindmilk. Allowing the infant to determine the length of sucking time ensures that this does not occur. This could be achieved by allowing the baby to complete the first breast before offering the second breast (this is not to be interpreted as one-sided feeding). Alternatively, the mother could offer one breast, and, when the baby indicates that he has had sufficient milk, the nappy could be changed; the second breast could then be offered. It is important to commence feeding on the opposite breast at the next feed.

Sucking needs

Sucking is a means of comfort, nourishment and love for a baby. In addition to being pleasurable, sucking also stimulates saliva, which contains enzymes that predigest the food before the stomach enzymes begin to work on it. Sucking may also have a soothing effect on the baby, and calm intestinal disorders by helping the baby to pass gas or use his bowels. Because sucking provides comfort as well as nourishment, sucking needs may depend on the baby's need to be comforted. The need for sucking is usually greater in the first 3 months than at any other time (Lauwers & Woessner 1990).

The usual response to a crying infant is to question whether the cause is hunger. As parents become tuned into patterns of sleeping and waking, they will be better able to decide whether the baby is hungry or crying for some other reason. They may also consider the length of time since the last feed, how well he nursed at the previous feed, his general disposition and whether he is easily soothed (Lauwers & Woessner 1990). (See also the mini sessions on infant crying below.)

MINI SESSION: INCREASING THE AMOUNT OF BREAST MILK

Objective

- New parents will understand how to increase the amount of breast milk available for the baby if necessary.

Important teaching point

- Discuss ways of increasing the amount of breast milk available for the baby.

Midwives' teaching notes

Increasing the milk supply

Women can use a number of strategies to increase the amount of breast milk at different times, for example during a 'growth spurt'. These include (Fisher 1983, Minchin 1985, Woolridge 1986b, Royal College of Midwives 1989, Lauwers & Woessner 1990):

- ensuring good attachment during feeds;
- for 24–48 hours concentrating only on feeding and resting; the mother should ask for help with other household tasks from her partner, friends or relatives;
- getting into bed with baby close by and sleeping as much as possible;
- nursing frequently: every 2 hours during the day (remembering that the supply increases according to demand);
- using relaxation techniques to encourage let-down;
- offering both breasts at each feeding;
- nursing long enough for the baby to receive hind milk;
- eating nutritious food, ensuring that meals and snacks include sufficient fruit, vegetables, carbohydrate and protein;
- if the baby is having complementary feeds, offering these after the baby has finished at the breast and *only* when necessary. As the milk supply increases, the complementary feeds should be reduced until they are no longer required.

MINI SESSION: MATERNAL SUPPORT

Objective

- The new mother will appreciate the importance of maternal support and continuous encouragement in maintaining breast-feeding.

Important teaching points

- Clarify and discuss the importance of maternal support.
- Emphasize the need for mothers to have a 'doula' or someone to 'mother the mother', who will offer continuous support and encouragement.
- If possible copy the pamphlet 'Your midwife's advice for surviving the early weeks' (see Chapter 10) and go through this with parents.

Midwives' teaching notes

Maternal support

(The new mother's needs and strategies to increase rest and relaxation are discussed more fully in Chapter 10.)

An important factor for successful breast-feeding is the support available in the mother's family and social environment. The mother herself is in need of support if she is successfully to continue breast-feeding (Raphael 1981, Bottorff 1990, Becker 1992, Freed et al 1992).

Raphael (1981) reviewed 278 anthropological reports on different cultures around the world and interviewed hundreds of American mothers who failed or succeeded at breast-feeding. She identified one critical element that seemed to facilitate success: the presence of someone who cared for the mother. Raphael described this person as a 'doula' or someone who literally 'mothers the new mother', offering continuous encouragement. Good candidates for the 'doula' role include the new mother's partner, sister, sister-in-law, older relative or friend. More recently, other researchers have emphasized the relationship between a mother's support and successful breast-feeding (Isabella & Isabella 1994).

Initially in the postnatal period, midwives and health visitors are the ideal people to assume a primary supportive role for new mothers while they learn to breast-feed. Satisfaction with midwifery care in the intrapartal and postpartal periods is related to successful breast-feeding (Rajan 1993).

MINI SESSION: COMMUNITY RESOURCES FOR BREAST-FEEDING WOMEN

Objective

- The new parents will be aware of available community resources that provide resources for breast-feeding women.

Important teaching points

- Inform women of all local community resources that promote breast-feeding and are available to help with breast-feeding problems.
- If possible, give women a written list of local resources.

Midwives' teaching notes

It is essential that midwives inform new mothers of all available community resources that may help with breast-feeding. These will vary from country to country but may include:

- La Leche League or Nursing Mothers
- National Childbirth Trust
- lactation consultants
- health visitors (UK)
- community (child health) nurses (Australia)
- public health nurses (USA).

CONCLUSION

In conclusion, there are several keys to successful breast-feeding. These include an early first feed, good position and attachment, and allowing the infant to determine how often and for how long he feeds. Again, it should be emphasized that these factors have the benefits of ensuring adequate milk for the infant, increasing emptying of the breasts and reducing the incidence of sore and cracked nipples and engorgement. In addition, adequate support for the mother and access to community resources, if required, are essential.

INFANT TEMPERAMENT

Introduction and rationale

New babies should obviously not be rigidly categorized or labelled. However, it is important for mothers to be aware that infants, like adults, have different temperaments and thus display different behaviours. This is particularly important for the mother of an 'active' or 'fussy' baby; she is more likely to feel positive if she views irritability as an indication of the baby's special need rather than as evidence of 'spoiling' or of her own incompetence (Crockenberg & McClusky 1986).

Similarly, it is important that midwives recognize babies who may have 'high needs' as such infants can also significantly affect the mother's responsiveness (Searle 1985). The daily experiences of parents whose child is predominantly good-natured and easy going are very different from those whose child reacts in an intensely negative manner to every minor irritation. Infants reported as 'difficult' have been associated with major concerns and large family adjustments (Cutrona & Troutman 1986).

Early referral can be made to the health visitor and the parents made aware of other appropriate community resources. Although the term 'difficult infant' is inappropriate, life is certainly more difficult for many parents of a 'high-needs' child as they learn to make necessary adjustments. Sears' (1985) book *The*

Fussy Baby may also be a valuable reference for parents of a 'high-needs' or 'active' baby.

In discussing infant temperament, key issues include the importance of:

- parents understanding that babies (like adults) have individual temperaments and therefore also have different needs;
- knowing about and being able to access community resources, particularly if they have a 'high-needs' child.

MINI SESSION: INDIVIDUAL TEMPERAMENT

Objective

- The new mother will appreciate that babies have individual temperaments and thus have different needs.

Important teaching points

- Emphasize that babies have individual temperaments and behaviour patterns.
- Include a description of an average, easy, placid, and 'active' or 'fussy' baby.

Midwives' teaching notes

Infant temperament

Temperament can be defined as 'a constitutionally based style of behaviour' (Thomas et al 1969, Buss & Plomin 1975): infants are born with a predisposition to respond to their environment in very different ways (Gross & Conrad 1995). These differences in temperament exist between individual neonates from birth (Korner 1974, McKim & Wiseman 1985).

Lauwers and Woessner (1990) described various behaviour patterns in infants that may be useful for mothers in helping them meet their own babies' needs. These included the average baby, easy baby, placid baby, and active or fussy baby.

Average baby. The 'average' breast-feeding infant sleeps between 12 and 20 hours a day, and nurses between 6 and 14 times. He may have one or two longer periods of sleep balanced by one or two fussy periods.

When awake, he is generally quiet, alert, listening and usually responsive when handled. He will attempt to soothe himself by sucking on his fist or displaying some other type of comfort measure. The mother may expect to spend 1 out of every 3 hours caring for her baby.

Easy baby. An 'easy baby' will sleep for longer periods and will be less demanding, with less fussiness. The nursing pattern is the same as an average baby. A conscious effort may need to be made to ensure that the baby receives the stimulation and attention he needs for his emotional and physical development.

Placid baby. These infants may sleep as much as 18–20 hours a day; they are quietly alert and tranquil when awake and make few demands for attention. A 'placid' baby may request as few as 4–6 feeds a day and must be monitored to guard against his becoming undernourished. In addition, it is essential to ensure that the emotional needs of these babies are fulfilled.

Active and fussy baby. An 'active', 'fussy' or 'high-needs' baby will sleep fewer hours than other infants and, when awake, will be active and unable to console himself, frequently fussing and crying. This infant has irregular sleep cycles and eating patterns, is slow to adapt, tends to withdraw from new situations and is intense in reaction. He may also nurse more frequently and greedily than the average baby (McKim & Wiseman 1985, Barr et al 1989). About 10% of infants fall into the category of being 'difficult' (McKim & Wiseman 1985). However, in more recent research, 20% of mothers described their infants as being 'difficult' (Jacobson & Melvin 1995).

While some researchers have categorized such infants as being 'difficult' (Thomas et al 1969, McKim & Wiseman 1985), others have argued against using the term 'difficult' because of its negative connotations; it can result in parental defensiveness or may become a self-fulfilling prophecy (Gross & Conrad 1995).

Conclusion

Like adults, infants have different temperaments. They can be loosely categorized into the 'average' baby, 'easy' baby, 'placid' baby, and 'active' or 'fussy' baby.

INFANT CRYING

Introduction and rationale

Crying is the infant behaviour that presents the greatest challenge to parents and midwives. Researchers have found that adults identify crying as a noxious sound (Rinne et al 1990, Hewat 1992).

Drummond et al (1993) found that first-time mothers had little knowledge about infant crying. At 6 weeks, mothers saw crying as a signal or noise of unknown meaning, and soothing was a matter of trial and error. At 10 weeks after the birth, infant crying

was seen as, among other things, a general communication of such things as 'bad temper', 'boredom' or 'being spoiled'.

As with breast-feeding, midwives and health visitors have an important teaching role to play. First, if new parents have more realistic expectations of how often and why babies cry, and are aware that infant crying is normal rather than being brought about by inadequate care on their part, they are more likely to cope with their new baby. They are also more likely to continue breast-feeding if they know that breast-fed babies do not cry more than artificially fed babies (Barr et al 1989) and that changing from breast milk to artificial milk does not lead to less crying (Keefe et al 1996). At 1 month after the birth, Keefe et al (1996) found that 40% of irritable infants were bottle-fed compared with only 15% of non-irritable infants.

Second, midwives have an important role to play in teaching parents how their newborns attempt to console themselves. In addition, parents can be helped to find other ways of soothing their newborns (Blackburn 1980). As is discussed below in more detail, infants vary in how well they can console themselves or be consoled by others. This is important because the parents' success or failure in calming their infant has a significant impact on their feelings of competence as parents.

Third, most parents want to fulfil their baby's needs but may be concerned about the 'right' or 'wrong' thing to do. Many face a common dilemma: should they pick up their crying infant or leave him to cry? Friends and relatives may insist that being attentive to a baby is 'spoiling' him. This fear of 'spoiling' may cause parents to refrain from consoling infants when they need help to regain control.

Finally, it is very important not to underestimate the effects of living with infants who cry excessively. Some women in Hewat's (1992) phenomenological study felt as if 'I'm going to drive her through this wall' or as if they 'were trapped in a nightmare'. They understood 'how people kill their children, how a woman can be so desperate that she will kill that child because its constantly at you. It never stops. It never goes away.'

(Possible midwifery actions in the presence of excessive crying are discussed in the section on infant temperament above.)

The family of a crying infant

The families of infants who cry excessively because of colic may experience high levels of stress. Similarly, as I discussed earlier, infants reported as having 'difficult' temperaments are associated with major family concerns and adjustments. Regardless of the underlying cause, the difficulty experienced by the families of 'colicky' or 'difficult' babies is one of excessive crying. Therefore, these two groups will be discussed together. Furthermore, there appears to be some overlap between the two groups of infants. Jacobson & Melvin (1995) found that 36% of colicky infants were clustered in the 'difficult' category compared with 20% of non-colicky infants.

Researchers have found a relationship between infant irritability and crying and maternal feelings of:

- distress and upset (Golton & St James Roberts 1991);
- depression (Brazelton 1962, 1985, Oberklaid 1979);
- personal inadequacy or inferiority (Brazelton 1962, Pinyerd 1992a), and the risk of decreased self-esteem (Elliot et al 1996);
- helplessness and rejection by the infant (Keefe 1988, Keefe & Froese-Fretz 1989, Carey 1990, Zuckerman et al 1990, Jacobson & Melvin 1995);
- guilt (Pinyerd 1992a);
- fatigue and exhaustion (Menahem 1978, Jones 1983, Pinyerd 1992a);
- anger tension (Waldman & Sarsgard 1983, Pinyerd 1992a) and resentment (Swaffield 1984);
- a more negative self-evaluation (Deutsch et al 1988);
- decreased parental competence (Blackburn 1980), as well as the mother's lower evaluation of herself in the maternal role (Reilly et al 1987);
- less satisfactory marital relationships (Levitt et al 1986) and increased marital tension (Brazelton 1962, 1985, Hinkley 1986, Berry 1988, Deutsch et al 1988);
- lower affect and life satisfaction regardless of the amount of support that women received from their husbands (Crockenberg 1981).

Researchers have also found:

- increased hostility, resentment and rejection of the infant (Pinyerd 1992a);
- that irritable infants were less responsive to their mothers (Keefe et al 1996);
- less responsive mothering (Jacobson & Melvin 1995), including less social and emotional growth-fostering behaviours (Keefe et al 1996);
- inadequate attachment and a lack of synchrony in parent–infant interaction (Hoffman & Drotar 1991, Keefe et al 1996);
- that persistent or relentless crying is a possible catalyst for child maltreatment (Frodi 1985, Mortimer & Kevill 1985, Berger 1986) and is the chief reason parents give for child abuse (Belsky 1980, Brazelton 1985);

- that early research suggests that fathers have more problems than mothers when babies are 'difficult' (Hobbs 1965, Russell 1974, Hobbs & Cole 1976, Wilkie & Ames 1986). Men rated themselves less powerful as husbands, and their wives as less powerful as wives and mothers (Wilkie & Ames 1986).

Key issues in teaching parents about infant crying include:

- parents being able to make decisions about how they will respond to infant crying that are based on up-to-date information and research;
- the amount that babies cry during the first few months of life;
- why babies under 6 months of age cry;
- that a newborn's 'needs' and 'wants' are the same;
- the importance of responding to the baby's cry;
- the pressures that others may exert on the parents;
- different ways to settle a restless and crying baby;
- infant colic;
- the importance of time away from a crying baby and of the mother resting when her infant is sleeping;
- knowing about and being able to access community resources.

MINI SESSION: CRYING PATTERNS
Objective

- The new parents will have realistic expectations about the amount that babies cry during the first few months of life.

Important teaching points

- New babies (on average) cry for about 2 out of 24 hours. This increases to about 3 hours a day and peaks at around 6 weeks.
- Emphasize that crying often occurs in the late afternoon and evening when the mother herself may be at her most tired.

Midwives' teaching notes

Crying patterns

Western cultures. An early study by Brazelton (1962) investigated the crying habits of 80 infants during the first 12 weeks of life:

- In the second week of life, infants cried for an average 1.75 hours daily.

- Crying increased to 2.75 hours daily at 6 weeks.
- There was a marked peak in crying in the evening between 6 and 10 pm.
- A reduction in crying occurred at 10 weeks, with peak crying times between 5 and 11 pm, and 6 and 11 am.

Since that time, other researchers in America have reported similar results. In the early weeks, babies cry for an average of about 2 hours, increasing to about 3 hours (and peaking at about 6 weeks). Most of the crying occurs in the late afternoon and evening when the mother's resources are lowest. These levels decline by 3–4 months and remain stable throughout the first year of life (Hunziker & Barr 1986, Barr 1990, Golton & St James-Roberts 1991, Acebo & Thoman 1992, Parkin et al 1993, St James-Roberts et al 1993). Some researchers have argued that first-time mothers are poorly prepared for the amount and timing of infant crying (Elliot et al 1996), and these figures will undoubtedly come as a shock to many mothers in the midwife's care.

Researchers have also reported the following:

- First-born infants are *not* more likely to be persistent criers (although the mothers of first-born infants are more likely to seek help for infant crying) (Golton & St James-Roberts 1991).
- Breast-fed babies do *not* cry more than artificially fed babies: no difference exists in the amount of crying over 24 hours or by period of the day between the two groups (Barr et al 1989).
- Changing from breast milk to artificial milk does *not* lead to less crying (Keefe et al 1996).
- At 2 months of age, babies who are fed more frequently and not kept waiting tend to fret less frequently (Elias et al 1986). (See also the breast-feeding mini sessions above).

Other cultures. Of particular interest to midwives and health visitors is that, although these figures represent the norm for countries such as North America, the UK and Australia, they are higher than those found in other cultures that have different care-giving practices. Early observations of the Kung San hunter-gatherers found that the duration of crying was about half that observed in Western societies. Babies in the Kung San culture are carried in an upright position that ensures constant close proximity and allows frequent feeding (De Vore & Konner 1974, Konner 1976, Konner & Worthman 1980).

Hunziker & Barr (1986) simulated some of the care-giving practices of other cultures by asking mothers in the experimental group to increase carrying and holding their babies for a minimum of 3 hours a day (spread over the whole day regardless of whether the baby was asleep or awake). This 'supplemental carrying' group held their babies for 4.2 hours (an increase of 1.8 hours) while the control group average was 2.7 hours. Six weeks after the birth (the time when infant crying peaks), babies in the 'supplemental carrying' group cried 43% less overall than control group babies and 54% less in the evening. The change was in the length of crying bouts rather than in their frequency. (See also the section below on strategies to reduce infant crying.)

Individual differences in infant consolability

Consolability is the ability of newborns to bring themselves to or be brought by others to a lower state (Wolff 1966, Parmalee & Stern 1972, Prechtl 1974, Blackburn 1980, Wenner & Barnard 1980). (Infant states are discussed in the mini session on infant sleep and activity states below.)

As was discussed in the section on infant temperament, researchers have identified that there are overall differences in infants from birth. Of particular interest for midwives is how newborns vary considerably in the ease or difficulty with which they can console themselves or be soothed by others (this is not influenced by infant feeding method).

There are significant differences in (Korner 1974, Blackburn 1980, McKim & Wiseman 1985):

- both the frequency of crying and its duration;
- how readily infants are soothed;
- how long they remain quiet after soothing;
- the amount of spontaneous oral activity and attempts at self-comforting;
- the success of this self-comforting through hand–mouth comforting;
- the infants' threshold for both auditory and visual, and other stimuli;
- their behavioural response to overstimulation.

Some infants make few or very brief attempts to console themselves and always need intervention on the part of their care-givers. A few infants consistently console themselves, needing minimal or occasional intervention. In addition, each individual infant may vary at times in his ability to console himself, sometimes trying and succeeding, at other times not trying at all (Blackburn 1980, Wenner & Barnard 1980).

MINI SESSION: WHY BABIES CRY
Objective

- The new parents will have a basic level of understanding of why babies under 6 months of age cry.

Important teaching points

- Discuss the various reasons why the newborn baby cries.
- Explain that crying is a means of communication for their baby and not just a way of telling his parents he is hungry.

Midwives' teaching notes

Possible reasons for infant crying

Infant crying is not only a distress signal, but also a powerful communicator used by the baby in order to interact with his environment. Crying is the only reliable way in which very young babies can signal to the adults who take care of them; it is their way of communicating their physical and emotional needs (Leach 1977).

Hunger.   In the early weeks of breast-feeding, it is common for the baby to sleep for short periods and to require frequent feeding. As discussed in the infant feeding section above, responding to hunger cries is likely to result in a more contented baby who cries less frequently than when a strict feeding schedule is maintained.

As parents become attuned to their infant's pattern of sleeping and waking, they will be better able to determine whether it is a hunger cry. If the baby has recently fed, other causes of crying could also be investigated. Unfortunately new mothers sometimes assume that hunger is the cause for a baby's fussy disposition and blame a low milk supply or 'poor-quality' milk (Lauwers & Woessner 1990).

Body discomfort.   A baby's body temperature on the surface of his skin has a direct effect on his comfort. Babies may cry from under- or overheating and should be dressed in the same quantity of clothing that an adult would wear. Similarly, the room temperature should be comfortable for adults.

A wet or dirty nappy will not cause crying but may lead to cooling and be a potential cause of discomfort. This cooling may make the baby more responsive to stimulation and thus more liable to cry for other reasons. Skin irritations such as heat or nappy rash may also be a cause of discomfort and crying.

Intestinal gas.   Gas in the intestines can also cause discomfort. Some babies also take in more milk than they are able to handle. This may cause pressure that can in turn make them uncomfortable (Lauwers & Woessner 1990).

External stimuli.   A baby may react unhappily to sensations such as movement, touch, smell, light, noise and excessive handling. Anything that happens suddenly can cause a baby to startle and result in crying. Unfamiliar or unpleasant smells may be disquieting to a baby, as are bright lights and loud or sudden noises.

Overhandling.   It has been argued that, at times, too much handling may cause a baby to cry: some infants certainly become very agitated when they are tired (see the mini session on infant temperament above). If the parents have ruled out hunger or discomfort and the baby lets them know he does not want to be held, they may choose to let him cry for a *few minutes only*. This is the only way in which some young babies can go to sleep (Lauwers & Woessner 1990).

Social and emotional needs.   A baby's cry often indicates some form of physical discomfort, for example hunger, or a reaction to his environment. However, a baby who is well fed, comfortable and in no pain may still cry simply to initiate intimate contact with the parents. In addition, babies may cry periodically as a way of releasing tension, many babies having a regular fussy time each day when it is difficult to console them.

MINI SESSION: THE NEWBORN BABY'S 'NEEDS' AND 'WANTS'

Objective

- The new mother will be aware that the 'needs' and 'wants' of a newborn baby are the same.

Important teaching points

- Clarify through discussion that a baby's 'needs' and 'wants' are the same. Explain that fulfilling a baby's needs is not 'spoiling' him.
- Emphasize that crying is an indicator of infant need rather than poor parenting.

Midwives' teaching notes

Needs versus 'wants'

Like all human beings, babies have needs that are necessary for their well-being. Some of these, for example physical needs, are obvious and simple to fulfil. Others may be less obvious, for example emotional and social needs, the need for close physical contact, love and attention, and the need for stimulation and social interaction.

The act of crying is sometimes misunderstood. Because it is used when the baby is hungry, uncomfortable or in pain, it is often assumed that these are the only messages it carries. If a baby cries, the parent may automatically conclude that one of these three problems must exist, but this is not necessarily so. If the baby is fed and then put down again, he or she may immediately start crying. In a healthy infant, this may well mean that the baby wants more intimate bodily contact.

Many parents will accept that crying because of hunger, cold and so on is a 'legitimate need' because physical needs are real: without food or warmth, the new baby would die. Researchers have found that it is easier for women to respond to hunger, pain and discomfort (Drummond et al 1993, 1994). However, without social interaction with adults, the baby may not be able to become a full human being. At times, a baby may cry because of the need to be picked up and held close for reassurance and comfort. This may be interpreted as 'just wanting attention', something that is not necessary.

One of the many myths about parenthood is the 'spoiling' myth. This particular myth states that if babies are picked up too often when they cry, cuddled too much or generally given too much attention, they will become 'spoilt'. It is almost as if the child is a cake, a flan or a piece of squid (that really can be spoilt by overhandling). For example, at 10 weeks after the birth, primiparas in Drummond et al's (1993) research saw infant crying as a general communication of such things as hunger, bad temper, boredom or 'being spoiled'.

However, for the infant, attention from adults is not a 'want'. Instead, it is a real need, one as important as his physical requirements. The baby needs his parents to provide not only for his bodily needs, but also for his comfort and reassurance.

MINI SESSION: RESPONDING TO CRYING

Objective

- The new parents will understand the importance of responding to the baby's cry.

Important teaching points

- Explain the importance of responding to infant crying.
- Briefly discuss the significance of the first relationship.
- Emphasize that babies whose cries are answered during the first year of life are less likely to use crying as a means of communication at 1 year of age.

Midwives' teaching notes

The importance of responding to a crying infant

(Theories of attachment are discussed in detail in Chapter 11.)

Parents need to know that their loving response to their baby's cry is both desirable and beneficial in the development of trust and positive self-concept: it will not lead to their child becoming 'spoilt' or manipulative.

Through crying, the infant learns that he has the ability to make things happen. When his parents respond, he learns that his needs will be met, and thus he cries less. When babies cries are answered during the first year of life, they are far less likely to use crying as a means of communication at 1 year of age (Ainsworth et al 1978). Conversely, when care-givers do not respond to infant crying, infants have been shown to cry louder and longer. Alternatively, a baby repeatedly left to cry alone may ultimately learn to give up and tune out the world (Sears 1988).

From a consistent response to his cries, a baby learns that he is loved and wanted, and can rely on someone to respond to his needs. This will in time lead to the development of a secure attachment to these special people and a sense of trust and positive self-concept.

MINI SESSION: PRESSURE FROM OTHERS

Objective

- Parents will be able to identify the pressures that others may exert to prevent them from responding to their crying baby.

Important teaching points

- Identify and discuss the pressures that others may use to prevent parents responding to their baby's cry.

Midwives' teaching notes

External pressures

As I said earlier, crying presents the greatest challenge that many new parents face. Most face a common dilemma: should they pick up their crying infant or leave him to cry? New parents will undoubtedly be offered a great deal of advice on how to look after their baby. This advice will usually be given in a positive way, and much of it may be useful. However, advice about not 'spoiling' their baby by picking him up or carrying him may have an adverse effect on some parents.

In my own research (Percival 1990), a number of women made comments about intrusive help from family and friends, for example 'All I want from family and outsiders is reassurance and support but they like to give inappropriate advice. Unfortunately, parenthood is riddled with self-appointed homemade experts.'

The information from these sessions and the reassurance of midwives and health visitors should help parents to withstand pressure from others. In addition, when people give unwanted advice, suggest that mothers do not waste energy arguing about the way they are going to do things. Instead, get them just to accept the advice, nod, smile and go their own way.

MINI SESSION: SETTLING A RESTLESS BABY

Objective

- The parents will be aware of different ways in which they can settle a restless baby.

Important teaching points

- Emphasize that, from birth, newborns vary a great deal in how they are able to console themselves or be consoled by others.
- Discuss ways of settling a crying infant.
- If possible copy the pamphlet 'Your midwife's advice on settling your crying baby' (below) and go through this with the parents.
- Where possible, use a doll to demonstrate holding and comforting.
- Demonstrate the tying and use of a baby sling.
- Show appropriate videos, for example relaxation baby bath techniques and baby massage.

Midwives' teaching notes

Infant-led settling strategies

As described above, newborns vary a great deal in how easily they can console themselves. A few infants almost always console themselves, needing little help to settle. Others make few or very brief attempts and always need help (Blackburn 1980, Wenner & Barnard 1980). When fussing or crying, most infants initiate any of several manoeuvres to quieten themselves. The baby's most commonly observed actions are (Blackburn 1980):

- bringing his hand to his mouth area;
- sucking on his fingers, fist or tongue;
- rooting movements;
- paying attention to sounds, visual objects or faces around him;
- postural change.

Care-giver-led settling strategies

Infants may also vary in their response to the consoling efforts of others. An infant may sometimes settle when talked to, while at other times he may need to be held and rocked. Most infants need periodic help from others in consoling themselves (Blackburn 1980, Wenner & Barnard 1980).

An initial reaction of parents to a crying baby is often to pick him up or feed him. However, other actions can sometimes be just as effective (Brazelton 1962). As parents get to know their baby, they will learn to distinguish types of cry and try different consoling methods to see what works best for their baby.

Many restless babies are helped to settle if they are held and moved in ways that copy the rhythms experienced in the uterus. Rocking and swinging movements have been found to be particularly effective (Elliot et al 1988). Where possible, advise the mother to use multiple soothing strategies at the same time, for example monotonous sounds, movement and swaddling, as this has been shown to be more effective (Korner 1974).

Pamphlet: 'Your midwife's advice on settling your crying baby'

Repeat the following steps until your baby settles

- Wait until the infant has been crying for at least 15 seconds in his cot.
- Lean over the infant and keep talking continuously.
- Place your hand on the infant's stomach, holding his arms against his chest.
- Pick him up and hold him in your arms.
- In addition to holding him, rock him in your arms.

These can be repeated with several episodes of crying (Blackburn 1980).

Other ways to settle your crying baby

Soothing movements

- Use slow, calm, deliberate movements in caring for your baby. A warm, firm touch tells your baby that you are confident and that he can relax, feel safe and secure, and trust you.
- Carry, hold and walk with your baby.

- Use a sling to carry your baby close to your body.
- Try monotonous, steady movement, for example rocking or swinging the baby.
- A bumpy pram ride or car ride may help.
- Hold or carry your baby in a position that puts gentle but firm pressure on his abdomen (placing him over your hip, arm or shoulder).
- Lie the baby on his stomach on your lap while you gently bounce your knees or move them back and forth.
- Rock in a rocking chair to relax you and your baby.
- Use a baby swing for times when individual attention is not possible.

Soothing touching

- Give your baby a warm relaxation bath, or take a bath together.
- Rub your baby's back.
- Massage the baby for 15 minutes (the baby may fuss during the massage but will usually become quiet afterwards).
- Close skin-to-skin contact with either parent can help to soothe the baby.
- Have the baby sleep or nap with you to gain comfort from your body warmth and heartbeat.

Soothing sounds

- Create a background of constant rhythmic stimulation such as constant, soft, soothing music. Alternatively, set up a monotonous sound by running a vacuum cleaner, dishwasher and so on, or play a tape recording of these sounds.
- Talk or sing to the baby in a soft voice.

Soothing feeding

- Feed your baby in a quiet, dark room.
- Use only one breast per feed to ensure that the infant receives the fat-containing hindmilk (as taught in your breast-feeding session).
- Burp the baby often during feeding, for example before offering the second breast. Take as long as necessary to burp after feeding.
- You may choose to use a dummy when feeding is well established and baby is well fed and still fussy.
- If the baby is still unsettled and crying and if you are breast-feeding, reduce the amount of caffeine in your diet (coffee, tea and cola). Chamomile tea is a soothing alternative.

Soothing sleep

- Ensure that your baby's room is dimly lit or dark. In winter, a lambskin or flannel sheet could be used and the bed warmed with a heating pad or hot water bottle before putting baby to bed (but *do not* allow baby to become overheated).
- As a last resort, allow baby to cry himself to sleep (for a very short time only).

(Hunziker & Barr 1986, Korner 1974, Blackburn 1980, Wenner & Barnard 1980, Fisher 1981, Minchin 1985, Sears 1985, Elliot et al 1988, Kitzinger 1989, Royal College of Midwives 1989, Barr 1990, Pinyerd 1992b, Drummond et al 1994).

MINI SESSION: INFANT COLIC
Objective

- Specifically, the parents will recognize the signs of infant colic and know where to get help.

Important teaching points

- Tell the parents that colic occurs in up to 25% of infants during the first 3 months.
- Emphasize that the cause is unclear and the condition improves over time.

Midwives' teaching notes

Infant colic

Infantile colic has also been called primary excessive crying or irritable infant syndrome and the infants described as relentless criers or incessantly crying infants. In diagnosing infant colic, the rule of three may be used: the crying occurs during the first 3 months of life, and the infant cries for more than 3 hours a day, for 3 days or more in 1 week, for more than 3 weeks (Wessel et al 1954).

Although colic occurs in up to 25% of infants, the cause remains unclear and the natural history is one of improvement over time. Some researchers have argued that a cause and cure for colic are unlikely to be found and have suggested that persistent crying may be something an infant 'does' rather than something it 'has' (Barr et al 1991).

Researchers have found the following:

- Babies with colic are no different from babies without colic in terms of the following: socio-economic status, birth order, gender, maternal anxiety rating, type of feeding (breast or artificial milk) or family history of allergy.
- On average, colic is present from 2 until 12 weeks of age, but in some infants it may persist until 6 months of age.
- The infant may be well nourished and otherwise healthy.

- Infants cry substantially more than is average for their age, prolonged crying bouts occurring particularly in the late afternoon and evening.
- In some infants, crying bouts last for more than 6 hours.
- Infants with colic spend more time in an awake/ alert state, sleep less, wake more at night and are much more difficult to console than other infants.
- The presence of symptoms that suggest pain may include drawing up the legs, kicking, holding the body stiff, clenching the fists, waving the arms purposelessly and passing gas rectally.

(Barr 1990, 1993, Carey 1990, Covington et al 1991, Hewat 1992, Pinyerd 1992b, Parkin et al 1993, Field 1994, Jacobson & Melvin 1995, Keefe et al 1996).

MINI SESSION: CRYING AND THE MOTHER'S NEEDS

Objective

- Specifically, the new mother will recognize the importance of time away from a crying baby and of resting when her infant is sleeping.

Important teaching points

- Emphasize the importance of the mother caring for herself.
- Discuss ways of increasing rest and relaxation opportunities.
- Encourage mothers to discuss their feelings about infant crying.
- If possible copy the pamphlet 'Your midwife's advice on surviving the early weeks' (see Chapter 10) and go through this with the parents.

Midwives' teaching notes

The mother's needs

(The new mother's needs and strategies to increase rest and relaxation are discussed more fully in Chapter 10.)

On occasions, there may be a need for physical distance from a crying infant while at the same time maintaining a presence. When a baby becomes upset, parents may sometimes become tense and frustrated by his behaviour. The sensitive baby may pick up on this tension and cry even more. If this occurs, there is a need to break the cycle. To do this, suggest that the mother go off in a room by herself for several minutes until she feels calmer.

As the mother is doubtless lacking sleep, insist that she sleeps or rests when the baby does. In addition, suggest that the father takes care of the baby while she goes to bed early in the evening (waking her for feeding as needed). Also, encourage the mother to leave the baby with other relatives or friends to give her some relief for several hours.

Where possible, give mothers the opportunity to talk about their feelings, for example anger, frustration and inadequacy. Encourage the mother to get together with other mothers so that she is aware that things will improve.

MINI SESSION: COMMUNITY RESOURCES FOR INFANT CRYING

Objective

- The new parents will be aware of community resources that help with infant crying, particularly when parents feel that it is excessive.

Important teaching points

- Inform women of all local community resources that help with infant crying.
- If possible, give women a written list of local community resources.

Midwives' teaching notes

Community resources

As with breastfeeding, it is essential to inform new mothers of all available community resources that help with infant crying. Again, these obviously vary from country to country but will include health visitors (community child health nurses/public health nurses).

When infant crying does not stop following the standard repertoire of cuddling, feeding and changing, help is essential for parents. As discussed earlier, infant crying can have far-reaching negative effects on parents.

CONCLUSION

In conclusion, there are several important things to remember about infant crying. On average, newborn crying takes up about 2 out of 24 hours, increasing to about 3 hours a day and peaking at around 6 weeks of age before decreasing. Babies have both physical and emotional needs: attention from adults is as important as having their physical needs met. Remember that when cries are answered during the first year of life, babies cry less at 1 year of age.

Babies, like adults, are all different, and newborns vary in how easily they can console themselves or be soothed by others. As described above, there are a number of ways to settle a crying baby. Rocking and swinging movements are particularly effective, and using multiple soothing strategies together is best.

Because being with a crying baby can be a tremendous strain, mothers should not feel guilty about leaving him with other relatives or friends while they have a break. After all, parents are only human. Community resources also exist to help mothers with a crying infant. Encourage parents to use these without feeling inadequate or guilty.

And finally, when people give unwanted advice, suggest that parents accept it, nod, smile and go their own way. Rest assured, it is not possible to 'spoil' a young crying baby by picking him up.

INFANT SLEEP AND ACTIVITY PATTERNS

During the early weeks after birth, the infant's age-appropriate, yet unusual, patterns of behaviour certainly change the lives of his parents (Wenner & Barnard 1980). In particular, sleep behaviour can effect the parent's sense of well-being and their views of their baby (Klinnert & Bingham 1994).

Providing information about their infant's sleep patterns will help exhausted parents to accept the disruptions that arrive with a new baby. Waking in the night (although still difficult for parents) will be seen as normal rather than evidence of a problem. Such information may also allow parents to understand and take pleasure in the progress as their baby matures (Wenner & Barnard 1980).

In addition, investigators have identified six sleep and awake states of the infant: deep sleep, light sleep, drowsiness, quiet alert, active alert and crying. Infants respond in a unique and predictable manner during each state.

Spending valuable time teaching parents about these infant states may seem like a luxury that midwives cannot afford (given the enormous demands on their time). However, knowing about these states really helps parents to meet their infants' needs (Wolff 1966, Parmalee & Stern 1972, Prechtl 1974, Blackburn 1980). At the very least, I would suggest that the midwife gives parents a brief written overview of these.

Sumner (1995) argued that when parents are able to understand and interpret their newborn infant's behaviour, they find that getting to know their infant is a marvellous experience. Sumner also discussed 'The Keys to

CaregivinG program', a video series for expectant parents (appropriate during the sixth and seventh months of pregnancy). Both first-time and experienced parents found the series helpful, experienced parents commenting 'If I had only known this when I had my first child.'

Key issues in discussing infant sleep include:

- normal infant sleep patterns during the early months of life;
- infant sleep and activity states and what these mean for parents as they care for their infants;
- being able to use different strategies to encourage sleep;
- the mother recognizing the importance of resting while her infant sleeps;
- knowing about and being able to access community resources.

MINI SESSION: NORMAL INFANT SLEEP PATTERNS

Objective

- The new parents will have an increased knowledge of normal infant sleep patterns during the early months of life.

Important teaching points

- Discuss normal sleep patterns in babies, in particular that average full-term newborns sleep for about 15–16 hours out of each 24 hours.
- Emphasize that individual sleeping patterns vary: a colicky baby may sleep for only 8 out of 24 hours, while a placid baby may sleep for 20 hours.
- Emphasize that longer periods of sleep ensue as the baby's central nervous system matures and that this is not affected by feeding type or solid foods.

Midwives' teaching notes

Infant sleep patterns

Several investigators have gathered information by asking mothers to record their babies' waking and sleeping patterns over the first year of life. These figures provide a very useful baseline for new parents. However, it is important to emphasize that individual sleeping patterns vary: an extremely colicky baby may sleep for as few as 8 hours out of each 24 hour period, while a placid baby may sleep as many as 20 hours (Lauwers & Woessner 1990).

Overall, the research has shown that, although the

total amount of sleep hardly decreases over the first year of life, the infant's sleep and activity patterns during the first few months of life are different from his behaviour after this time. These researchers reported the following:

- Infants younger than 3 months of age sleep an average 15–16 hours out of 24 h. About 35% sleep for 6 hours continuously at night.
- In newborns, sleep/wake states alternate in 3–4 hour cycles, and wakefulness is the same regardless of day or night.
- Within the first month, sleep/wake states begin to adapt to the light/dark cycle and to regularly recurring social cues from care-givers.
- Sleeping through the night requires neurological growth (nervous system development). On average, infants can be expected to waken at least twice a night for the first 3 months.
- During the first 16 weeks of life, infants show a steady ability to sleep for longer periods. By 3–4 months old, more sleep for 6 hours at night.
- By 6 months of age, the longest continuous sleep period is 6 hours at night. The infant may sleep for two 6-hour periods interrupted by a brief awakening.
- As the central nervous system matures, the length of continuous sleep increases to about 10–11 hours at night. There is no relationship between the increased length of sleep and the commencement of solid foods or type of feeding.
- Infants also showed a steady but slower increase in staying awake for longer. Wakeful periods shift to the daytime and lengthen, being interrupted by brief periods of sleep.
- The earlier fragmented patterns of sleep and wakefulness are gradually replaced by patterns more like those of an adult. Waking time increases during daylight hours, and sleep increases at night until most sleep is at night, except for one or two daytime naps.
- The total amount of sleep decreases relatively little and gradually during the first year of life. By 12 months of age, the average infant still sleeps for 14–15 hours out of 24.

(Parmalee et al 1964, Blackburn 1980, Anders & Keener 1985, Michelsson et al 1990, Anders 1994, Sumner 1995).

Premature infants

The sleep patterns of prematurely born infants are very different from those of term infants. The parents of these infants are even more at risk of exhaustion from interrupted sleep patterns and need special consideration. Researchers have suggested that sleep may be very important in showing the level of maturity of the infants' central nervous systems: as gestational age increases, sleep patterns become more organized (Wenner & Barnard 1980, D'Apolito 1991).

News flash for later in the first year!

Although the amount of parental sleep increases after the first few months, some parents of typically developing new babies have interrupted sleep patterns caused by child awakenings during most of the first year after the birth. Although there is a decrease in the number of night awakenings at 3–6 months, there may well be an increase at 9 months.

Scher (1991) found that regular night wakening was a common characteristic during the first year. At 3 months, 46% of babies woke during the night. This decreased to 39% at 6 months but increased to 58% at 9 months, remaining at 55% at 12 months.

MINI SESSION: SLEEP AND ACTIVITY STATES

Objective

- Parents will be aware of normal infant sleep and activity states and how these influence care.

Important teaching points

- Discuss the six different sleep and activity states.
- Emphasize that the way in which infants respond and what they can do (e.g. feed or play) is strongly influenced by their state of consciousness.

Midwives's teaching notes

Sleep and activity states

Investigators have identified six sleep/awake states of the infant. These states are deep sleep, light sleep, drowsiness, quiet alert, active alert and crying (Wolff 1966, Parmalee & Stern 1972, Prechtl 1974, Blackburn 1980, Sumner 1995).

During these different states, body activity, eye movements, breathing pattern and the infant's level of response all differ. The way in which infants respond to their parents is strongly influenced by their state of consciousness.

Deep sleep. During deep or quiet sleep, infants lie nearly still except for occasional startles or twitches. There are no facial or eye movements, respiration is smooth and regular, and infants may have occasional bursts of sucking in which there are several sucking movements in a row at regular intervals.

In this state infants are unresponsive, and only very intense and disturbing stimuli can arouse them. The baby should not be fed at this time as, even if he is aroused briefly, he will not suck or swallow well, so feeding will not be a positive experience.

Light sleep. Light sleep accounts for the highest proportion of newborn sleep and usually precedes wakening. This state is also called active sleep or REM sleep because of the rapid eye movements that occur. During light sleep, infants display more body and face movements than in deep sleep, with irregular respiration and occasional smiles. They also may make brief fussing or crying sounds.

In this state, infants are more responsive to stimuli such as hunger or being handled than when they are in deep sleep. Because of this, parents may think that their infants are awake and try to feed them before they are ready to eat.

Drowsiness. In the drowsy state, infants' eyes may flutter and occasionally open, but they are usually closed, with a glazed, heavy-lidded and dull appearance. Breathing patterns are irregular and activity level is variable, with mild occasional startles.

From the drowsy state, infants may return to sleep or awaken further. If infants are left alone, they may return to a sleep state. If parents wish to wake the infant, they can provide something for infants to see, hear or suck. These activities may arouse them to a quiet alert state when they will be more responsive to feeding.

Quiet alert. During the quiet alert state, body activity is minimal and breathing regular. The infant's face has a bright, shining, sparkling look, with brightening and widening of the eyes. As infants become older, they will spend more and more time in this state.

During this state, infants give much pleasure and positive feedback. They are most attentive to their surroundings and open to play and stimulation. Infants will focus their attention on any stimuli that are present, for example the nipple, voices, a face or moving objects. If parents provide something for them to see, hear or suck, this will often maintain a quiet alert state or help infants to enter a quiet alert state from either a drowsy or an active alert state.

Active alert. During the active alert state, infants' eyes are open, but their eyes and faces are not as bright as in quiet alert. Infants are more fidgety, with increased body activity and facial movement. Their breathing patterns are irregular. Infants may become more active and start to cry.

In the active alert state, infants are more sensitive to hunger, fatigue, noise, excessive handling and stimulation. To avoid crying, they need the parent to interrupt this state in a quite calm way, allowing them to return to a state of lower arousal.

Crying. Crying is an infant state that is easily recognized. It is characterized by intense crying for at least 15 seconds. During this state, infants cry, grimace, change colour and display increased motor activity.

Crying is a communication signal and is often a response to such things as fatigue, hunger or discomfort. It tells us that the infants' limits have been reached. Sometimes, infants can console themselves and return to a lower state; at other times, they need help.

MINI SESSION: ENCOURAGING INFANT SLEEP

Objective

- The parents will be able to use different strategies to encourage infant sleep.

Important teaching points

- Discuss strategies to encourage sleep, particularly at night.
- If possible, give parents a copy of the pamphlet 'Your midwife's advice on helping your baby sleep' to refer to while you are speaking.
- Emphasize the importance of not overheating the baby (see the mini session on SIDS below).
- If available, show a video on the relaxation baby bath technique or baby massage (if it has not been used in a previous session).

Midwives' teaching notes

Pamphlet: 'Your midwife's advice on helping your baby sleep'. Other information is found in Parmalee & Stern (1972), Prechtl (1974), Blackburn (1980), Sears (1985, 1988) and Lauwers & Wessner (1990).

Sleeping area

- Your baby's room can be dimly lit or dark. In winter, flannel sheets could be used and the bed warmed *before* putting the baby in. *However, it is very important that your baby does not become overheated while sleeping.*
- Overtiredness or overstimulation can cause fretfulness.

- Loud sounds, bright lights, a room that is too hot or cold and too much bedding can interfere with sleep.

Feeding

- As hunger is satisfied, infants often move to a quiet alert state.
- Milk is the ideal food for encouraging a baby to sleep well. When adults experience restless sleep, warm milk is usually suggested.
- Do not give cereal at night: it does not encourage baby to sleep for longer but it can cause indigestion and further encourage wakefulness.
- Changing from breast milk to artificial milk will not help your baby to sleep through the night; this happens as your baby matures.

Reduce your caffeine intake

- If you are breast-feeding and your baby still seems to have trouble sleeping, you may need to reduce the amount of caffeine in your diet (from coffee, tea and soft drinks). Chamomile tea is a soothing alternative.

Encourage night sleep

- During the first month, your baby will begin to adapt to the light/dark cycle and to things that usually happen at different times of the day and night.
- However, some babies still confuse day and night, sleeping for longer periods during the day and staying awake at night.
- Gradually get your baby to reverse this pattern by encouraging more frequent feeds during the day and reducing all activity and stimulation during nighttime feeds.
- At night, feed in a dim, warm room, and avoid disturbance at the end of the feed by changing the nappy before feeding on the second breast.
- As your baby develops and has fulfilled sucking needs during the day, he or she will find it easier to sleep for longer periods at night.

Routine

- Quiet soothing activities just before bedtime, for example a bath, rocking and nursing, may help your baby to sleep.
- As your baby gets older, a bedtime ritual such as a bath or story can help him or her to go to sleep at about the same time every night.

Swaddling

- Infants often react with calmness and drowsiness to total body restraint.

MINI SESSION: MOTHER'S SLEEP AND REST
Objective

- The new mother will recognize the importance of resting when her infant is sleeping.

Important teaching points

- Emphasize the importance of the mother caring for herself.
- Discuss ways of increasing rest and relaxation opportunities.
- If possible, copy the pamphlet 'Your midwife's advice on surviving the early weeks' and go through this with the parents.

Midwives' teaching notes

The mother's rest needs

(The new mother's needs and strategies to increase rest and relaxation are discussed more fully in Chapter 10.)

Remind mothers of strategies to ensure that they have some sleep. The sleep patterns of new babies usually result in sleep deprivation for parents, with resulting ongoing fatigue. Recommend strongly that the mother sleeps when the baby does during the day. In addition, suggest that the father cares for the baby while the mother goes to bed early in the evening, awakening her for feeding. Also, encourage the mother to leave the baby with other relatives or friends to give her a break.

MINI SESSION: COMMUNITY RESOURCES FOR INFANT SLEEP DIFFICULTIES
Objective

- The parents will know of and be able to access community resources that can help with sleep difficulty.

Important teaching points

- Inform women of all local community resources that are available to help with infant sleep problems.
- If possible, give women a written list of resources in their area.

Midwives' teaching notes

Community resources

As with breast-feeding and infant crying, it is essential that you, the parents' midwife, inform them of all available community resources that may help with infant sleep problems. Again, these obviously vary from country to country but will include health visitors (or community child health nurses/public health nurses).

CONCLUSION

In conclusion, newborn babies sleep for on average about 15–16 hours in a 24 hour period. However, a baby with colic may sleep as few as 8 hours and a placid baby as many as 20. Although the amount of sleep does not vary much during the first year, the infant's sleep patterns during the first months of life are quite different from those later in the first year. As their nervous system develops, infants learn to distinguish between day and night, and also gradually sleep for longer periods.

Infants also pass through several different infant sleep and awake states (deep sleep, light sleep, drowsiness, quiet alert, active alert and crying). These states affect infant response; for example, in deep sleep, they will not feed well, but while in the quiet alert state they are most attentive and responsive, and give much pleasure to parents.

There are several ways of encouraging infant sleep. These include feeding or swaddling the infant and ensuring that his room is warm and dimly lit or dark. When telling parents about these strategies, it is very important to emphasize the importance of not overheating the baby (see the mini session on SIDS below for more detail). It is also essential that the mother rests and sleeps when the baby is sleeping during the day.

SUDDEN INFANT DEATH SYNDROME

'Reducing the risks of SIDS' programmes were introduced in many countries during the early 1990s, resulting in a change from prone to side- or back-sleeping. This change was associated with the predicted reduction in SIDS rates by about 50–70% (Dwyer & Ponsonby 1996).

However, such deaths remain the largest single group of deaths in infants between 1 week and 1 year old (Wigfield & Fleming 1995). A study of infants in the UK born since the development of the recommendations against prone sleeping indicate that this is still a major risk factor (Fleming et al 1996). In Western Australia, SIDS remains the principal cause of death for indigenous infants (Alessandri et al 1996).

It appears that most midwives and health visitors already incorporate the following teachings into their work with new parents. To assist in this, I have provided a summary of the latest findings on SIDS from around the world. This review includes recommendations from:

- The 1996 Third Annual Report of the United Kingdom Confidential Enquiry into Stillbirths and Deaths in Infancy (CESDI) (CESDI 1996);
- The 1997 multidisciplinary forum convened by the National SIDS Council of Australia to review recent evidence concerning risk factors of SIDS and to revise the guidelines where appropriate (Henderson-Smart et al 1998).

MINI SESSION: SUDDEN INFANT DEATH SYNDROME

Key issues in encouraging preventing SIDS include the importance of:

- putting the infant on his back to sleep;
- making sure that the infant's head remains uncovered during sleep;
- not allowing the baby to become too hot or too cold;
- keeping baby in a smoke-free zone before and after the birth;
- the parents not bed-sharing (sleeping with) baby if they smoke;
- breast-feeding in relation to SIDS;
- knowing about and being able to access community resources.

Objective

- The parents will know the positive things that they can do to reduce the risk of their baby experiencing SIDS.

Important teaching points

- Discuss and provide parents with written information on reducing the risk of SIDS.
- If possible, use a doll to demonstrate the best way for baby to sleep.
- Inform women of community resources that can advise on the prevention of SIDS and give parents a pamphlet (or a copy of Fig 17.8 below) that shows these preventive measures.

Midwives' teaching notes

Back sleeping position

It is very important that you recommend that parents place the baby *on his back* for sleeping as there is strong evidence that the risk of SIDS is higher when infants sleep prone. Reviews of SIDS research by Beal & Finch (1991) and Dwyer & Ponsonby (1996) (including more than 19 retrospective case-control studies) found a threefold or greater increased risk of SIDS when infants slept in the prone position.

Many parents may need to be reassured that placing their baby on his back to sleep is safe. They may, for example, be concerned about vomiting and choking. Parents can be reassured that:

- in Asian countries, where babies traditionally sleep on their backs, aspiration is not a problem (Beal & Porter 1991);
- in England, there has been no increase in the number of aspiration deaths following the change in sleeping position from prone to supine (Fleming 1994);
- infants are at the greatest risk of choking if they vomit when sleeping face down (Fleming 1994, Katwinkel et al 1994);
- in Tasmania, infants with an increased risk of SIDS (who sleep supine) do not have increased rates of apnoea or cyanosis (Ponsonby et al 1997).

Side-sleeping. There is a smaller but significantly increased risk of SIDS when infants are placed on their sides rather than their backs to sleep. The following evidence is of relevance here:

- Ponsonby et al (1995) found no difference in the risk of SIDS between the side- and back-sleeping positions.
- However, Mitchell et al (1992, 1997) and Fleming et al (1996) reported a significantly higher risk of SIDS with the side-sleeping position.

The side-sleeping position is only safe if parents are certain the baby cannot roll into the prone position while sleeping. If parents decide to place baby on his side, they must make sure that his lower arm is well forward to prevent him rolling onto his tummy.

Foot to foot with head uncovered

The next important recommendation for parents is to make sure their *baby's head does not become covered* during sleep. In teaching this section, a practical demonstration using a doll is ideal. It is also beneficial to refer parents to an appropriate SIDS brochure or to Figure 17.8 and go through this with them.

Suggest that parents (CESDI 1996, Henderson-Smart et al 1998):

1. place their baby with his feet close to or touching the bottom of the cot;
2. tuck their baby in firmly so that he cannot move around freely and slip under the covers (as loose bedding can cover the baby's head);
3. avoid quilts, duvets, pillows, soft toys and cot bumpers during the first year;
4. do not cover baby's head with a hat or bonnet while sleeping;
5. use a firm, clean and well-fitting mattress;
6. do not place the baby to sleep on a beanbag or water bed.

Researchers have found that:

- a proportion of SIDS infants are discovered with their faces covered by bedding (Wilson et al 1994, Beal & Byard 1995, Fleming et al 1996);
- covering infants with duvets or quilts has also been associated with a higher risk of SIDS (Fleming et al 1996);
- firm wrapping was protective among infants sleeping in their own cot (who were not bed-sharing) (Wilson et al 1994);
- swaddling was not associated with an increased SIDS rate for side- or back-sleeping babies but had an adverse effect on prone-sleeping infants (Ponsonby et al 1993).

Baby being too hot or too cold

It is also important that parents make sure their baby *does not become either too hot or too cold*: both hyperthermia and hypothermia increase the risk of SIDS in young babies. Parents can be advised to clothe their babies very much as they would themselves, so that they are comfortably warm but not hot.

Researchers have reported the following:

- When thick clothing and bedding are used, the head (particularly the face), becomes the main route for heat loss (Nelson et al 1989). Sleeping in the prone position makes it more difficult for this to happen, and infants are more likely to become overheated.
- Two early studies found that heavy clothing and bedding, and room heating, were associated with SIDS when prone-sleeping was more common (Fleming et al 1990, Ponsonby et al 1992).
- In Williams et al's (1996) research, infants in the prone position were more vulnerable to the effects

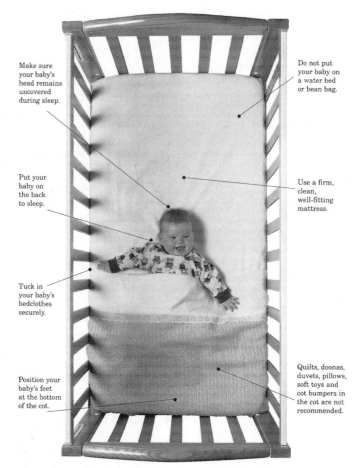

Make sure your baby's head remains uncovered during sleep.

Do not put your baby on a water bed or bean bag.

Put your baby on the back to sleep.

Use a firm, clean, well-fitting mattress.

Tuck in your baby's bedclothes securely.

Position your baby's feet at the bottom of the cot.

Quilts, doonas, duvets, pillows, soft toys and cot bumpers in the cot are not recommended.

Figure 17.8 Recommended sleeping position. (National SIDS Foundation of Australia, with permission.)

of overinsulation and SIDS, while for infants who slept supine, there was a relationship between SIDS and underinsulation.

Smoke-free zone

It is extremely important that parents are informed that *cigarette smoking increases the risk of SIDS*. The risk is increased if the mother smokes during pregnancy, and if fathers smoke while the mother is pregnant, the risk increases again. If both parents smoke, the risk is doubled.

As with parents who chose not to breast-feed, it is also very important not to criticize or judge parents who smoke. It is quite likely that they may already feel ill at ease if they smoke; certainly in Australia, smoking has become an 'antisocial' activity. Nevertheless, it is important that parents make an *informed* decision about

the effects of smoking on their baby that is based on up-to-date information and research. It is also important to provide parents with details of structured supportive programmes that can help them to stop smoking.

Research evidence is as follows:

- Reviews of SIDS research by Mitchell et al (1995) and Golding (1997) (including more than 30 case-control and cohort studies) found an increased risk of SIDS when babies were exposed to cigarette smoke.
- A recent UK study (Blair et al 1996) found that the incidence of SIDS was greater when mothers smoked during pregnancy. This increased further if fathers smoked, and increased again if the parents smoked in the house after the birth.
- The proportion of risk attributed to smoking is now higher than that reported before the reduction of prone-sleeping (Mitchell et al 1995).

Bed-sharing and SIDS

Co-sleeping, or bed-sharing, is associated with an increased risk of SIDS *when mothers smoke* (Mitchell et al 1992, Blair et al 1996, Fleming et al 1996). At the present time, there has not been shown to be a significantly increased risk of SIDS when the parents do not smoke. However, it is important that adult pillows or bedclothes do not cover the baby's head as this could cause overheating or asphyxia.

Breast-feeding and SIDS

At the present time, the research findings on the relationship between breast-feeding and the risk of SIDS are not consistent, and it is up to the midwife to decide whether to include this portion of the mini session when teaching parents.

The following evidence has been reported:

- The findings of one USA study (Hoffman et al 1988) and one New Zealand study (Ford et al 1993) suggested that breast-feeding was protective for SIDS.
- However, Kraus et al (1989) found that the protec-

Pointers for practice

- Of all health professionals, midwives have most to do with women before and after the birth and are ideally placed to help men and women get to know their baby.
- As you help men and women to become parents at the dawn of the new century, emphasize 'the time after the birth is over' as much as the birth itself, and try to get prospective parents to do the same.
- Anticipate the needs of new mothers in your care and volunteer information as new parents may not know what to ask.
- Enable parents to make decisions about different aspects of their baby's care by giving them the information they need to do this.
- As far as possible, base your advice on normative data with respect to breast-feeding, infant crying and infant sleeping and activity states.
- Try not to give parents inconsistent advice; giving information that is based on research findings helps to keep things more consistent. Present alternatives not as being 'right' or 'wrong' but instead as different things that can be tried.
- Where possible, provide continuity of care when teaching parents how to care for their baby.
- Work smarter not harder; groups are a really cost-effective way of teaching parents as well as helping parents to get to know each other.

Activities

1. Identify community resources available to assist with problems related to breast-feeding, crying or colic and sleep, particularly outside health visiting (community child health/public health nurse) clinic hours. These may include child health residential facilities, outreach or day programmes, and after-hours emergency telephone lines.
2. Obtain information on structured support programmes that can help parents to stop smoking.
3. Make a list of these community resources for your area that includes the telephone number and address. Give this list to parents before they are discharged from midwifery care.
4. Contact your local SIDS service and obtain appropiate leaflets on the prevention of SIDS if these are available. Such pamphlets usually include a contact telephone number to call in the event of SIDS.
5. Find out where to buy a baby sling and its cost. If a cheaper alternative is needed, investigate how to make one. Learn how to demonstrate the tying and use of a baby sling.
6. Identify appropriate videos on breast-feeding, settling crying infants, relaxation baby bath techniques and baby massage.
7. Find out whether your hospital has dolls that can be used in antenatal classes to allow demonstrations of the positioning and attachment of the baby on the breast or of holding and comforting an unsettled baby. Are there sufficient dolls to allow individual parents to practise these skills while being supervised?
8. If you are a student, get together with colleagues and practise using the dolls to help your practical skills at teaching breast-feeding and settling strategies.
9. Ask someone whether you and a colleague can review the 'preparation for parenthood' component of your antenatal classes. Could you use or adapt some of the mini sessions included in this chapter?
10. If you are a student midwife, negotiate with your lecturers to do some of the above as an assignment.

---

tive effect of breast-feeding was reduced after adjustment for maternal education or birth weight, and in a UK study (Fleming et al 1996), breast-feeding was not associated with a significantly altered risk of SIDS after socio-economic status and other factors were taken into account.

- Breast-feeding was not found to be protective in a Tasmanian study (Ponsonby et al 1995) and a UK study (Gilbert et al 1995).

However, I agree with Henderson-Smart et al's (1998) observations as follows:

1. The first two studies (that found breastfeeding protective) had larger samples and were therefore able to detect quite small effects of breastfeeding on SIDS.

2. The smaller size of the latter two studies (Gilbert et al 1995, Ponsonby et al 1995) may have led to inadequate statistical power to detect slight protective effects of breast-feeding (at $P < 0.05$).

CONCLUSION

In this chapter, I have not attempted to cover all aspects of caring for a baby. Instead, I have included those topics which are of most concern to many parents during the first few months after the birth. With respect to breast-feeding, infant crying, sleeping and activity states, I have provided information about normal infant behaviour during the first year of life. This information should be particularly valuable to new parents during the early weeks as they struggle to get to know the puzzling new little person in their lives (one who arrived without an instruction manual).

Although there is a broad range of normal behaviour, and all infants (like adults) are individuals, giving parents some idea of what to expect can only be positive. Armed with this knowledge, they are less likely to be the victims of the many myths about parenthood that we discuss in Chapter 10. They are also less likely to feel guilty when their baby feeds frequently, cries frequently and wakes frequently.

SIDS has been included because teaching parents a few simple things about their infant's care can reduce the number of deaths. Moreover, it remains the principal cause of death for Indigenous infants in Western Australia.

REFERENCES

Acebo C, Thoman E B 1992 Crying as social behaviour. Infant Mental Health Journal 13(1): 67–82
Ainsworth M D S, Blehar M C, Waters E, Wall S 1978 Patterns of attachment: a psychological study of the strange situation. Lawrence Erlbaum, Hillsdale, NJ
Alessandri L M, Read A W, Eades S, Gurrin L, Cooke C 1996 Recent sudden infant death syndrome rate in aboriginal and non-aboriginal infants. Journal of Sudden Infant Death Syndrome and Infant Mortality 1: 315–19
Aloia J F, Cohn S H, Vaswani A 1985 Risk factors for postmenopausal osteoporosis. American Medical Journal 78: 95–100
Anders T F 1994 Infant sleep, nighttime relationships, and attachment. Psychiatry 57(1): 11–21
Anders T, Keener M 1985 Developmental course of nighttime sleep–wake patterns in full-term and pre-term infants during the first year of life. Sleep 8: 173–92
Anderson A M 1996 The father–infant relationship: becoming connected. Journal of the Society of Pediatric Nursing 1(2): 83–92
Aniansson G, Alm B, Andersson B et al 1994 A prospective cohort study on breastfeeding and otitis media in Swedish infants. Pediatric Infectious Disease Journal 13: 183–8
Astbury J, Brown S, Lumley J, Small R 1994 Birth events, birth experiences and social differences in postnatal depression. Australian Journal of Public Health 18(2): 176–84
Bailey V F, Sherriff J 1992 Reasons for the early cessation of breastfeeding in women from lower socio-economic groups in Perth, Western Australia. Australian Journal of Nutrition and Dietetics 49(2): 40–3
Ball J A 1982 Stress and the postnatal care of women. Nursing Times 78(45): 1904–7
Ball J A 1984 Adaptations to motherhood. Nursing (London) 2(21): 623–4
Ball J A 1987 Reactions to motherhood: the role of postnatal care. Cambridge University Press, Cambridge
Barclay L, Everitt L, Rogan F, Schmied V, Wyllie A 1997 Becoming a mother – an analysis of women's experience of early motherhood. Journal of Advanced Nursing 25: 719–28
Barnett B 1991 Coping with postnatal depression. Lothian, Port Melbourne
Barr R G 1990 The 'colic' enigma: prolonged episodes of a normal predisposition to cry. Infant Mental Health Journal 11(4): 340–8
Barr R G 1993 Normality: a clinically useless concept: the case of infant crying and colic. Developmental and Behavioral Pediatrics 14(4): 264–70
Barr R G, Kramer M S, Pless I B, Boisjoly C, Leduc D 1989 Feeding and temperament as determinants of early infant cry/fuss behavior. Pediatrics 84: 514–21
Barr R G, McMullan S J, Spiess H et al 1991 Carrying as colic 'therapy': a randomized controlled trial. Pediatrics 87: 623–30
Beal S M, Byard R W 1995 Accidental death or sudden infant death syndrome? Journal of Paediatric Child Health 31: 269–71
Beal S M, Finch C F 1991 An overview of retrospective case-control studies investigating the relationship between prone sleeping position and SIDS. Journal of Paediatric Child Health 27: 334–9
Beal S M, Porter C 1991 Sudden infant death syndrome related to climate. Acta Paediatrica Scandinavica 80: 278–87
Beck M 1989 Breast-feeding: the midwife's role. Midwives Chronicle and Nursing Notes (December): 412–14
Becker G E 1992 Breastfeeding knowledge of hospital staff in rural maternity units in Ireland. Journal of Human Lactation 8(3): 137–42
Belsky J 1980 Child maltreatment: an ecological integration. American Psychologist 35: 320–35

Bennett V R, Brown L K (eds) 1993 Myles' textbook for midwives, 12th edn. Churchill Livingstone, Edinburgh

Berger R G 1986 Psychology in paediatrics and childcare. In: Rachman S (ed.) Contributions to medical psychology, vol. 1. Pergamon Press, Oxford

Berry S J 1988 The role of maternal expectations and infant characteristics in the transition to parenthood. Dissertation Abstracts International 48 (12-B, part 1): 3669

Blackburn S 1980 Individual differences in infant behaviour. In: Barnard K E (ed.) NCAST II learner manual. NCAST Publications, Seattle, Washington

Blair P S, Fleming P J, Bensley D et al 1996 Smoking and the sudden infant death syndrome: results from 1993–5 case-control study for confidential inquiry into stillbirths and deaths in infancy. British Medical Journal 313: 195–8

Bono B 1992 Assessment and documentation for the breastfeeding couple by health care professionals. Journal of Human Lactation 8: 17–22

Bottorff J L 1990 Persistence in breastfeeding: a phenomenological investigation. Journal of Advanced Nursing 15: 201–9

Bragg M 1991 The effect of delivery room routines on success of first breastfeed. MIDIRS Midwifery Digest 1(1): 73

Brazelton T B 1962 Crying in infancy. Pediatrics 29: 579–88

Brazelton T 1985 Application of cry research to clinical perspective. In: Lester B, Boukydis C (eds) Infant crying: theoretical and research perspectives. Plenum Press, New York

Buchko B, Pugh L, Bishop B, Cochran J, Smith L, Lerew D 1994 Comfort measures in breastfeeding, primiparous women. Journal of Obstetric, Gynaecological and Neonatal Nursing 23(1): 46–51

Buss H, Plomin R 1975 A temperament theory of personality development. Wiley-Interscience, New York

Carey W B 1990 Infantile colic: a pediatric practitioner-researcher's point of view. Infant Mental Health Journal 11: 334–9

Carter D, Mason L 1989 Health visitors' perceptions of normal infant behaviour. Health Visitor 62(2): 56–7

CESDI (Confidential Enquiry into Stillbirths and Deaths in Infancy) 1996 Third annual report concentrating on the first two years of combined studies on: sudden unexpected deaths in infancy. Department of Health, London

Coles E R 1983 A study of sleeping patterns and its results. Midwife, Health Visitor and Community Nurse 19(8): 322, 324–6

Cooke M 1996 Mothers' experience of infant feeding: a new theory. In Barclay L, Jones L (eds) Midwifery: trends in clinical practice. Churchill Livingstone, Melbourne

Covington C, Cronenwett L, Loveland-Cherry C 1991 Newborn behavioral performance in colic and noncolic infants. Nursing Research 40(5): 292–6

Cox S G, Turnbull C J 1994 Choosing to breastfeed or bottlefeed: an analysis of factors which influence choice. Breastfeeding Review 2(10): 459–64

Crockenberg S B 1981 Infant irritability, mother responsiveness, and social support influences on the security of infant mother attachment. Child Development 52: 857–65

Crockenberg S, McCluskey K 1986 Change in maternal behaviour during the baby's first year of life. Child Development 57(3): 746–53

Cummings R G, Klineberg R J 1993 Breastfeeding and other reproductive factors and the risk of hip fractures in elderly women. International Journal of Epidemiology 22(4): 684–91

Cunningham A S 1979 Morbidity in breastfed and artificially fed infants, II. Pediatrics 95: 685–9

Cunningham A, Jelliffe D 1991 Breastfeeding and health in the 1980's: a global epidemiologic review. Journal of Pediatrics 118: 659–66

Cutrona C E, Troutman B R 1986 Social support, infant temperament, and parenting self-efficacy – a mediational model of postpartum depression. Child Development 57(6): 1507–18

Dahlen H 1993 Lactation mastitis. Nursing Times 89(36): 38–40

D'Apolito K 1991 What is an organized infant? Neonatal Network 10(1): 23–9

De Chateau P 1980 The first hour after delivery, its impact on synchrony of parent–infant relationship. Paediatrician 9: 151–68

Deutsch F M, Ruble D N, Fleming A, Brooks-Gunn J 1988 Information-seeking and maternal self-definition during the transition to motherhood. Journal of Personality and Social Psychology 55(3): 420–31

De Vore I, Konner M J 1974 Infancy in the hunter-gatherer life: an ethological perspective. In: White N F (ed.) Ethology and psychiatry. University of Toronto Press, Toronto

Dewey K G, Heinig M J, Nommsen L A, Peerman J M, Lonnerdal B 1993 Breast-fed infants are leaner than formula-fed infants at 1 year of age: the Darling study. American Journal of Clinical Nutrition 57: 140–5

Drewett R F, Woolridge M W 1981a Milk taken by human babies from the first and the second breast. Physiology and Behaviour 26: 327–9

Drewett R, Woolridge M 1981b Sucking patterns of human babies on the breast. Early Human Development 3(15): 320

Driscoll J W 1992 Breastfeeding success and failure: implications for nurses. NAACOG's Clinical Issues: Perinatal Women's Health 3(4): 565–9

Drummond J E, McBride M L, Wiebe C F 1993 The development of mothers' understanding of infant crying. Clinical Nursing Research 2(4): 396–413

Drummond J E, Wiebe C F, Elliott M R 1994 Maternal understanding of infant crying: what does a negative case tell us? Qualitative Health Research 4(2): 208–223

Duffy E P, Percival P, Kershaw E 1997 Positive effects of an antenatal group teaching session on postnatal nipple pain, nipple trauma and breast feeding rates. Midwifery 13: 189–96

Duncan B, Ey J, Holberg C J, Wright A L, Martinez F D, Taussig L M 1993 Exclusive breastfeeding for at least 4 months protects against otitis media. Pediatrics 90: 228–32

Dwyer T, Ponsonby A L 1996 The decline in SIDS: a success story for epidemiology. Epidemiology 7: 323–5

Elias M F, Nicholson N A, Konner M 1986 Two sub-cultures of maternal care in the United States. In: Taub D M, King F A (eds) Current perspectives in primate social dynamics. Van Nostrand Reinhold, New York

Elliott M R, Fisher K, Ames E W 1988 The effects of rocking on the state and respiration of normal and excessive criers. Canadian Journal of Psychology 42: 163–72

Elliott M R, Drummond J, Barnard K E 1996 Subjective appraisal of infant crying. Clinical Nursing Research 5(2): 237–50

Ellis D 1983 Needs of the breastfeeding dyad: how nurses

can assist. Australian Journal of Advanced Nursing 1(1): 38–43

Fahy K, Holschier J 1988 Success or failure with breastfeeding. Australian Journal of Advanced Nursing 5(3): 12–18

Family Health International 1988 Breastfeeding as a family planning method. Lancet ii(8621): 1204–5

Fetherston C 1995 Factors influencing breastfeeding initiation and duration in a private Western Australian maternity hospital. Breastfeeding Review 3(1): 9–11

Field P A 1985 Parents' reactions to maternity care. Midwifery 1: 37–46

Field P A 1987 Maternity nurses: how parents see us. International Journal of Nursing Studies 24(3): 191–9

Field P A 1994 A comparison of symptoms used by mothers and nurses to identify an infant with colic. International Journal of Nursing Studies 31(2): 201–15

Fisher C 1981 Breastfeeding: a midwife's view. Maternal and Child Health (February: 52–7

Fisher C 1983 Positions of success. New Generation 3: 20–1

Fisher C 1994 Resolving and preventing mothers' problems with breastfeeding. Modern Midwife (February): 17–19

Fisher C 1995 Attachment and position: a 'hands off' approach. Lecture: Chloe Fisher Tour, April, QE11 Centre, Perth, Western Australia

Fleming P J 1994 Understanding and preventing sudden infant death syndrome. Current Opinion in Pediatrics 6: 158–62

Fleming P J, Gilbert R, Azaz Y et al 1990 Interaction between bedding and sleeping position in the sudden infant death syndrome: a population based case-control study. British Medical Journal 301: 85–9

Fleming P J, Blair P S, Bacon C 1996 Environment of infants during sleep and risk of the sudden infant death syndrome: results of 1993–5 case control study for confidential inquiry into stillbirths and deaths in infancy. British Medical Journal 313: 191–5

Flint C 1984 Midwives and breastfeeding. Nursing Times 11: 30–1

Ford R P K, Taylor B J, Mitchell E A et al 1993 Breastfeeding and the risk of sudden infant death syndrome. International Journal of Epidemiology 22(5): 885–90

Forsyth S, Fowlie P 1995 Caring for the future. Modern Midwife 5(7): 23–6

Frank D 1994 Nipple pain. Journal of Obstetric, Gynecological and Neonatal Nursing 23(5): 375–6

Freed G, Fraley J K 1993 Effect of expectant mothers' feeding plan on prediction of fathers' attitudes regarding breastfeeding. American Journal of Perinatology 10: 300–3

Freed G L, Jones T M, Schanier R J 1992 Prenatal determination of demographic and attitudinal factors regarding feeding practice in an indigent population. American Journal Perinatal 9(5–6): 420–4

Frodi A 1985 When empathy fails: aversive infant crying and child abuse. In: Lester B M, Boukydis C E (eds) Infant crying: theoretical and research perspectives. Plenum Press, New York

Garcia J, Garforth S, Ayers S 1987 The policy and practice of midwifery study: introduction and methods. Midwifery 3: 2–9

Gay J T, Edgil A E, Douglas A B 1988 Reva Rubin revisited. Journal of Obstetric, Gynecological and Neonatal Nursing (Nov/Dec): 394–9

Gilbert R E, Wigfield R E, Fleming P J, Berry P J, Rudd P T 1995 Bottle feeding and the sudden infant death syndrome. British Medical Journal 310: 88–90

Glover R 1991 The key to successful breastfeeding. Midwife/lactation consultant. Allen & Unwin, Australia

Glover R 1997 Pamphlet: The key to successful breastfeeding. Copies can be obtained from Rebecca Glover, 6 Finlay Court, Lesmurdie, Western Australia 6076. Email: REBLACT @ WANTREE. COM.AU, Phone and Fax 08 92917319

Golding J 1997 Sudden infant death syndrome and parental smoking: a literature review. Paediatric and Perinatal Epidemiology 11: 67–77

Golton F, St James Roberts I 1991 Crying rates in infancy. Health Visitor 64(6): 188–90

Green J M, Coupland V A, Kitzinger J V 1990 Expectations, experiences and psychological outcomes of childbirth: a prospective study of 825 women. Birth 17(11): 15–24

Gross D, Conrad B 1995 Temperament in toddlerhood. Journal of Pediatric Nursing 10(3): 146–51

Hammer R L, Babcock G, Fisher A G 1996 Breastfeeding Review 4(1): 29–34. In: MIDIRS Midwifery Digest 6(4): 462

Hamosh M, Freed L M, Jones J B et al 1985 Enzymes in milk. In: Jensen R G, Neville M C (eds) Human lactation: milk components and methodologies. Plenum Press, New York

Hanson J 1996 Breastfeeding education: meeting the needs of the expectant parent. Breastfeeding review 4(2): 65–8

Harris H 1994 A solution to breastfeeding attachment through co-bathing. Breastfeeding Review 11(11): 465–8

Hartge P, Schiffman M H, Hoover R 1989 A case-control study of epithelial ovarian cancer. American Journal of Obstetrics and Gynecology 161(1): 10–16

Hartmann P 1995 Changes in the breast. Presentation to the Nursing Mothers Association of Western Australia, Department of Health, Perth, Western Australia

Hartmann P E, Kent J C 1988 The subtlety of breast milk. Breastfeeding Review 13: 14–18

Hartmann P E, Prosser C G 1984 Physiological basis of longitudinal changes in human milk yield and composition. Federation Proceedings 43(9): 2448–53

Hauck Y L, Dimmock J E 1994 Evaluation of an information booklet on breastfeeding duration: a clinical trial. Journal of Advanced Nursing 20(5): 836–43

Hauck Y, Reinbold J 1996 Criteria for successful breastfeeding: mothers' perceptions. Australian College of Midwives Incorporated Journal (March): 21–7

Health Department of Western Australia 1991 The information needs of new mothers. Health Department of Western Australia, Perth

Health Department of Western Australia 1995 Consumer views of maternity services: a survey for mothers. Health Department of Western Australia, Perth

Henderson-Smart D J, Ponsonby A L, Murphy E 1998 Reducing the risk of sudden infant death syndrome: a review of the scientific literature. Journal of Paediatric Child Health 34: 213–19

Hewat R 1992 The experience of living with an incessantly crying infant. Phenomenology and Pedagogy 10: 160–71

Hill P D 1987 Effects of education on breastfeeding success. Maternal Child Nursing 16(2): 145–56

Hinkley K R 1986 An interdisciplinary approach to the transition to parenthood. Dissertation Abstracts International 47(6-A): 2332

Hobbs D F 1965 Parenthood as crisis: a third study. Journal of Marriage and the Family 37(3): 367–72

Hobbs D F, Cole S P 1976 Transition to parenthood: a decade

replication. Journal of Marriage and the Family 38(3): 723–31

Hoffman H J, Damus K, Hillman L, Krongrad E 1988 Risk factors for SIDS: results of the National Institute of Child Health and Human Development SIDS Cooperative Epidemiological Study. New York Academy of Science 533: 13–30

Hoffman Y, Drotar D 1991 The impact of postpartum depressed mood on mother–infant interaction: like mother like baby? Infant Mental Health Journal 12(1): 65–80

Houston M R, Field P 1991 Teaching and support: nursing input in the postpartum period. International Journal of Nursing Studies 28(2): 131–44

Houston M, Howie P, McNeilly A 1983 Midwifery forum: breastfeeding. Nursing Mirror 156(suppl): i–viii

Howie P W 1985 Breastfeeding: a new understanding. Midwives Chronicle 98(1170): 184–92

Howie P W, Forsyth J S, Ogston S A, Clark A, Forey C du V 1990 Protective effect of breastfeeding against infection. British Medical Journal 300: 11–16

Hunziker U A, Barr R G 1986 Increased carrying reduces infant crying: a randomized controlled trial. Pediatrics 77: 641–8

Inch S 1990 Postnatal care relating to breastfeeding. In: Alexander J, Levy V, Roach S (eds) Postnatal care: a research-based approach. Macmillan, London

Isabella P H, Isabella R A 1994 Correlates of successful breastfeeding: a study of social and personal factors. Journal of Human Lactation 10(4): 257–64

Jacobson D, Melvin N 1995 A comparison of temperament and maternal bother in infants with and without colic. Journal of Pediatric Nursing 10(3): 181–8

Jacobson S W, Jacobson J L 1992 Breastfeeding and intelligence. Lancet 339: 926

Jenner S 1988 The influence of additional information, advice and support on success of breastfeeding in working class primiparas. Child: Care, Health and Development 14: 319–28

Jensen D, Wallace S, Kelsay P 1994 LATCH: A breastfeeding charting system and documentation tool. Journal of Obstetric, Gynecological and Neonatal Nursing 23(1): 27–32

Johnson N W 1986 Breastfeeding at one hour of age. American Journal of Maternal and Child Nursing (Jan/Feb): 12–16

Jones S 1983 Crying baby, sleepless nights. Warner Books, New York

Katwinkel J, Brooks J, Keenan M E, Malloy M 1994 Infant sleep position and sudden infant death syndrome (SIDS) in the United States: joint commentary from the American Academy of Pediatrics and selected agencies of the federal government. Pediatrics 93: 820

Keefe M R 1988 Irritable infant syndrome: theoretical perspectives and practice implications. Advances in Nursing Science 10(3): 70–8

Keefe M R, Froese-Fretz A 1989 Living with an irritable infant: the maternal perspective. Maternal Child Nursing 16: 255–9

Keefe M R, Kotzer A M, Froese-Fretz A, Curtin M 1996 A longitudinal comparison of irritable and nonirritable infants. Nursing Research 45(1): 4–9

Kennedy H P 1995 The essence of nurse-midwifery care: the woman's story. Journal of Nurse-Midwifery 40(5): 410–17

King F T 1913 Feeding and care of the baby. Macmillan, London

Kitzinger S 1989 Breastfeeding your baby. Doubleday, Sydney

Klein J O 1982 Prevention of persistent middle ear infusion: immunoprophylaxis. Pediatric Infections Disease Journal 1(suppl. 1): 99–106

Klinnert M D, Bingham R D 1994 The organizing effects of early relationships. Psychiatry 57: 1–10

Koldovsky O, Bedrick A, Pollack P, Rao R K, Thornburg W 1987 Hormones in milk: their presence and possible physiological significance. In: Goldman A S, Atkinson S A, Hanson L A (eds) Human lactation 3: The effects of human milk on the recipient infant. Plenum Press, New York

Koniak-Griffin D 1993 Maternal role attainment. IMAGE: Journal of Nursing Scholarship 25(3): 257–62

Konner M J 1976 Maternal care, infant behavior and development among the Kung. In: Lee R B, DeVore I (eds) Kalahari hunter-gatherers: studies of the Kung San and their neighbors. Harvard University Press, Cambridge

Konner M J, Worthman C 1980 Nursing frequency, gonadal function, and birth spacing among Kung hunter-gatherers. Science 207: 788–91

Korner A F 1974 Individual differences at birth: implications for childcare practices. Birth Defects 10(2): 51–61

Kramer M S, Barr R G, Leduc D G 1985 Determinants of weight and adiposity in the first year of life. Journal of Pediatrics 81: 365–71

Kraus J F, Greenland S, Bulterys M 1989 Risk factors for sudden infant death syndrome in the US collaborative perinatal project. International Journal Epidemiology 18: 113–20

Ladden M, Damato E 1992 Parenting and supporting programs. NAACOG's Clinical Issues 3(1): 174–87

Laufer A B 1990 Breastfeeding: towards resolution of the unsatisfying birth experience. Journal of Nurse-Midwifery 35(1): 42–5

Lauwers J, Woessner C 1990 Counselling the nursing mother: a reference handbook for health care providers and lay counsellors, 2nd edn. Avery Publishing, Garden City Park, NY

Lawson K, Tulloch M 1995 Breastfeeding duration: prenatal intentions and postnatal practices. Journal of Advanced Nursing 22: 841–9

Layde P M, Webster L A, Boughman A L 1989 The independent associations of parity, age at first full term pregnancy, and the duration of breastfeeding with the risk of breast cancer. Journal of Clinical Epidemiology 42(10): 963–73

Leach P 1977 Baby and child. Penguin Books, Ringwood, Australia

Leff E W, Gagne M P, Jefferis S C 1994 Maternal perceptions of successful breastfeeding. Journal of Human Lactation 10(2): 99–104

Leff E W, Jefferis S C, Gagne M P 1994 The development of the maternal breastfeeding evaluation scale. Journal of Human Lactation 10(2): 105–11

L'Esperance C 1980 Pain or pleasure: the dilemma of early breastfeeding. Birth and Family Journal 7: 21–5

Levitt M J, Weber R A, Clark M M 1986 Social network relationships as sources of maternal support. Developmental Psychology 22(3): 310–16

Lewis P R, Brown J B, Renfree M B 1991 The resumption of ovulation and menstruation in a well nourished population of women breastfeeding over an extended period of time. Fertility and Sterility 55: 529–36

Libbus M K, Kolostov L S 1994 Perceptions of breastfeeding and infant feeding choice in a group of low income mid-Missouri women. Journal of Human Lactation 10: 17–23

Littman H, Medendorp S V, Goldbarb J 1994 The decision of breastfeed: the importance of the fathers' approval. Clinical Pediatrics (April): 214–19

Locklin M, Naber S 1993 Does breastfeeding empower women? Insights from a select group of educated low income, minority women. Birth 20: 30–5

Lowe T 1994 Breastfeeding – what happens during the first 12 months? Breastfeeding Review 2(10): 487–90

Lucas A, Morley R, Cole T J, Lister G, Leeson-Payne C 1992 Breastmilk and subsequent intelligence quotient in children born preterm. Lancet 339: 261–4

McIntosh J 1993 The experience of motherhood and the development of depression in the postnatal period. Journal of Clinical Nursing 2: 243–9

McKim E, Kenner C, Flandermeyer A, Spangler L, Darling-Thompson P, Spiering K 1995 The transition to home for mothers of healthy and initially ill newborn babies. Midwifery 11: 184–94

McKim M, Wiseman B E 1985 Parent–infant clinic. Cry 1(1): 20–6

McNatt M H, Freston C N M 1992 Social support and lactation outcomes in postpartum women. Journal of Human Lactation 8(2): 73–7

Martell L K, Imle M, Horwitz S, Wheeler L 1989 Information priorities of new mothers in short-stay programs. Western Journal of Nursing Research 11(3): 320–7

Martin J, White A 1988 Infant feeding 1985. Department of Health and Social Services, London

Maxwell N I, Burmaster D E 1993 A simulation model to estimate a distribution of lipid intake from breastmilk during the first year of life. Journal of Environment and Epidemiology 3(4): 383–406

Menahem S 1978 The crying baby – why colic? Australian Family Physician 7: 1262–6

Mercer R T 1986a First-time motherhood: experiences from teens to forties. Springer, New York

Mercer R T 1986b Predictors of maternal role attainment at one year postbirth. Western Journal of Nursing Research 8(1): 9–32

Michelsson K, Rinne A, Paajanen S 1990 Crying, feeding and sleeping patterns in 1 to 12 month old infants. Child: Care, Health and Development 16: 99–111

Minchin M 1981 About breast and nipple problems. Nursing Mother's Association of Australia, Victoria

Minchin M 1985 Breastfeeding matters: what we need to know about infant feeding. Alma Publications, Victoria

Minchin M 1989a Breastfeeding matters. George Allen & Unwin, Sydney

Minchin M 1989b Positioning for breastfeeding. Birth 16: 67–73

Mitchell E A, Taylor B J, Ford R P K et al 1992 Four modifiable and other major risk factors for cot death: the New Zealand study. Journal of Paediatric Child Health 28(1): S3–S8

Mitchell E A, Stewart A W, Clements M, New Zealand Cot Death Study Group 1995 Immunisation and the sudden infant death syndrome. Archives of Disease in Childhood 13(73): 448–501

Mitchell E A, Tuohy P, Brunt J M et al 1997 Risk factors for sudden infant death syndrome following the prevention campaign in New Zealand: a prospective study. Pediatrics 100: 335–40

Morris S F H 1985 Methods for investigating the presence and physiologic role of growth factors in milk. In: Jensen R G, Neville M C (eds) Human lactation: milk components and methodologies. Plenum Press, New York

Mortimer P, Kevill F 1985 Frustration and despair. Community Outlook 22: 19–20

Moss P, Bolland G, Foxman R, Owen C 1987 The hospital inpatient stay: the experience of first-time parents. Child Care and Health Development 13(3): 153–67

Murphy-Black T 1987 Postnatal care at home: the experience of some Scottish mothers. Unpublished manuscript, Nursing Research Unit, Department of Nursing Studies, University of Edinburgh

Murphy-Black T 1990 Antenatal education. In: Alexander J, Levy V, Roch S (eds) Antenatal care: a research-based approach. Macmillan Books, London

Nash L 1913 Breastfeeding, its management and mismanagement. Lancet (June 14): 1657–9

National Health and Medical Research Council 1987 Nutrition policy statement, 1987. Commonwealth Department of Health, Canberra

Nelson E A S, Taylor B J, Weatherall I L 1989 Sleeping position and infant bedding may predispose to hyperthermia and the sudden infant death syndrome. Lancet 1: 199–201

Newcomb P A, Storer B E, Longnecker M P 1994 Lactation and a reduced risk of premenopausal breast cancer. New England Journal of Medicine 330(2): 81–7

Newman J 1994 Nipple pain. Journal of Obstetric, Gynecological and Neonatal Nursing 23(1): 12

NSW Women's Consultative Committee 1994 If motherhood is bliss why do I feel so awful? Community consultations in postnatal stress and depression in NSW. NSW Ministry for the Status and Advancement of Women, New South Wales

Oberklaid F 1979 Letter. Medical Journal of Australia 2: 486–7

Office of Population Censuses and Surveys 1992 Infant feeding. HMSO, London

O'Meara C 1993 A diagnostic model for the evaluation of childbirth and parenting education. Midwifery 9: 28–34

Parkin P C, Schwartz C J, Manuel B A 1993 Randomized controlled trial of three interventions in the management of persistent crying of infancy. Pediatrics 92: 197–201

Parmalee A H, Stern E 1972 Development of states in infants. In: Clements C, Purpura D, Mayer F (eds) Sleep and the maturing nervous system. Academic Press, New York

Parmalee A H, Wenner W H, Schulz H R 1964 Infant sleep patterns: from birth to 16 weeks of age. Journal of Pediatrics 65: 576–82

Percival P 1998 Research in progress. Edith Cowan University, Western Australia

Percival P 1990 The relationship between perceived nursing care and maternal adjustment for primiparae during the transition to motherhood. Unpublished Doctoral dissertation, Curtin University of Technology, Western Australia

Percival P, Duffy E D 1998 Research in progress. Edith Cowan University, Western Australia

Peterson C E, Da Vanzo J 1992 Why are teenagers in the United States less likely to breastfeed than older women? Demography 29(3): 431–50

Pinyerd B J 1992a Infant colic and maternal mental health: nursing research and practice concerns. Issues in Comprehensive Pediatric Nursing 15: 155–67

Pinyerd B J 1992b Strategies for consoling the infant with colic: fact or fiction? Journal of Pediatric Nursing 7(6): 403–11

Ponsonby A-L, Dwyer T, Gibbons L E, Cochrane J A, Jones M E, McCall M J 1992 Thermal environment and sudden infant death syndrome: case control study. British Medical Journal 304: 277–82

Ponsonby A-L, Dwyer T, Gibbons L E, Cochrane J A, Wang Y G 1993 Factors potentiating the risk of sudden infant death syndrome associated with the prone position. New England Journal of Medicine 329: 377–82

Ponsonby A-L, Dwyer T, Kasl S V, Cochrane J A 1995 The Tasmanian SIDS case-control study: univariable and multivariable risk factor analysis. Paediatric Perinatal Epidemiology 9: 256–72

Ponsonby A-L, Dwyer T, Cooper D 1997 Sleeping position, infant apnea and cyanosis: a population based study. Pediatrics 99: 1–7

Prechtl H F R 1974 The behavioral states of the newborn. Brain Research 6: 185–212

Pugh L C, Buchko B L, Bishop B A et al 1996 Birth 23(2): 88–93. In: MIDIRS Midwifery Digest 6(4): 463

Pukander J S, Sipila M M, Kataja M J, Karma P H 1993 The Bayesian approach to the evaluation of risk factors affecting the prolongation of middle ear effusion after acute otitis media. In: Lim D J, Bluestone C D, Klein J O, Nelson J D, Ogra P L (eds) Recent advances in otitis media. Decker, Philadelphia

Quarles A, Williams P D, Hoyle D A, Brimeyer M, Williams A R 1994 Mothers' intention, age, education and the duration and management of breastfeeding. Maternal Child Nursing Journal 22(3): 102–8

Rajan L 1993 The contribution of professional support, information and consistent correct advice to successful breast feeding. Midwifery 9: 197–209

Rajan L 1994 The impact of obstetric procedures and analgesia/anaesthesia during labour and delivery on breastfeeding. Midwifery 10: 87–103

Raphael D 1981 The midwife as doula: a guide to mothering the mother. Journal of Nurse-Midwifery 26(6): 13–15

Rassin D K, Markides K S, Baranowski T, Richardson C J, Mikrut W D, Bee D E 1994 Acculturation and the initiation of breastfeeding. Journal of Clinical Epidemiology 47(7): 739–46

Redman S, Watkins J, Evans L 1995 Evaluation of an Australian intervention to encourage breastfeeding in primiparous women. Health Promotion International 10(2): 101–13

Reilly T W, Entwisle D R, Doering S G 1987 Socialization into parenthood: a longitudinal study of the development of self-evaluations. Journal of Marriage and the Family 49: 295–308

Renfrew M, Fisher C, Arms S 1990 Bestfeeding: getting breastfeeding right for you. Celestial Arts, California

Rider A 1985 Postnatal care. Midwifery after birth. Nursing Times 81(32): 24–26

Righard L, Alade M 1990 Effect of delivery room routines on success of first feed. Lancet 336: 1105–7

Rinne A, Saenz A H, Michelsson K 1990 Amount and perception of baby crying in Finland and Colombia. Early Child Development and Care 65: 139–44

Rossi A S 1968 Transition to parenthood. Journal of Marriage and the Family 30(1): 26–9

Royal College of Midwives 1989 Successful breastfeeding. Royal College of Midwives, London

Royal College of Midwives 1991 Successful breastfeeding, 2nd edn. Royal College of Midwives, London

Rubin R 1967a Attainment of the maternal role. Part 1: Processes. Nursing Research 16(3): 237–45

Rubin R 1967b Attainment of the maternal role: Part 2: Models and referents. Nursing Research 16(3): 346–74

Rubin R 1968 Body image and self esteem. Nursing Outlook: 20–3

Rubin R 1975 Maternity nursing stops too soon. American Journal of Nursing 75: 1680–8

Ruchala P L, Halstead L 1994 The postpartum experience of low-risk women: a time of adjustment and change. Maternal–Child Nursing Journal 22(3): 83–9

Russell C S 1974 Transition to parenthood: problems and gratifications. Journal of Marriage and the Family 36(2): 294–301

Saarinen U M 1982 Prolonged breastfeeding as a prophylaxis for recurrent otitis media. Acta Paediatrica Scandinavica 71: 567–71

Saint L, Maggiore P, Hartmann P E 1986 Yield and nutrient content of milk in 8 women breastfeeding twins and 1 woman breastfeeding triplets. British Journal of Nutrition 56: 49–58

St James-Roberts I, Hurry J, Bowyer J 1993 Objective confirmation of crying durations in infants referred for excessive crying. Archives of Disease in Childhood 68: 82–4

Salariya E M, Easton P M, Carter J I 1987 Duration of breastfeeding after early initiation and frequent feeding. Lancet 2(8100): 1141–3

Samuel J, Balch B 1985 Maternity care in action. Part III: Care of the mother and baby. Midwives Chronicle 98 (1169): 161–2

Sassen M L, Brand R, Grote J J 1994 Breastfeeding and acute otitis media. American Journal of Otolaryngology 15: 351–7

Scher A 1991 A longitudinal study of night waking in the first year. Child: Care, Health & Development 17(5): 295–302

Schy D S, Maglaya C M, Mendelson S G, Race E H, Ludwig-Beymer P 1996 The effects of in-hospital education on breastfeeding practice. Journal of Human Lactation 12(2): 117–22

Scott J A, Binns C W 1995 Breastfeeding practices amongst Perth women. Proceedings of Nutrition Society of Australia 19: 115

Searle A 1985 The effects of postnatal depression on mother–infant interaction. Australian Journal of Sex, Marriage and Family 8(2): 79–86

Sears W 1985 The fussy baby. La Leche League International, Franklin Park, IL

Sears W 1988 Growing together. Collins Dove, Melbourne

Sethi S 1995 The dialectic in becoming a mother: experience a postpartum phenomenon. Scandinavian Journal of Caring Science 9: 235–44

Slaven S, Harvey D 1981 Unlimited sucking time improves breastfeeding. Lancet 392–3

Smith M P 1989 Postnatal concerns of mothers: an update. Midwifery 5: 182–8

Stamp G E, Crowther CA 1994 Women's views of their postnatal care by midwives at an Adelaide women's hospital. Midwifery 10: 148–56

Sumner G 1995 Keys to CaregivinG: a new NCAST program for health care providers and parents of newborns. Zero to Three 16(1): 33–5

Swaffield L 1984 Crying babies. Nursing Times 80: 16–17

Taylor A 1986 Maternity services: the consumer's view. Journal of the Royal College of General Practitioners 36(285): 157–60

Thapa S, Short R V, Potts M 1988 Breastfeeding, birth spacing and their effects on child survival. Nature 335(6192): 679–82

Thomas A, Chess S, Birch H 1969 Temperament and behavior disorders in children. New York University Press, New York

Thomsen M E, Hartstock T G, Larson C 1979 The importance of immediate postnatal contact: its effects on breastfeeding. Canadian Family Physician 25: 1374–8

Toffler A 1970 Future shock. Bodley Head, London

United Kingdom National Case-Control Study Group 1993 Breastfeeding and the risk of breast cancer in young women. British Medical Journal 307(6895): 17–20

Victora C, Smith P G, Vaughn J P et al 1989 Infant feedings and deaths due to diarrhea: a case control study. American Journal of Epidemiology 129(5): 1032–51

Virden S F 1988 The relationship between infant feeding method and maternal role adjustment. Journal of Nurse-Midwifery 33(1): 31–5

Waldman W H, Sarsgard D 1983 Helping parents to cope with colic. Pediatric Basics 33: 12–14

Walker M 1989 Management of selected early breastfeeding problems seen in clinical practice. Birth 16(3): 148–58

Weber F, Woolridge M, Baum J 1986 An ultrasonographic analysis of sucking and swallowing in newborn infants. Developmental Medicine and Child Neurology 28: 19–24

Wenner W, Barnard K E 1980 The changing infant: sleep and activity patterns during the first months of life. In: Barnard K E (ed.) NCAST II learner manual. NCAST Publications, Seattle, Washington

Wessel M A, Cobb J C, Jackson E B, Harris G S Jr, Detwiler A C 1954 Paroxysmal fussing in infancy, sometimes called 'colic'. Pediatrics 14: 421–34

Widstrom A M, Ransjo-Arvidson A B, Christensson J K, Mattieson A S, Winberg J, Uvanas-Moberg 1987 Gastric suction in healthy newborn infants: effects on circulation and developing feeding behaviour. Acta Paediatrica Scandinavica 76: 566–72

Wigfield R, Fleming P J 1995 The prevalence of risk factors for SIDS: the impact of an intervention campaign. In: Rognum T O (ed.) Sudden infant death syndrome: new trends in the nineties. Scandinavian University Press, Oslo

Wilkie C F, Ames E W 1986 The relationship of infant crying to parental stress in the transition to parenthood. Journal of Marriage and the Family 48(3): 545–50

Williams S M, Taylor B J, Mitchell E A, New Zealand Cot Death Study Group 1996 Sudden infant death syndrome: insulation from bedding and clothing and its effect modifiers. International Journal of Epidemiology 25: 366–75

Wilson C A, Taylor B J, Liang R M, Williams S M, Mitchell E A 1994 Clothing and bedding and its relevance to sudden infant death syndrome: further results from the New Zealand Cot Death Study. Journal of Paediatric Child Health 30: 506–12

Wolff P H 1966 The causes, controls, and organization of behavior in the neonate. Psychological Issues 5, Monograph 17. International Universities Press, New York

Woolridge M 1986a The aetiology of sore nipples. Midwifery 2: 172–6

Woolridge M 1986b The 'anatomy' of infant sucking. Midwifery 2: 164–71

Woolridge M W 1990 Do changes in pattern of breast usage alter the baby's nutrient intake? Lancet 336: 385–97

Woolridge M W, How T V, Drewett R F, Rolfe P, Baum J D 1982 A method for the continuous measurement of milk intake at a feed. Early Human Development 6: 365–72

World Health Organization and United Nations Children's Fund 1989 Protecting, promoting, and supporting breastfeeding: the special role of maternity services. A joint WHO/UNICEF statement. World Health Organization, Geneva

Ziemer M, Pigeon J 1993 Skin changes and pain in the nipple during the first week of lactation. Journal of Obstetric, Gynecological and Neonatal Nursing 22(3): 247–56

Zuckerman B, Bauchner H, Parker S, Cabral H 1990 Maternal depressive symptoms during pregnancy and newborn irritability. Developmental and Behavioral Pediatrics 11(4): 190–4

FURTHER READING

CESDI (Confidential Enquiry into Stillbirths and Deaths in Infancy) 1996 Third annual report concentrating on the first two years of combined studies on: sudden unexpected deaths in infancy. Department of Health, London

Henderson-Smart D J, Ponsonby A L, Murphy E 1997 Reducing the risk of sudden infant death syndrome: a review of the scientific literature. Journal of Paediatric Child Health 34: 213–19

Royal College of Midwives 1991 Successful breastfeeding, 2nd edn. Royal College of Midwives, London

UK Baby Friendly Initiative 1994 The baby friendly initiative in the UK. UK Baby Friendly Initiative, London

UNICEF UK Baby Friendly Initiative 1993 Practical steps in promoting breastfeeding. UNICEF, London

Index